The Sociology of Medicine

The International Library of Critical Writings in Sociology

Series Editor: Howard Newby
Professor and Vice-Chancellor of the University of Southampton, UK

1. The Sociology of the Environment (Volumes I, II and III)
   Michael Redclift and Graham Woodgate
2. The Sociology of Development (Volumes I and II)
   Bryan R. Roberts, Robert G. Cushing and Charles Wood
3. The Sociology of Religion (Volumes I and II)
   Steve Bruce
4. The Sociology of Medicine
   William C. Cockerham

Future titles will include:

Economic Sociology
Richard Swedberg

The Sociology of Urban Communities
Michael Harloe

The Sociology of Rural Communities
Graham Crow

The Sociology of the Sciences
Helga Nowotny and Klaus Taschwer

Social Stratification
John Holmwood

The Sociology of Industry
Richard K. Brown

The Sociology of Politics
William Outhwaite and Luke Martell

The Sociology of Welfare
Alan C. Walker

The Sociology of Education
Robert Burgess

The Sociology of the Family
Colin Bell

The Sociology of Gender Relations
Christine Delphy

The Sociology of Medicine

Edited by

William C. Cockerham

Professor of Sociology, Medicine and Public Health
Chair of the Department of Sociology
University of Alabama at Birmingham, US

THE INTERNATIONAL LIBRARY OF CRITICAL WRITINGS IN SOCIOLOGY

An Elgar Reference Collection
Aldershot, UK • Brookfield, US

Published by
Edward Elgar Publishing Limited
Gower House
Croft Road
Aldershot
Hants GU11 3HR
UK

Edward Elgar Publishing Company
Old Post Road
Brookfield
Vermont 05036
US

British Library Cataloguing in Publication Data
Sociology of Medicine. – (International
Library of Critical Writings in Sociology;
Vol. 4)
I. Cockerham, William C. II. Series
306.461

Library of Congress Cataloguing in Publication Data
The Sociology of medicine / edited by William C. Cockerham.
p. cm. — (The International library of critical writings in sociology; 4)
Includes bibliographical references and index.
1. Social medicine. I. Cockerham, William C. II. Series.
RA418.S6744 1996
306.4'61—dc20 95–24273
CIP

ISBN 1 85898 021 6

Printed in Great Britain by Galliard (Printers) Ltd, Great Yarmouth

Contents

Acknowledgements

The editor and publishers wish to thank the following who have kindly given permission for the use of copyright material.

American Public Health Association for articles: Dean T. Jamison and W. Henry Mosley (1991), 'Disease Control Priorities in Developing Countries: Health Policy Responses to Epidemiological Change', *American Journal of Public Health*, **81** (1), January, 15–22; Marilyn A. Winkleby, Darius E. Jatulis, Erica Frank and Stephen P. Fortmann (1992), 'Socioeconomic Status and Health: How Education, Income, and Occupation Contribute to Risk Factors for Cardiovascular Disease', *American Journal of Public Health*, **82** (6), June, 816–20.

American Sociological Association for articles: William C. Cockerham, Gerhard Kunz and Guenther Lueschen (1988), 'Social Stratification and Health Lifestyles in Two Systems of Health Care Delivery: A Comparison of the United States and West Germany', *Journal of Health and Social Behavior*, **29**, June, 113–26; Donald W. Light (1988), 'Toward a New Sociology of Medical Education', *Journal of Health and Social Behavior*, **29**, December, 307–22; Peter Conrad (1988), 'Learning To Doctor: Reflections on Recent Accounts of the Medical School Years', *Journal of Health and Social Behavior*, **29**, December, 323–32; Steven C. Martin, Robert M. Arnold and Ruth M. Parker (1988), 'Gender and Medical Socialization', *Journal of Health and Social Behavior*, **29**, December, 333–43; Eugene B. Gallagher (1988), 'Convergence or Divergence in Third World Medical Education? An Arab Study', *Journal of Health and Social Behavior*, **29**, December, 385–400; Sarah Rosenfield (1989), 'The Effects of Women's Employment: Personal Control and Sex Differences in Mental Health', *Journal of Health and Social Behavior*, **30**, March, 77–91; Barry Glassner (1989), 'Fitness and the Postmodern Self', *Journal of Health and Social Behavior*, **30**, June, 180–91; Howard Waitzkin (1989), 'A Critical Theory of Medical Discourse: Ideology, Social Control, and the Processing of Social Context in Medical Encounters', *Journal of Health and Social Behavior*, **30**, June, 220–39; Leonard I. Pearlin (1989), 'The Sociological Study of Stress', *Journal of Health and Social Behavior*, **30**, September, 241–56; Rose Weitz (1989), 'Uncertainty and the Lives of Persons with AIDS', *Journal of Health and Social Behavior*, **30**, September, 270–81; Charles W. Hunt (1989), 'Migrant Labor and Sexually Transmitted Disease: AIDS in Africa', *Journal of Health and Social Behaviour*, **30**, December, 353–73; Stella R. Quah (1989), 'The Social Position and Internal Organization of the Medical Profession in the Third World: The Case of Singapore', *Journal of Health and Social Behavior*, **30**, December, 450–66; Mark La Gory, Ferris J. Ritchey and Jeff Mullis (1990), 'Depression among the Homeless', *Journal of Health and Social Behavior*, **31**, March, 87–101.

Basil Blackwell Ltd for articles: A. d'Houtaud and Mark G. Field (1984), 'The Image of Health: Variations in Perception by Social Class in a French Population', *Sociology of Health & Illness*, **6** (1), March, 30–60; Deborah C. Glik (1990), 'The Redefinition of the Situation: The Social Construction of Spiritual Healing Experiences', *Sociology of Health & Illness*, **12** (2), 151–68; Keith Bakx (1991), 'The "Eclipse" of Folk Medicine in Western Society', *Sociology of Health & Illness*, **13** (1), 20–38; Sam Porter (1992), 'Women in a Women's Job: The Gendered Experience of Nurses', *Sociology of Health & Illness*, **14** (4), 510–27; Simon J. Williams, Michael Calnan, Sarah L. Cant and Joanne Coyle (1993), 'All Change in the NHS? Implications of the NHS Reforms for Primary Care Prevention', *Sociology of Health & Illness*, **15** (1), January, 43–67; Karen K. Yoshida (1993), 'Reshaping of Self: A Pendular Reconstruction of Self and Identity among Adults with Traumatic Spinal Cord Injury', *Sociology of Health & Illness*, **15** (2), March, 217–45.

Baywood Publishing Company Inc. for article: William A. Glaser (1991), 'Paying the Hospital: American Problems and Foreign Solutions', *International Journal of Health Services*, **21** (3), 389–99.

Elsevier Science Ltd, Pergamon Imprint for articles: Isabelle Baszanger (1985), 'Professional Socialization and Social Control: From Medical Students to General Practitioners', *Social Science and Medicine*, **20** (2), 133–43; Sally Macintyre (1986), 'The Patterning of Health by Social Position in Contemporary Britain: Directions for Sociological Research', *Social Science and Medicine*, **23** (4), 393–415; Johannes Siegrist, Richard Peter, Astrid Junge, Peter Cremer and Dieter Seidel (1990), 'Low Status Control, High Effort at Work and Ischemic Heart Disease: Prospective Evidence from Blue-Collar Men', *Social Science and Medicine*, **31** (10), 1127–34; Hiroyuki Hattori, Stephan M. Salzberg, Winston P. Kiang, Tatsuya Fujimiya, Yutaka Tejima and Junji Furuno (1991), 'The Patient's Right to Information in Japan – Legal Rules and Doctor's Opinions', *Social Science and Medicine*, **32** (9), 1007–16; Marie R. Haug, Hiroko Akiyama, Georgeanna Tryban, Kyoichi Sonoda and May Wykle (1991), 'Self Care: Japan and the U.S. Compared', *Social Science and Medicine*, **33** (9), 1011–22; Christine Obbo (1993), 'HIV Transmission Through Social and Geographical Networks in Uganda', *Social Science and Medicine*, **36** (7), 949–55; Joel M. Hanna and Maureen H. Fitzgerald (1993), 'Acculturation and Symptoms: A Comparative Study of Reported Health Symptoms in Three Samoan Communities', *Social Science and Medicine*, **36** (9), 1169–80.

InformationsZentrum Sozialwissenschaften, Bonn, for excerpts: Uta Gerhardt (1993), 'The Sociological Relevance of Chronic Illness' in Thomas Abel, Siegfried Geyer, Uta Gerhardt, Johannes Siegrist and Wim van den Heuvel (eds), *Medical Sociology: Research on Chronic Illness*, 11–36; Sara Arber (1993), 'Chronic Illness over the Life Course: Class Inequalities among Men and Women in Britain' in Thomas Abel, Siegfried Geyer, Uta Gerhardt, Johannes Siegrist and Wim van den Heuvel (eds), *Medical Sociology: Research on Chronic Illness*, 39–64.

JAI Press Inc. for article: William C. Cockerham, Thomas Abel and Günther Lüschen (1993), 'Max Weber, Formal Rationality, and Health Lifestyles', *Sociological Quarterly*, **34** (3), 413–28.

Routledge for article: Bryan S. Turner (1989), 'Ageing, Status Politics and Sociological Theory', *British Journal of Sociology*, **40** (4), December, 588–606.

Sage Publications Inc. for article: Eliot Freidson (1985), 'The Reorganization of the Medical Profession', *Medical Care Review*, **42** (1), Spring, 11–35.

Society for the Study of Social Problems for article: Marianne A. Paget (1990), 'Life Mirrors Work Mirrors Text Mirrors Life ... ', *Social Problems*, **37** (2), May, 137–48.

Taylor & Francis for excerpts: Ursula M. Sharma (1990), 'Using Alternative Therapies: Marginal Medicine and Central Concerns' in Pamela Abbott and Geoff Payne (eds), *New Directions in the Sociology of Health*, Chapter 9, 127–39, references; Nicki Thorogood (1990), 'Caribbean Home Remedies and their Importance for Black Women's Health Care in Britain', in Pamela Abbott and Geoff Payne (eds), Chapter 10, *New Directions in the Sociology of Health*, Chapter 10, 140–52, references.

University of North Carolina Press for article: George Ritzer and David Walczak (1988), 'Rationalization and the Deprofessionalization of Physicians', *Social Forces*, **67** (1), September, 1–22.

Every effort has been made to trace all the copyright holders but if any have been inadvertently overlooked the publishers will be pleased to make the necessary arrangement at the first opportunity.

In addition the publishers wish to thank the Library of the London School of Economics and Political Science and the Photographic Unit of the University of London Library, for their assistance in obtaining these articles.

Introduction

The international collection of articles contained in this reader presents ideas, concepts and findings that reflect many of the current directions in the sociology of medicine. Compared to other subdisciplines in sociology, the sociology of medicine is a relatively new field. It was established in the aftermath of World War II, initially in the United States and Great Britain, and subsequently spread to many other nations. Medical sociologists analyse the social causes and consequences of health and illness. They do this by studying the social aspects of health and disease, the social functions of health organizations and institutions, patterns of health care delivery, the social behaviour of health personnel and patients, social policies towards health, and other health matters with a sociological component.

The readings presented in this book are divided into ten sections covering a variety of topics, ranging from theory to health care delivery and social change. The papers were selected to provide a contemporary overview of the field that illustrates both the scope and depth of the subdiscipline. The initial section is on 'Sociological Theory and Health'. At its inception, the sociology of medicine was largely atheoretical because much of its focus was on producing knowledge that could be applied to medical practice. In time, however, as medical sociology matured, work in the field became increasingly theoretical. This development is reflected in the papers in Part I, in the first of which the German medical sociologist Uta Gerhardt reviews the development of sociological theory in relation to chronic illness since the 1950s. Gerhardt details the manner in which chronic illness has affected sociological thinking with respect to concepts of equality and individuality.

Chapter 2, by the editor and his German colleagues Abel and Lüeschen, applies Max Weber's concept of formal rationality (one of the central paradigms of sociological thought) and his ideas about lifestyles in general to current trends in health lifestyles. Weber's work offers a theoretical background which both enriches our understanding of health lifestyles and overcomes the initial theoretical challenges posed by research in this specific field. In Chapter 3, American physician and medical sociologist Howard Waitzkin applies a Marxist approach to an analysis of discourse between physicians and their patients, noting the routine use of language by physicians supportive of the prevailing social order, the element of social control in the encounter, and the exclusion of criticism about society. Besides the presentation of his findings, Waitzkin provides a review of contemporary Marxist approaches in sociology for analysing medical ideology. The section concludes with Australian sociologist Bryan Turner's paper on ageing, status politics and sociological theory. Turner, who has published extensively on theory and the human body, rejects both structural-functionalist activity theory and Marxist perspectives on ageing, adopting instead an exchange theory approach to explain the politics of ageing.

Following this introduction to the use of sociological theory in medical sociology, we turn in Part II to 'Social Factors and Disease'. This section begins with a paper published in the *American Journal of Public Health* by Marilyn Winkleby and her associates (Jatulis, Frank and Fortmann) on socioeconomic status and health. Sociologists typically measure socioeconomic status (SES) by determining an individual's income, occupational status and level of education. Winkleby *et al.* studied the effects of each determinant of SES on health risk factors and found that education is the strongest and most consistent predictor of healthy behaviour. This paper explains why. Chapter 6 by Joel Hanna and Maureen Fitzgerald compares the health effects of modernization on young adults in American Samoa and Honolulu (Hawaii), followed in Chapter 7 by a report on depression among the homeless in the US by American sociologists Mark La Gory, Ferris Ritchey and Jeff Mullis. Both papers are concerned with the relation between social change and health.

The section concludes with three papers on AIDS. American medical sociologist Rose Weitz examines feelings of uncertainty in the lives of people with AIDS and notes how having AIDS can become a 'master status', largely determining the nature and extent of the infected person's social relationships. Another American sociologist, Charles Hunt, explains how the migrant labour system in central, eastern and southern Africa has promoted the transmission of AIDS. Long absences and increased family breakdowns have encouraged an increase in numbers of sexual partners among a population which has historically suffered from epidemics of sexually transmitted diseases. The final paper in this section is by Christine Obbo who works in France and has likewise examined the transmissions of AIDS in Africa. Focusing on Uganda, she targets long-distance truck drivers and prostitutes as major sources of the spread of the HIV virus. Her study helps us to understand why people, especially female prostitutes, continue their risky sexual practices with knowledge of the consequences of their behaviour. Often, the women simply have no choice as to how they are to earn a living.

Part III on 'Social Demography' features papers by two British medical sociologists, Sally Macintyre and Sara Arber, and one American, Sarah Rosenfield. Macintyre provides an extensive analysis of British health patterns by social class, while Arber focuses on health inequalities between classes and gender with respect to chronic illness in Britain. Both papers provide an excellent review of class differences in health, with Arber including a gender dimension as well. Rosenfield examines gender differences in mental health in the US from the standpoint of the effects of women's employment. Her paper explores the relationship between personal control over work in relation to sex differences in analysing symptoms for anxiety and depression.

Part IV ('Social Stress') consists of two articles. Chapter 14, by American medical sociologist Leonard Pearlin, contains an in-depth review of the sociological literature on stress and an overview of current concepts. Chapter 15 is an account of a study conducted in Germany by Johannes Siegrist and his colleagues (Peter, Junge, Cremer and Seidel) investigating the relationship between high effort at work by male blue-collar employees and ischemic heart disease. This study, which was conducted over a period of six years, found that factors such as status inconsistency, job insecurity, work pressure and a need for control over one's work, independently predicted a higher risk of heart disease.

Part V ('Health Behaviour') contains three papers dealing with the social behaviour of healthy people who wish to stay healthy. The first is a study of variations in perceptions of health by social class in France, conducted by French medical sociologist Alphonse d'Houtaud and his American counterpart Mark Field. Whereas persons in the working class tended to view health as a means to an end (the capability to work), the middle class wanted health for the purpose of enjoying life and having a sense of physical vitality. Chapter 17 reports the results of a cross-national study conducted in the US and West Germany by the editor and two German colleagues (Kunz and Lueschen). Utilizing a Weberian perspective, this study found no major differences between Americans and Germans participating in healthy lifestyles. The more paternalistic system of state-sponsored health benefits in Germany did not undermine personal incentives to stay physically fit in comparison to persons living in the more individualistic system in the US. Finally, Chapter 17 by American sociologist Barry Glassner examines contemporary fitness activities in relation to postmodern concepts of self. Fitness activities are treated as a social movement and scrutinized by postmodern theory.

Part VI ('Illness Behaviour') is concerned with the social activities of the ill. Chapter 19 by Marie Haug and her colleagues (Akiyama, Tryban, Sonoda and Wykle) compares the self-care activities of Americans and Japanese, with the Japanese found to perform more self-care in lieu of visiting a medical doctor than the Americans. The reasons for this cross-cultural difference are discussed. Chapter 20 by Canadian medical sociologist Karen Yoshida explores the impact of chronic illness (spinal cord injuries) on the self-concepts of a sample of men and women in southern Ontario. Lastly, there is the account of American medical sociologist Marianne Paget's experience in coping with her own diagnosis of terminal cancer.

Part VII ('Alternative Medicine') contains four papers on the use of non-physician healers, the first three by British medical sociologists. Ursula Sharma investigates some of the major concerns associated with the use of alternative therapies in modern societies, while Nicki Thorogood explores the use of Caribbean home remedies among black women in Britain. Keith Bakx associates the use of contemporary folk medicine with postmodern conditions. In a postmodern society, traditional centres of authority become fragmented and individuals are left more on their own. Chapter 25 by American Deborah Glik examines spiritual and religious healing in Baltimore (Maryland). The majority of respondents in her study reported some degree of healing, primarily associated with the alleviation of symptoms rather than cures.

The next section ('Health Professions and Occupations') presents eight studies from the extensive literature on health practitioners in medical sociology. Chapters 26 and 27 are by American medical sociologists. Donald Light examines the dimension of change in medical practice in the US from more of a seller's market (dominated by physicians) to more of a buyer's market (dominated by patients and their decisions). Light discusses how this change is likely to be reflected in future medical education. Peter Conrad, in turn, shows how the demands of medical training adversely impact on the humanistic orientation of medical students. Those doctors who maintain such an orientation through medical school are likely to have developed this attitude prior to their medical training. In a similar study, French sociologist Isabelle Baszanger investigates how the French medical profession socializes general practitioners and describes the marginal status in medicine held by GPs once they leave hospital training and begin working in the community.

The remaining paper in Part VIII is from Americans Steven Martin and his co-workers (Arnold and Parker) who analyse the socialization of men and women medical doctors, gender differences in career choices and styles of practice. Stella Quah, a medical sociologist in Singapore, discusses the social position of physicians in the Third World, noting that their relatively high status reflects that held in the First World. Next, the research by Hiroyuki Hattori and his colleagues (Salzberg, Kiang, Fujimiya, Tejima and Furono) on the patient's right to information in Japan discloses that physicians typically do inform the family – but not the patient – of a cancer diagnosis. The Hattori study explains this cross-cultural difference. In Chapter 32, American medical sociologist Eugene Gallagher studies the impact of Islamic culture on medical education in Saudi Arabia, while in Chapter 33 Northern Ireland medical sociologist Sam Porter investigates gender inequality in nursing.

Part IX ('Hospitals') consists of American social scientist William Glaser's analysis of hospital financing in the US, Canada and Western Europe. The focus of the final section ('Health Care Delivery and Social Change') is on the changing social conditions of medical practice. Simon Williams (with Calnan, Cant and Coyle) investigates Britain's National Health Service reforms for primary care prevention, while Eliot Freidson examines the potential for reorganization of the medical profession in the US. In Chapter 37, George Ritzer and David Walczak present their analysis of the deprofessionalization (defined as a decline in status and professional autonomy) of physicians in American society. The book concludes with international policy recommendations by Americans Dean Jamison and W. Henry Mosley on dealing with changing patterns of diseases among children and adults. They note that most developing countries do not have an information base about many major diseases because they lack the capacity to collect and analyse relevant data.

In sum, this book contains a selection of articles from scholars in different parts of the world analysing many of the most important health issues in human society today. The intention is to provide readers with insight into each of these issues and the manner in which they are explored by an international group of scholars. As society moves into the 21st century, work in the sociology of medicine is likely to become increasingly important because many social conditions – whether they be poverty, AIDS or unhealthy lifestyles – affect health. The socialization of health practitioners and their relationships with patients, together with the operation of health care delivery systems, remain critical issues in providing quality care. Research and analysis in medical sociology contribute significantly to decision making about these issues. The articles included in this book provide a background to current debates on the relationship between health and society and present the reader with authoritative analyses by scholars working in the field of the sociology of medicine.

Part I
Sociological Theory and Health

[1]

Uta Gerhardt

The Sociological Relevance of Chronic Illness

Introduction

This introductory essay focuses on the intersection between general sociology/social theory and medical sociology, on the one hand, and medicine and medical sociology, on the other hand. In what way has chronic illness become or been a thematic point of intersection between the two areas of sociology? Frequently social theory is being placed in the arcane realm of conceptual generalization whereas medical sociology is being located in the profane realm of practice detail. Often theory passes by the mundane facts of empirical research whereas special sociologies such as medical or urban or educational sociology disdain the generalizations of social theory. How can the two be intertwined? This question is answered by looking at the field of chronic illness as a topic that has been discussed since the 1950s.

How can medicine and medical sociology work together to supplement each other's approach as relevant to the various sides of an illness? Does not medicine claim an exclusive right to understand illness, and sociology must deny this in order to establish its own right of existence? Has not professional dominance and medicalization drawn a line of demarcation between medicine and sociology such that the twain shall never meet on common ground? This question is addressed inasmuch as chronic illness represents an area of intersection where medicine and sociology can collaborate.

The "discovery" of chronic illness

Medical sociology "discovered" chronic illness as a topical focus in the late 1950s. It became an antidote against Talcott Parsons's social-systems theory of medical practice, undermining the latter's contested plausibility. Although the criticism may have been ill-founded, it established chronic illness as a viable theme for medical sociology refusing to align itself with medicine's professional standpoint.

In Chapter 10 of *The Social System*, published in 1951, Parsons juxtaposed the role of the physician and that of the sick under the auspices that they denoted the same pattern-variable orientations. He focused on the status of sickness as "in the type case temporary" [1]. The idea was that medical therapy, "in the type case", restored the individual to normal role capacity using "unconscious psychotherapy". [2] The four stages of treatment dynamics were pictured similar to those of other social-control processes, namely, permissiveness, support, denial of reciprocity, and manipulation of rewards. [3] The aim of medical practice was, therefore, to return society's members to their duties and responsibilities, i.e. restore them to health or an equivalent state of social normality.

The idea was challenged by David Mechanic at the end of the 1950s. He charged that Parsons had unduely emphasized the patient's return to normal roles, focusing exclusively on his or her overcoming the state of sickness. This meant, Mechanic stated, that Parsons looked at the acutely sick but disregarded the chronically ill whereas medical sociology had to account for the course and outcome of all sickness in society. Since Parsons excluded the chronically sick from his analysis, Mechanic contended, his conceptual analysis was insufficient. [4] Citing Mechanic's argument, other critics wrote that emphasis on normality or return to work or family roles as outcome of spells of sickness underestimated how many patients with chronic diagnoses were exposed to negative experiences such as loss of job, or being blamed for their illness; those who lost their job were ostrasized by their families, or were deemed responsible for and stigmatized because of illness that was permanent. [5] Until today, Mechanic's claim that Parsons cannot account for chronic illness has remained a credo for many medical sociologists. This unwarranted criticism was remarkably immune against Parsons's own demonstration in a paper presented to the 1974 World Congress of Sociology in Toronto how chronic illness can be reconciled with the social-system view of medical practice. [6]

The role of advocate of the chronically sick befitted medical sociologists inasmuch as sociologists became spokespersons for the underprivileged in the 1960s. Equal opportunity was an icon of the better society, and the chronically sick were recognized as one of the groups to whom equal opportunity was denied. This made them a conspicuous victim of exploitation and discrimination which sociology wished to stem. Democracy became the goal toward which sociologists intended to move society, and it meant that the normal and the deviant, the ablebodied and the incapacitated, the healthy and the sick had to have the same or at least similar chances of self-realization and uncontested social and personal identities. Sociology's interest in humane living conditions for every individual citizen spurred identification with the plight of the chronically sick, particularly those in mental institutions.

Erving Goffman published *Asylums* in 1961, castigating the "custodial care" rendered to the mentally ill in psychiatric hospitals and other "total institutions". He further clarified in *Stigma*, published in 1963 and subtitled The *Management of Spoiled Identity*, how the dismal lives of the chronically ill or handicapped were the infamous underside of the dichotomy between wellness and sickness, normality and stigma. Goffman argued that stigma was not due to sickness in a vast number of cases but rather followed upon social labelling of a person as a deviant. Therefore, not bizarre behaviour or mental incapacity led to a citizen's stigmatization as chronically ill but, rather, contingencies such as visibility of one's "defect", availability of a physician or hospital to diagnose and admit a patient, etcetera. [7] From a similar standpoint, Howard Becker, focusing on drug addicts, alcoholics, and mental patients in *Outsiders* (1963), posed the provocative question, "Whose Side Are We On?" [8] He suggested that sociology was a partisan endeavour, where the sociologist could take sides either with society's power-wielding establishment, or with the underclass citizen whose rights were spurned.

Chronic illness thus became a focus for sociological research endorsing the human condition in the interest of all-pervasive democracy. The topic of chronic illness helped to immunize sociology against inadvertently conforming with the policies of groups or organizations wielding power or representing wealth in society. Sociological research thereby meant to protect itself against naïvité that blinded the researcher against the inequalities resulting from capitalism's known as well as intrinsic inequalities. [9]

From this vantage point, professional practice became a target for criticism launched from a position partisan to the needs of the chronically ill. Goffman's empirically based treatises, and also Thomas Scheff's *Being Mentally Ill* (published in 1966), focused on the process of medical labelling. Doctors' diagnoses, it was shown, marked the beginning of indefinite careers of psychiatric or other chronic sickness(es). Seeking professional help, accordingly, proved a trap rather than a boon. Medical care was recognized as the point of entrance into a status of unending stigmatization. Goffman as well as Scheff identified three stages of the process, namely, *first*, an inconspicuousness stage where the person functioned more or less satisfactorily in a normal world (world of normals) where strange behaviours and also hallucinations were all but common; *second*, a crisis or labelling stage when experts made the person a patient by means of diagnosis; and, *third*, an illness stage spurring a career of spoiled identity exacerbating stigma. [10] In a similar vein, Eliot Freidson (1966) equalled disability with permanent deprivation and degradation. The status of sickness was revealed to entail a role of relentless subordination to medical and welfare-state authorities. Chronic illness made the patient a victim of the power of the profession, and disease came to represent powerlessness confining the person to the disenfranchised status of patient. [11]

Along this line of argument lay the conclusion that medical practice as such - at least as how it prevailed in modern western society - was flawed. What was wrong with medical practice, and could be observed particularly well inasmuch as the chronically sick were but an unwanted clientele of technical care geared to the acutely ill, was its professionalism. That is, the very structure of medicine was revealed as detrimental to the needs of patients epitomized by what was essential for those with chronic conditions.

In the early 1970s, Freidson launched his denouement of professional medicine. In two books both published in 1970, *Profession of Medicine* and *Professional Dominance*, he attacked the medical construction of illness. It served mainly the professional politics of organized medicine, he ventured, whereas the lay construction of illness reflected the sick person's need and capacity to manage his or her everyday life. The aim was to shatter professional medicine's claim that it alone could realize and fulfil patients' needs. In fact, professional medicine was charged to conspicuously deviate from the standards of morality and humaneness. The implicit reproach was that the Hippocratic principle was violated and frequently even abandoned by modern medicine. Its technology was said to harm or maim more than could be justified by the purpose of healing, and its communicative patterns were attacked as hegemonic and patient-aversive. [12] On a similar note, Anselm Strauss edited a collection of essays dealing with the topic of *Where Medicine Fails* (1970, 1979[3]), and he and a collaborator devoted a volume to issues of *Humanizing Health Care*. [13]

At the end of the 1970s, self-assertiveness vis-à-vis medicine was challenged unsuccessfully. Phil Strong (1979) castigated sociologial imperialism as a misguided response to professional dominance. His argument was that sociology erected a straw man when it criticized medicine for its hegemony concerning health care, and that sociology's praising its own approach as viable alternative to medicine's allegedly imperialistic definition of health and illness could only lead to equally unsubstantiated sociological imperialism. Strong's criticism was contradicted by Howard Waitzkin (1979) and repeatedly by Peter Conrad and Joseph Schneider (1979, 1980) who insisted that medicine lacked humanistic and egalitarian motives. The medicalization process of modern society, they stressed, meant that the world was in danger to be manipulated by all-powerful professional groups who camouflaged their self-centered actions as therapy. [14]

The medicalization argument, to be sure, had surfaced early in the 1970s. Irving Zola had warned of the risk of medicalization of intrinsically political or social phenomena such as radicalism or unemployment. [15] Ivan Illich, diagnosing triple iatrogenesis in the modern world, had derived the destruction of personal, social, and cultural independence of modern man from a process of alienation produced by hegemonic technological medicine. He concluded medical nemesis, as indicated by the dramatic increase of the prevalence rates for chronic illness(es) in contemporary industrial societies. [16] This underscored what Thomas McKeown had argued in several books since the middle 1960s, namely, that modern health care appeared less and less able to forestall chronic illness(es). Modern technological medicine, he proved, was not responsible for the decrease of infectious and acute diseases over the last one and a half centuries. Despite its inability to prevent chronic disease(s) and irrespective of its stagnating or decreasing effectiveness and efficiency, modern medicine's financial requirements had risen to historically unprecendented levels, McKeown warned. [17]

McKeown's argument has become common ground of medical sociology disregarding its ideological clout. However, the argument may nevertheless be flawed. Ernest Gruenberg (1977) raised a counter-argument which makes high prevalence rates of chronic illness a sign of high instead of low performance levels of modern medicine. He maintains that increasing prevalence for chronic illness(es) during the four or five most recent decades indicates two obvious successes of medicine. One is that infectious diseases have all but vanished due to antibiotics (introduced on a mass basis in the 1930s and thereafter) and the other is that surgical and drug treatments of non-infectious diseases have dramatically improved since the Second World War. The reduction of infections, particularly of pneumonia as a cause of mortality, and also the introduction of sophisticated surgery such as, for instance, coronary artery bypass grafting or renal transplantation, had two effects on the chronically ill, Gruenberg argues. One is that they have all but ceased to die from secondary infections such as pneumonia that was extremely common among diabetics, stroke or heart-attack victims and others chronically sick up to the first half of the twentieth century. The improvement of treatment makes such patients more likely to eventually die of their main condition which is chronic. The other effect is that they tend to live far longer than ever in the past history of humankind.

Improvement of life expectancy after diagnosis, Gruenberg maintains, is partly due to improved surgical and/or drug treatment. For instance, insulin therapy for diabetics has considerably lengthened their life span such as has dialysis or transplantation for end-stage renal failure, or anti-hypertensive drug treatment or bypass surgery or percutaneous transluminal coronary angioplasty (PTCA) for heart disease or vascular occlusion. Years and often decades of symptom-free or medically contained chronic sickness may thus be added to a person-patient's life span; therefore, quality of life as well as life expectancy are greatly improved. It goes without saying that this increase of patients' length and quality of life raises prevalence rates for chronic diseases as measured by socio-medical statistics. [18]

The place of the patient's view

In the middle 1970s, "grounded theory" made the experience of the chronically ill a topic of medical sociology in its own right. Permanent and/or varying incapacity but also management of everyday activities became an explicit object of study. Until the end of the 1960s, "grounded theory" had mainly focused on the social problems of dying but in 1975, Anselm Strauss and Barney Glaser edited a collection of essays elucidating the problems of patients' coping with chronic disease. Their collection entitled *Chronic Illness and the Quality of Life* elucidated how the chronically handicapped or the permanently incapacitated used strategies of managing their activities and interpersonal relations, and their extended introductory essay explained in the framework of "symbolic interactionism" theory how thus is established a semblance of normality. [19]

Contrary to Goffman who castigated the normal population for unduely expecting the disabled to hide or gloss over their stigma when participating in social life, Strauss and his collaborators insisted that the chronically sick themselves are keen to appear as normal as possible and to participate in a wide range of normal activities. For the purpose of identity management, "grounded theory" researchers showed, the chronically ill develop elaborate techniques of bodily or self control that help them keep up the appearance of normality in most interpersonal settings. These strategies of management are aided by a circle of family and friends, "grounded theory" research proved, who chaperone a patient's appearance of normality but may also be drawn into a relationship invoking overprotection or exhaustion.

For nearly two decades, "grounded theory" has continued to depict how the shared and managed "definitions of the situation" shape the conduct of the chronically ill, and how they and their interaction partners use negotiation to constantly adapt and readapt their levels of competence and compassion. [20] Inherent in this research is a philosophy of human dignity apt to pervade each and every encounter. The rationale behind exploring and mapping the stages and strategies of illness management is that the sick should be equally equipped as the well to conduct their public and personal activities in a manner preserving their dignity. It is from this vantage point that patient power has become an issue for symbolic interactionist medical sociology. [21]

The message has been heeded widely that chronic illness means deliberate or unavoidable construction of socially negotiated normality. In this vein, illness experience has become a legitimate topic pervading large parts of medical sociological research. In the middle 1980s, Joseph Schneider and Peter Conrad's *Having Epilepsy: The Experience and Social Control of Illness* set the stage for nearly a decade of exploration of how specific illnesses shape the person-patient's suffering as well as mastery. [22] Two collections of essays published in the middle 1980s epitomize the line of work started by Conrad's epilepsy study. Ray Fitzpatrick et al.'s *Experience of Illness* (1984) combines description of symptoms with analysis of personal feelings and accounts of suffering and coping. [23] Julius Roth and Peter Conrad's *The Experience and Management of Chronic Illness* (1987) links patients' and their relatives' private worlds with time structures and illness trajectories, focusing on chronic conditions such as multiple sclerosis, end-stage renal disease, hypoglycemia, or diabetes. [24] Another more recent volume focuses on *The Illness Experience* concentrating on patients' interpretations of symptoms in the light of their outlook into the future shaped by the expectable trajectory of their disease. [25]

The focus on patients' experience has been introduced as an antidote against a medically informed perspective viewing the patient from an outside standpoint. Conrad, in the introduction to the collection of essays on the experience and management of chronic illness, distinguishes between an insider's perspective that "focuses directly and explicitly on the subjective experiences of living with and in spite of chronic illness", and an outsider's perspective that identifies with physicians' views of their patients' diagnosis; the latter, Conrad maintains, neglect patients' personal suffering and overlook the reduction of the scope of their life-worlds.[26] Whereas Parsons's notion of sick role represents the outsider's perspective, Conrad contends, authentic research in the sociology of the experience and management of chronic illness must embrace the insider's perspective. Such authenticity is believed to be the only safeguard for sociological honesty that benefits what Becker called society's "underdog", emulating partisanship with disenfranchised groups as in the 1960s.

The emphasis on experience has developed into a focus on biography. Michael Bury using qualitative data in a study of patients' coping with rheumatoid arthritis finds that a three-stage process of disruption and subsequent re-normalization of biography reconciles the patient's chronic illness with his or her life-world(s).[27] Gareth Williams, using detailed accounts from three cases, emphasizes the moral quality of a person's social identity that is threatened by a diagnosis of chronic disease; the patient's making sense of his or her illness is also an attempt to account for his or her life such that the moral value of the person is preserved.[28] With an audience of clinicians in mind, Williams and Philip Wood point out that to understand patients' lay explanations of their illness could mean for the physician that he or she might ease communication with the patient and adapt treatment or its explanation to the latter's own understanding of the disease.[29]

A special issue of "Social Science and Medicine" in 1990, discussing "Qualitative Research On Chronic Illness", distinguishes between three different approaches that partly go beyond analysing the patients' experience. Using non-statistical data (qualitative research), revised "grounded theory", ethnomethodology/narrative analysis, and the biographical approach,[30] are to represent more sociological depth than the literature focusing on experience. The idea is that structures of experience, not their individual representation, are the sociological issue. This opens up a new perspective for sociology in medicine. Reconciling the patient's view with medicine's progress, medical sociology's findings on chronic illness are shown to be of crucial value to modern clinical practice: "Sociology might help to sensitize physicians to, by giving them detailed information on, potentially hazardous corollaries of home or work life of what might be technically or pharmaceutically unproblematic treatment." [31]

Along similar lines, using material about the history of public health and community medicine, David Armstrong has proved that since the early twentieth century medicine's prevalent paradigm has become biographical. Doctors together with their patients, Armstrong argues, form a unit of discourse evoking a social relationship and drawing every aspect of the patient's biography into a realm of potentially medically relevant facts. Nothing is excluded from the grip of medical surveillance, and community medicine epitomizes a medical gaze intent on prevention as an alternative to cure or rehabilitation. In this setting, Armstrong clarifies in an article entitled *The Patient's View*, no contrast exists between the doctor's professional dominance and the patient's lay-person powerlessness. Rather, the patient's view has itself become a part of the medical paradigm. The latter, a newly inclusive image of medical practice, has arisen in modern society over the last six decades or more. Consequently no hidden agenda of patient-aversive medical definition of an illness prevails in a practice setting, and no tacit conflict exists between doctor and patient. Rather, both form a new albeit skewed unity. The patient's perspective has itself become an element of the doctor's understanding, and the physician must make sure to ascertain the patient's view, and incorporate it into his diagnostic and therapeutic judgments. [32]

This analysis draws medical sociology's interest in the experience and management of chronic illness closer to medicine's work. The issue is no longer to contrast the physician's alleged outsider's perspective with the patient's presumed insider's perspective. The conflict is no longer between the medical profession's suspected interest in power and domination and medical sociology's avowed effort to promote a program of humanist values. The new paradigm merges the two under the auspices of medicine that caters for a growing number of chronically sick individuals. Their increasing prospect of living a relatively normal life for decades, possibly comparable to that of anyone else, makes them normals as social actors and puts medicine among the conditions that make their lives possible. From this vantage point, the relevance of chronic illness for sociology must also be re-ascertained. If the theoretical salience of chronic illness is no longer that of the place of the individual in society - as was held in the 1960s -, the question must be raised anew what makes chronic illness a viable sociological topic.

The two hinges of theory

To root the interest in and importance of chronic illness in the canon of explanatory concepts of society and social action in sociological theory, is a somewhat speculative undertaking. The argument ventured here cannot but be unfolded in what is a non-direct manner, often seemingly losing sight of the problem of the sociological relevance of chronic illness and only eventually coming back to its point. The latter, to be sure, is how the conceptual heritage of classical sociological thought may embrace the realities of the all too mundane lives of those who are chronically sick. That is, from the perspective of what it entails to live with chronic illness, the question is what are the theoretical key issues under which sociology could or should sensibly conceptualise its structural as well as contextual connotations. In other words, what are the general points of sociological interest which are raised explicitly or implicitly by medical sociology's focussing on chronicity of sickness?

Over the three decades of medical sociology's concern with chronic illness, two such issues of theoretical impact have emerged. One is *equality*, the other is *individuality*.

In what way does the topic of equality matter with respect to chronicity of sickness? In 1978, summing up a life-time's insights on the health-disease divide, Parsons insisted that powerlessness was one of humankind's predicaments whereas sickness was another. The World Health Organization's definition of health established after World War II, he stated, had obfuscated the issue of wellbeing. Equating health not just with the absence of disease but with physical, psychological, and social wellbeing, WHO had inadvertently set itself an end that could not be reached by the means it commanded. This had stalled rather than facilitated efforts toward worldwide improvement of the human condition. [33]

To be sure, Parsons's sociology has always been concerned with health rather than illness. In 1951, he explained how health was the basic prerequisite of system formation in society establishing equality between all individual members in terms of their capacity to compete in the educational and occupational realms. Competition between equals was the pre-requisite of stratification allowing for division of labour but also for reciprocity in interactive exchange system(s). [34] In this way, he stated, health meant capacity of the individual to take advantage of equality of opportunities as offered in Western democracies, and medicine made it the outcome or target of clinical work. Medical practice, therefore, helped to avail every citizen of the equality of opportunities as guaranteed by modern liberalism. It contributed decisively to society's integration inasmuch as it fostered the ability for voluntary commitment; this, in turn, could best be directed to goals benefiting the community if citizens were not hindered or handicapped by lack of capacity or self-control. [35]

Invoking health as the icon of equality, Parsons focused on psychological more than on physical functioning. Since society's reciprocity relations depended more on the flexible adaptation of actors to the expectations of others with whom they interacted - within the confines of given sets of morally imperative values and norms -, Parsons deemed deficiencies of psychological make-up a more serious source of deviance than lack of physical prowess. Therefore, as long as the individual could function in his or her occupational and other roles such that others' sensible response could ensue and was appreciated, it did not matter whether one or both of the actors had only restricted functioning of, say, a limb or an organ such as their liver. It was from this perspective that normalization accomplished by someone chronically sick - in a non-psychiatric sense - who tried to act as healthy-like as possible, and normality of a non-sick person who acted as he or she felt fit, were sociologically equivalent. As long as the precarious web of interrelationships persisted in everyday life, producing a climate of interpersonal sensitivity where gratification was adjusted to achievement or performance, those with a long-term chronic condition controlled by treatment, and those not jeopardized by an impairment of function, could contribute just as well to the give-and-take in the social system. [36]

Parsons's focus on health facilitating equality of opportunity, therefore, encompasses both those who are normal (non-sick) and those who normalize (that is, whose chronic illness is under medical care). Although the latters' condition might render more difficult their adaptation to competition in our industrial society, they nevertheless often manage to abide by the rules of occupational life. In a way, lack of health can thus be understood as one among a range of difficulties or disadvantages hampering an individual's progress in his or her occupational or private life - presumably comparable to a stigmatized racial origin, an inadequate educational background, "wrong" age or sex, or any other non-mainstream or prejudiced attribute of the person.

The issue raises the more general question whether the chronically ill are social actors like everyone else. Is it true that handicap or disability make a person a less-than-normal actor in the social world? This leads back to the classic theory of social action, namely, that of Max Weber. He lay the groundwork for the most widely used ideas about what social action is, not only because Talcott Parsons based his own analytical "action frame of reference" on Weber's conception, but also because his notions reach beneath and beyond those of Parsons. What can Weber's sociology contribute to the understanding of (chronic) illness? To be sure, Max Weber did not distinguish between disease and well-being as what characterizes the normal actor; nor were they mentioned as conditions of rationality that supposedly was typical for the social actor in general. In a way, it seems that Weber took for granted that every actor in society is healthy. That is, Weber did not explicitely consider a person's reduced action capacity or orientation due to physical or psychological handicap of any kind.

This presupposition of Weberian action theory may, in fact, seem unrealistic - if only because Weber himself suffered from a chronic condition which made him unable to hold down his professorship for some two decades. [37] But, as is well known, apart from an interlude of relative unproductiveness, despite his incapacitating illness Weber managed to read, write and debate passionately about the issue how he felt one ought to adequately analyse and understand society. In this vein, he was not a theoretician who overlooked variations of capacity of the social actor, but an example of how the chronically sick person may function in healthy-like fashion.

The theoretical problem involved here makes it visible that chronic illness need not be an impediment to rational action. However, it may be an aggravating condition of an individual's life situation comparable to, say, a disenfranchised racial or ethnic background, poverty as a deprived socio-economic status, etcetera. In a society characterized by equality of opportunity as its basic principle, chronic illness may be said to jeopardize one's chances inasmuch as it represents disadvantage. It may or may not be coupled with other attributes unfavourable to achievement and upward social mobility (such as, for instance, low education or foreign nationality). It makes equality with others so much harder but not impossible. Whereas it makes rational goal attainment more difficult in a world of occupational and personal competition, it is far from rendering impossible participation as a full-fledged citizen in the life of the community.

Of course, some life situations may be difficult enough without the added burden of chronic illness. Accordingly, a chronic condition may make nearly impossible taking advantage of society's equality of opportunity. Among the various realms of disadvantaged status, low social-class origin affects a person's life chances particularly badly. Since low socio-economic status often means lack of sufficient income, lack of educational knowledge and proficiency, insecure job situation, and poor housing condition, and since lower-class mentality typically favours physical strength over intellectual capacity as a means of power and prestige, lower-class persons seem to find it particularly hard to normalize in the face of chronic disease or disablement. [38] The reasons have been discussed under the theme of coping and its antecedents from two opposite standpoints. One claims that a lack of resources deprives the lower-class person's life situation of potentially protective agents and energies, including psychological capacities of coping ensuring flexibility which could help use whatever scarce resources are available. [39] The other argument emphasizes that higher exposure to noxious work conditions often connected with unhealthy life-style due to lower income in the lower social strata makes them more vulnerable to severe diseases. [40] To be sure, during the last thirty years evidence has become overwhelming that low or very low socio-economic status means increased morbidity from chronic conditions. Moreover, it also means higher mortality from a wide range of chronic illnesses including neoplasms (except breast cancer), heart disease, liver cirrhosis, and emphysema, to name but a few. [41]

This situation appears less tolerable than fifty years ago because the focus on equality and freedom has shifted from economic opportunity to bodily self-expression in the modern world. In the eighteenth century, democracy meant political freedom based on *habeas corpus*. In the nineteenth century, after the French Revolution had spurred abolition of traditional institutions and ushered in an era of industrial growth, political equality needed to be supplemented by economic well-being. Mass poverty combined with exploitative labour conditions characterized the lives of large parts of the population who were too powerless to assert their right to live. The welfare state, first introduced in Germany as a measure against the Socialist Workers' Party, became an effective antidote against economic inequality. By the middle of the twentieth century, health care has become a part of the welfare state in nearly all industrialized countries. But it also dawned on many critical analysts that the problem of economic opportunities has been insufficiently solved by the welfare state. [42]

At the same time, since the 1960s, a new topic has arisen epitomizing society's failure to foster freedom and equality in yet another respect. Focusing on the body, to be sure, invoked illness as a condition calling for medical help since almost every sick citizen nowadays has access to medical treatment in most industrial societies. Claudine Herzlich and Janine Pierret stress that the problem is no more whether or not a sick person can afford treatment. Since state-funded or insurance-based health-care systems have eased the individual's financial burden connected with health care, and since everybody in most Westernized countries is entitled to medical care irrespective of socio-economic position, access to health care is taken for granted, Herzlich and Pierret maintain. The concern nowadays has shifted to issues of mode of medical work, such as informed consent, patients' rights, personal dignity during treatment, and protection against exploitation or impoverishment for people with disabilities. [43]

The topic of the "social body", its equality and individuality has also been raised by another French author. In what he called an archaeological approach to understanding the medical perspective, Michel Foucault has shown that medicine as an egalitarian scientific endeavour has had a social-control function hitherto unnoticed. The clinic or hospital itself, he argued, and also the nosological system of categories providing medicine's knowledge base, are themselves repressive inasmuch as they submit the body to an all-pervasive code of right and wrong. [44] He claimed that "docile bodies" are being created not so much by medicine but by penitentiaries and prisons. [45] David Armstrong, however, elaborated Foucault's argument from *Discipline and Punish* into one about medicine. In *The Political Anatomy of the Body* (1983), Armstrong argues that "docile bodies" are being created and maintained by medicine in the twentieth century. Since public health has become a part of the "medical gaze", he contends, individuals have come to understand their bodies in the terms of its medical connotations and they have learned that health is but a state of potential illness open for control by an all-powerful medical profession. [46] In this way, medicine and illness - particularly chronic illness that extends until one's death - acquire a new interface, namely, that of producer and product, creator and creation of "docile body".

The book's title, "Political Anatomy of the Body", refers to two issues. On the one hand, Armstrong wishes to emphasize that whereas as a student he took for granted that dissecting bodies in anatomy lessons established medicine's groundwork, he later came to realize how historically relative is the notion of the body thus represented.[47] At the same time, anatomy as a political endeavour means production of relevant knowledge about what medicine is or what it is not doing. In modern times, he suggests, medicine must also comprise the social sciences representing the interpersonal dimensions of illness etiology, experience, and treatment. The message, in short, is that medicine in its modern social and survey extension means near-total power.[48]

Chronic illness, from this perspective, is the constant object of all pervasive surveillance. Bryan Turner has emphasized in various books and articles that chronic illness under the proviso of more or less all-pervasive medical power wielded through clinical knowledge raises the issue of how much freedom the body is granted. In our society, Turner maintains, only to be healthy means to be free from treatment and control; otherwise, powerful therapeutic agencies feel entitled to encroach upon a person's nutrition, life-style, or other aspects of physical or psychological integrity. Turner advocates that the individual should genuinely *be* his or her body rather than only *have* it - emulating a distinction originally made by the German philosopher Hellmuth Plessner. Turner's criticism is that the difference between being and having a body is whether or not medicalization of bodily expressions has driven a wedge between the person and his or her embodied self.[49]

This criticism takes the standpoint that the body has come to signify the human condition in contemporary society but under circumstances of more rather than less inequality than two centuries ago. The chronically ill are seen as a group representing best an apparently characteristically deprived human condition, namely, that of the politically and economically independent individual who is nevertheless under constant medical surveillance and also non-medical control curtailing freedom of the body in our era of public health. Surveillance monitors on individuals' healthy or adequate social functioning. The individual is expected to submit himself or herself to any kind of treatment deemed necessary to improve his or her bodily condition. The argument is, that the chronically ill functioning under constant medicalized control in an utmost normalizing fashion, reflect the human condition that is typical for modern "therapeutic-state" society. [50] Medicine, in this scenario, is seen to provide the diagnostic epistemology and the treatment technology that allow for the body to become a locus of all-pervasive manipulation.

In this debate, the issue is individuality. Whereas the body has long been disregarded in sociological literature, Turner observes, its relevance is beyond doubt. The reason for Turner is that misrepresentation of "the social body" in modern medicine destroys the body's authentic capacities. Realizing such alienation can help to free the body from its dependency on fads and fashions making it liable to social control, Turner states. His view of individuality in society is that it is embodied, and he clarifies that in modern - if not postmodern - society this means that a new role of sociology is called for. The unity of body and mind must be sociology's basic postulate, Turner demands. He opts for uniting suffering and healing as expressions of the self of the social actor. [51] Turner wishes sociology to accomplish a denouement of medicine and re-establishment of the body as a physical cum cognitive and evaluative endowment of the individual. He claims that the freedom of the actor is to be secured better in the future than at present or in the past, if sociology makes embodiment its main conceptual focus.

Individuality epitomizing freedom of expression is a traditional value of Western democratic culture. Now the idea of individuality has come to be extended to incorporate the body, and illness, particularly chronic illness, comes into the picture in this vein. Sociological theory concerned with individuality has traditionally been occupied with problems such as identity, authenticity, or autonomy. Now the perspective on the body is to pervade these more or less cognitive dimensions.

Whether a viable sociological approach will eventually result from this equating embodiment with individuality, is as yet an open question. It is, however, clear that the new focus on the body has brought to the fore that in contemporary society the body has become an incarnation of the ideas of equality, liberty, and maybe even fraternity. The body encompasses personhood and integrity. It is now the body where these values are to be realized, not any longer mainly the economic sphere (where inequality still prevails), nor just the political realm (where inequality also still occurs).

To summarize: The two hinges of theory where chronic illness touches upon traditional sociological thought, are equality and individuality. Although these connecting points between medical sociological thought focusing on chronic illness and sociological theory may so far remain vague and certainly require further clarification, it may be said that these are obvious intersections. Issues of quality and individuality motivate research into a wide range of empirical phenomena of chronic illness. In a direct or indirect manner, however, the area of medical sociology's research on chronic illness owes its baseline to these theoretical concerns.

Concluding remark

What, then, is the sociological relevance? The question has been given three answers. First, contrary to the credo of the 1960s that chronic illness contradicts modern medicine's claim to efficiency, it was argued that chronic illness testifies to medicine's professional viability under a biographical paradigm. Second, from a social-order point of view, healthy normality was shown to be equal to healthy-like normalization, which incorporates the chronically sick into the world of work and family, public and private life. Third, the philosophical problems addressed by classical sociological theory that also matter for health-illness issues are equality and individuality, epitomized in the discussions on "Health for All" and the body.

Notes

1 Parsons adds to his explaining the two right-two duty-structure of the sick role: "It is, in the first place, a 'contingent' role into which anyone, regardless of his status in other respects, may come. It is, furthermore, in the type case temporary. One may say that it is in a certain sense a 'negatively achieved' role, through failure to 'keep well',

Medical Sociology: Research on Chronic Illness

though, of course positive motivations also operate, which by that very token must be motivations to deviance." Parsons, *The Social System*, London: Free Press of Glencoe 1951, p. 438

2 The respective text refers to what since ancient times has been invoked as the 'art of medicine'. "The structure of the physician's role", writes Parsons, "must have some effect on the mental state of the patient whether it is used for deliberate psychotherapy or not...The general conclusion is that a very important part of non- and prepsychiatric medical practice is in fact 'unconscious psychotherapy'". *Social System*, p. 462. For further discussion of the 'unconscious psychotherapy' see: U. Gerhardt, *Ideas About Illness*, London: Macmillan 1989, pp. 52-56

3 T. Parsons and R. Fox: "Illness, Therapy, and the Modern Urban Family", *Journal of Social Issues*, Vol. 4, 1952, 31-44; T. Parsons, E.A. Shils and R. Bales, *Working Papers in the Theory of Action*, Glencoe, IL: Free Press, 1953, esp. pp. 238-245; T. Parsons: "Definitions of Health and Illness in the Light of American Values and Social Structure", in: E. Jaco (ed): *Patients, Physicians, and Illness*, 3rd edition, New York: Free Press 1979, pp. 120-144 (originally 1958)

4 D. Mechanic: "Illness and Social Disability: Some Problems of Analysis." *Pacific Sociological Review*, Vol. 2, 1959, pp. 37-41; the argument is taken up in A. Twaddle: "Aging, population growth and chronic disease", *Journal of Chronic Disease*, Vol. 21, 1968, pp. 417-422

5 R. Sobel and A. Ingalis: "Resistance to treatment: explorations of the patient's sick role", *American Journal of Psychotherapy*, Vol 18, 1964, pp. 562-573; B. Bursten and R. d'Esopo: "The obligation to remain sick", *Archives of General Psychiatry*, Vol. 12, 1965, pp. 402-407; G.G. Kassebaum and B.O. Baumann "Dimensions of the sick role in chronic illness", *Journal of Health and Social Behaviour*, Vol. 6, 1965, pp. 16-27

6 T. Parsons: "The sick role and the role of the physician reconsidered", *Milbank Memorial Fund, Health and Society*, Vol. 53, 1975, pp. 257-278 (reprinted in T. Parsons: *Action Theory and the Human Condition*. New York: Free Press 1978)

7 E. Goffman: *Asylums*. Essays on the Social Situation of Mental Patients and other Inmates. New York: Anchor/Doubleday 1961; E. Goffman: *Stigma*. Notes on the Management of Spoiled Identity. Englewood Cliffs: Prentice Hall 1963

8 H. Becker: *Outsiders*. Studies in the Sociology of Deviance. New York: Free Press 1963; H. Becker: "Whose sick are we on?", *Social Problems*, Vol 14, 1967, pp. 239-247

9 See, for instance, A. Gouldner: "The sociologist as partisan: sociology and the welfare state", *American Anthropologist*, Vol. 3, 1968, pp. 103-116; W. Ryan: *Blaming the Victim*, London: Orbach & Chambers 1971; M. Rossdale: "Health in a sick society", *New Left Review*, Vol. 34, 1965, pp. 82-90

10 T. Scheff: *Being Mentally Ill*. A Sociological Theory. Chicago: Aldine 1966, in: U. Gerhardt: *Ideas About Illness*, op.cit., pp. 91-122

11 E. Freidson: "Disability as social deviance", in: M. Sussman (ed): *Sociology and Rehabilitation*, Washington: American Sociological Association 1966, pp. 71-99

12 E. Freidson: *Profession of Medicine*. A Sociology of Knowledge of Applied Science. New York: Dodd, Mead 1970; E. Freidson: *Professional Dominance*. The Structure of Medical Care. Chicago: Aldine 1970. Freidson's argument spurred the discussion throughout the 1970s and into the 1980s, for instance in: B.S. Turner: *Medical Power and Social Knowledge*, London: Sage 1987

13 A. Strauss (ed): *Where Medicine Fails*. New Brunswick: Transaction Books 1970; J. Howard and A. Strauss (eds): *Humanizing Health Care*. New York: Wiley 1975

14 P. Strong: "Sociological imperialism and the profession of medicine". *Social Science and Medicine*, Vol. 13 A, 1979, pp. 179-215; H. Waitzkin. "Medicine, superstructure and micropolitics", *Social Science and Medicine*, Vol. 13 A, 1979, pp. 613-619; P. Conrad and J.W. Schneider: "Looking at levels of medicalization: A comment on Strong's critique of the thesis of medical imperialism". *Social Science and Medicine*, Vol. 14 A, 1980, pp. 75-79

15 I.K. Zola: "Medicine as an institution of social control". *Sociological Review*, Vol. 220, 1979, pp. 487-503; I.K. Zola "In the name of

health and illness: On some socio-political consequences of medical influence", *Social Science and Medicine*, Vol. 9, 1975, pp. 83-87

16 I. Illich: *Medical Nemesis*. London: Calder & Boyars 1975

17 T. McKeown and C.R. Lowe: *An Introduction to Social Medicine*. Oxford: Blackwell Scientific 1965; T. McKeown: *The Modern Rise of Population*. New York: Academic Press 1976; T. McKeown: *The Role of Medicine: Dream, Mirage or Nemesis?* London: Nuffield Provincial Trust 1979. See also: J. McKinlay and S. McKinlay: "The questionable contribution of medical measures to the decline of mortality in the United States in the twentieth century". *Milbank Memorial Fund Quarterly*, Vol. 55, 1977, pp. 451-465

18 E.M. Gruenberg: "The failures of success". *Milbank Memorial Fund Quarterly Health and Society*, Vol. 55, 1977, pp. 3-24; for an appreciation of Gruenberg see: U. Gerhardt: "Probleme der Medizinkritik", in: F. Wagner (ed): *Medizin - Momente ihrer Veränderung*. Berlin: Springer 1989, pp. 23-33

19 A. Strauss and B. Glaser: *Chronic Illness and the Quality of Life*. St. Louis: Mosby 1975, 19842

20 See, for instance, J. Corbin and A. Strauss: "Accompaniments of chronic illness: Changes in body, self, biography, and biographical time", in: *Research in the Sociology of Health Care*, Vol. 6 (ed. by J. Roth and P. Conrad) Greenwich, CT: JAI Press 1986, pp. 249-281; and in the same volume: C. Charmaz: "Struggling for a self: Identity levels of the chronically ill", pp. 283-328; also C. Charmaz: *Good Days, Bad Days*. The Self in Chronic Illness and Time. New Brunswick: Rutgers University Press 1991

21 C. Wiener, A. Strauss, S. Fagerhaugh and B. Suszek: "Patient power: Complex issues need complex answers". *Social Policy*, Vol. 11, 1980, pp. 31-38

22 J. Schneider and P. Conrad: *Having Epilepsy: The Experience and Social Contact of Illness*. Philadelphia: Temple University Press 1983; for further accounts of living experience see, for instance, R. Anderson and M. Bury (eds): *Living with Chronic Illness*. London: Unwin Hyman 1988; R. Weitz: *Life with AIDS*. New Brunwick. Rutgers University Press 1991

23 R. Fitzpatrick, J. Hinton, S. Newman, G. Scambler, and J. Thompson: *The Experience of Illness*. London: Tavistock 1984

24 J. Roth and P. Conrad (eds): *The Experience and Management of Chronic Illness*. Greenwich, CT: JAI Press 1987

25 J.M. Morse and J.L. Johnson: *The Illness Experience*. Dimensions of Suffering. Newbury Park: Sage 1991

26 P. Conrad: "The experience of illness: Recent and new directions", in: J. Roth and P. Conrad (eds), *op.cit.*, p. 2

27 M. Bury, "Chronic illness as a biographical disruption". *Sociology of Health and Illness*, Vol. 4, 1982, pp. 167-182

28 G. Williams: "The genesis of chronic illness: Narrative reconstruction". *Sociology of Health and Illness*, Vol. 6, 1984, pp. 175-200

29 G.H. Williams and P.H.N. Wood: "Common-sense beliefs about illness: A mediating role for the doctor". *Lancet*, 1986, ii, pp. 1435-1437

30 *Qualitative Research on Chronic Illness*. Guest editor: U. Gerhardt. *Social Science and Medicine*, Vol. 30, No. 11, 1990, containing, among other contributions: G. Scambler and A. Hopkins: "Generating a model of epileptic stigma: The role of qualitative analysis", pp. 1187-1194; U. Gerhardt: "Patient careers in end-stage renal failure", pp. 1211-1224; D. Armstrong: "Use of the genealogical method in the exploration of chronic illness. A research note", pp. 1225-1228

31 U. Gerhardt: "Qualitative research on chronic illness: The issue and the story". *Social Science and Medicine*, Vol. 30, 1990, p. 1149

32 D. Armstrong: "The Patient's View". *Social Science and Medicine*, Vol. 18, 1984, pp. 737-744; for interpretation of the model of medicine see U. Gerhardt: "Gesundheit - Was hat sie mit Medizin zu tun?", in: P. Novak (ed): *Lebensweisen und Gesundheitsorientierungen* (forthcoming 1992)

33 T. Parsons: "Health and Disease: A Sociological and Action Perspective", in: *The Human Condition*, op. cit., p. 81

34 See U. Gerhardt: "The Parsonian paradigm and the identity of medical sociology". *Sociological Review*, Vol. 27, 1979, pp. 229-254, esp. p. 231

35 Parsons's famous consideration that health is one of the prerequisites of adequate motivation of social actors who constitute (i.e. act within) social system is expressed in, for instance, the following statement: "The distinction between the negative and positive aspects of the problem of adequate motivation is relative and gradual. Both present functional problems in terms of the operation of the social system, which focus attention on the mechanisms which fit into the relevant context. But in spite of this relativity there is an important distinction between action which is positively disruptive of a going system of social relationships, and simple withdrawal of the individual from performance of his obligations. The principal criterion would be that in the latter case the only interference with others would consist in forcing them to do without the benefits expected from a person's actions. The possibility of withdrawal in fact defines one of the most important directions of deviant behaviour, and enters as we shall see in most important ways into the structure of the problems and mechanisms of social control. Illness is for example one of the most important types of withdrawal behaviour in our society." *Social System, op. cit.*, p. 30-31

36 How much reciprocity characterizes Parsons's basic idea of social action has been stressed by W.C. Mitchell: *Sociological Analysis and Politics*: The Theories of Talcott Parsons. Englewood Cliffs, N.J.: Prentice Hall 1967, whereas A. Gouldner completely misconceived the issue in *The Coming Crisis of Western Sociology*. London: Heinemann 1970

37 Regarding Weber's biography and illness of N. Fügen: *Max Weber*. Reinbek: Rowohlt 1978; also M. Weber: *Max Weber*. Ein Lebensbild. Tübingen: Mohr 1926

38 To be sure, higher rates of early retirement among lower class patients with, say, heart disease have frequently been interpretated as proof that they are at a disadvantage regarding normalization chances. But data from an ongoing study at the Giessen Medical Sociology Unit suggest that higher likelihood of lower-class coronary artery bypass patients to retire postoperatively may be due to their perception

that after return to work they have no guarantee whatsoever that their employment can be kept up until normal retirement age; therefore, they seize the opportunity offered by the German welfare state to retire early on medical disability benefits. In this way, lower-class patients normalize in a way that upper-class observers might evaluate as disenfranchisement. See: U. Gerhardt: "Frühberentung und Handlungsrationalität. Zur Statusdynamik bei Arbeitern nach koronarer Bypassoperation". *Soziale Welt*, Vol. 44, 1992 (forthcoming); B. Borgetto and U. Gerhardt: "Soziale Statuslage und Alternsdynamik bei koronarer Bypassoperation". *Sozial- und Präventivmedizin* (under consideration).

39 B.P. Dohrenwend and B.S. Dohrenwend: "Class and race as status-related sources of stress", in: S. Levine and N.A. Scotch (eds): *Social Stress*, Chicago: Aldine 1970, pp. 111-140; S.L. Syme and L.F. Berkman, "Social Class, susceptibility, and sickness". *American Journal of Epidemiology*, Vol. 104, 1976, pp. 1-8

40 R.G. Wilkinson (ed): *Class and Health*. Research and Longitudinal Data. London: Tavistock Publications 1986

41 P. Townsend and N. Davidson: *Inequalities in Health: The Black Report*. Harmondsworth: Penguin 1982; based on N. Hart: Health and Inequality. University of Essex. *mimeo* 1978

42 Cf. U. Gerhardt: "Preface", in: S. Platt, H. Thomas, S. Scott, and G. Williams (eds), *Locating Health*. London: Tavistock (forthcoming)

43 C. Herzlich and J. Pierret: *Illness and Self in Society*. Baltimore: John Hopkins University Press 1987 (originally in French, 1984). It ought to be noted, however, that the United States is not among the countries guaranteeing equal access to care provided or bolstered by the welfare state. On the contrary, some forty million population seem to have little if any access to care that they are able to afford in case of major sickness.

44 M. Foucault: *The Birth of the Clinic*. An Archaeology of Medical Perception. New York: Vintage 1975 (originally in French, 1963)

45 M. Foucault: *Discipline and Punish*. The Birth of the Prison. New York. Vintage 1979 (originally in French, 1975)

46 D. Armstrong: *The Political Anatomy of the Body*. Medical Knowledge in the Twentieth Century. Cambridge: Cambridge University Press 1983

47 *op. cit.*, p. xi

48 He writes: "Political anatomy unifies those various sciences which have as their common object the human body and its surrounding space. In political anatomy those disparate knowledges, which have offered seemingly diverse or contradictory explanations of the body or its behaviour, can be seen as components of a single apparatus of power. The great debates of the twentieth century which oppose the individual and the social, the citizen and the state, the biological versus the environmental, are various manifestations of the same underlying dream, the same pervasive diagram of power." *op. cit.*, p. 117

49 B.S. Turner: *Regulating Bodies*. Essays in Medical Sociology. London: Sage 1992, esp. p. 57, 84, 95

50 The polemical thrust of the argument is obvious in T. Szasz: *The Therapeutic State*: Psychiatry in the Mirror of Current Events. Buffalo: Prometheus 1984; J. O'Neill: *Five Bodies*: The Human Shape of Modern Society. Ithaca and London: Cornell University Press 1985; D. Cohen (ed), Challenging the Therapeutic State. Critical Perspectives on Psychiatry and the Mental Health System. *The Journal of Mind and Behaviour*, Vol. 11, No. 3-4 (special issue).

51 Turner summarizes his argument as follows: "Essentially, the argument behind the sociology of the body is, first, that sociology is genuinely a sociology of action, and that the social actor is not a Cartesian subject divided into body and mind but an embodied actor whose practicality and knowledgeability involve precisely this embodiment." *Regulating Bodies*, p. 170

[2]

MAX WEBER, FORMAL RATIONALITY, AND HEALTH LIFESTYLES

William C. Cockerham
University of Alabama at Birmingham
Thomas Abel
University of Marburg
Günther Lüschen
University of Düsseldorf

Max Weber's concept of formal rationality and ideas about lifestyles in general are applied to current trends in health lifestyles. The central contribution of Weber's thinking is recognition of the dialectical interplay between formal versus substantive rationality, consumption versus production, choice versus life chances, class similarities versus distinctions, and self-control versus conformity in shaping health lifestyles and the reality of their operationalization in the postmodern world. In a largely applied subdiscipline like medical sociology, Weber's work offers a theoretical background on which to enrich our understanding of health lifestyles and grapple with the initial theoretical challenges posed by lifestyle research.

The usefulness of classic sociological theory in explaining social change in today's world has not always been apparent, despite the fact that, as Parsons (1981) observed, one can often learn something new by returning to the classics. The goal of this article is to apply Weber's theory of formal rationality—one of the major paradigms of sociological thought—and his general ideas about lifestyle to the concept of health lifestyles. This approach allows us to acquire new insights into an important emerging feature of postmodernity, namely, the growing dominance of formal rationality in health matters.

We argue that formal rationality (the purposeful calculation of the most efficient means to an end) is a more dominant aspect of health-lifestyle participation in postmodern society than substantive rationality (an orientation toward ideal values and ends). Whereas the rationality behind health lifestyles in the past tended to be more substantive (reflecting the value of health as an ideal state), it has become more formal (the most effective method for individuals to look better, enjoy increased vitality, and enhance life expectancy). What this trend signifies is that a distinctive aspect of postmodernity is greater personal control over one's health and—consistent with Ritzer and Walczak's (1988)

*Direct all correspondence to: Dr. William C. Cockerham, Department of Sociology, University of Alabama at Birmingham, UAB Station, Birmingham, AL 35294.

The Sociological Quarterly, Volume 34, Number 3, pages 413-425.

ISSN: 0038-0253.

analysis of formal rationality and the deprofessionalization of American physicians—a lessening dependence upon physicians as authority figures.

Consequently, we see Weber's concept of formal rationality, as do others (Alexander 1987; Löwith 1982; Mommsen 1987, 1989; Roth 1987; Tenbruck 1975), also depicting a potentially liberating circumstance for the individual, not just irreversibly locking people into a bureaucratic "iron cage" of dehumanization and overwhelming dependence on technical procedures administered by experts. Whereas most Weberian scholarship in the past emphasized loss of freedom via the "iron cage" interpretation of formal rationality, more recent insight reminds us of the potential for creativity and freedom such rationality also provides (cf. Alexander 1987; Roth 1987; Whimster and Lash 1987).

Before examining the evidence concerning the expansion of formal rationality in health lifestyles, we will establish the context for our analysis by selectively reviewing Weber's theory of rationality and his views on lifestyles. Since Weber was sometimes ambiguous and inconsistent in his use of particular terms (Brubaker 1984; Kalberg 1980; Wiley 1987), our discussion will draw not only on Weber's own writings, but also on those of others who have recently interpreted his work.

WEBER ON RATIONALITY

The essence of Weberian theory, as Jaspers (1988) comments, is that Weber's ideas stand between a vanishing and rising era. This is especially true with respect to his idea of rationality and the unifying theme it provided for his explanation of the transition to modernity in Western society (Alexander 1983; Brubaker 1984; Hennis 1987, 1988; Kalberg 1980; Käsler 1988; Schluchter 1981; Spinner 1989; Whimster and Lash 1987). In analyzing the origins and characteristics of a particular form of rationalism most evident in Western culture, Weber (1922, 1978) focused on two distinct types of rationality: formal and substantive. Kalberg (1980) identifies two other types of rationality, practical and theoretical, in Weber's theory, but the key factor in the development of modernism was the ascendance of formal over substantive rationality.

Weber does not claim that formal rationality characterizes modern Western society as a whole; rather, he notes the continued and irreconcilable conflict in modernity between the merits of a rational behavior that is formal (logically calculated, efficient, and objective) in achieving goals as opposed to rational behavior that is substantive (based on personal devotion, tradition, piety, and custom). In the West, substantive rationality has been increasingly dominated but not destroyed by its formal counterpart. Rather, it is the disregard of substantive values and ends in favor of efficiency that makes Western rationalism "specific and peculiar." Formal rationality provided "a freedom to inquire, to dispute, to experiment, a belief in the possibilities of improvement, a concern for the practical rather than the abstract, a rationalism which defied mandarin codes, religious dogma, and traditional folklore" (Kennedy 1987, p. 30). This gave the West the opportunity to be the first to industrialize, to develop an advanced state of capitalism, and to become the center of world power beginning in the 19th century.

Weber's concept of formal rationality at the macro level and his notion of *zweckrationalität* (purposeful goal-oriented action) at the micro level, along with his observation of the replacement of traditional and charismatic forms of authority in Western society by rational-legal systems, are all part of a general process of rationalization constructed on the principles of efficiency and calculation. The rise of the bureaucracy, with its inherently impersonal (though theoretically more efficient) form of social organization, led Weber to warn of a future in which rationalization could impose itself on individuals in the form of an "iron cage." Weiss (1987) claims this process is irreversible, not because Weber viewed the unfolding of Western rationalization as an irresistible historical development but because human beings have deliberately chosen this course of action as their best alternative. Weiss (1987, p. 159) states that Weber, without a doubt, "was convinced that the process of progressive rationalization would lead increasingly to the restriction of the free play of action and have an obligatory character independent of the will of individuals." But this does not mean, notes Weiss, that Weber was forced to draw a fatalistic conclusion about the future direction of modern society. Rather, Weiss points out that Weber's final conclusion was that the individual's freedom of action needed to be strengthened and developed as part of the overall process of formal rationalization.

Others (Roth 1987; Tenbruck 1975, 1980) suggest that Weber's analysis appears to be more of a warning than a certainty, since his writings contain evidence that he also viewed rationality as a force to enhance human freedom. Weber (1949, pp. 124–25) states, for instance, that "we associate the strongest empirical 'feeling of freedom' with precisely those actions which we know ourselves to have accomplished rationally, i.e. in the absence of physical or psychic 'compulsion;' actions in which we 'pursue' a clear conscious 'purpose' by what to our knowledge are the most adequate means."

Consequently, Löwith (1982) points out that Western rationalism, as depicted by Weber, also represents a countertendency toward the freedom of self-responsibility. Löwith explains that the individual's capacity for self-responsibility is the positive meaning of rationality, since it provides the means by which people can break the iron cage and assume control over their circumstances. Alexander (1987) likewise notes that rationalization is the only human path for liberation. Roth (1987) argues, in turn, that Weber did not consider bureaucratic rationalization to lead to dehumanization; instead, he claims that Weber's work explains the amalgamation of tradition and modernity in ways that open new directions for rationalization.

Mommsen (1989) indicates that Weber considered the bureaucratic aspects of formal rationalism as an inevitable phenomenon that people in modern societies simply have to endure, but nevertheless viewed the rational techniques associated with modernity as providing new opportunities for creative action. Mommsen (1989, p. 195) suggests that Weber's primary interest was to give concrete answers to the question how and under what political and social conditions in the course of history did a *Lebensführung* (life conduct) prevail which allowed for responsibility and creativity, in spite of institutional forces that tend to stifle individual initiative. In essence, what Weber principally tries to explain with his theory of rationality is the evolution of a way of life that changed society.

The merit of Weber's concept of formal rationality for this discussion is to recall attention to the relationship between freedom and constraint which his original work intended. The notion of the constraining effects of the "iron cage" of rationality has, until recently, been considered the ultimate outcome of modernity, but it is now clear that, for serious Weber scholars, there is an emerging view that his concept of formal rationality includes the idea that such rationality also provides freedom and the capacity for action that promotes creativity. As Scaff (1989, p. 70) explains, Weber attributed a paradox to historical development by finding it constrained by "structure" yet "open to living." Hence, the dominance of formal over substantive rationality in Western society does not just consist of the imposition of rationally calculated rules and regulations on people, but opens, as Alexander (1987) observes, a path for liberation by which people can logically determine the most effective means to reach their objectives in life.

It is also apparent that Weber did not intend an evolutionary theory of rationality, nor wish to make global generalizations (Ritzer and Walczak 1988; Weber 1981; Weiss 1987). Also, he did not exhaust the systematic scope of his theoretical approach, but largely restricted his investigation to the emergence of the Protestant Ethic (Habermas 1984). Nevertheless, Weber (1922, 1946, 1978) recognized that the process of rationalization was a universal phenomenon that assumed various forms. We would argue that health lifestyles in Western society constitute a particular form or expression of formal rationality because they involve the exercise of efficiency and calculability as a means to achieve a preferred end state—a healthy body. This process includes demystification of medical knowledge as such knowledge becomes increasingly available to the lay public (Cassell 1986). Health-lifestyle participation can be considered liberating rather than dehumanizing, since it symbolizes the personal assumption of greater control and self-responsibility for one's own health. After all, it was Weber's (1920, p. 114; see also Scaff 1989, p. 227) position that formal rationality disenchants the world and sustains a culture that devalues "mysterious incalculable forces" in favor of knowledge "that [allows] one in principle, [to] *master* all things by *calculation*."

WEBER ON LIFESTYLES

The concept of lifestyle has played a role in sociological theory since the 19th century. In his political writings in the 1850s, Marx (1960) mentions lifestyle differences between social classes, while Veblen (1899) used the concept of lifestyle as a basis for his theory of the leisure class. But it remained for Weber (1922, 1946, 1978) to produce a more thorough accounting than Marx or Veblen of the role of lifestyle in relation to socioeconomic status. Weber maintained that a distinguishing characteristic of status was "status honor" or prestige which was normally expressed by the fact that a particular lifestyle could be expected from all who wished to belong to a certain group. Weber made the particularly pertinent observation that lifestyles were based not so much on what a person produced, but on what he or she consumed. Thus, for Weber, the difference between status groups did not lie in their relationship to the means of production but in their relationship to the means of consumption.

In the case of health lifestyles, a person is attempting to produce good health according to his or her degree of motivation and capabilities. The aim of this activity, however, is ultimately one of consumption. People attempt to maintain or enhance their health in order to use it for some end, such as work, a longer life, or enhanced enjoyment of their physical being. For example, d'Houtaud and Field (1984) found in France that health was viewed as something to be cultivated for increased vitality and enjoyment of life among the upper and middle classes, and for the ability to continue to work among working-class respondents. But in both situations, health was something that was to be consumed, not simply produced.

Weber used three distinct terms in the original German to express his concept of lifestyles. These terms are *Lebensstil* or *Stilisierung des Lebens*, which mean lifestyles, and *Lebensführung* (life conduct) and *Lebenschancen* (life chances), which comprise the two basic components of lifestyles. *Lebensführung* refers to the choices people have in their selection of lifestyles and *Lebenschancen* is the probability of realizing these choices. The link between choice and lifestyles appears to have been overemphasized in most interpretations of Weber, while the connection between lifestyles and life chances has received little attention. However, it is clear that Weber did not regard lifestyles simply as a matter of choice, nor did he ignore the structural conditions necessary to support a particular lifestyle.

This crucial distinction in Weber's conceptualization of lifestyles has been obscured in English language translations of his *Wirtschaft und Gesellschaft* (1922). In the section in chapter IX titled "Machtverteilung innerhalb der Gesellschaft. Klassen, Stände, Parteien" ("The Distribution of Power within the Political Community: Class, Status, Party"), *Stilisierlung des Lebens and Lebensführung* are both translated simply as "lifestyles" in Gerth and Mills (Weber 1946) and Roth and Wittich (Weber 1978)—the two most frequently cited English language translations. Moreover, the idea that *Lebensführung* and *Lebenschancen* are the two components of *Stilisierlung des Lebens* or *Lebensstil* is not brought forward. The result, as Abel and Cockerham (1993) point out, is that Weber's distinctly different terms *Lebensführung* (life conduct) and Lebensstil (lifestyles) have essentially the same meaning in Anglo-American literature. Translated literally, *Lebensführung* means life conduct and refers to choice and self-direction in a person's behavior, not lifestyles. Consequently, *Lebensführung* is the element of choice within Weber's overall concept of *Lebensstil* (lifestyles) and joins with Lebenschancen (life chances) as one of *Lebensstil*'s two basic components. To use *Lebensführung* to mean simply lifestyles, overlooks the depth of Weber's thinking on the subject. Weber's original concept of lifestyles is depicted in Figure 1.

Weber's intent with respect to conceptualizing lifestyles appears to be that of recognizing that people have choices in the lifestyles they wish to adopt, but the actualization of these choices are influenced by their life chances. Dahrendorf (1979, p. 73) notes that Weber is ambiguous about what he really means by life chances, but one particularly insightful meaning he found suggested by Weber is that life chances are: "the crystallized probability of finding satisfaction for interests, wants and needs, thus the probability of the occurrence of events which bring about satisfaction." For Weber, the notion of life chances therefore refers to the probability of acquiring satisfaction which is anchored in structural conditions. These structural conditions are depicted by Weber (1922, 1978) as strongly economic—involving income, property, the opportunity for profit, and the like—

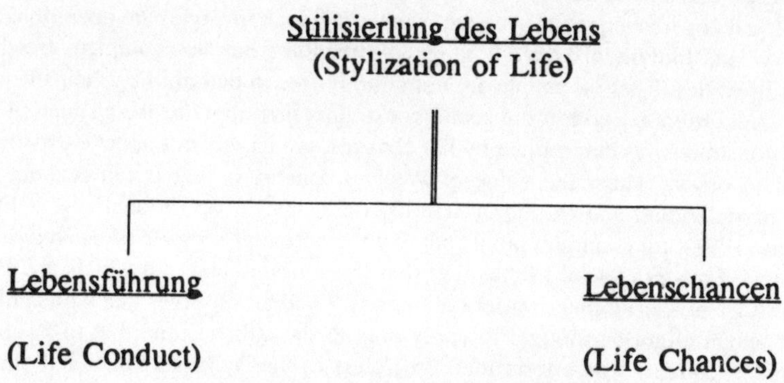

Figure 1. Weber's Concept of Lifestyles

but also involving rights, norms, and social relationships (the probability that others will respond in a certain manner). Thus, Weber's thesis is that chance is socially determined and social structure is an arrangement of chances (Dahrendorf 1979).

Of course, the life chances that enhance participation in health lifestyles are greatest among upper and middle socioeconomic groups who have the best resources to support their choices. Clearly, social stratification is an important determining factor in the operationalization of health lifestyles. Yet, it was also Weber's position, as Bendix (1960, pp. 260–261) reminds us, that lifestyles frequently spread beyond the groups in which they originate. The best example is Weber's analysis of the spread of the Protestant Ethic into the general culture of Western society. One result is that, in the modern world, the Protestant Ethic is no longer distinctive to Protestants (Jaspers 1988). While lifestyles set people apart, Weber demonstrates that aspects of a particular group's lifestyle can also gain widespread influence in the larger society.

Additionally, the Weberian concept of *Lebensführung* denoting individual choice does not imply complete disregard of substantive values. Rather, beginning with Tenbruck (1975) and noted by other Weberian scholars (Habermas 1984; Hennis 1987, 1988; Mommsen 1989; Schluchter 1981) is the association of an "ethics of responsibility" with *Lebensführung*. As explained by Mommsen (1989), such ethics require the individual to "weigh-up" the possible consequences of his or her actions with a view toward optimal possible realization of ideal values. Thus, if good health is a valued end-state for an individual, a person's conduct (*Lebensführung*) will be guided by a set of ethics influencing the choices made to realize this end. Hence, lifestyles (health or otherwise) are not random behaviors lacking structural anchors, but typically are deliberate (formal) choices influenced by life chances.

It is here that we find one of Weber's most important contributions to enhancing our understanding of health lifestyles. Our reading of what Weber meant by the term *Stillisierlung des Lebens* is to impose a dialectical capstone over the interplay of choice and structure in lifestyles. Münch (1988), for example, has previously noted that Weber's theory of rationalization is "dialectic." Münch (1988, p. 211) rejects Schluchter's (1979) contention that Weber's rationalization theory reflects paradoxes and argues instead that Weber's true achievement is his conceptualization of modern Western development "as being intrinsically and uniquely determined by the interpenetration of opposing spheres." The recognition of Weber's concept of rationalization as a dialectic theory and the identification of life chances as the dialectic opposite of choice in his lifestyle scheme, provide the theoretical key to conceptualizing the manner in which lifestyles are operationalized in the real world. Individuals have a range of freedom, but not complete freedom, in choosing lifestyles. That is, people are not entirely free in determining their lifestyle but have the freedom to act within the social constraints that apply to their situation in life. Lifestyle constraints, as determined by life chances, are largely but not exclusively socioeconomic in origin. Thus, the value of Weber's concept is that it can account for the problem of individual choice and structural constraints in operationalizing a lifestyle.

Giddens (1991), for example, points out that the notion of lifestyle takes on a particular significance in modern social life, as tradition loses ground and individuals are forced to make lifestyle choices among a variety of options. Giddens observes that while "lifestyle" is a term which might be thought to apply only to the affluent, and that to a substantial degree this is correct, it is a term that also refers to the decisions taken and courses of action followed under conditions of severe material constraint. Lower-class life involves distinctive cultural styles and modes of activity that still require choices. Lifestyle patterns across social strata also include deliberate rejection as well as acceptance of various forms of behavior and consumption. No culture, indicates Giddens (1991, p. 80), eliminates choice altogether in day-to-day affairs.

Yet, Giddens also recognizes that a tradition of habit tends to order life within established channels; consequently, individuals not only follow certain lifestyles but in many cases may be pressured by convention to do so. Group influence, socioeconomic circumstances, and available knowledge push people to make certain choices. As Giddens (1991, p. 81) puts it, "we have no choice but to choose." On balance, the context of Weber's concept of lifestyles emphasizes choice; however, external influences like life chances clearly structure the options available.

HEALTH LIFESTYLES

Health behavior refers to the activity undertaken by people who believe themselves to be healthy for the purpose of preventing illness or injury (Kasl and Cobb 1966). Drawing upon the work of Milo (1981) and McQueen (1988), and consistent with Weberian theory, we suggest that the term "health lifestyles" refers to patterns of voluntary health behavior based on choices from options that are available to people according to their life situations. Health lifestyles include contact with the medical profession in the case of checkups and preventive care, but the majority of activities take place outside the health care delivery system. These activities typically consist of choices and practices, influenced by the individual's probabilities for realizing them, that range from brushing one's teeth and using automobile seat belts to relaxing at health spas. For most people, health lifestyles involve decisions about food, exercise, relaxation, personal hygiene, risk of accidents, coping with stress, use of cigarettes, alcohol, and drugs, and having medical checkups. Unfortunately, there is not an abundance of research on participation in health lifestyles because, as Kickbusch (1989, p. 125) observes, it was only "about ten years ago academics discovered the fact that people actually take care of themselves." Nonetheless, there is enough evidence to determine whether formal rationality is a more dominant aspect of health lifestyle participation in the United States than substantive rationality.

Historically, it would appear that substantive rationality largely influenced public participation in health lifestyles in the United States. Green's (1986) work, consisting of an extensively documented history of health and fitness activities between 1830–1940, supports this conclusion. He found that early in the 19th century, a strong religious sentiment was associated with health. Various religious reformers argued that the second coming of Christ might be advanced if humankind could achieve a state of grace and perfection, which included a healthy body. "Good health—the avoidance of disease, debility, and premature death—thus took on extraordinary importance," states Green (1986, p. 10). Physical degeneration became regarded by many not only as a medical problem, but a spiritual one as well.

Other developments identified by Green during the 19th and 20th centuries included: linking health with the vitality of the nation; the emergence of romantic notions about the peasantry of supposedly healthier (and poorer) cultures, depicting them as simple people who lived innocently, worked hard, and were physically strong; associating health with beauty; athletics as a foundation for a "muscular Christianity"; sports as a method to instill "team spirit" and an outlook necessary for success in business and war; health as vital to upward social mobility for immigrants because of its close association with Americanism; and, finally, fitness activity as an expression of a desire for community. Health lifestyles were also advocated by some groups and individuals along more formal lines as a means to avoid illness, reduce the chances of dying early, and gain an "edge" on competition in the workplace, but, on balance, the rationality that was expressed about health in Green's study is more substantive than formal.

Gillick (1984) agrees that early participation by Americans in health and fitness activities was strongly influenced by religion and other substantive concerns. However, Gillick, who focuses exclusively on jogging, argues that after a period in the 1970s when popular interest in running was largely due to a desire to improve the body's cardiovascular functions, the jogging movement took a new turn. It changed to emphasizing the effect of running on a person's overall sense of well-being, especially mental health. Hence, Gillick maintains that jogging can now be associated, like it was in the past, with upright living or what she (Gillick 1984, p. 379) calls "save our souls." Gillick adds that the pursuit of physical fitness by some people is also seen as a means to improve America.

Gillick's work suggests that when it comes to jogging, substantive rationality remains more prevalent today than formal rationality. However, her data in this regard comes largely from accounts in running magazines written by jogging enthusiasts who stress the spiritual nature of running. Consequently, these data may not be representative of the mass population of joggers, nor of persons who practice healthy lifestyles but do not necessarily jog. Gillick does provide some support for a more formal or instrumental rationality for jogging by noting that Americans also jog for reasons of cardiovascular fitness and control over their health. The merit of Gillick's paper is its reminder that substantive values remain an important aspect of exercise, but the data utilized are too selective to support a general conclusion that substantive rather than formal rationality is dominant today in jogging in particular or in fitness activities in general.

Rather, it falls to Crawford (1984) to explain why formal rationality emerged in recent years to dominate its substantive version for reasons of health promotion. First, suggests Crawford, there has been a growing recognition on the part of the lay public that major-disease patterns have changed from infections to chronic illnesses that medicine cannot cure. Second, numerous health disasters—like AIDS and cigarette-induced lung cancer—have been caused by particular styles of living. Third, there has been a virtual campaign by the mass media and health professionals emphasizing lifestyle change and individual responsibility for health. The result has been an increased awareness that medicine is no longer the automatic answer to dealing with health problems. Consequently, strategies on the part of individuals for healthier lifestyles have gained in popularity. As Crawford explains, when the environment cannot be controlled to stop sickness and medicine cannot provide a cure, self-control over the range of personal behaviors that affect health is the remaining option.

Crawford also suggests that health is a metaphor for consumption; that is, good health is a form of release in that it provides a person with the freedom to consume in order to satisfy individual needs. Furthermore, Crawford argues that an abundance of news and commentary in the media on lifestyles and health have reduced complacency about staying healthy, and he notes media declarations that health and fitness have themselves been declared a lifestyle. An important response to this situation is the virtual flood of commercial products intended to help the individual "manufacture" health. Thus, states Crawford (1984, p. 76), "the complex ideologies of health are picked up, magnified, and given commodity form by the image-makers." Commercial activities associated with physical fitness not only produce profits, but also reinforce an instrumental approach to health and fitness.

Empirical data supporting the ascendancy of formal over substantive rationality in health lifestyles is found in a series of community, state, and national surveys. Analyzing a national sample, Ransford (1986) determined that lower-class blacks were especially likely to practice health-protective behavior because of concern about heart disease. Well-educated whites were found to participate in health lifestyles because of a more general concern about health. But the end result was the same: health behavior cut across class and racial lines.

In Ohio, Harris and Guten (1979) found that practically everyone in their survey did something to protect his or her health. A series of studies in Illinois found a distinct lack of difference among races, social classes (to include cross-national comparisons with West Germans), and occupational groups in participation in health lifestyles (Abel 1991; Abel, Cockerham, Kunz, and Lueschen 1989; Cockerham, Kunz, and Lueschen 1988; Cockerham, Lueschen, Kunz, and Spaeth 1986). Although the quality of participation may vary, health lifestyles in these studies appeared widely accepted and practiced. Other research in South Carolina determined that socioeconomic factors were not significant variables in predicting changes in health practices among government employees in a health promotion project; there were simply not enough socioeconomic differences between groups practicing good health habits (Kronenfeld, Jackson, Davis, and Blair 1988). What these studies suggest is that even though the origin of health lifestyles can be traced to the middle and upper-middle social classes in American society (Crawford 1984; Gillick 1984; Glassner 1989), they appear to be spreading across class lines in a manner similar to that suggested by Weber in his analysis of the spread of the Protestant Ethic (Cockerham, Kunz, and Lueschen 1988).

However, it should not be said that social class does not matter in health lifestyle participation. The current economic recession clearly impacts adversely on the health lifestyles of the poor. This is seen in U.S. Department of Agriculture reports showing weekly food spending per person among the poorest one-fifth of the population dropping 13.1 percent between 1980–1988, as well as in studies of garbage in New York City showing the poorest neighborhoods with the heaviest meat, regular soda, and high-fat, high-salt chips remains, and affluent neighborhoods with more diet soda and low-salt peanuts remains (O'Neill 1992; Rothschild 1990). A link between light foods, like salads and vegetables, and higher social status persists in American society (Weaver 1989). None of the major sociological surveys in the United States claim equity in health lifestyles, but all show a general pattern of diminishing class differences with respect to efforts to participate in accordance with one's life chances. The exception would be the poorest of the poor and the homeless (Rossi 1989).

Findings from the existing health lifestyle surveys (Abel 1991; Abel et al. 1989; Cockerham, Lueschen, Kunz, and Sapeth 1986; Cockerham, Kunz, and Lueschen 1988; Harris and Guten 1979; Kronenfeld et al. 1988; Ransford 1986) suggest that individual self-control over one's health is the principal rationale given for participating in various types of health and fitness activities in contemporary American society. The same theme is found in broadly based literature reviews and essays on fitness and the postmodern self (Glassner 1988, 1989). "By becoming fit," states Glassner (1989, p. 187), "persons are said to achieve a degree of independence from medical professionals and medical technology." Thus, the majority position is that health lifestyles are pursued because they allow a person to assume greater control over their life course.

Studies of corporate wellness programs uncover a related theme. Relevant research shows that the respondents participated in fitness activities sponsored by their employers because they wanted to stay in shape, lose weight largely to just look better, and socialize with other people (Conrad 1988; Kotarba and Bentley 1988). That is, their health goals were limited to participating in workouts that would result in a positive body image and level of physical conditioning which would allow them to get more out of life (Conrad 1988). The fact that it was a collective activity with friends was also important (Kotarba and Bentley 1988). Participation was not determined by religious ideology nor by working for a better America, but simply by a desire on the part of the individual to look and feel good through exercise and dieting by working out with friends.

Therefore, as Kotarba and Bentley (1988, p. 558) explain, workplace wellness programs "illustrate a more general trend in our culture that is transforming health from a status—something an individual has—to an accomplishment—something an individual does." In this context, health, as Kotarba and Bentley point out, becomes an accomplishment to the degree that an individual can rationally and systematically attempt to seek, nurture, and prolong it.

The motivation to be healthy either for greater self-control or enjoyment of life clearly suggests an enhanced role for formal rationality in health lifestyles among Americans. According to Glassner (1988), greater self-control over a person's quality of life through the medium of the body has emerged as a major component of modernism. The rationality underlying this development is predominately formal since it reflects the purposeful calculation of the most efficient means to achieve health so it can be used for something. Health is not valued so much as a substantive, idealized end state; rather, health is valued because it has a practical and utilitarian function to perform. As Turner (1984, 1987) explains, religion dominated ideas about the physical use of the body (i.e., control of emotions, sexual restraint) in past Western history, but rationalization and secularization have produced a modern emphasis on the use of the outer surface of the body for desirable feelings and personal significance.

This development runs counter to Foucault's (1980) view of the body as a passive object and something to be acted upon by social institutions. Foucault's genealogy, as Lash (1990) suggests, may, in the end, be of greatest use to feminists in accounting for the manner in which modernity imposed a familial structure on female sexuality. Gender differences in health-related behavior are beyond the scope of this paper but represent a critically important area for future health lifestyle research. Books on weight control, for instance, appear to be written primarily for women, while health self-help groups are largely feminist in origin (Withorn 1986). The strong possibility exists that gender differences in health lifestyles may be as important or more important than socioeconomic distinctions.

As Giddens (1991) suggests for lifestyles in general, there may also be normative and group pressures forcing choices in health lifestyles. Workplace norms and employer policies are capable of pushing employees into fitness programs, while the opportunity to socialize in working out with others can provide further collective incentives (Conrad 1988; Kotarba and Bentley 1988). The volume of mass-media information on health, public health campaigns, and advice from medical professionals likewise establish and reinforce normative health behavior. Thus, there is irony in the liberating potential of health lifestyles from subordination to physicians in that much of the knowledge behind the activity is medical in origin and context.

But regardless of whether people are pushed into health lifestyles or are pulled into them by choice, such lifestyles have become a normative activity in American society (Crawford 1984; Goldstein 1992). Public restrictions on smoking and legal requirements to list ingredients, calories, fat content and the like in prepared foods illustrates this fact. Baudrillard (1988a) goes so far as to depict dieting, jogging, and body-building as a new form of involuntary servitude in American culture.

Moreover, in Baudrillard's own France, Herzlich and Pierret (1987) identify a current shift in French thinking toward a norm of a "duty to be healthy." Herzlich and Pierret find that the normative "duty to be healthy" is most pervasive in the middle class, but provide accounts of less socially-advantaged persons espousing the same orientation and imply that this norm is spreading in French society. They describe health as both an exigency of society, requiring effort and discipline, and the means by which an individual achieves personal self-realization. Herzlich and Pierret (1987, p. 231) state, "Today, the 'right to health' implies that every individual must be made responsible for his or her health and must adopt rational behavior in dealing with the pathogenic effects of modern life."

Yet, the decision to participate in health lifestyles ultimately falls to the individual, not society. It is the individual who makes the choices about his or her diet, smoking, exercise, and other health-promoting actions and whether or not to follow through on those decisions. People who reject such lifestyles despite the widespread dissemination of health information show that freedom of choice is not only operative but paramount in lifestyle selection. Normative situations pressure, shape, and reinforce these choices and life chances constrain them but, in a Weberian framework of analysis, *Lebensführung* or choice in one's life conduct is decisive. It was Weber's (1968, pp. 507–508) view that in the final analysis, every important action and life as a whole signifies a chain of ultimate decisions through which the individual chooses his or her own fate (see also Scaff 1989, p. 92).

CONCLUSION

Regardless of whether modern society is in a state of postmodernity, featuring cultural dedifferentiation (Lash 1990), or high modernity in which a diversity of lifestyle options are available (Giddens 1991), it is clear that most of human society has entered an advanced stage of modernity on a global scale. According to Giddens (1990, 1991), at this point in human development, social relations cross wide spans of time and space, social life is propelled away from preestablished practices, and knowledge—continuously revised on the basis of new findings—is used regularly to shape social interaction. Giddens (1991, p. 5) thus finds that "in modern social life, the notion of lifestyle takes on a particular significance" as a major key to understanding individual self-identity and behavior. All indications are that, as sociology moves into the 21st century, research on lifestyles is going to be a major focus of the discipline.

We suggest that Weber's central contribution to our understanding of health lifestyles in the postmodern/high-modernity period lies in his conceptual recognition of the dialectical forces contained within such lifestyles. Health lifestyles are derived from formal rationality, yet involve an admittedly weaker but enduring substantive rationality; are modes of consumption requiring production; are based on choice yet constrained by life chances; feature broad similarities but distinct differences between social classes; and promote self-control as well as conformity. To overlook the interplay of these elements in shaping health lifestyles fails to capture the reality of their operationalization in a postmodern world. A Weberian perspective on health lifestyles and rationality has some limits, however, as nonrational aspects of lifestyles, like addictions and habits, can also determine health behavior. But overall, it would seem that Weberian theory captures the essence of most health lifestyle experiences.

Our position with respect to the application of Weberian theory to health lifestyles in the context of the modernity/postmodernity debate is one that emphasizes the creative and liberating aspects of formal rationalization. Although there is not total agreement on the exact meaning of postmodernity, the term can nevertheless be generally conceptualized as a form of reaction to, or departure from, modernism. According to Harvey (1990), modernism is a belief in progress, absolute truths, rational planning, and the standardization of knowledge; postmodernism, in contrast, is redefinition, fragmentation, indeterminacy, and distrust of universal discourses. We would see the dependence of individuals on physicians and medical knowledge as modernist and efforts to demedicalize one's approach to health behavior, reduce dependency in the patient-physician relationship, and take control of one's health situation as postmodernist. This is consistent with Crawford's (1984) assertion that when environments cannot be controlled to eliminate sickness and medicine cannot find a cure, self-control over personal behavior is an only remaining health option. When limits are reached, such as medicine's capacity to cure, postmodernity, as Baudrillard (1988b) comments, is the attempt to reach a point where one can live with what is left. Thus, taking control of one's health situation to the greatest extent possible appears as a postmodernist act.

This position contrasts with that of Holton and Turner (1989), who suggest that Weber's version of modernity is optimistic and accepting of the inevitability of rationalization, secularization, and the spread of bureaucratic management, while Weber's postmodernist view is pessimistic and holds that modernization is self-defeating because it ultimately leads to the iron cage of rationalization. We would say, as stated earlier by Alexander (1987), Roth (1987), Tenbruck (1980), and others, that the iron cage is but one alternative of formal rationalization and greater freedom is the other. The postmodernist seems most likely to adopt a view that responsibility for a person's health should not fall routinely on experts but on the self to the fullest extent possible. This means redefining one's health situation and taking control over one's physical status through strategies that include a healthy lifestyle. Many Weberian theorists have, in our view, tended to overemphasize Weber's iron cage concept and neglect the liberating potential of rationalization in anticipating the future. Current scholarship should rectify this trend.

Our intent in this paper has been not to modify Weberian theory but to clarify and extend the depth of Weber's thinking on lifestyles generally to health lifestyles. Weber did not address the subject of health lifestyles, but in a relatively atheoretical subdiscipline like medical sociology, the work of classical theorists like Weber offers a theoretical foundation upon which to enrich our understanding and help us to grapple with the initial theoretical challenges posed by lifestyle research.

ACKNOWLEDGEMENT

This article is a revision of a paper presented to the 1990 American Sociological Association meeting, Washington, D.C., and the European Society of Medical Sociology meeting, Marburg, Germany, and the basis for a panel discussion at the 1992 joint meeting of the British Sociological Association Medical Sociology Group and the European Society of Medical Sociology, Edinburgh, Scotland. The authors wish to thank Andrea Fontana, Joseph Kotarba, and Virginia Olesen for their insightful comments. A conversation with Richard Münch was very helpful as well.

REFERENCES

Abel, Thomas. 1991. "Measuring Health Lifestyles in a Comparative Analysis: Theoretical Issues and Empirical Findings." *Social Science and Medicine* 32: 899–908.

Abel, Thomas and William C. Cockerham. 1993. "Lifestyle or Lebensführung? Critical Remarks on the Mistranslation of Weber's 'Class, Status, Party.'" *Sociological Quarterly* 34: 551–556.

Abel, Thomas, William C. Cockerham, Guenther Lueschen, and Gerhard Kunz. 1989. "Health Lifestyles and Self-Direction in Employment Among American Men: A Test of the Spillover Effect." *Social Science and Medicine* 28: 1269–1274.

Alexander, Jeffrey C. 1983. *The Classical Attempt at Theoretical Synthesis: Max Weber, Theoretical Logic in Sociology*, Vol. 3. Berkeley: University of California Press.

———. 1987. "The Dialectic of Individuation and Domination: Weber's Rationalization Theory and Beyond." Pp. 185–206 in *Max Weber, Rationality and Modernism*, edited by S. Whimster and S. Lash. London: Allen & Unwin.

Baudrillard, Jean. 1988a. *America*. London: Verso.

———. 1988b. *Selected Writings*, edited by M. Poster. Stanford: Stanford University Press.

Bendix, Reinhard. 1960. *Max Weber: An Intellectual Portrait*. New York: Doubleday.

Brubaker, Rogers. 1984. *The Limits of Rationality: An Essay on the Social and Moral Thought of Max Weber*. London: Allen & Unwin.

Cassell, Eric J. 1986. "The Changing Concept of the Ideal Physician." *Daedalus* 115: 185–208.

Cockerham, William C., Gerhard Kunz, and Guenther Lueschen. 1988. "Social Stratification and Health Lifestyles in Two Systems of Health Care Delivery: A Comparison of the United States and West Germany." *Journal of Health and Social Behavior* 29: 113–126.

Cockerham, William C., Guenther Lueschen, Gerhard Kunz, and Joe L. Spaeth. 1986. "Social Stratification and Self-Management of Health." *Journal of Health and Social Behavior* 27: 1–14.

Conrad, Peter. 1988. "Health and Fitness at Work: A Participant's Perspective." *Social Science and Medicine* 26: 545–550.

Crawford, Robert. 1984. "A Cultural Account of Health: Control, Release, and the Social Body." Pp. 60–103 in *Issues in the Political Economy of Health Care*, edited by J. McKinley. New York: Tavistock.

Dahrendorf, Ralf. 1979. *Life Chances*. Chicago: University of Chicago Press.

d'Houtaud, A. and Mark G. Field. 1984. "The Image of Health: Variations in Perception by Social Class in a French Population." *Sociology of Health and Illness* 6: 30–59.

Foucault, Michel. 1980. *History of Sexuality*, Vol 1. New York: Pantheon.

Giddens, Anthony. 1990. *The Consequences of Modernity*. Stanford, CA: Stanford University Press.

———. 1991. *Modernity and Self-Identity*. Stanford, CA: Stanford University Press.

Gillick, Muriel R. 1984. "Health Promotion, Jogging, and the Pursuit of the Moral Life." *Journal of Health Politics, Policy and Law* 9: 369–387.

Glassner, Barry. 1988. *Bodies*. New York: G.P. Putnam.

———. 1989. "Fitness and the Postmodern Self." *Journal of Health and Social Behavior* 30: 180–191.

Goldstein, Michael S. 1992. *The Health Movement: Promoting Fitness in America*. New York: Twayne.

Green, Harvey. 1986. *Fit for America: Health, Fitness, Sport and American Society*. New York: Pantheon.

Habermas, Jurgen. 1984. *The Theory of Communicative Action*, Vol. 1, *Reason and the Rationalization of Society*, translated by T. McCarthy. Boston: Beacon.

Harris, Daniel M. and Sharon Guten. 1979. "Health-Protective Behavior: An Exploratory Study." *Journal of Health and Social Behavior* 20: 17–29.

Harvey, David. 1990. *The Condition of Postmodernity*. Cambridge, UK: Blackwell.

Hennis, Wilhelm. 1987. "Personality and Life Orders: Max Weber's Theme." Pp. 52–74 in *Max Weber, Rationality, and Modernism*, edited by S. Whimster and S. Lash. London: Allen and Unwin.

———. 1988. *Max Weber, Essays in Reconstruction*, translated by K. Tribe. London: Allen & Unwin.

Herzlich, Claudine and Janine Pierret. 1987. *Illness and Self in Society*. Baltimore: Johns Hopkins University Press.

Holton, Robert J. and Bryan S. Turner. 1989. *Max Weber on Economy and Society*. New York: Rutledge.

Jaspers, Karl. 1988. *On Max Weber*, edited by J. Dreijmans. New York: Paragon House.

Kalberg, Stephen. 1980. "Max Weber's Types of Rationality: Cornerstones for the Analysis of Rationalization Processes in History." *American Journal of Sociology* 85: 1145–1179.

Kasl, S. and S. Cobb. 1966. "Health Behavior, Illness Behavior, and Sick Role Behavior." *Archives of Environmental Health* 12: 246–266.

Käsler, Dirk. 1988. *Max Weber: An Introduction to His Life and Work*. Chicago: University of Chicago Press.

Kennedy, Paul. 1987. *The Rise and Fall of the Great Powers*. New York: Random House.

Kickbusch, Ilona. 1989. "Self-Care in Health Promotions." *Social Science and Medicine* 29: 125–130.

Kotarba Joseph A. and Pamela Bentley. 1988. "Workplace Wellness Participation and the Becoming of Self." *Social Science and Medicine* 26: 551–558.

Kronenfeld, Jennie J., Kirby L. Jackson, Keith E. Davis, and Steven N. Blair. 1988. "Changing Health Practices: The Experience from a Worksite Health Promotion Project." *Social Science and Medicine* 26: 515:524.

Lash, Scott. 1990. *Sociology of Postmodernism*. London: Routledge.

Löwith, Karl. 1982. *Max Weber and Karl Marx*, edited by T. Bottomore and W. Outhwaite. London: Allen & Unwin.

Marx, Karl. 1960. *Politische Schriften* (*Political Writings*), edited by H. Lieber. Stuttgart: Enke.

McQueen, David V. 1988. "Research in Health Behaviour." In *Health Behaviour Research and Health Promotion*, edited by R. Anderson, J. Davies, I. Kickbusch, and D. V. McQueen. Oxford: Oxford University Press.

Milo, Nancy. 1981. *Promoting Health Through Public Policy*. Philadelphia: Davis.

Mommsen, Wolfgang. 1987. "Personal Conduct and Societal Change." Pp. 35–51 in *Max Weber, Rationality and Modernism*, edited by S. Whimster and S. Lash. London: Allen & Unwin.

———. 1989. *The Political and Social Theory of Max Weber*. Cambridge: Polity Press.

Münch, Richard. 1988. *Understanding Modernity*. London: Routledge.

O'Neill, Molly. 1992. "As the Rich Get Leaner, The Poor Get French Fries." *New York Times* (March 18): B1, B5.

Parsons, Talcott. 1981. "Revisiting the Classics Throughout a Long Career." Pp. 183–194 in *The Future of the Sociological Classics*, edited by B. Rhea. London: Allen & Unwin.

Ransford, H. Edward. 1986. "Race, Heart Disease Worry, and Health Protective Behavior." *Social Science and Medicine* 12: 1355–1362.

Ritzer, George and David Walczak. 1988. "Rationalization and the Deprofessionalization of Physicians." *Social Forces* 67: 1–22.

Rossi, Peter H. 1989. *Down and Out in America*. Chicago: University of Chicago Press.

Roth, Guenther. 1987. "Rationalization in Max Weber's Developmental History." Pp. 75–91 in *Max Weber, Rationality, and Modernism*, edited by S. Whimster and S. Lash. London: Allen & Unwin.

Rothschild, Nan A. 1990. *New York City Neighborhoods*. New York: Academic Press.

Scaff, Lawrence A. 1989. *Fleeing the Iron Cage: Culture, Politics, and Modernity in the Thought of Max Weber*. Berkeley: University of California Press.

Schluchter, Wolfgang. 1979. "The Paradox of Rationalization: On the Relation of Ethics and World." Pp. 11–64 in *Max Weber's Vision of History*, edited by G. Roth and W. Schluchter. Berkeley: University of California Press.

———. 1981. *The Rise of Western Rationalism: Max Weber's Developmental History*. Berkeley: University of California Press.

Spinner, Helmut. 1989. "Weber gegen Weber: Der ganze Rationalismus einer> >Welt von Gegensätzen> >Zur Neuinterpretation des Charisma als Gelegenheitsvernunft." (Weber versus Weber: The Whole Rationalism of a< <World of Contradictions> >Toward a New Interpretation of the Charisma of the Reason of Opportunity.") Pp. 250–295 in *Max Weber heute* (*Max Weber Today*), edited by J. Weiss. Frankfurt am Main, Germany: Suhrkamp.

Tenbruck, Friedrich. 1975. "Wie gut kennen wir Max Weber?" ("How Well Do We Know Max Weber?) *Kölner Zeitschrift für Soziologie und Sozialpsychologie* 27: 663–702.

———. 1980. "The Problem of Thematic Unity in the Works of Max Weber." *British Journal of Sociology* 31: 316–351.

Turner, Bryan S. 1984. *The Body and Society*. Oxford: Blackwell.

———. 1987. "The Rationalization of the Body: Reflections on Modernity and Discipline." Pp. 2124–2141 in *Max Weber, Rationality, and Modernity*, edited by S. Whimster and S. Lash. London: Allen & Unwin.

Veblen, Thorstein. 1899. *Theory of the Leisure Class*. New York: Macmillan.

Weaver, William Woys. 1989. *America Eats*. New York: Harper & Row.

Weber, Max. 1920. *Gesammelte Aufsätze zur Religionssoziologie* (*Collected Essays on the Sociology of Religion*), Vol. 1. Tübingen, Germany: Mohr.

———. 1922. *Wirtschaft und Gesellschaft* (*Economy and Society*). Tübingen, Germany: Mohr.

———. 1946. *From Max Weber: Essays in Sociology*, edited and translated by H. Gerth and C. Mills. New York: Oxford University Press.

———. 1949. *The Methodology of the Social Sciences*, translated and edited by E. Shils and H. Finch. New York: Free Press.

———. 1958. *The Protestant Ethic and the Spirit of Capitalism*, translated by T. Parsons. New York: Scribner.

———. 1968. *Gesammelte Aufsätze zur Wissenschaftslehre* (*Collected Essays on the Theory of Science*), 3rd ed., edited by J. Winckelmann. Täbingen, Germany: Mohr.

———. 1978. *Economy and Society*, 2 Vols., edited and translated by G. Roth and C. Wittich. Berkeley: University of California Press.

———. 1981. *General Economic History*. New Brunswick, NJ: Transaction Books.

Weiss, Johannes. 1987. "On the Irreversibility of Western Rationalization and Max Weber's Alleged Fatalism." Pp. 154–163 in *Max Weber, Rationality and Modernity*, edited by S. Whimster and S. Lash. London: Allen & Unwin.

Whimster, Sam and Scott Lash (eds.). 1987. *Max Weber, Rationality, and Modernity*. London: Allen & Unwin.

Wiley, Norbert. 1987. "Introduction." Pp. 7–27 in *The Max Weber Debate*, edited by N. Wiley. Beverly Hills, CA: Sage.

Withorn, Ann. 1986. "Helping Ourselves." Pp. 416–428 in *The Sociology of Health and Illness: Critical Perspectives*, edited by P. Conrad and R. Kern. New York: St. Martin's.

[3]

A Critical Theory of Medical Discourse: Ideology, Social Control, and the Processing of Social Context in Medical Encounters*

HOWARD WAITZKIN
University of California, Irvine

Journal of Health and Social Behavior 1989, Vol. 30 (June):220–239

The personal troubles that patients bring to doctors often have roots in social issues beyond medicine. While medical encounters involve "micro-level" interactions between individuals, these interpersonal processes occur in a social context shaped by "macro-level" structures in society. Examining prior theories pertinent to medical discourse leads to the propositions: (a) that medical encounters tend to convey ideologic messages supportive of the current social order; (b) that these encounters have repercussions for social control; and (c) that medical language generally excludes a critical appraisal of the social context. The technical structure of the medical encounter, as traditionally seen by health professionals, masks a deeper structure that may have little to do with the conscious thoughts of professionals about what they are saying and doing. Similar patterns may appear in encounters between clients and members of other "helping" professions. Expressed marginally or conveyed by absence of criticism about contextual issues, ideology and social control in medical discourse remain largely unintentional mechanisms for achieving consent.

Why look at medical encounters from a theoretical point of view?

More than a quarter century ago, C. Wright Mills analyzed the relationships between "personal troubles" and "social issues." Mills pointed out that the troubles a person experiences arise in the context of broader social problems. According to Mills, an individual's difficulties are almost always interconnected with structures in society, although these links may not be obvious on the surface. Mills argued that an important goal for people concerned with social problems—those with what he called the "sociological imagination"—is to clarify how personal troubles and social issues relate to one another (1959, pp. 3–24).

In the intimacy of the medical encounter, patients present to their doctors a variety of personal troubles. From Mills' perspective, these troubles often have roots in social issues that go beyond the individual level. Yet the social issues themselves tend not to receive critical attention in conversation between patients and doctors. In trying to help their patients, doctors often find ways that patients can adjust to troubling social conditions.[1]

* Direct all correspondence to Howard Waitzkin, UCI/North Orange County Community Clinic, 300 West Romneya Drive, Anaheim, CA 92801.

This article is one of a series of papers from an ongoing research project on medical discourse. The research has been supported in part by grants from the National Center for Health Services Research (HS-02100), the Robert Wood Johnson Foundation (through the Clinical Scholars Program), the Fulbright Program, the National Institute on Aging (1-F32-AG05438), and the Academic Senate of the University of California, Irvine (Honorary Faculty Research Fellowship). During a span of many years, John Stoeckle, Elliot Mishler, Sam Bloom, members of the primary care research discussion group at the University of California, Irvine, and participants in the Society of General Internal Medicine have given me constructive suggestions about the project. Stephany Borges, Theron Britt, J. Hillis Miller, Mark Poster, Leslie Rabine, and John Carlos Rowe have helped in my attempts to negotiate the terrain of critical theory in the humanities. My errors are no fault of theirs.

MEDICAL DISCOURSE

Seen from this vantage point, medical encounters are "microlevel" processes that involve the interaction of individuals. These interpersonal processes, however, occur in a social context, which is shaped by "macro-level" structures in society. For example, when patients and doctors discuss problems at work, they take their bearings from the organization of work in society, social expectations about work, social class relations pertaining to work, and so forth. Similarly, when problems pertaining to family life arise in medical encounters, the conversation must deal in some way with such issues as women's and men's roles in the family, expectations about reproduction and the maintenance of households, and social patterns affecting children, elderly people, and individuals at different stages of the life cycle. Patients also raise other kinds of social problems when they talk with their doctors, and macrolevel structures in the society shape the context of those problems as well.

One challenge for social theory has been to clarify how macrolevel social structures and microlevel processes affect one another. Many schools of thought have dealt with this theoretical challenge. Some theorists have argued for the importance of macrolevel structures like social class and political power in determining what happens in interpersonal processes at the micro level. Others have claimed that microlevel processes are primary, and that macrolevel structures emerge only as a reflection (similar terms include integration, aggregation, gloss, repetition, and transformation) of microlevel processes occurring routinely in everyday life. A compromise position holds that macrolevel structures profoundly influence interpersonal processes, but that microlevel processes cumulatively reinforce social structures at the macro level as well (for a critical review, see Knorr-Cetina and Cicourel 1981).

In this paper, I do not hope to resolve this theoretical debate, but rather to explore how the macro and micro levels impinge on each other in the single institutional sphere of medicine. When patients and doctors talk with each other about social problems, their words have much to do with the social order around them. Structures of society help generate the specific social context in which patients and doctors find themselves. The talk that occurs in medical encounters also may reinforce broader social structures. Similar patterns probably occur in the communication between clients and members of other helping professions, such as law, psychology, and social work. Clarifying these patterns in medicine therefore sheds light on professional-client discourse more generally. In exploring the interconnections between personal troubles and social issues, and between the micro and macro levels, I first build on the work of prior theorists to deal with the issue of medical ideology. I then examine social control by professionals in their encounters with clients. Afterward, I ask how the language of medical encounters pertains to the social context of medicine.

MEDICAL IDEOLOGY

Ideology, while difficult to define, is in general an interlocking set of ideas and doctrines that form the distinctive perspective of a social group. Through such ideas and doctrines, ideology represents—on an imaginary level—individuals' relationship to the real conditions of their existence (cf. Al thusser 1971, pp. 162–165; a critical appraisal of Althusser's contribution follows later in this paper). This imaginary quality of ideology, which patterns how individuals perceive and interpret their experience, contributes to ideology's impact in society. Because it helps shape a population's perceptions and interpretations, ideology can achieve a most profound effect on social life.

As a macrolevel structure in society, ideology impinges on patients and doctors as part of the social context of medical encounters. At the micro level of interpersonal interaction, elements of ideology appear in doctor-patient communication. What patients and doctors say when they meet reinforces their particular ideologic conceptions about social life. Although ideology has received wide attention in social theory, several previous theoretical contributions are helpful for clarifying ideology in medicine. In presenting these perspectives on ideology, I emphasize those theoretical strands that shed light on ideologic processes in medical encounters.

Ideology, work, and the family: perspectives from early Marxist theory. In classic Marxist theory, ideology is an important though inconsistently developed notion. According to the principle of economic determinacy, the events of history emerge chiefly from economic forces and the conflicting relations of social class. From this viewpoint, economic forces affect the ideologies of a specific historical period. Despite the primacy of economic forces, ideology is crucial in sustaining and reproducing the social relations of production, especially patterns of domination. Marx called attention to the mechanisms by which ideology reinforces capitalist relations of production and the interests of the capitalist class (1894, pp. 370–90, 790–94). While ideologies arise in many different areas, including religion, aesthetics, and politics, early Marxist analyses did not discuss in depth the ideologic components of medicine (Marx and Engels 1846, pp. 3–78).

The Marxist perspective, however, leads to questions about how elements of ideology in medical encounters relate to economic behavior. Ideologic conceptions of work, as they are transmitted in doctor-patient interaction, reflect more general ideologic notions about economic activities in a given society. When they are spoken in medical encounters, these notions reinforce a society's dominant ideologic conceptions about the nature of work and of economic production.

For instance, among the many definitions of "health" that have appeared during the twentieth century, modern medicine has emphasized in practice an interpretation of health as ability to work. There are several ways that this definition of health has been reinforced and diffused in the population. The public health policies that large philanthropies and government agencies have initiated in the United States and other countries consistently have emphasized the importance of a healthy work force (Brown 1979, pp. 112–34; Franco-Agudelo 1983). Images of health conveyed by the mass media also have supported the symbolism of health as the capacity to do productive work (Kelman 1975). These images have communicated a message that the healthy person is one who produces economically. Moreover, a widely touted standard by which to judge medicine's cost-effectiveness is its contribution to patients' subsequent work productivity (Weinstein and Stason 1977).

Doctor-patient interaction, I will argue, reinforces this same definition of health as the ability to work. In certain encounters with patients, doctors communicate explicitly or subtly a message that work is preferable to idleness. When people become sick, they often stop working, and doctors get involved in this process in several ways. Frequently doctors certify that a patient is physically disabled and thus unable to work. By the certification of disability, a doctor in effect decides when a patient must return to the job. When judging the seriousness of a patient's complaints, a doctor investigates whether the patient's problems interfere with work. Doctors write letters to employers, insurance companies, and government agencies about patients' work limitations and discuss this correspondence to a greater or lesser degree with the patients themselves. During their routine talk with patients, doctors inevitably convey attitudes about work, usually to encourage patients' continued performance on the job. In these instances and many others, the impact of the doctors' words is to define health as the capacity to work productively.

The family becomes a second important focus for ideologic elements in medical encounters, and theorists in the Marxist tradition have emphasized the connections between the family and economic production. For example, Engels claimed that the family, by "propagation of the species," plays a key role in reproducing the labor force. Women's subordinate position in the family, according to Engels, helps maintain the family's reproductive role (1891). However, the family's importance goes beyond the physical reproduction of labor. The family also helps reproduce the ideologic framework of the economic system. For instance, patterns of sexuality and child rearing in the family reinforce personality characteristics and attitudes that tend to accept hierarchies of class and authority. By sustaining such patterns, Engels argues, the family becomes an important institution for ideologic reproduction, which helps achieve the population's acquiescence to and participation in current relations of economic production.

Medicine also mediates the family's reproductive role. As noted already, medicine tends to define health as the ability to work. However, a secondary and related definition is that health is the ability to reproduce labor. Women's activities as homemakers, wives, and mothers are crucial in the family's reproductive activities. Even when women do not work outside the home, they often care for working husbands and for children who later will take part in production and reproduction. Although a greater proportion of women have entered the labor force since World War II, they still face the social expectation that they remain primarily responsible for these reproductive activities. That is, "healthy" women do these things, and doctors predictably help many women in sustaining their reproductive capabilities. For their male clients, doctors also may interest themselves in the stability of family relations. For both men and women, adequate functioning in familial responsibilities thus becomes another criterion in doctors' assessment of health. As discussed later in this paper, doctors are among the expert professionals who increasingly have regulated family life during the twentieth century. How doctor-patient interaction conveys ideologic notions about family life is a question of some interest.

Later theories of ideology. The examples of work and the family lead to a consideration of how certain other theorists—Gramsci, Lukacs, Althusser, and Habermas—have treated the question of ideology. A unifying theme among these theoretical positions, all of which are influenced by classical Marxism, is that ideology serves as a subtle mechanism which helps win a population's consent to the ways a society is organized. These theorists also emphasize that ideology helps maintain the economic system and that supporting institutions like the family are key elements in reproducing a society's dominant ideologic patterns. Although the theorists to be considered do not deal specifically with medical encounters, one purpose of reviewing these theories is to apply them to the question of ideology in medicine.

From Gramsci's viewpoint, groups in power use two types of sociopolitical control to maintain and reproduce relations of economic production (1971, p. 123–202, 375–77, 406–7). In the first place, there is direct coercion; by holding the legal means of violence—in the armed forces, police, prisons, courts, and related institutions—the state protects the established order partly through force and repression. However, Gramsci claims, no regime can hold power for long periods of time strictly by authoritarian rule.

Ideologic hegemony, according to Gramsci, is a second and ultimately more important mechanism of control. Such institutions as the schools, churches, mass media, and family inculcate a system of values, attitudes, beliefs, and morality. This ideologic system supports the established order and the class interests that dominate it. The same ideologic forces achieve consent and mute resistance from disadvantaged groups.

While Gramsci did not consider medicine's ideologic impact, a similar theoretical perspective would ask to what extent medicine reinforces the dominant ideologic system of a society. When doctors convey ideologic notions about desirable behavior, especially as these notions help shape patients' roles in work and the family, medical encounters contribute to the broader hegemonic impact of ideology. In this sense, medicine exerts ideologic effects that parallel those of such institutions as schools, churches, and the mass media.

Lukacs' conceptions of class consciousness and reification also are pertinent to medicine's ideologic impact. Regarding class consciousness, Lukacs, like Gramsci, explores how a society's dominant ideologies are conveyed and reinforced. In discussing literature and other forms of cultural expression, Lukacs emphasizes the ways that these materials both reflect and strengthen broad ideologic patterns (1971a, pp. 46–222; 1971b; Jameson 1971b; Taussig 1980). According to Lukacs, such ideologic patterns shape the consciousness of individuals and, cumulatively, of social classes. In this process, the *totality* of social relations in an entire society becomes mystified and blocked from conscious thought. Reification, Lukacs argues, involves the transformation of social relations into things or thing-like beings that take on their own separate reality in people's consciousness. Shaped by ideology, consciousness focuses on the concrete problems and objects of everyday life, especially economic commodities, rather than on the totality of social relations that lies behind these routine concerns. Attention becomes focused on the concrete objects of daily life, and in this process of reification the totality of social relations escapes conscious attention.

Reification contributes to medicine's impact. In medical encounters, technical statements help direct patients' responses to objectified symptoms, signs, and treatment. This reification shifts attention away from the totality of social relations and the social issues that are often root causes of personal troubles. Instead, attention gets paid to problems of individual pathophysiology and personality.

By reifying problematic social relations, medicine reduces the potentiality for effectively criticizing those relations. Symptoms, signs, and treatment take on an aura of scientific fact, rather than subjective manifestations of a troubled social reality. The medical processing of social problems invests them with the symbolism of objects, relatively immune from criticism or change. This same process constricts the level of attention to the disturbed individual, rather than social structures impinging on the individual. For instance, when the organization of work or tension in the family creates personal distress, expression of that distress in a medical encounter tends to reify the social structural roots of the problem. Under these circumstances, it is the objectified symptom or sign that requires treatment—not the institutional sources of individual distress.

Influenced by Gramsci and Lukacs, Althusser further analyzes the structures of control in modern societies. Althusser considers the interconnections among repressive and ideologic institutions, as well as their relationships to government (1971). Repressive state apparatuses (RSAs), Althusser argues, include the army, police, prisons, courts, and other institutions that maintain control through violence or repression. Ideologic state apparatuses (ISAs) are institutions that instill dominant ideologies in the population. In Althusser's analysis, ISAs include the family, legal system, electoral politics, mass media and communication systems, education, and cultural systems. RSAs are not purely repressive, nor are ISAs purely ideologic. Ideologies often legitimate the actions of RSAs. For example, justice and equality are ideologic notions that legitimate the functioning of the courts. Similarly, ISAs may use punishment for discipline, such as physical force or other forms of sanctioning that occur in the family or school system. Althusser argues that ISAs are especially important in reproducing class structure and the relations of economic production. According to Althusser, many social institutions—particularly the educational system—promulgate ideologies that assure the population's acquiescence and participation in productive work.

Althusser's analysis of the wide-ranging repressive and ideologic effects of many institutions in society, though controversial, pertains to medicine as well. In rare instances, medicine exerts directly repressive effects—as when physicians helped implement policies of genocide in Nazi concentration camps. Less obvious instances of medicine's repressive impact include doctors' roles in involuntary mental hospitalization, prison health care, capital punishment (in some cases administering lethal injections or otherwise assisting in executions), involuntary sterilization, and so forth.

Medicine's ideologic impact, however, is doubtless much more important than its repressive role. In their encounters with patients, doctors may interpret personal problems and encourage individual behaviors in directions that are consistent with the society's dominant ideologic patterns. From the perspective of Althusser's theory, when medical encounters convey a definition of health as the ability to work, they encourage workers' participation in economic production. Doctor-patient interaction also predictably transmits notions about family life that strengthen the family's ideologic impact. In these ways, medicine exerts ideologic effects consistent with those of other institutions like the educational system and mass media.

Another quite different theoretical approach also pertains to medical ideology. The "critical theory" of Habermas and other analysts of the Frankfurt School provides a link between ideology and science—and by extension, scientific medicine. Although Habermas's and Althusser's theories both have roots in classical Marxism, these two schools of thought diverge in fundamental ways. In particular, the Frankfurt School usually assumes that individuals have the capacity to reflect critically about society and to take "purposive" political action; Althusser diminishes the potentiality for effective criticism and political action by individuals. Both approaches, however, emphasize the impact of ideology. While Althusser focuses on the ideologic effects of various social institutions in reproducing the relations of production, Habermas stresses the ideologic components of science.

For Habermas, science is ideology par excellence precisely because it claims to be above ideology, that is, objective and value neutral (1970). Habermas argues that scientific ideology has defined an increasing range of problems as amenable to technical solutions. In this way, scientific ideology tends to depoliticize these social issues by removing them from critical scrutiny. According to

Habermas, science legitimates current patterns of domination, including the class relations of production:

> Technocratic consciousness is, on the one hand, "less ideological" than all previous ideologies. . . . On the other hand today's dominant, rather glassy background ideology, which makes a fetish of science, is more irresistible and farther-reaching than ideologies of the old type. For with the veiling of practical problems it not only justifies a *particular class's* interest in domination and represses *another class's* partial need for emancipation, but affects the human race's emancipatory interest as such (1970, p. 111).

What are the specific processes by which scientific ideology provides legitimation? One problem in Habermas' account is that it remains on an abstract level and rarely grounds theoretical claims in empirical reality. Habermas conveys an impression that scientific ideology creates legitimation through cultural symbols in the mass media, educational system, and technical organization of the workplace. He also argues that ideology and domination appear in the face-to-face interaction of individuals. Distorted communication, Habermas argues, arises in both the macrolevel realm of politics and the microlevel realm of interpersonal relationships. Domination creates distortion in communication, and undistorted communication is impossible, according to Habermas, under conditions of domination (1970, p. 113; 1971, pp. 214–73; 1974, pp. 1–40, 195–282; 1975, pp. 33–96; 1985, pp. 273–337). In a major part of his project, Habermas encourages resistance against domination and aims toward the creation of new, less distorted forms of communication. Concrete examples of scientific ideology, however, rarely appear in Habermas' work; for this reason, his account remains abstract and utopian regarding directions of change. On the other hand, his analysis causes one to look for specific instances of scientific legitimation and distorted communication in face-to-face interactions.

These considerations are pertinent to medical encounters to the extent that doctor-patient interactions convey ideologic messages under the rubric of scientific medicine. From Habermas' perspective, such messages legitimate current problems in society and further depoliticize these issues by deflecting critical attention from them. In addition, medical interactions show features of distorted communication, fostered for instance by devices of language that reinforce professional domination. In actual encounters between patients and doctors, then, one can ask how and to what extent medical discourse transmits scientific ideology.

PROFESSIONAL SOCIAL CONTROL

Social control—again to offer a simple definition of a complex concept—refers to mechanisms that achieve people's adherence to norms of appropriate behavior. In medicine, ideology and social control are closely related. When doctors transmit ideologic messages that reinforce current social patterns—at work, in the family, and in other areas of life—they help control behavior in ways that are defined as socially appropriate.

Dealing with problems outside the narrow realm of technical medicine tends to "medicalize" a wide range of psychological, social, economic, and political problems. Historically, numerous areas gradually have fallen under medical control. Examples include sexuality and family life, work dissatisfaction, problems of the life cycle (including birth, adolescence, aging, dying, and death), difficulties in the educational system (learning disabilities, maladjustment, and students' psychological distress), environmental pollution, and many other fields. By participating in these areas, practitioners often believe that they are extending the caring function of the medical role.

On the other hand, medicalization has become the subject of a critique that focuses on heath professionals' expanding role in social control (Conrad and Schneider, 1980; Ehrenreich and Ehrenreich 1978; Fox 1977; Illich 1975; Waitzkin 1971, 1983; Waitzkin and Waterman, 1974; Zola 1972, 1975, 1983). As medical management of social problems has increased, the societal roots of personal troubles become mystified and depoliticized. That is, by responding in limited ways to some of patients' nontechnical problems, medical practitioners tend to shift the focus of attention from societal issues to the troubles of individuals.

The history of professional social control: Foucault. The intrusion of the scientific discourse into many areas of social life has preoccupied Foucault in his work on the history of the professions. Through his studies of what he calls the human sciences, Foucault has conveyed the connections between knowledge and power (1980). According to Foucault, as such professions as medicine, psychology, law, and social work have developed, they have taken on positions of control in everyday life. By describing the political role of the human sciences, Foucault has clarified how professional social control emerged historically.

While Foucault's early work traces the history of medicine's diagnostic and therapeutic ideas (1975), his more recent studies emphasize how professional control has widened into everyday life (1977). Although modern punishment is more hidden than prior techniques like torture and public execution, Foucault argues, it orients itself to surveillance and professional control over the deviant population. Through new technologies of power, according to Foucault, the criminologic profession could create what appeared to be a humane reform over prior forms of gross corporal punishment. Further, he argues, the administrators of penal institutions have achieved surveillance of people who deviate from society's expectations about appropriate behavior.

Most important from Foucault's viewpoint, criminology has become a standard for professional practices throughout society. According to Foucault, similar technologies of surveillance also have emerged to achieve professional power in mental institutions, hospitals and clinics, workplaces, and schools. Foucault's examples show that social control has become more subtle, professionalized, and oriented to surveillance of deviant behavior.

Although Foucault's studies of prisons touch on medicine mainly by analogy, his work on sexuality pertains directly to medical encounters (1978). Foucault's colorful account of modern sexuality begins in the seventeenth century. Until that time, Foucault argues, religious institutions took an interest in sexuality, mainly through the confessional. When people confessed their sexual activities, priests commented on what liaisons and positions were appropriate and what actions required penance. After the Reformation and Counter Reformation, according to Foucault, concern gradually shifted from bodily activities to thoughts, fantasies, intentions, and other mental processes related to sexuality. Especially during the nineteenth century, Foucault notes, surveillance and regulation of mental processes pertaining to sex became a preoccupation of science and particularly medicine. Professional practitioners then assumed a measure of control over the activities and psychological meanings of sexual life.

In discussing sexuality, Foucault emphasizes professional discourse and links discourse to power. That is, what professionals have said about sexuality has deepened professional power in everyday life (1978, pp. 101–102). What previously was a concern for the clergy has become a challenge for professionals, who assume various degrees of control over their clients' sexual expression. Medical doctors mediate sex, according to Foucault, but so do psychoanalysts, social workers, educators, bureaucrats in social welfare agencies, and other professionals who lay claim to expert knowledge. The discourse through which professionals communicate their special knowledge, from Foucault's perspective, enhances their ability to intervene in and to control others' behavior.

Where does one find such professional discourse? Foucault of course looks for discourses on sex in the books, articles, and other documents that professionals have written and published. However, for Foucault, unpublished discourse becomes as important as publications in achieving professional power, if not more so. For this reason, a variety of materials are appropriate sources for study. These sources include the brochures and files of medical institutions treating sexual disorders, the records of public welfare bureaucracies, therapists' notes, and professional correspondence concerning individuals who are considered deviant. Perhaps most important for the purposes here, one also may look for such discourse, whenever possible, in the face-to-face talk of professionals and their clients. Predictably, for instance, what doctors say to their patients about sex comprises a concrete expression of professional discourse and its power in daily life, probably to a greater extent than what doctors write about sex in textbooks and scientific articles (Poster 1984, pp. 131–32). Although Foucault alludes to the usefulness of oral materials, however, he does not use them himself in developing his arguments.

On the unintentionality of medical social

control. As noted earlier, social control in medicine is generally an unintended process, dimly if at all perceived by participants in doctor-patient encounters. Health professionals seldom consciously view their activities as contributing to social control. In listening to words of distress from their clients, doctors usually do not see their responsibility as preserving the current organization of economic production or the stability of the family. Nonetheless, by focusing on individual troubles rather than social issues, doctor-patient encounters may reinforce the social order as presently constituted. Why do these processes tend to occur without the participants' conscious awareness?

To help explain the unintentionality of medical social control, one may look first to the class origins and position of health professionals. Since the beginning of the twentieth century, the vast majority of doctors have come from upper-middle-class families. In 1920, 12 per cent of North American medical students came from working-class families, and this percentage has stayed almost exactly the same until the present time (Ziem 1977). The extremely limited recruitment of doctors from working-class families has persisted despite recent increases in the proportion of women and racial minorities entering the profession. For the small numbers with working-class roots, as for the rest of the profession, the acquired class position of physicians is one of relative privilege. Their predominantly comfortable lifestyle does not encourage professionals to criticize the social structural roots of their clients' distress, especially the sources of suffering in class structure. Instead, professionals' life experiences predictably leads them to help clients adjust to things as they are.

Professional education and socialization further contribute to the unintentionality of medical social control. A critique of power in society is, needless to say, seldom part of the medical school curriculum. On the contrary, professionals in training receive many lessons about individual pathophysiology and treatment. Within progressive instructional programs, trainees hear information about emotional disturbance and social problems. This training, however, consistently emphasizes the importance of psychological and social knowledge in responding to the needs of the individual patient. Such an approach seeks to help the patient cope with stresses arising in work, the family, and other key institutions. It does not, even in its more progressive and enlightened versions, foster social criticism or social change as part of the medical mission.

There are also situational constraints that leave medical social control below the level of consciousness. When a client is in trouble, a professional usually feels that something should be done. Yet the professional also senses the limits of what he or she as an individual can do. For instance, when a patient's symptoms reflect stress at work, a doctor tends to feel that changing the workplace is beyond the responsibility or even the capability of the medical role. With rare exceptions, such as those involving physical abuse, disruption of familial relations is not an appropriate goal of medical intervention. Wanting to help but unable personally to change the social structure, a health professional typically seeks a solution within the existing institutional context. Relaxation techniques, tranquilizers, counselling, family therapy, and related methods are all feasible approaches for the professional who wants to do something. For a patient in crisis, a doctor cannot do everything. What can be done tends to encourage coping and accommodation. Conscious recognition of these choices, or consideration of more critical alternatives, seldom occurs.

These situational constraints contribute to the generally conservative effects of the medical role. On the one hand, medical discourse usually does not attend to institutional causes of suffering. This orientation leads health professionals to overlook social change as a possible therapeutic option. On the other hand, when doctors do consider institutional problems in their encounters with patients, this intervention frequently serves to support the status quo. When a professional encourages mechanisms of coping and adjustment, such communication conveys a subtle political content. By seeking limited modifications in social roles—at work and in the family, for instance—which preserve a particular institution's overall stability, the practitioner exerts a conservative political impact. Despite the best conscious intentions, the practitioner thus helps reproduce the same institutional structures that form the roots of personal anguish. This contradiction is one source of pathos in the helping professions.

Medical social control also involves the management of potentially troublesome emotions. Doctors, for instance, regularly deal with patients' anger, anxiety, unhappiness, social isolation, loneliness, depression, and other emotional distress. Often these feelings derive in one way or another from patients' social circumstances, such as economic insecurity, racial or sexual discrimination, occupational stress, and difficulties in family life. Such emotions, of course, are one basis of political outrage and organized resistance. How health professionals manage these sentiments is an interesting question. One of medicine's effects may be the defusing of socially caused distress. Medicine is not the only institution in which such processes occur, nor do these phenomena necessarily occupy a major part of medical encounters. Still, it is worth asking how such largely unintentional microlevel processes take place. This question leads us to an analysis of the structure of doctor-patient interaction.

THE TRADITIONAL FORMAT OF THE MEDICAL ENCOUNTER

The traditional format of the medical encounter is as follows:

> Chief complaint (CC) → present illness (PI) → past history (PH) → family history (FH) → social history (SH) → systems review (SR) → physical examination (PE) → other investigations (OI) → diagnosis (Dx) → plan (P).

During a typical encounter, the doctor tries to cover some or all of these components in his or her spoken interaction, and by examination of the patient. In addition, the doctor provides a written version of the encounter, in the medical record. There, the doctor usually labels each component of the encounter with the same abbreviations that I am using here. This traditional format appears in most textbooks that provide instruction on clinical methods for trainees and practitioners of medicine. Research on doctor-patient communication, reported previously, has confirmed that medical practitioners actually do use the traditional structure as an organizing framework for their encounters with patients (Waitzkin 1985).[2]

To define and to comment on each of these elements, I will focus first on the components of the medical history (Hx), which comprises CC, PI, PH, FH, SH, and SR in the above scheme. In the chief complaint (CC), the physician elicits what is bothering the patient, in the briefest possible terms. The physician leads into the chief complaint usually with an opening question like: "Hello, what brings you in today?" or "Well, what's bothering you today?" or "How can I help you?" To these or similar questions, the patient might answer, "Headaches" or "My back hurts" or "I've got pain in my chest" or "I can't sleep" or "I want a check-up" and so forth. In asking for the CC, the physician seeks to elicit the patient's foremost concern.

Through the present illness (PI), the patient elaborates on the chief complaint. He or she tells the doctor when the problem began, what the specific characteristics of the symptom might be, which medications or other measures relieve the symptoms, what prior medical attention he or she has received for the problem, and similar details that may contribute to the doctor's attempts to reach a diagnosis. Guiding the patient to elicit the CC and PI purportedly is the greatest skill that doctors develop in taking a medical history; some commentators argue that this is the most important skill in medicine. Doctors in training presumably learn a comfortable and effective balance between open-ended listening to the patient's story and more directive questioning that clarifies the patient's problem in terms of medical diagnoses.

Interruptions by doctors commonly begin to occur during the PI. Such interruptions basically are attempts to cut off story-telling by patients, for the following reasons (among others): the story may not contribute to a doctor's cognitive process of reaching a diagnosis; the patient's version of the story may be confusing or inconsistent; telling the story may take more time than is perceived to be available; or parts of the story may create feelings that are uncomfortable for the doctor, the patient, or both. The circumstances under which the doctor interrupts the patient's story to focus the PI (that is, what is interrupted, when it is interrupted, what reason is given for the interruption, and so forth) are important, especially to the extent that they cut off concerns about the social context of the medical encounter. Predictably, the PI is a critical juncture, during which certain elements, though they may be quite important in the patient's experience, come to be excluded from discourse, while other elements are included.

What is the relationship between the spoken PI and the version that the doctor writes in the medical record? While writing a comprehensible PI may involve skillful effort by a doctor, its orderliness invariably gives a false sense of what happens during the spoken PI. For example, the doctor never writes, "I interrupted the patient at this point," or "I thought the patient's comments about his family here weren't pertinent to his pain, so I asked him about what medications he was taking," or "I was in a hurry to get my daughter from child care so I cut off the patient at this point," and so forth. Instead, the written PI represents the doctor's interpretation of a disorderly series of spoken exchanges. The orderliness of the written version belies what actually gets said during the PI, which is my chief focus here. This is not to say that the written PI is uninteresting, and others have documented the enormous differences in content between the spoken and written versions (Zuckerman, Starfield, Hochreiter and Kovasznay 1975). I am mainly concerned, however, with the spoken PI in all its disorderliness.

While the CC and PI are almost always present in medical encounters (assuming the patient is awake and conversant), other components may appear or not, depending on time, the doctor's desire to complete a comprehensive evaluation, financial issues such as the patient's insurance and how extensive an evaluation it permits, and other situational constraints. A doctor may choose to defer some or all the remaining components to future visits, or not cover them at all, although there is usually some attempt initially to develop a diagnosis and plan.

In the past history (PH), the doctor gathers information about past medical events in the patient's life that are not directly pertinent to the PI. These events typically include prior hospitalizations and surgery, other major illnesses, medications, allergies, immunizations, smoking, drinking habits, and recreational substance use.

The family history (FH) includes data about illnesses and deaths in the patient's immediate family: mother, father, sisters, brothers, spouse, and children. Additionally, in this section many doctors routinely elicit information about family occurrences of cancer, heart disease, hypertension, diabetes mellitus, and other common problems that may carry an increased risk in certain families.

Although one might expect the social history (SH) to be important for a contextual analysis of medical encounters, it is usually a perfunctory listing of demographic data. For instance, the doctor typically asks about birthplace, occupation, educational attainment, living situation, and insurance status. The contextual concerns that pertain to a patient's distress usually appear, subject to interruption and cut-off, during the PI, rather than the SH. In the SH itself, the doctor traditionally tends not to pursue in much depth how the patient's social circumstances might relate to the difficulties for which he or she is seeking medical attention.

Presumably, the systems review (SR) elicits any additional information about the patient that might be left out or missed by other parts of the history. The SR is sometimes very brief and sometimes quite lengthy; scuttlebutt among medical practitioners has it that the SR's length is inversely related to clinical experience. The expectation, however, is that the doctor will ask the patient whether he or she has experienced symptoms in more or less each of the following organ systems: skin, lymph nodes, head, eyes, ear, nose, throat, neck, respiratory system, cardiovascular system, gastrointestinal system, genitourinary system, reproductive system, neurologic system, endocrine system, and bones and joints. For instance, under the gastrointestinal system, the doctor would question about symptoms of the esophagus (principally swallowing), stomach (heartburn, ulcers, cancer, and so forth), duodenum, small intestine, large intestine (irregularity in bowel habits, bleeding, infections), rectum (hemorrhoids, fissures, bleeding), liver (jaundice, hepatitis, toxic exposures), and pancreas. In other words, the SR can be quite exhaustive, even more so if the patient happens to be a "yea-sayer." Then, doctor and patient enter potentially endless labyrinths of questions and answers, leading to frustrating excursions through a welter of symptoms and diseases that have little to do with the current purposes of the medical encounter. Gradual recognition of these pitfalls during a medical career accounts for the exhaustive efforts that medical students devote to the SR, while their supervising physicians often truncate the SR to a very brief series of questions, for which they do not expect to hear "yes" as a frequent answer.

The physical examination (PE) involves the laying on of hands, whose impact in medicine has been so highly touted. Without intimate touch, medical encounters would not differ nearly so much from other types of professional-client interactions. If time is available and if it has not already been done, a doctor will examine the body's entire external surface during the PE, as well as its internal orifices. When time is not available, or if the doctor is not inclined toward comprehensiveness, he or she does a more focused PE, concentrating on those parts of the body that might be related to the CC and PI.

After the PE, the doctor sometimes initiates one or more other investigations (OI)—lab tests, x-rays, electrocardiograms, and so forth—whose purported aim is to clarify the diagnosis or to gather data that may be useful for treatment or prevention. OIs also seem to communicate something. They may convey an impression of thoroughness and concern. A scientifically oriented intervention may be reassuring because of the technical knowledge it presumably reflects. Further, when an OI leads to a negative finding, it doubtless produces a feeling of relief and well-being. In fact, one research study has shown that normal lab results lead to improvement in symptoms, even when OIs are not ordered for a specific clinical reason from a doctor's point of view (Sox, Margulies and Sox 1981). Thus, a doctor's act of recommending an OI may have several meanings in a medical encounter, aside from the specific results that are obtained.

With the data gleaned from the various components of the medical history, the PE, and the results of OIs, the doctor reaches a diagnosis (Dx), that may be provisional or confirmed. The cognitive operations involved in making a diagnosis undoubtedly are complex and poorly understood. Essentially the doctor takes the patients' comments in the medical history, observations made during the PE, and data from OIs, and shapes this information into one or more diagnostic categories.

The drive to reach a diagnosis is extremely strong. Practitioners and doctors in training view the facility of diagnostic categorization as one of the most important professional skills in medicine. The "differential diagnosis" involves a list of all possible categories into which a patient's physical problems might fall. Most practitioners would acknowledge that the tendencies to interrupt, cut off, or otherwise redirect the patient's story during the PI derive at least partly from the drive to make a diagnosis. That is, a doctor wants to hear those words that are consistent with previously defined diagnostic categories. Parts of patients' stories that do not fit neatly into these categories function as unwanted strangers in medical discourse and tend to be shown to the door (Beckman and Frankel 1984; West 1984).

While the drive to make a diagnosis is strong, diagnostic reasoning tends to be both limited and exclusionary. True, doctors and doctors-in-training must learn to deal with an awesome number of diagnostic categories and subcategories. Yet this set of diagnoses corresponds to no more than a tiny fraction of human experience. In large part, the cognitive process of reaching a diagnosis involves excluding a substantial part of a patient's experience that—no matter how relevant to the patient—is not relevant to the diagnosis. Features of patients' social context may be very troubling to patients and actually may affect their physical conditions in fairly direct ways. These contextual issues, however, are almost always difficult to define with precision, are loaded with ambiguity, and are not completely consistent with the technical categories of differential diagnosis. The exclusionary drive, so much a part of reaching a medically proper diagnosis, profoundly affects what is spoken and recorded during medical encounters. Contextual concerns that do not lend themselves to the technical lexicon of diagnostic possibilities tend to gravitate toward the margins of medical talk.

The medical plan (P) constitutes the interventions that the doctor suggests, usually toward the end of an encounter. Traditional teaching about the medical plan holds that it contains two components. First, there is a diagnostic plan, which involves the OIs that the doctor wishes to obtain after the present encounter ends. Second, in the therapeutic plan, the doctor recommends the medication, surgery, diet, rest, exercise, counselling, relaxation, attitude change, and so forth that he or she believes the patient's diagnosis warrants. A substantial part of medical education involves learning and keeping up with current vogues of preferred diagnostic and therapeutic plans.

Just as it affects diagnostic reasoning, the exclusionary drive also shapes the plan that is formulated. Among the infinitely varied possibilities for human action, the limited range of medical diagnoses encourages relatively few options. Usually these options involve OIs that create more technical data, or treatments that use medication, surgery, or similar technical intervention. Alternatively, a doctor may suggest nonintervention, which involves reassurance that a problem is not serious enough to require technical action, or a schedule of follow-up to be sure that the problem does not become worse. Sometimes, a doctor recommends other maneuvers such as dietary improvement, changes in habits such as smoking and alcohol consumption, counselling, psychotherapy, or behavioral change. In such situations, the problems under consideration often have roots in the social context of the encounter.

Partly because the medical diagnosis rarely provides a technical name for such contextual problems, the plan does not generally call for a contextual intervention. Instead, the medical plan tends to accept the social context as a given. Even the limited behavioral changes that doctors may encourage generally aim at a patient's less troublesome reconciliation with his or her context, rather than change in the context itself. For the medical plan, given the power and limits of the diagnostic process, the range of the possible becomes quite restricted.

Where does giving information to the patient fit in the traditional format of the medical encounter? Remarkably, this format—as taught to generations of doctors in training—lacks a specific niche for providing information. It is probably for this reason that giving information has often been catch-as-catch-can in medicine. Similarly, the absence of a specific place to give information in the encounter's format doubtless has contributed to the very problematic deficiencies and dissatisfactions that have arisen in this arena (Waitzkin 1984, 1985). Suffice it to say, the traditional format also does not guide the doctor in communicating information about contextual issues.

BENEATH THE TRADITIONAL FORMAT: PROCESSING IDEOLOGY AND CONTEXT

By questioning, by interrupting, and by otherwise shifting the direction of conversation from nontechnical problems to technical ones, doctors *exclude* certain topics from talk and *include* others. Of particular interest here are the verbal techniques that divert attention from sources of personal distress in the social context. Such techniques cut off the possibility of considering the context critically, let alone changing it. How medical encounters convey ideologic messages, and how they invoke social control, sometimes involve doctors' explicit pronouncements about what patients should or should not do. It is also likely that ideology and social control emerge from what doctors and patients exclude from their talk, and how it comes to be excluded.

Several studies of communication in medicine have suggested that medical encounters contain common structural features. In a sociolinguistic analysis of doctor-patient conversations, West has found typical "troubles" that arise in encounters (1984). When patients express concerns about events in their lives that are not amenable to doctors' technical intervention, West argues, questions and interruptions are mechanisms by which doctors steer patients'. concerns back to a technical track. As West notes, other studies also have observed that doctors interrupt patients frequently and initiate more questions than patients do (Beckman and Frankel 1984; Fisher 1986; Fisher and Todd 1983; Frankel 1986). In West's tape-recorded sample of medical interactions, male doctors tended to interrupt patients more often than did female doctors. West interprets interruptions and frequent questioning as gestures of dominance, by which doctors control the flow of conversation. She also postulates a connection between social power and sexual differences in language use, in conversations generally, and more specifically in professional-client encounters.

Further, in his study of medical encounters, Mishler demonstrates how medical discourse cuts off contextual issues and redirects the focus to technical concerns (1984). Mishler presents detailed transcripts from recordings of doctor-patient communication (Waitzkin 1985) and describes two "voices" that compete with each other. The "voice of medicine" involves the technical topics (of physiology, pathology, pharmacology, and so forth) which concern doctors in their professional work. Alternatively, the "voice of the lifeworld" comprises the everyday, largely nontechnical problems that patients carry with them into the medical encounter. According to Mishler's analysis of transcripts, patients often try to raise contextual issues through the voice of the lifeworld. Doctors, however, are ill-equipped to deal with such issues and therefore repeatedly return to the voice of medicine. For instance, patients raise personal troubles that do not pertain to technical problems. Or, although related to technical problems, these personal troubles do not seem amenable to technical solutions. Or, the raising of personal troubles leads to discomfort for the professional, the client, or both. Under these circumstances, doctors typically introject questions, interrupt, or otherwise change the topic, to return to the voice of medicine.

Although Mishler's approach conveys how medical language encourages the saying of some things and the leaving unsaid of others, the "lifeworld" remains rather general. Mishler implies that patients' concerns about contextual issues in the lifeworld are very important to them and that cutting off these concerns is undesirable. When the voice of medicine gains sway, however, this achievement also has much to do with ideology and social control. Diverting critical attention away from the lifeworld, doctors subtly reinforce the ideas that pattern the lifeworld and may help win acquiescence to those features of the lifeworld that patients find most disconcerting. In short, a re-reading of Mishler's materials might emphasize that the voice of medicine not only tends to suppress the voice of the lifeworld but also reinforces the reasonableness and acceptability of the lifeworld in its present form.

What is left silent, unsaid, or hidden in medical encounters has fascinated other researchers, who have interpreted rich textual materials but with little or no contextual theory. For instance, Katz provides an extensive account of the "silent world" of the doctor-patient relationship (1984). He shows how medical language overlooks or downplays some important features of doctors' and patients' experience. Thus, Katz argues, doctors often gloss over their patients' concerns, and patients tend to leave these concerns unsaid. In Katz's account, doctors and patients tend to remain silent about many topics, especially those that would require patients' informed consent. Similarly, Cassell interprets the confusions, misunderstandings, insensitivities, and communication lapses in transcripts of doctor-patient interaction (1985). He reiterates a viewpoint frequently expressed, that doctors in training should learn better communication skills to avoid such gaffes in practice. Commenting on the unsaid socioemotional content of medical encounters, Cassell urges that health practitioners pay more attention to what is excluded from conversation, as well as the reasons why.

These accounts of the unsaid in medical language do not emphasize enough the pertinence of the unsaid for the context of professional encounters. Doctors do not simply overlook or downplay or suppress patients' contextual concerns. The exclusion of social context from critical attention is a fundamental feature of medical language, a feature closely connected to ideology and social control. Inattention to social issues, especially when these issues lie behind patients' personal troubles, can never be just a matter of professional inadequacy, or the inadequacy of professional training. Instead, this *lack* is a basic part of what medicine *is* in our society.

What elements of social context help shape the ideologic content of discourse? Social class, of course, is a key contextual element. Relationships of social class are crucial parts of the context in which discourse arises and in which ideology is transmitted. To the extent that doctors and patients occupy different class positions, this class difference patterns the ideologic content of their discourse. Predictably, doctors sometimes voice explicit ideologic messages that legitimate the current class structure of society; or the transmission of ideology occurs more subtly, conveyed by the absence of criticism about class structure and its various injuries. In medical encounters, marginalization constrains an oppositional voice, perhaps that of a patient in distress, through interruption, cut-off, or de-emphasis. This way of looking at medical discourse provides a slightly different theoretical prism to see the same problems uncovered by sociolinguists who observe a "diffidence" of working-class patients in medical encounters, or who note contention between the "voice of medicine" and the "voice of the lifeworld" (Waitzkin 1985; Mishler 1984). Such observations confirm that social class relations, as an element of context, pattern ideology within discourse.

But social class is not the only contextual element that affects discourse; other crucial elements include gender, age, and race. All these contextual elements can become the basis of dominance and subordination, and they are closely linked to social class. Ideologies of gender pertain in large part to the roles men and women occupy in the family and at work. Through ideologies of gender, expectations about what men and women appropriately should and should not do enter everyday language. Arising in the context of discourse, these ideologies profoundly affect what is or can be said, what appears at the center of discourse, and what slips in at the margins. Similarly, as people age, they encounter a changing set of expectations and demands, which vary a great deal among societies. In the United States, for instance, ideologies of aging can convey the image of a trash heap, where elderly people actually or symbolically move when their productivity, or reproductivity, is used up. Other societies tend to be more lenient, or even respectful, in ideologies of aging. Ideologies of race have entered discourse whenever societies have encountered the contrast between majority and minority groups. Expressions of racial ideologies have ranged from the master-slave vernacular to the only slightly more subtle versions of modernity.

Why highlight these contextual elements here? Class, gender, age, and race are some of the contextual elements that pattern ideologic language in face-to-face discourse, as well as medical discourse. It is not enough to acknowledge that ideology may be reproduced in medical discourse; the question is *how* this happens. That is, in concrete examples of discourse, the critical reader needs to seek specific places where ideologic reproduction occurs, and where context impinges on discourse. I propose that these places may become apparent as part of an underlying structure that is not obvious or consciously appreciated in surface meanings. Further, I expect to find these places, at least partly, in the margins of discourse—in what is left unsaid, interrupted, cut off, or deemphasized.[3]

CONCLUSION: A CRITICAL THEORY OF MEDICAL DISCOURSE

Now let me turn to three summaries of actual doctor-patient encounters. Transcripts of these encounters were prepared as part of a large study of doctor-patient communication that involved random sampling from private practices and hospital outpatient departments. The encounters are summarized here because they illustrate typical patterns in the sampled interactions (Waitzkin 1985). In each encounter, doctors and patients deal with personal troubles that derive largely from broader contextual issues (cf. Mills 1959, pp. 3–24). After the summaries, I try to reorganize the elements of discourse so that an underlying structure may become apparent. Then, after reviewing the three encounters, I present a general structural view of medical discourse. The structural analysis of these particular materials also points ahead to other papers in this series, which provide the full transcripts and more detailed analyses of these and other encounters.

—A man comes to his doctor several months after a heart attack. He is depressed. His period of disability payments will expire soon, and his union is about to go on strike. His doctor tells him that he is physically able to return to work and that working will be good for his mental health. The doctor also prescribes an antidepressant and a tranquilizer.

—A woman visits her doctor because of irregularities in her heart rhythm. She complains that palpitations and shortness of breath are interfering with her ability to do housework. The doctor checks an electrocardiogram while she exercises, changes her cardiac medications, and congratulates her in her efforts to maintain a tidy household.

—A man goes to his doctor for a premarital blood test. The doctor questions him closely about his drinking problem, his smoking, his job, his family, and his plans for married life. Then the doctor encourages attendance at Alcoholics Anonymous and orders a test of liver function, in addition to the premarital blood test that the patient requested.

Figure 1 shows some structural elements of discourse in the first encounter. Seen in this way, the contextual issue of uncertain employ-

FIGURE 1. Structural Elements of Medical Encounter with a Man Anticipating Return to Work After a Heart Attack

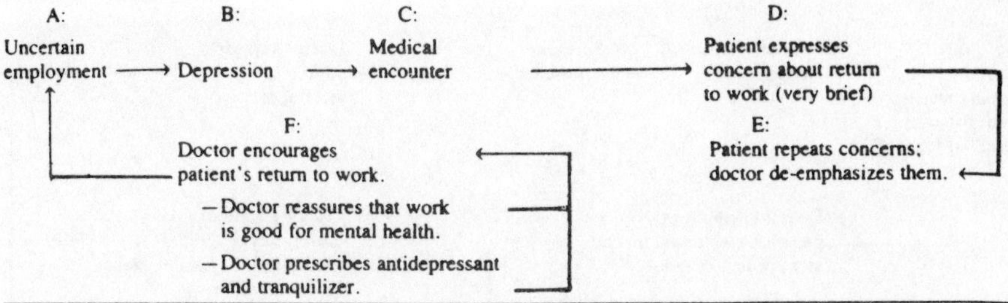

ment initially presents itself (A). Depression is a personal trouble that the patient experiences in anticipation of a return to uncertain employment (B). Coming to the medical encounter (C), the patient tentatively and briefly expresses concern about his impending return to work when his union intends to go on strike (D). He repeats these concerns at several points, but the doctor de-emphasizes them (E). Rather than pursuing the contextual problem, the doctor reassures the patient that work is good for his mental health; further, the doctor prescribes both an antidepressant medication and a tranquilizer (F). After the encounter, one assumes, the patient continues to prepare himself for a return to work.

Structural elements of the second encounter appear in Figure 2. Here the contextual issue involves expectations about women's social role in the family (A). Housework, as many have noted, is an important activity in economic "reproduction," which traditionally is the responsibility of women. Because this patient's heart symptoms interfere with her housework, she experiences emotional distress (B). When she sees her doctor (C), the patient mentions this concern (D). Rather than exploring her concern in depth, the doctor does an electrocardiogram while the patient exercises (E). Based on the results, the doctor changes the patient's cardiac medications. He also encourages her efforts in at least trying to maintain a tidy household (F). The patient thus returns to her personal challenge of doing housework in the face of serious heart disease.

Figure 3 gives some structural elements of the third encounter. This patient faces a contextual issue that derives from the patterning of role expectations that affect men (A). Like most men, this patient finds that he must hold a job steadily to support himself and his family—to use a convenient term, he must earn the "means of subsistence." Further, as he approaches marriage, he also faces an expectation that he stably perform as "head" of a family. Such expectations about work and the family, however, are not simple ones, since the patient is something of a lush. The patient therefore experiences a personal trou-

FIGURE 2. Structural Elements of Medical Encounter with a Woman Whose Heart Symptoms Interfere with Her Housework

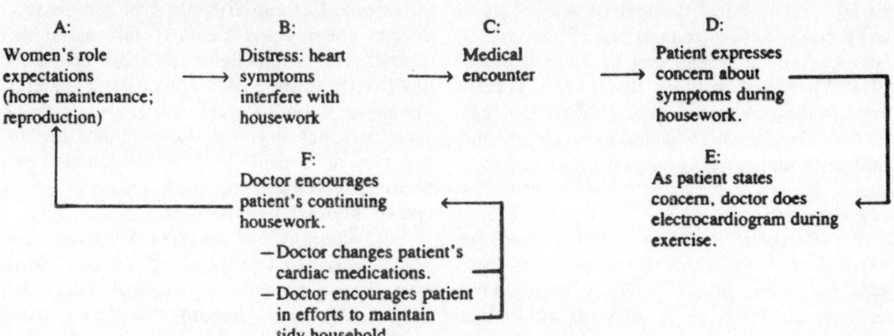

FIGURE 3. Structural Elements of Medical Encounter with a Man Whose Alcohol Problem Potentially Interferes with Work and Family Relations

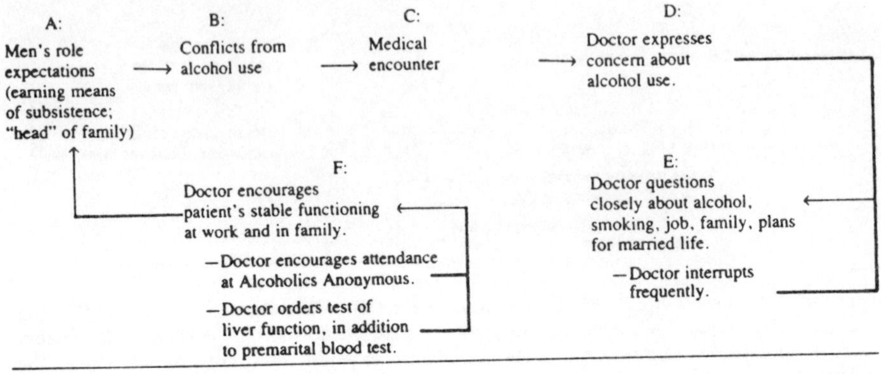

ble that pertains to actual or potential conflicts deriving from alcohol use (B). During the medical encounter (C), the doctor takes the lead in expressing concern about alcohol (D). The doctor questions the patient closely about alcohol, as well as his heavy smoking, his job, family, and plans for married life. In pursuing these questions, the doctor interrupts the patient frequently (E). Beyond voicing strong encouragement that the patient attend Alcoholics Anonymous, the doctor also orders a test of liver function. In this discourse, the doctor encourages the patient's stable functioning at work and in the family (F).

In the paragraphs that follow, reasoning from these and other encounters, I map some islands around which medical discourse seems to flow (Figure 4). I interpret these islands as underlying structures in the flow of medical discourse, rarely discerned consciously by the doctors and patients who travel there.

A. *Social issue as context:* The economic, social, and political context of society contains many difficult conditions. These social issues often lie behind and help create some of the personal troubles that clients experience in their everyday lives (Mills 1959, pp. 3–24). (In the three encounters above, the pertinent social issues are: uncertain employment, women's role expectations, and men's role expectations.)

B. *Personal trouble:* Clients tend to experience these troubles privately, as their own individual problems. They are unlikely to recognize consciously the social issues that lie behind their personal troubles. (In the same three encounters, personal troubles include: depression, distress that heart symptoms interfere with housework, and conflicts from alcohol use.)

C. *The medical encounter:* Clients come to medical professionals with complaints that very often (though not always) have economic, social, and political roots. Such contextual sources of personal troubles include class structure and the organization of work; family life, gender roles, and sexuality; aging and the social role of the elderly; the patterning of leisure and substance use; and limited resources for dealing with emotional distress.

D. *Expression of contextual problems in medical discourse:* The traditional and technical sequence of the medical encounter does not facilitate the expression of contextual concerns. Regarding patients' own characteristics, the relations between language and social structure predictably make the expression of contextual concerns more difficult for working-class people, women, and racial minorities. Certain humanistic or progressive doctors encourage patients to talk about the nontechnical components of their problems that pertain to their lifeworlds. These patients can express concerns and vent emotions about such personal troubles. Less humanistic or progressive doctors tend to discourage patients from expressing such concerns or to ignore them when expressed.

E. *Countertextual tensions deriving from social context:* Contextual problems, however, create tensions in medical discourse. Periodically such tensions that derive from troubling social issues erupt into the dis-

FIGURE 4. The Micropolitical Structure of Medical Discourse

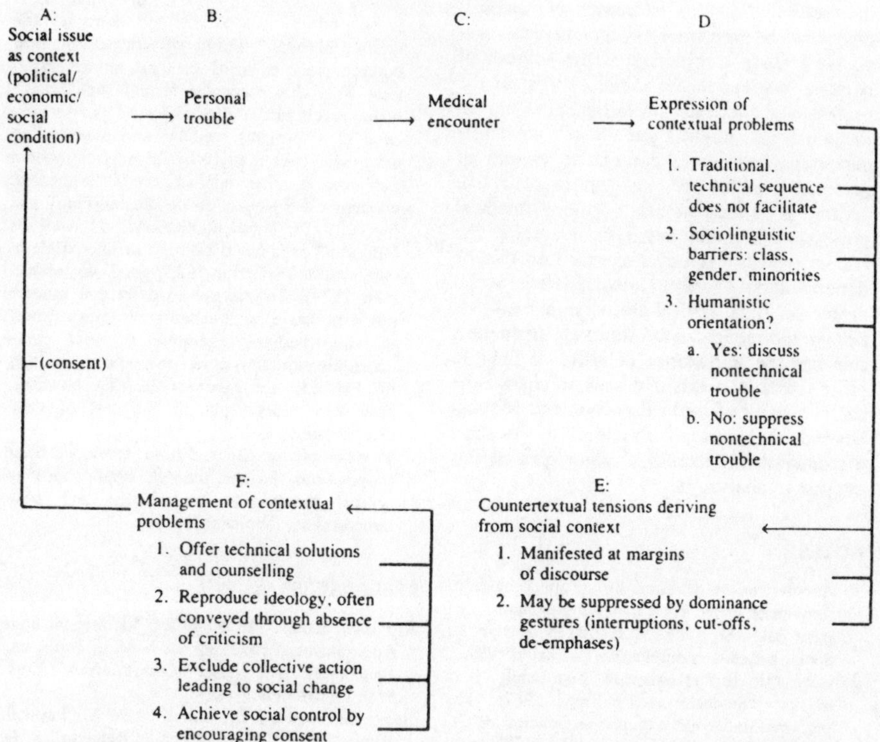

course, or appear at its margins, and create a countertextual reality that cannot be resolved in the framework of a medical encounter. Doctors tend to suppress such tensions by dominance gestures like interruptions, cut-offs, and de-emphases that get the discourse back on a technical track.

F. *Management of contextual problems:* Whether such tensions are expressed or suppressed, the language of medicine leaves few options for action. Limited options for action apply to both humanistic encounters, when doctors encourage patients to talk about nontechnical components of their personal troubles, and to less humanistic encounters, where such concerns are discouraged. Generally, doctors respond with technical solutions and counsel patients how best to adjust to their previous roles. The language of medical science can convey ideologic content, especially when it converts social problems into technical ones. Ideologic language also arises at the margins of medical discourse or achieves its impact through absence. That is, by a lack of criticism directed against sources of distress in the social context, medical discourse ideologically reinforces the status quo. The discourse of medicine thus tends to exclude basic social change as a meaningful alternative. In accepting the present context as given, and in remaining silent about collective political action, medical discourse encourages consent by rendering social change unthinkable. This latter accomplishment of medicine may be its main contribution to social control.

Further studies will show how this structure helps us understand what is happening as doctors and patients deal with problems of work, the family and gender roles, aging, sexuality, leisure, substance use, other "vices," and troublesome emotions. In addition, medical discourse in which this structure is not apparent will become a matter of particular interest.

To whatever extent this theory is persuasive, other questions immediately suggest themselves: Can the structure of medical discourse be reformed? Can medical discourse include a criticism of the sources of personal distress in the social context of the professional encounter? A critical discourse in medicine, one might argue, would no longer encourage consent to contextual sources of personal troubles. By suggesting collective action as a meaningful option, medical professionals might begin to overcome the impact that its exclusion exerts. Can this be done without further medicalizing social problems? If so, critical discourse in medicine also would recognize the limits of medicine's role and the importance of building links to other forms of praxis that seek to change the social context of medical encounters. Moving beyond the current structure of medical discourse then becomes a major goal of this attempt to analyze it.

NOTES

1. Another article develops this proposition from summaries of recorded medical encounters that were randomly sampled as part of a study of doctor-patient communication (Waitzkin 1989a).
2. How this format emerged historically is a mystery (Stoeckle and Billings 1987). The preferred and widely taught sequencing of CC → PI → PH → FH → SH → SR → PE → OI → Dx → P probably goes back to late nineteenth century Europe. Many of these components appeared in textbooks of clinical medicine published in Germany during that period. While Foucault and others who have studied the history of medicine in Europe do not deal with this specific question, a similar format of the encounter presumably arose in France and Britain as well. As with most of the other features of laboratory-based "scientific" medicine, North Americans probably brought the medical encounter's format to the Eastern seaboard in the late nineteenth or early twentieth century. To what extent similarities existed between this format and those used earlier in North America is unknown. Also mysterious are the formats of medical encounters in most pre-modern societies. For instance, although much anthropologic data are available on "ethnomedical" beliefs, little is known about how encounters between so-called primitive healers and their clients are organized. What little is known indicates that some kind of history taking, physical examination, diagnostic categorization, and medical plan does appear in most ethnomedical encounters (cf. Good and Good 1981).

   While elaborating the medical encounter's history and pre-history is a worthy enterprise, it is beyond my scope here and there is little doubt that the traditional format is now commonplace in many or most human societies. That this particular format should have arisen is remarkable partly because its effectiveness in improving medical conditions is so unproven. Like many other aspects of modern medicine, the beneficial impact of the medical encounter's organization on the morbidity and mortality of large populations, as well as individual patients, is difficult or impossible to demonstrate (Waitzkin 1983, pp. 3–43; McKeown 1979). This is not to deny that modern medicine has accomplished great things. Many of the medical encounter's most time-consuming and thus costly components (such as the FH, SR, and much of the PE), however, have never been put to the test of cost-effectiveness.
3. In a companion paper, I have developed these propositions further through applications of critical theory in structuralism and post-structuralism (Waitzkin 1989b).

REFERENCES

Althusser, Louis. "Ideology and Ideological State Apparatuses." 1971. Pp. 127–86 in *Lenin and Philosophy and Other Essays*. New York: Monthly Review Press.

Beckman, Howard B., and Richard M. Frankel. 1984. "The Effect of Physician Behavior on the Collection of Data." *Annals of Internal Medicine* 101:692–696.

Brown, E. Richard. 1979. *Rockefeller Medicine Men*. Berkeley: University of California Press.

Cassell, Eric J. 1985. *Talking With Patients*, 2 volumes. Cambridge: MIT Press.

Conrad, Peter. 1975. "The Discovery of Hyperkinesis: Notes on the Medicalization of Deviant Behavior." *Social Problems* 23:12–21.

Conrad, Peter, and J.W. Schneider. 1980. *Deviance and Medicalization: From Badness to Sickness*. St. Louis: Mosby.

Ehrenreich, Barbara, and John Ehrenreich. 1978. "Medicine and Social Control." Pp. 39–79 in *The Cultural Crisis of Modern Medicine*, edited by John Ehrenreich. New York: Monthly Review Press.

Ehrenreich, Barbara, and Deirdre English. 1973. *Complaints and Disorders: The Sexual Politics of Sickness*. Old Westbury, NY: Feminist Press.

______. 1978. *For Her Own Good*. New York: Anchor/Doubleday.

Engels, Friedrich. 1891 [1942]. *The Origin of the Family, Private Property and the State*. New York: International.

Fisher, Sue. 1986. *In the Patient's Best Interest*. New Brunswick, N.J.: Rutgers University Press.

Fisher, Sue, and Alexandria Dundas Todd, eds. 1983. *The Social Organization of Doctor-Patient Communication*. Washington, D.C.: Center for Applied Linguistics.

Foucault, Michel. 1975. *The Birth of the Clinic: An Archaeology of Medical Perception*. New York: Vintage.

______. 1977. *Discipline and Punish*. New York: Pantheon.

______. 1978. *The History of Sexuality*, volume 1. New York: Pantheon, 1978.

______. 1980. *Power/Knowledge: Selected Interviews and Other Writings*. New York: Pantheon.

Fox, Renée C. 1977. "The Medicalization and Demedicalization of American Society," *Daedalus* 106:9–22.

Franco-Agudelo, Saul. 1983. "The Rockefeller Foundation's Anti-Malarial Program in Latin America." *International Journal of Health Services* 13:51–57.

Frankel, Richard M. 1986. "Talking in Interviews: A Dispreference for Patient-Initiated Questions in Physician-Patient Encounters," in *Interaction Competence*, edited by George Psathas. Norwood, N.J.: Ablex.

Good, Byron J., and Mary-Jo Delvecchio Good. 1981. "The Meaning of Symptoms: A Cultural Hermeneutic Model for Clinical Practice." Pp. 165–96 in *The Relevance of Social Science for Medicine*, edited by Leon Eisenberg and Arthur Kleinman. Boston: Reidel.

Gramsci, Antonio. 1971. *Prison Notebooks* New York: International.

Habermas, Juergen. 1970. "Technology and Science as 'Ideology.' " Pp. 81–122 in *Toward a Rational Society*. Boston: Beacon.

______. 1971. *Knowledge and Human Interests*. Boston: Beacon.

______. 1974. *Theory and Practice*. Boston: Beacon.

______. 1975. *Legitimation Crisis*. Boston: Beacon.

______. 1985. *The Theory of Communicative Action, Volume One: Reason and the Rationalization of Society*. Boston: Beacon.

Illich, Ivan. 1975. *Medical Nemesis*. London: Calder & Boyars.

Jameson, Frederic. 1971a. "The Case for George Lukacs." Pp. 160–205 in *Marxism and Form*. Princeton: Princeton University Press.

______. 1971b. *Marxism and Form*. Princeton: Princeton University Press.

______. 1981. *The Political Unconscious: Narrative as a Socially Symbolic Act*. Ithaca: Cornell University Press.

Katz, Jay. 1984. *The Silent World of Doctor and Patient*. New York: Free Press.

Kelman, Sander. 1975. "The Social Nature of the Definition Problem in Health." *International Journal of Health Services* 5:625–642.

Knorr-Cetina, Karin, and Aaron V. Cicourel, eds. 1981. *Advances in Social Theory and Methodology: Toward an Integration of Micro- and Macro-Sociologies*. Boston: Routledge & Kegan Paul.

Lukacs, George. 1971a. *History and Class Consciousness*. Cambridge: MIT Press.

______. 1971b. *The Theory of the Novel*. Cambridge: MIT Press.

Marx, Karl, 1894 [1971]. *Capital*, volume 3. Moscow: Progress Publishers.

Marx, Karl, and Friedrich Engels. 1846 [1939]. *The German Ideology*. New York: International.

McKeown, Thomas. 1979. *The Role of Medicine: Dream, Mirage, or Nemesis?* Princeton: Princeton University Press.

Mills, C. Wright. 1959. *The Sociological Imagination*. New York: Oxford University Press.

Mishler, Elliot G. 1984. *The Discourse of Medicine: Dialectics of Medical Interviews*. Norwood, N.J.: Ablex.

Poster, Mark. 1984. *Foucault, Marxism, and History*. New York: Basil Blackwell.

Sox, Harold C., Iris Margulies, and Carol Hill Sox. 1981. "Psychologically Mediated Effects of Diagnostic Tests." *New England Journal of Medicine* 95:680–85.

Stoeckle, John D., and J. Andrew Billings. 1987. "A History of History-taking: the Medical Interview." *Journal of General Internal Medicine* 2:119–27.

Taussig, Michael T. 1980. "Reification and the Consciousness of the Patient." *Social Science & Medicine* 14B:3–13.

Waitzkin, Howard. 1971. "Latent Functions of the Sick Role in Various Institutional Settings." *Social Science & Medicine* 5:45–75.

______. 1978. "The Informative Process in Medical Care: Terminal Progress Report." Submitted to National Center for Health Services Research (HS-02100, Working Paper #32).

______. 1983. *The Second Sickness: Contradictions of Capitalist Health Care*. New York: Free Press.

______. 1984. "Doctor-Patient Communication: Clinical Implications of Social Scientific Research." *Journal of the American Medical Association* 252:2441–46.

______. 1985. "Information Giving in Medical Care." *Journal of Health and Social Behavior* 26:81–101.

______. 1989a. "A Critical Theory of Medical Discourse: How Health Professionals Deal With Social Problems." *International Journal of Health Services*. Forthcoming.

______. 1989b. "A Critical Theory of Medical Discourse: Text, Context, and the Structure of Medical Encounters." In *Current Research on Occupations and Professions*, forthcoming.

Waitzkin, Howard, and John D. Stoeckle. 1972. "The Communication of Information About

Illness: Clinical, Sociological, and Methodological Considerations." *Advances in Psychosomatic Medicine* 8:180–215.

______. 1976. "Information Control and the Micropolitics of Health Care." *Social Science & Medicine* 10:263–76.

Waitzkin, Howard, and Barbara Waterman. 1974. *The Exploitation of Illness in Capitalist Society*. Indianapolis: Bobbs-Merrill.

Weinstein, Milton C. and William B. Stason. 1977. "Foundations of Cost-Effectiveness Analysis for Health and Medical Practices." *New England Journal of Medicine* 296:716–721.

West, Candace. 1984. *Routine Complications: Troubles With Talk Between Doctors and Patients*. Bloomington: Indiana University Press.

Ziem, Grace. 1977. "Medical Education Since Flexner," *Health/PAC Bulletin* 76:8–14, 23.

Zola, Irving Kenneth. 1972. "Medicine as an Institution of Social Control." *Sociological Review* 20:487–504.

______. 1975. "In the Name of Health and Illness: On Some Socio-political Consequences of Medical Influence." *Social Science & Medicine* 9:83–87.

______. 1983. "The Medicalizing of Society." Pp. 243–96 in *Socio-Medical Inquiries*. Philadelphia: Temple University Press.

Zuckerman, A., B. Starfield, C. Hochreiter, and B. Kovasznay. 1975. "Validating the Content of Pediatric Outpatient Medical Records by Means of Tape Recording Doctor-Patient Encounters." *Pediatrics* 56:407–11.

HOWARD WAITZKIN *is Professor of Medicine and Social Sciences, and Chief of the Division of General Internal Medicine and Primary Care, at the University of California, Irvine. His research interests focus on doctor-patient communication and health policy. Currently, he is finishing a book, tentatively titled* At the Margins of Medicine: A Critical Study of How Patients and Doctors Deal With Social Problems (Yale University Press, Forthcoming).

[4]

Bryan S. Turner

Ageing, status politics and sociological theory*

ABSTRACT

As a feature of social change and as an aspect of social stratification, ageing and age groups have been seriously neglected by sociological theory. This article attempts to conceptualise age groups in a multi-dimensional model of stratification which considers ageing in relation to economic class, political entitlement, or citizenship, and cultural life-styles. This multi-dimensional model provides an analytical basis for rejecting functionalist theories of ageing, which emphasize the positive functions of social disengagement, activity theories, which show that self-esteem in ageing is an effect of continuing social involvement, and Marxist social gerontology, which argues that retirement is determined by labour-market requirements in capitalism. The article concludes by developing a reciprocity-maturation curve of ageing which explains age stigmatization through exchange theory as an effect of declining social reciprocity. Both young and elderly social groups in a period of economic recession are perceived to be socially dependent, and become the targets of 'the politics of resentment'. The processes of social ageing can be located in the core of sociological theory, because they are connected fundamentally to the conditions of social solidarity.

INTRODUCTION

The problems of incorporating ethnicity into any theory of social stratification are well known.[1] While ethnicity is clearly directly related to various types of social inequality, ethnicity appears to cross-cut many conventional dimensions of social stratification, specifically cross-cutting social class divisions. Ethnic divisions and gender divisions stand in a similar relationship to classical theories of stratification. While in general it has proved difficult to incorporate ethnic and gender divisions within a general sociological theory of social stratification, the problems are somewhat compounded within a Marxist framework on economic class divisions.

Although there have been a number of attempts to resolve the difficulties,[2] there is at present no parsimonious solution to these analytical problems.

In this article I draw attention to a parallel problem, namely the absence of a coherent sociological theory of ageing and age groups as features of social stratification.[3] Indeed, it can be argued that neither contemporary nor classical sociological theory has ever fully addressed these issues. There are of course a number of interesting and important approaches to generational differences and generational groups.[4] There are also a number of valuable contributions to the historical analysis of age categories within the development of Western society.[5] The fact remains that an interest in social gerontology is a recent development within the social sciences.

The absence of a coherent perspective on ageing and age groups in classical sociology may be related to two separate issues. First, the primary anxiety of political economy was the Malthusian legacy, namely anxieties about the overcrowding of urban space and the threat of infectious diseases. The economic problems of ageing populations and population decline did not become significant political issues until in Britain in the 1930s it appeared that the population was no longer being replaced. Secondly, classical sociology became theoretically and morally distant from both Darwinistic theory and from eugenics, emphasising instead the importance of values and culture in the explanation of human action and social organisation. For example, Talcott Parsons' *The Structure of Social Action* regarded any use of biological causality as a form of positivistic reductionism in the theory of voluntaristic action.[6] Parsonian action theory gave a particular emphasis to the idea of choice guided by norms towards ends which were determined by values, thereby precluding any discussion of the biological conditions of action. While Parsons provided an interesting essay on the problems of ageing in a society based upon the value of activism,[7] ageing as a social process and age groups as a feature of social stratification did not become issues within mainstream Parsonian functionalism or its derivative theoretical perspectives. For both historical-empirical and conceptual-theoretical reasons, therefore, ageing has not featured as a significant focus of debate in mainstream sociology.

In this article I describe a three-dimensional theory of social stratification as a model which can incorporate ageing and age groups within a more analytical and comprehensive approach to social stratification. I then provide an analysis of the politics of ageing in contemporary capitalist societies in a period of economic recession; I describe this political context as 'the politics of resentment'. Finally, I outline a theory of ageing, stigmatisation and social reciprocity as an alternative to current Marxist or political-economy approaches to age as a feature of social inequality.

A THEORY OF SOCIAL STRATIFICATION

Following Weber and T. H. Marshall, we can conceptualise the social structure of society in terms of three inter-related dimensions, namely economic class, political inequalities and cultural life-styles.[8] I shall not elaborate on the idea of economic class as a major feature of social stratification, since this aspect of social inequality is probably the most developed and extensively defended as a theoretical perspective.[9] Following Marshall's analysis of citizenship, we can identify a second dimension of social structure, namely status or citizenship as socio-political entitlement. For example, age groups make claims against the state as a status group on the basis of a right of citizenship, independently of their social class position. While political entitlement is clearly influenced by economic class, political rights cannot be simply reduced to economic conditions.[10] However, by elaborating the work of Pierre Bourdieu, we can develop a third dimension of social stratification, namely the idea of status as cultural life-style.[11] Ageing and age groups are demarcated not only by economic and political practices, but also by specific life-styles, a cultural habitus and by dispositions which differentiate them from other, competing social groups.

The social stratification system is structured by an economic dimension (the ownership and control of the means of production), by a political or citizenship dimension (the control of various political and legal resources, which structure the distribution of rights and obligations), and by a cultural dimension (the monopolisation of various forms of cultural capital which at the level of life-style differentiate and demarcate social groups). The relationship between these three dimensions of social stratification is historically contingent, and the dominance of any particular dimension can only be ascertained by historical and empirical research. For example, historically one might argue that in early capitalism the economic dimension of stratification was dominant, but with the emergence of mass culture there is much stronger and more prominent emphasis on cultural competition for goods of distinction. Within state socialist societies, there is some general agreement that the political dimension is the most significant feature in the general distribution of resources.[12]

Marshall saw capitalism as a social system in which there was a permanent contradiction or tension between economic class and citizenship, since there were tensions between an economic system that necessarily generated social inequality and a political system based upon democracy which emphasised universalistic rights. The result is that in a liberal, capitalist system individuals constantly experience a contradiction between their formal rights of equality of opportunity and their everyday experiences of deprivation and exploitation. To Marshall's classical account, I have added a third dimension, namely the notion that with the growth of a mass society, there are rising expectations of general access to consumer goods through new forms of credit and distribution. The deprivations of the market place and the exploitation of work are compensated by the benefits of mass consumption, which has been made possible in the post-war period by the availability of credit. Consumption is the 'positive' side of work, just as citizenship is the 'positive' side of social membership.[13] Insofar as mass society brings about a certain democratic levelling of tastes, there may be further tensions or contradictions between rising expectations of consumption, political expectations of equality and economic inequalities in the market place.[14]

In the post-war period when in the West there was considerable economic expansion and social reconstruction, many of these tensions in the system of social stratification could be managed in societies experiencing high rates of social mobility, high levels of employment and some redistribution of wealth through the welfare system. Dramatic improvements in the infantile mortality rates in Britain after 1945 are a simple but compelling illustration of this assertion. Economic class differences in mortality rates continued of course to be important.[15] The result was a relatively optimistic wave of social theory, because the liberal democracies appeared to have resolved many of the problems of political representation, ideology and technological growth. Parsons, who had been in many respects pessimistic about the possibility of democratic capitalism in the fascist period, turned in the post-war period towards 'a theory of successful modernity'.[16] With the sharp downturn in economic growth, increasing unemployment and instability in the financial markets since 1973, problems of political management have increased, and there are sharper contradictions between the democratic implications of universal citizenship and the ongoing, and to some extent deepening, inequalities between classes and status groups. In a period of recession, the problems of a 'greying' population become particularly prominent, given the economic dependency of the aged on the general (employed) population. The potentially negative implications of ageing populations for economic recovery and economic growth along with the global problems of population 'exchanges' between societies are now widely discussed and widely recognised.[17] The explosive combination of political citizenship with economic decline generates a politics of resentment whereby various social groups compete for diminishing resources leading in the case of ageing to a new category of discrimination in ageism (Levin and Levin, 1980). The politics of ageing therefore can be conceptualised as a series of conflicts along the economic, political and cultural dimensions of the system of social stratification. The actual experience of ageing and inequalities related to retirement are structured by a differential location along these three dimensions of stratification, but I am assuming considerable interaction between these dimensions.

These social conflicts typically assume a competition between social groups to coerce the state into recognising the presence of a welfare need. Since the aged experience ageing as a form of discrimination which negates or conflicts with their universalistic rights as citizens, the aged become clients of the state in order to enforce their social entitlements.[18] In so far as the state, as it were, accepts their legitimate right to political clientship, we may refer to 'state-administered status groups', which are groups constituted by the state's response to citizenship claims. The expanding expectations of entitlement and political clientism are also associated with a new service demand, contributing to the growth of the service sector. Contemporary politics have changed from a politics of class to a politics of status, as various competing groups attempt to improve their position in terms of welfare and tax distributions.[19] We can see the recent political history of Britain as a shift from social Keynesianism to monetarism, which is essentially an attempt to reduce the state's share of gross national product in the interests of various status columns. Monetaristic politics is an attempt to reassert the privileges of the employed and the welfared against various dependent sectors of the society who are forced to rely upon the continuity of a welfare system. These general policies of the state are the effect of social struggles over economic, political and cultural resources in which politically disunited sectors of the population such as the aged are marginalized in citizenship terms. These struggles in contemporary society have produced a number of complex paradoxes in social and political life.

Any attempt to achieve greater equality between status groups is likely to produce greater bureaucratic surveillance of the individual. This dilemma involves the classical contradiction between a liberal view of individual freedoms and a socialist idea of egalitarianism as the primary moral and political value. While I do not subscribe to the view that freedom and equality are mutually exclusive. there are clearly tensions between individual rights and personal freedoms and the political regulation of the economic process in order to achieve greater equality, especially equality of outcome.[20] One underlying theme of this discussion is therefore a moral implication concerning the function of status-group conflicts within a democratic system as opposed to a regulated society based upon an absolutist ideal of equality of outcome. Behind this moral debate is yet another moral and sociological theme, namely the relationship between social stability and moral autonomy. These classical dilemmas are particularly relevant to a sociology of ageing, since the process of ageing implies increasing dependency and bureaucratic management with the loss of employment and mobility.

While I emphasise the conflictual and competitive struggle between social groups over resources as the essential feature of a sociology of status, I also recognise that this competition for a position within society can in a complex way produce new forms of social solidarity and identity. Social struggles over cultural capital have, at least in the past, also assumed some broad social agreement over what will count as worthy of distinction. Combative status groups are in any case internally cohesive.[21] While the competitive struggle for status is one of conflict, the underlying notion here is that contemporary societies are based upon an extensive concept of citizenship which is a way of defining social membership and personal identity.[22] The expansion of social membership as a solidaristic principle is the unintended effect of status competition and conflict within a society in which social mobility and enhanced social membership are in principle always possible. Intra-social competitions may be perfectly compatible with higher order societal integration. My view of status conflicts is in this limited sense 'positive', since I treat this competitive struggle as a process which brings about various forms of social solidarity and group membership. Social welfare rights as consequences of political struggle are also mechanisms for the integration of oppositional and marginal groups within the political community. Inflationary wage spirals may be unintentionally a safety valve against more violent forms of political protest.[23]

While within a democratic system status politics make possible incremental change thereby incorporating groups within the wider socio-political framework, these political adjustments may often have negative economic consequences, at least for the profitability of private investment. For example, small companies often find it difficult to adjust to the economic climate which is dominated by the corporatist system of multinational corporations, the state and the unions.[24] In short, the relationship between the conditions of integration and disintegration of the political system is variable and complex, and again the analysis of these relations has to be an empirical one. The outcome of political struggles between classes and status groups is a contingent effect of social conflicts; it is not a subject amenable to general law-like statements.

The argument here parallels that presented by Bell[25] that social and political conflicts over entitlements (citizenship rights) are the essential core of modern political life, often contributing to a fiscal crisis which the state cannot manage adequately, because the economic demands of status communities, status blocs and classes tend to be permanently expansionary, producing various negative economic outcomes. However, this political situation and its economic consequences should not necessarily be described as a 'crisis', since these tensions are permanent or at least long-term structural features of democratic, capitalist, welfare systems. While Marxist sociology typically treats the doctrines of democratic equality and individualism as producing ideological incorporation and the stabilisation of capitalist relations, there is an equally strong argument which can be traced back to Alexis de Tocqueville *Democracy in America* in 1844 that the concept of egalitarian citizenship is revolutionary and essentially modern in its implications. The problem with equality (of income for example) is that it 'is affected to only a limited degree by the institutional arrangements and policies of a society'.[26]

AGE AND STATUS ENTITLEMENTS

Classical social theory saw the historical emergence of modern society in terms of a transition from fixed status positions to open, contractual relationships in the market. Within this paradigm, the emergence of the market and the development of free labour relations were indeed crucial aspects of modern civilisation. This model has many ramifications in terms of classical views about culture, religion and law, especially in relation to the dominance of the market. Within both political economy and sociology, the market was seen to have revolutionary consequences for culture and social structure in the emergence of capitalism. The contractual relationship was corrosive of traditional hierarchies and conventional beliefs.[27] For various historical reasons the 'pure' market situation did not emerge without modification. While Marx expected economic class to be the main feature of the labour market in contemporary society, for reasons which are closely related to the continuity of status, labour markets are for example often structured in terms of inequalities between ethnic communities and age groups. While Weber expected the market to be dominated by associational (*gesellschaft*) relations, again for reasons connected with status closure, communal (*gemeinschaft*) relations are characteristic of the structuring of the market. The organisation of class sytems and economic relations in terms of status and cultural divisions also represents a major deviation away from Weber's conception of a rationally organised market place and Marx's concept of capitalism in which labour power is freely bought and sold like any other commodity. These illustrations point to the continuity of ascriptive criteria in societies dominated by a formal doctrine of achievement and universalism.

For Parsons the two primary illustrations of ascriptive criteria in social stratification systems were sex and age (or more precisely the particular position of a person within the biological life-cycle).

Parsons drew attention to these two dimensions 'because of their universality and their relevance to certain intrinsic functional problems of social systems'.[28] While Parsons acknowledged age grading as an important feature of status (especially in the USA where early retirement often leads to extreme isolation of the aged), he also argued that, given the emphasis on activism in the USA, the importance of ascriptive components in the stratification system would be eventually eroded. However, the reduction of ascriptive components (such as age grading) has also 'opened up important new potentialities for inequality'.[29] These new sources of inequality derive from the bureaucratisation of social welfare systems, creating new inequalities in authority and power. The second source of inequality is derived from the increasing differentiation of social functions within contemporary society, which creates new levels of and expectations for competence and performance.

The issue of age as a basis for status and entitlement is important not simply because ageing has been neglected by theorists of social stratification, but because an examination of age and ageing helps to throw analytical light upon the more general problem of status differences in contemporary society. While within medical science ageing is properly understood in terms of bio-chemical explanations of the pathological deterioration of the human organism through time, the social sciences take a different view of ageing as a cultural and sociological process by which human beings are classified and ranked by reference to their chronology. The sociological view is that age and ageing are socially constructed categories for the classification of persons. The notions of age and age groups are historically and culturally specific, which means that we must regard the problem of age and ageing as relative to various social and historical contexts. For example, it is possible to argue that in European societies there has been a gradual differentiation of age groups, giving rise to distinctive generational groupings with specific lifestyles and culture. Following the work of Ariès,[30] the cultural notion of childhood emerged gradually through the seventeenth and eighteenth centuries, with the result that children came to be regarded as a special social group with individual needs and problems. Furthermore, it was thought that children needed to be protected from the moral and sexual dangers of contact with adults. One indication of this specialisation of childhood was the development of specific forms of caring for children to denote and distinguish them from adults. Children were eventually separated in the schooling system into different age groups and, with the development of legal regulations for the control and protection of children, children were no longer exploited on the labour market because they were no longer regarded as mature persons. Within the English context, the Factory Acts of the nineteenth century gave some legal protection for children as a specific age group within the labour market. Therefore, unlike preindustrial societies, contemporary communities identify a range of transitional age groups between early infancy and adulthood, including childhood, adolescence and youth.

Clearly age and ageing as criteria of honour and prestige change through historical time. For example, in early colonial America, a gerontocratia dominated society and the elderly were venerated for their wisdom and maturity. In the revolutionary period (1770–1820) there were important changes in American attitudes which became more positive toward youthfulness and youth.[31] In American culture, various derogatory and pejorative labels emerged for defining the elderly as less important than younger people. For example, the notion of 'old gaffer' and 'old fogy' were in common use by the 1830s. In American society there is along with activism a high evaluation of youth and youth culture which are associated with enjoyment, hedonism, activity and beauty. Youthfulness has become a desirable attribute of all social groups almost regardless of their actual age. Indeed Parsons[32] has argued that Western societies are characterised as a whole by what he referred to as 'the romantic idealization of youth patterns' and youth cultures. Age has become profoundly downgraded as a value in the culture of western societies. In an age of narcissism, our society 'defines them (the elderly) as useless, forces them to retire before they have exhausted their capacity for work, and reinforces their sense of superfluity at every opportunity'.[33]

Changing attitudes towards age, ageing and retirement in contemporary societies however have often produced contradictory situations, which have in turn been reinforced by legislative change. Because of the general emphasis on youthfulness and activity, early retirement or compulsory retirement typically have traumatic and negative consequences for self-image, social involvement and social status for older age groups. On the other hand, early retirement is often claimed to offer certain positive advantages; for example, it prevents the continuous exploitation of the workforce by the open labour market and in principle provides opportunities for creative leisure and enjoyment after the hard labour of employment. By contrast, it is possible to argue that compulsory retirement at the age of sixty-five years for men is an entirely arbitrary decision, based upon particularistic, ascriptive criteria rather than upon egalitarian, universalistic and activist principles.

The question of retirement raises various moral and economic problems. For example, should we regard early retirement on the basis of age as a reward for long service, or should we regard retirement as a mechanism for increasing the employment possibilities of younger workers? Should retirement be a welfare benefit, or is it in practice a punitive measure for constraining workers within the labour market? These questions are also related to problems of retirement and unemployment through economic recession based upon the principle of seniority (particularly the principle of 'first in, last out'). Within the contemporary period of economic recession, these principles of employment and unemployment by seniority have become the basis of complex political issues. The seniority principle can be regarded initially as the outcome of successful trade-union pressure for a period of respite from work in which the benefits of employment can be enjoyed by those currently retired

> seniority is a claim-right that exists when employers acknowledge the claims of employees that they deserve to have length of service taken into account when personnel decisions are made. Two kinds of rights emerged from acknowledgement of such claims: competitive status seniority and benefits seniority. Competitive status seniority ties lay-off, recall from lay-off, and promotion decisions to length of service on the grounds that those who have served longer deserve preference. Benefits seniority means that paid vacations, pensions and severance pay are proportional to length of service.[34]

Seniority rules are an essential part of the whole industrial-relations system, providing negotiators with at least one potentially effective rule for making judgements between the conflicting claims of different sectors within the workforce. However, the potential conflict between preference on the basis of performance and merit versus benefits on the basis of an ascriptive principle such as age and length of service indicate more general conflicts in the notions of age, ageing and retirement as aspects of the distribution of entitlements. Age very clearly indicates the conflict between ascription and achievement in the ranking of individuals, but it also points to highly divisive status differences with the working class.

Contradictory views of the nature of ageing and retirement in Western societies are reflected in different sociological theories of ageing. Broadly speaking there are two important but contradictory theories of ageing which have dominated recent social gerontology. In so-called disengagement theories, it is argued that with ageing people begin to relinquish certain social responsibilities and expectations in order to engage more fully in personally rewarding leisure activities.[35] As the elderly withdraw from social roles, society as it were disengages from the ageing in order to bring about a neutral process of declining reciprocity. It may be noted[36] that disengagement theory in gerontology is the obverse of the functionalist theory of social stratification, which has been a prominent theory of social differentiation in American sociology.[37]

There are two crucial aspects of functionalist theories of stratification. The first is a theory of motivation which suggests that, in order for difficult but important positions in society to be filled by the most technically competent people, it is necessary to have a system of inducements to reward such individuals, not only to fill these positions, but to undertake the training necessary to acquire the competence for these social roles. The rewards for filling these complex and difficult social tasks include not only high wages, but considerable social prestige, honour and the satisfactions of rewarding occupations. This theory attempts to explain why income differentials are, along with status and job satisfaction, unequally distributed in society. Secondly, the functionalist theory argues that stratification is socially functional for the continuity of society and therefore some forms of inequality may be not only necessary but positively advantageous to society. Disengagement theory of ageing parallels the arguments of the functionalist theory of stratification, but it suggests that the ageing need some motivation to relinquish their social roles in order thereby to create new niches in the system for younger generations to secure social standing through educational attainment. Retirement benefits, leisure and the 'golden handshake' are the principal components of these motivational inducements to disengage. Disengagement theory can be criticised on grounds rather similar to general criticisms of functionalism.[38] First, it is not self-evident that the aged in powerful social positions do in fact easily or voluntarily give up their authority, power and prestige with ageing. The political elites of most contemporary democratic and socialist systems are characteristically dominated by men who are well past the normal retirement age. Secondly, retirement and disengagement, far from permitting the personal enjoyment of new forms of leisure, tend to usher in a period of increasing impoverishment and declining social status. In the USA in the late 1970s, the federal government reported that approximately fourteen per cent of the population over sixty-five were classified as poor compared with a seven per cent poverty rate for those between the ages forty-five and fifty. It has been suggested in Britain that retirement results in an average decline in disposable income of almost fifty per cent.[39]

Against disengagement theory, the engagement theory of ageing suggests that experiences after retirement tend to be closely related to previous life-styles and socio-economic status. Studies in the United States have also noted that the single most important cause of social disengagement is illness rather than a 'natural' process of diminishing participaton in pursuit of leisure.[40] Engagement or activity theories come to conclusions which are more or less the obverse of disengagement theory, namely that personal satisfaction and self-esteem are consequences of continuing rather than declining social activity with retirement.[41]

The implication of both theories is that the problems of the ageing and the elderly in contemporary society cannot be analysed independently of the economic context of the ageing in relation to the labour market, or of the whole political environment of ageing with respect to welfare benefits, retirement funds and health-care systems, or of the general cultural values which are ascribed to youth and age. However, some writers wish to make a strong connection, not only between ageing and economic class, but more generally between ageing as a process and the labour requirements of industrial capitalism. Given the emphasis on activism and achievement in modern societies, compulsory retirement for men and women appears to define arbitrarily a person as no longer productive and therefore no longer of social value. Furthermore, retirement patterns are clearly associated with the specific character of the economic and political conditions of a capitalist economy, since early retirement brings about a restriction in the supply of labour, thereby enabling younger persons to enter the workforce, while also bringing about reductions in the cost of labour since younger workers are generally paid lower wages. Retirement and ageing rather than simply being 'natural' processes are bound up with struggles between labour and capital, alongside the political representation of the elderly as voters. Because retirement is an important aspect of industrial relations, some writers adopting a Marxist perspective have tried to suggest that the elderly worker rather than being retired should be regarded as having been abandoned, because he or she can no longer provide effective or efficient economic service to capital.[42] The loss of social status and the stigmatisation of the elderly can within this perspective be seen as more directly a consequence of the character of capitalist production rather than as a consequence of the stratification system as such.

There are a number of problems with a Marxist interpretation of ageing and the elderly. First, the stigmatisation of the elderly has been common to many societies over a long historical period and is therefore not peculiar to capitalism.[43] Secondly, there is evidence to suggest that in state-socialist societies attitudes towards the aged are not particularly different in terms of stereotypes than attitudes found commonly in capitalist societies.[44] Thirdly, the implications of the ageing of populations for welfare benefits, economic growth and the labour market are more complex than a Marxist framework would suggest, and we need to consider the issue of ageing within capitalism from the perspective of citizenship, status politics and welfare because age groups as status blocs cannot be assimilated analytically to economic class analysis.

A MODEL OF STIGMATIZATION

We have seen that we cannot explain the stigmatization of the elderly or negative attitudes towards the process of ageing simply by reference to certain economic or political needs of a capitalist mode of production. We need an alternative perspective which would locate the stigmatization of the aged in some fundamental social processes which are common to all societies, regardless of their rather different historical processes and modes of production. In this section I argue that we can explain the stigmatization of the aged through an analysis of dependency within a framework of social exchange and reciprocity. We can regard all social interactions as forms of endless exchange which generate the norm of reciprocity.[45] We can therefore define dependency as unequal exchange within the network of social reciprocities, and following R. Pinker[46] we may regard all forms of social service as part of a macro-system of societal exchange. Within this paradigm, dependency is socially acceptable only where it is a return on previous social contributions or where it is given in anticipation of a contribution in the future. The outcome is that an absence of reciprocity (as a consequence of prolonged unemployment, extreme poverty or life-long disability) has significant social and moral implications for the status of a dependent person, family or group. It is this lack of social reciprocity in social exchange which is the basic explanation of the stigma which is associated with the recipients of charity, taxation benefits or social welfare. Dependency without anticipation of some future reciprocity gives rise to stigmatised labels and descriptions such as 'scrounging' or 'chiselling'.[47] Because compulsory retirement creates a condition of extended and in principle probably unlimited dependence on welfare, the aged become stigmatized as parasitic recipients of social benefits in a situation where they are forced to compete for scarce resources with unemployed youth.

Indeed there is an interesting parallel between the stigmatization of the young and of the aged as marginal, dependent groups who are perceived to be either no longer or unable to contribute to the common good. Because the adolescent and the elderly have a number of shared characteristics (such as dependency, the absence of social obligations and the absence of paid work), they are often described within the same pejorative, stigmatizing vocabulary. While we often describe the elderly as childish or irresponsible, we may also refer to the elderly as undergoing a second childhood. Stigmatization is an effect of lack of social reciprocity, long-term dependency and an ideology of normative obligations. We can express this idea of stigmatization in terms of a reciprocity-maturation curve[48] in Figure I.

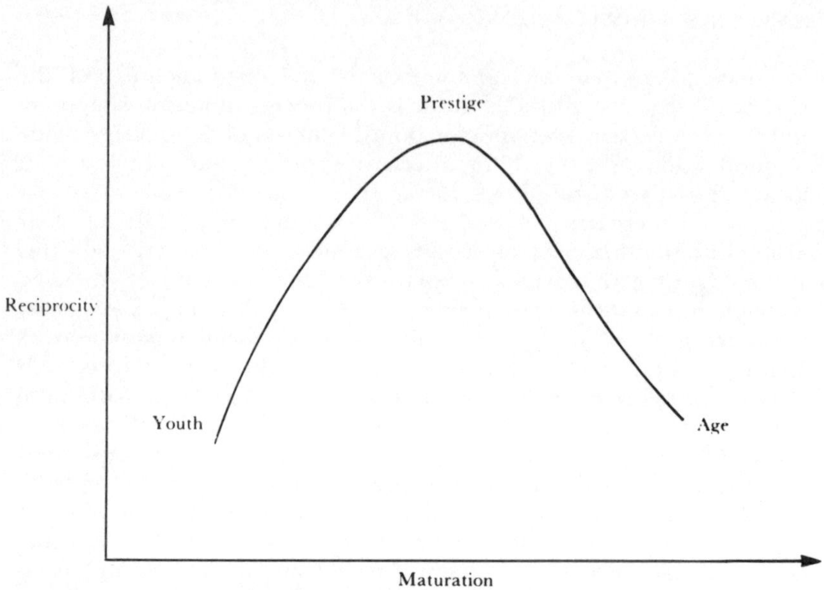

FIGURE I: *The reciprocity-maturation curve*

As individuals mature they characteristically take on new social obligations and responsibilities, by occupying new social roles which are demanding and tie them both in time and resources into the core of the social system. For example, as people mature, become married, have children and enjoy the benefits of employment, they become more reciprocally bound into the social system. As their reciprocity with and integration into the society increases, so their social status and personal self-esteem within the community also rise. This reciprocity-maturation curve can incorporate engagement and disengagement theories. As the reciprocity of individuals increases, they move up the prestige curve becoming increasingly engaged in the social system. Ageing and retirement bring about a necessary disengagement from the social system; while in principle bringing about certain rewards in terms of leisure, retirement also threatens the self-image of an individual by increasing their dependence and hence the threat of stigmatization. In a period of significant unemployment and economic recession, many sectors of the young population may never in fact enter the formal labour market or they may only enter it on a casual basis. The result is that some young groups today will never enter the pattern of increasing reciprocity moving instead from youth to old age in a permanently stigmatized social role.

In addition we need to see this curve moving through time since as the total population undergoes a process of ageing the high point of the prestige curve may move, as it were, upwards into older age groups as the whole society experiences 'greying'. Following the work of Bourdieu,[49] there will be a significant social struggle over life-styles indicating and protecting the prestige core of the system. These two processes — the demographic greying of the population and cultural struggles over the values of activism and autonomy — will also bring about continuous redefinitions of 'middle age'. While I have defined stigmatization as a function of low reciprocity, I do not thereby exclude the idea of ideological struggle over what counts as 'a contribution' to the social system. While this explanation of stigmatization therefore has some parallel in the Durkheimian explanation of suicide,[50] my explanation does not ignore historical change or rule out social conflict and social struggle. On the contrary, the model assumes that the experience of ageing will be determined by struggles in three fields (the field of economic practices, the field of cultural life-style and the political field of citizenship entitlements). The impact of the reciprocity-maturation curve will be mediated by class position, by the accumulation of cultural capital and by the ability of aged groups to mobilise for political action.

CONCLUSION

The ageing of the populations of the industrial societies has important social and economic implications, because of the growth of the so-called dependent populations consequent upon retirement. Ageing has become politically significant because of the introduction of compulsory retirement in a wide range of occupations. For example, by 1980 in the UK approximately eighty per cent of the male population over the age of sixty-five was retired and therefore in formal terms dependent. Almost nine-tenths of all elderly people are economically dependent on some form of state benefit for all or some of their household income. The political and economic problems associated with the ageing of populations had become obvious by the 1970s.[51] However, in this discussion I have argued that sociological theory has yet to come to terms with these empirical changes in the social structure.

In the European industrial societies at least thirteen per cent of the population was over the age of sixty-five by the 1970s. Sweden had fourteen per cent of its population over the age of sixty-five by 1971 and similar degrees of ageing were also common in France,

Germany and the UK. To take another example, government old-age pensions account for almost thirty-three per cent of all social welfare benefits in the Netherlands, and it is anticipated that by year 2030 these benefits will amount to half of all social welfare benefits. The decline in fertility and the ageing of the population results in a sharp decline in the number of workers in comparison to retirees, which of course has major economic and political implications. Government based old-age pensions represent a significant subtraction from national income. For example, in the Netherlands pensions absorb almost twelve per cent of national income, whereas in West Germany fourteen per cent and in Japan twelve per cent of national income is absorbed by pensions. Given the current recession which characterises the world economy, the ageing of the human population poses not only serious economic implications for economic growth, but also raises the spectre of significant political conflict between different age groups. I have suggested that we can refer to such struggles as a politics of resentment between welfare clients.

The political issue can be stated simply by noting that while retirement may severely restrict economic rights and privileges, retirement has in principle no direct implication for voting or more generally for political rights. The aged populations of liberal democracies are increasingly politically organised to protect their interests against government policies which might seek either to diminish welfare benefits to the elderly or to privatise many government-run agencies for the elderly. In the USA, the Gray Panthers represent an important lobby within the political arena and similar institutions or social movements exist in other Western societies. Age is a status position which cannot be explained exclusively in terms of economic class analysis. Furthermore, the status politics of the elderly cannot be regarded simply as a form of class politics, since ageing as an ascriptive process cuts across class or other economic divisions. The elderly within liberal democratic societies are increasingly organised into status blocs which, appealing to the notions of universal citizenship, seek to promote and protect their status interests against other age groups. Furthermore, gerontologists and other welfare professionals associated with the care of the elderly have paradoxically an interest in the preservation of age as a social or health problem. The state by responding to the political and economic claims of the aged as a status bloc in one sense guarantees the continuity of age as an ascriptive label which brings about entitlements. The state in responding to the problems of ageing and the demands of the aged becomes the patron of the elderly. It is for this reason that it has been argued that age can be properly conceptualised as an issue within a three dimensional theory of status stratification. We can therefore refer to the aged as 'a state-administered status bloc' within the system of stratification of Western societies.

(Date accepted: March 1988)

Bryan S. Turner
Faculty of Social Sciences
The State University of Utrecht
The Netherlands

NOTES

* The research for this article was made possible by a fellowship from the Alexander von Humboldt Foundation. It was first given as a public lecture to the Centre for the Study of Adult Life, Teesside Polytechnic, England. I am grateful to the participants for their criticism.

1. J. Rex, *Race and Ethnicity*, Milton Keynes, Open University Press, 1986.

2. O. C. Cox, *Caste, Class and Race*, New York, Monthly Review Press, 1970.

3. The contours of such a theory and its general importance for sociology are discussed in M. W. Riley, 'On the Significance of Age in Sociology', *American Sociological Review*, vol. 52 (1), 1987, pp. 1–14.

4. K. Mannheim, 'The Problem of Generations', *Essays on the Sociology of Knowledge*, London, Routledge and Kegan Paul, 1952, pp. 276–322; S. N. Eisenstadt, *From Generation to Generation, Age Groups and Social Structure*, Glencoe, Illinois, Free Press, 1956.

5. P. Ariès, *Centuries of Childhood*, Harmondsworth, Penguin Books, 1962.

6. T. Parsons, *The Structure of Social Action*, New York, McGraw-Hill, 1937. The development of Parsons' analysis of the biological conditions of action is presented in J. C. Alexander *Theoretical Logic in Sociology, Volume Four, The Modern Reconstruction of Classical Thought: Talcott Parsons*, London, Routledge and Kegan Paul, 1984.

7. T. Parsons, 'Age and Sex in the Social Structure of the United States', *American Sociological Review*, vol. 7, 1942, pp. 604–16.

8. For a commentary on Weber's analysis of social stratification, V. Burris, 'The Neo-Marxist Synthesis of Marx and Weber' in N. Wiley (ed.), *The Marx-Weber Debate*, Newbury Park, Sage, 1987, pp. 67–90. Marshall's sociology of citizenship in relation to social stratification was developed in *Sociology at the Crossroads*, London, Heinemann, 1963 and summarized in *The Right to Welfare and Other Essays*, London, Heinemann, 1981.

9. J. L. Elster, *Making Sense of Marx*, Cambridge, Cambridge University Press, 1985.

10. This argument is defended in B. S. Turner, *Citizenship and Capitalism, The Debate over Reformism*, London, Allen and Unwin, 1986 and in *Equality*, Chichester, Ellis Horwood and London, Tavistock, 1986.

11. P. Bourdieu, *Distinction, a social critique of the judgement of taste*, London, Routledge and Kegan Paul, 1984.

12. For example, see the discussion in M. Matthews, *Privilege in the Soviet Union, a study of elite lifestyles under communism*, London, Allen and Unwin, 1978 and F. Parkin, 'Class stratification in capitalist societies', *British Journal of Sociology*, vol. 20, 1969, pp. 355–74.

13. This argument was developed in B. S. Turner, 'Marx, Weber and the Coherence of Capitalism, the problem of ideology' in N. Wiley (ed.), *ibid.*, pp. 169–204.

14. L. R. Della-Fave, 'On the structure of egalitarianism', *Social Problems*, vol. 22, 1974, pp. 199–213, and E. Gellner 'The social roots of egalitarianism', *Dialectics and Humanism*, vol. 4, 1979, pp. 27–43.

15. R. G. Wilkinson (ed.), *Class and Health, research and longitudinal data*, London and New York, Tavistock, 1986.

16. J. C. Alexander, *Twenty Lectures, sociological theories since World War II*, New York, Columbia University Press, 1987, p. 73.

17. The longterm implications are considered by D. Bell 'The world and The United States in 2013', *Daedalus*, vol. 116 (3), 1987, pp. 1–31.

18. For an analysis of the concept of entitlements, D. Bell, *The Cultural Contradictions of Capitalism*, New York, Basic Books, 1976.

19. F. Parkin, *Marxism and Class Theory, a bourgeois critique*, London, Allen and Unwin, 1979.

20. Some features of this paradox are outlined in N. Abercrombie, S. Hill and B. S. Turner, *Sovereign Individuals of Capitalism*, London, Allen and Unwin, 1986.

21. The idea that status groups are both combative and cohesive was crucial to Weber's contrast between economic class and status groups. On this issue, see F. Parkin, *Max Weber*, Chichester, Ellis Horwood and London, Tavistock, 1982.

22. The historical relationship between social solidarity and citizenship was examined in T. Parsons, *The System of Modern Societies*, Englewood Cliffs, Prentice-Hall, 1971.

23. J. H. Goldthorpe, 'The Current Inflation, towards a sociological account', in F. Hirsch and J. H. Goldthorpe (eds), *The Political Economy of Inflation*, Oxford, Martin Robertson, 1978, pp. 186–214.

24. J. O'Connor, *The Fiscal Crisis of the State*, New York, St. Martins Press, 1973.

25. Bell, 1976, *ibid*.

26. P. L. Berger, *The Capitalist Revolution, fifty propositions about prosperity equality and liberty*, Aldershot, Wildwood House, 1987, p. 219.

27. On the relationship between exchange, markets and individualism, see, L. Goldmann, *The Philosophy of the Enlightenment, the Christian Burgess and the Enlightenment*, London, Routledge and Kegan Paul, 1973.

28. T. Parsons, *The Social System*, London, Routledge and Kegan Paul, p. 89.

29. T. Parsons, 'Equality and inequality in modern society, or social stratification revisited', *Sociological Inquiry*, vol. 40, 1970, p. 18.

30. Ariès, 1962, *ibid*.

31. D. H. Fischer, *Growing Old in America*, Oxford, Oxford University Press, 1978.

32. Parsons, 1942, *ibid*.

33. C. Lasch, *The Culture of Narcissism, American Life in an age of diminishing expectations*, New York, W. W. Norton, 1978, p. 209.

34. C. Gersuny, 'From contract to status: perspectives on employment seniority', *Sociological Inquiry*, vol. 54, 1984, p. 45.

35. E. Cumming, 'Further thoughts on the theory of disengagement', *International Social Science*, vol. 15, 1963, pp. 377–93.

36. The relationship is discussed in W. C. Cockerham, *Medical Sociology*, Englewood Cliffs, New Jersey, Prentice-Hall, 1982.

37. On the functionalist theory of social stratification, K. Davis and W. Moore, 'Some priniciples of stratification', *American Sociological Review*, vol. 10, 1945, pp. 242–9.

38. The critical debate around functionalism can be found in M. M. Tumin (ed.), *Readings on Social Stratification*, Englewood Cliffs, New Jersey, Prentice-Hall, 1970.

39. A. Walker, 'Dependency and old age', *Social Policy and Administration*, vol. 16, 1982, pp. 115–35.

40. E. Palmore, 'The effects of ageing on activities and attitudes', *Gerontologist*, vol. 17, 1968, pp. 315–20, and E. Palmore, *Social Patterns in Normal Ageing, findings from the Duke Longitudinal Study*, Durham, NC, Duke University Press, 1981.

41. C. F. Longino and G. S. Kart 'Explicating activity theory, a formal replication', *Journal of Gerontology*, vol. 37, 1982, pp. 713–22.

42. C. Phillipson, *Capitalism and the Construction of Old Age*, London, Macmillan Press, 1982.

43. S. de Beauvoir, *Old Age*, London,

Weidenfeld and Nicolson, 1972.
44. D. Willcocks, 'Stereotypes of old age, the case of Yugoslavia' in D. Jerrome (ed.), *Ageing in Modern Society, Contemporary Approaches*, London and Canberra, Croom Helm, 1983, pp. 104–23.
45. A. W. Gouldner, 'The norm of reciprocity', *American Sociological Review*, vol. 25, 1960, pp. 161–78.
46. R. Pinker, *Social Theory and Social Policy*, London, Heinemann, 1971.
47. These labels are considered in P. Spicker, *Stigma and Social Welfare*, London and Canberra, Croom Helm, 1984.
48. The reciprocity-maturation curve was first developed in B. S. Turner *Medical Power and Social Knowledge*, London, Sage, 1987, pp. 122–5.
49. Bourdieu, 1984, *ibid.*
50. E. Durkheim, *Suicide, a study in sociology*, Glencoe, Illinois, Free Press, 1951.
51. C. Russell, *The Ageing Experience*, Sydney, Allen and Unwin, 1981.

Part II
Social Factors and Disease

[5]

Socioeconomic Status and Health: How Education, Income, and Occupation Contribute to Risk Factors for Cardiovascular Disease

Marilyn A. Winkleby, PhD, Darius E. Jatulis, MS, Erica Frank, MD, MPH, and Stephen P. Fortmann, MD

ABSTRACT

Background. Socioeconomic status (SES) is usually measured by determining education, income, occupation, or a composite of these dimensions. Although education is the most commonly used measure of SES in epidemiological studies, no investigators in the United States have conducted an empirical analysis quantifying the relative impact of each separate dimension of SES on risk factors for disease.

Methods. Using data on 2380 participants from the Stanford Five-City Project (85% White, non-Hispanic), we examined the independent contribution of education, income, and occupation to a set of cardiovascular disease risk factors (cigarette smoking, systolic and diastolic blood pressure, and total and high-density lipoprotein cholesterol).

Results. The relationship between these SES measures and risk factors was strongest and most consistent for education, showing higher risk associated with lower levels of education. Using a forward selection model that allowed for inclusion of all three SES measures after adjustment for age and time of survey, education was the only measure that was significantly associated with the risk factors ($P < .05$).

Conclusion. If economics or time dictate that a single parameter of SES be chosen and if the research hypothesis does not dictate otherwise, higher education may be the best SES predictor of good health. (*Am J Public Health.* 1992;82:816–820)

Introduction

One of the strongest and most consistent predictors of a person's morbidity and mortality experience is that person's socioeconomic status (SES).[1–5] This finding persists across all diseases with few exceptions, continues throughout the entire life span,[5] and extends across numerous risk factors for disease.[6–9]

The significant impact of SES on disease makes its definition and measurement of critical importance. SES is a complex phenomenon predicted by a broad spectrum of variables that is often conceptualized as a combination of financial, occupational, and educational influences.[10–13] Although these dimensions of SES are interrelated, it has been proposed that each reflects somewhat different individual and societal forces associated with health and disease. For example, income reflects spending power, housing, diet, and medical care; occupation measures prestige, responsibility, physical activity, and work exposures; and education indicates skills requisite for acquiring positive social, psychological, and economic resources.[9,14]

Much has been written about the underlying mechanisms through which SES may operate to affect disease. Many authors have suggested that certain dimensions of SES are more predictive of health than others;[1,14–16] however, such proposals tend to be theoretically based, without substantiating data. Over time, education has become the most commonly used measure of SES in epidemiological studies,[17] yet no investigators in the United States have conducted an empirical analysis quantifying the relative contributions of different measures of SES to risk factors or disease outcomes. (This paper does not suggest which component of SES may be the most reliable and valid measure because this question has been examined, with a variety of conclusions, in previously published reports.)[10–13, 17–18]

The present study examines the association between income, education, occupation, and a set of risk factors for cardiovascular disease—namely, cigarette smoking, systolic and diastolic blood pressure, and total and high-density lipoprotein (HDL) cholesterol. Our study objectives are to (1) examine the impact of each separate dimension of SES on cardiovascular risk factors, (2) use a forward stepwise selection model to evaluate if one measure of SES is the strongest predictor of risk factors, and (3) offer guidance to researchers about selection of SES measures. This guidance is critical because nearly all epidemiological studies use SES as an explanatory or a control variable, or for the selection of subjects or matching criteria.

Methods

Subjects aged 25 to 64 were drawn from the two control cities of the Stanford Five-City Project,[19] a communitywide cardiovascular disease intervention study that contains data from four separate

The authors are with the Stanford Center for Research in Disease Prevention, Stanford University School of Medicine, in Palo Alto, CA.

Requests for reprints should be sent to Marilyn A. Winkleby, Stanford Center for Research in Disease Prevention, Stanford University School of Medicine, 1000 Welch Road, Palo Alto, CA 94304-1885.

This paper was submitted to the Journal April 19, 1991, and accepted with revisions September 13, 1991.

Editor's Note. See related editorial on p 785 of this issue.

cross-sectional surveys, conducted from 1979 to 1986. Participants who were unemployed (n = 98), students (n = 130), or retirees (n = 146) were excluded because they had no occupation that could be ranked. Data from the four cross-sectional surveys were pooled because demographic characteristics, including measures of SES, showed no significant interactions over time.[7] As previously reported,[20] the educational attainment of respondents from the control cities were well matched to those from the treatment cities. A nonrespondent questionnaire indicated that participants were generally more educated than those in both treatment and control communities who refused to participate.[20]

Information on education, income, and occupation was ascertained through questionnaires. Education was recorded as the highest number of years of schooling completed. It was used as a continuous variable in regression analyses and was divided into the following four categories in stratified analyses: less than 12 years, 12 years, 13 to 15 years, and 16 years or more. Income information, defined as gross annual household income, was collected in intervals of $5000. For multivariate analyses, the midpoint of the income categories was used; for the remaining analyses, income was divided into five categories ranging from less than $10 000 to $40 000 or more per year.

Current occupation was collected as an open-ended variable and coded using the 1980 US Bureau of the Census occupational scaling system, which creates a hierarchy of occupations ordered on the basis of education and income.[21] To examine associations between separate occupations and risk factors, we coded each occupation, including homemaker, as an indicator variable, with executives as the reference category. In multivariate models, we excluded homemakers and used occupation as a ranked variable ranging from executives to unskilled workers.

Participants were considered cigarette smokers if they reported ever smoking on a daily basis and had smoked one or more cigarettes in the last week. Participants whose plasma thiocyanate exceeded 100 μmol/L and whose expired-air carbon monoxide level exceeded 8 ppm were classified as smokers regardless of their self-reported responses.[22] Total and HDL plasma cholesterol were derived from nonfasting venous samples, analyzed fresh by standard methods established by the Lipid Research Clinics Program.[23] Three blood pressure measurements were taken on the right arm using a semiautomatic recorder, and the average of the second and third readings were used for analyses.[24]

Results

An overall response rate of 69% was achieved. Approximately 600 individuals participated in each survey, resulting in a total of 2380 participants for all surveys combined. Because the study population was predominantly White, non Hispanic (85%), findings are not generalizable to populations representing a broad spectrum of racial groups.

All pairwise correlations between education, income, and occupation were positive and were stronger for men than for women (Table 1). The lowest correlation was between education and income, indicating that education is not a primary determinant of wage. Higher correlations were shown for education and occupation, suggesting that skills acquired during education may help determine occupation. Although correlations ranged from .23 to .67, their relatively low magnitude (highest adjusted R^2 = 45%) indicates that the three dimensions are not redundant measures of SES.

Although the study population had relatively high educational and financial levels, individuals from all education, income, and occupation categories were well-represented (Table 2). However, while men were represented fairly evenly across occupations, approximately 75% of women employed outside the home held nonprofessional white-collar jobs. Men tended to have more years of education than women and to be from higher-income households.

In general, those with the lowest educational attainment exhibited the highest prevalence of risk factors (Table 3). Clear gradients were seen between educational level and smoking for both sexes, and between education and total and HDL cholesterol for women. Across all risk factors, men consistently exhibited higher risk than did women.

Income and occupation were less consistent risk predictors. Higher risk was associated with lower incomes for smoking and HDL cholesterol in both sexes but with higher incomes for total cholesterol in men. Within occupations, men and women white-collar executives and managers exhibited the lowest levels of smoking. Among men, executives and managers showed the lowest mean levels of blood pressure.

TABLE 1—Correlation Coefficients for Education, Income, and Occupation

	Men	Women
Education/income	+.32	+.23
Income/occupation	+.41	+.30
Education/occupation	+.67	+.66

Note. Table excludes homemakers. All correlations are significant at $P \leq .0001$.

TABLE 2—Distribution of Study Population by Education, Income, and Occupation

	Men, % (n = 1108)	Women, % (n = 1272)
Education, y		
<12	9.7	13.1
12	23.9	31.8
13–15	24.9	27.8
≥16	41.5	27.4
Household income		
<$10 000	6.2	13.3
$10 000–$19 999	21.1	25.6
$20 000–$29 999	26.6	25.6
$30 000–$39 999	20.6	17.8
≥$40 000	25.5	17.8
Occupation		
Unskilled	6.1	5.4
Semiskilled	10.7	6.8
Skilled	17.3	3.5
Clerical	13.4	25.1
Administrators	19.9	9.3
Managers	17.8	12.7
Executives	14.7	1.7
Homemakers	0.0	35.7

Note. Table includes homemakers, all of whom were women.

TABLE 3—Prevalence of Risk Factors by Education, Income, and Occupation, Adjusted for Age and Time of Survey

	% Cigarette Smokers		Mean Systolic Blood Pressure		Mean Diastolic Blood Pressure		Mean Total Cholesterol		Mean HDL Cholesterol	
	Men	Women	Men	Women	Men	Women	Men	Women	Men	Women
Education, y										
<12	47	41	126	117	76	73	198	201	44	52
12	41	34	127	118	77	74	198	194	44	55
13–15	31	23	126	116	77	73	203	192	44	58
≥16	18	14	125	114	76	71	196	190	46	61
Household income										
<$10 000	50	32	124	116	77	72	190	192	43	54
$10 000–$19 999	30	31	126	117	76	72	193	197	45	57
$20 000–$29 999	31	25	126	115	75	73	200	195	45	55
$30 000–$39 999	26	24	126	118	76	74	200	193	46	59
≥$40 000	25	19	126	116	77	72	202	187	46	59
Occupation										
Unskilled	36	33	128	115	78	72	191	199	46	50
Semiskilled	39	22	126	117	76	74	198	187	44	56
Skilled	37	44	127	117	77	71	195	195	46	58
Clerical	41	31	126	117	77	74	206	194	42	57
Administrators	27	25	126	115	77	72	201	190	44	58
Managers	21	18	125	114	76	70	195	190	45	61
Executives	16	20	124	115	75	74	200	192	48	58
Homemakers	n/a	25	n/a	117	n/a	73	n/a	195	n/a	56

Note. Tables includes homemakers. A logistic regression model was used for smoking; a multiple regression model was used for blood pressure, total cholesterol, and HDL cholesterol. Lower mean levels of HDL cholesterol indicate higher risk.

TABLE 4—Partial Correlations and *P* Values from Univariate and Forward Selection Regression Models for Three Dimensions of SES and Disease Risk Factors

	Cigarette smoking		Systolic Blood Pressure		Diastolic Blood Pressure		Total Cholesterol		HDL Cholesterol	
	Men	Women	Men	Women	Men	Women	Men	Women	Men	Women
Univariate Model[a]										
Education	–.23***	–.18***	–.05	–.08*	–.06	–.12***	–.02	–.07*	+.11***	+.21***
Income	–.08**	–.11**	–.00	–.03	+.02	+.02	+.05	–.04	+.06*	+.08*
Occupation	–.18***	–.08*	–.06	–.05	+.05	+.06	+.02	–.03	+.04	+.16***
Forward Selection Model[b]										
Education	–.23***	–.18***	...	–.08*	...	–.12***	...	–.07*	+.11***	+.21***
Income	...	...	...	...	...	...	...	...	...	...
Occupation	...	...	...	...	...	...	...	...	...	...

Note. Table excludes homemakers. Two-tailed significance values are coded as *$P < .05$, **$P < .01$, and ***$P < .001$.

[a]Adjusted for age and time of survey.

[b]Model allowed for inclusion of education, income, and occupation after adjusting for age and time of survey. Ellipses indicate not selected for inclusion in model at $P < .05$.

To compare the strength of the interrelationships between the three dimensions of SES, we conducted regression analyses (Table 4), adjusted for age and time of survey. Partial correlations are presented with two-tailed P values, with significance defined as $P < .05$. The univariate relationship between SES and risk factors was strongest and most consistent for education, showing higher risk associated with lower levels of education. Using a forward selection model that allowed for inclusion of all three measures of SES after adjustment for age and time of survey, education was the only measure of SES that was significantly associated with the risk factors. This finding is consistent with a previously conducted multivariate analysis, which showed that the strength and significance of the associations between education and a set of disease risk factors remained virtually unchanged after adjustment for income and occupation.[7]

When stratified by White, non-Hispanic and Hispanic ethnicities (not shown), education remained the strongest SES predictor but became nonsignificant for smoking, possibly because of the small sample of Hispanics.

Discussion

Strengths and Limitations of Using Education as the Marker for SES

We caution that, in some studies, using only one indicator of SES may yield misleading results or provide less information than using multiple measures. However, using multiple or composite measures[10–14] requires the cost and time of collecting data on several SES parameters and may not significantly explain more about a population than would a single, well-chosen parameter. As noted by a recent working group of the National Heart, Lung, and Blood Institute, use of composite measures may obscure important differences in associations.[25]

Based on our findings, education may be the most judicious SES measure for use in epidemiological studies (unless the study hypothesis dictates which dimension of SES is to be chosen). In studies that have a cost or time restraint but need a measure of SES as a potential confounding variable, education is an expeditious choice. In addition, education is available for all individuals regardless of employment status, has high reliability and validity,[17] is generally stable after early adulthood, is easily reported, and can be collected as a continuous variable. Furthermore, because education is often available in epidemiological studies,[17] it also permits opportunities for meta-analyses and interstudy comparisons.

However, there are potential limitations to using education as a sole indicator of SES. Its stability can mask important changes in individuals' circumstances. There may also be a cohort effect distorting differences between populations of various ages. For example, the percent of the population obtaining at least a high school education has increased nearly threefold since 1940.[17] This has led to increasing homogeneity in the amount of education obtained, making differentiation between educational strata more difficult. Other potential problems include regional differences in education, the question of whether degrees or certification are better measurement parameters than years of schooling,[17,26,27] and the possibility that other dimensions of SES are more sensitive markers for health in some population subgroups. (For example, for foreign-born female Hispanics, acculturation may be a stronger measure of SES.)[13]

Comparison with Past Studies

To our knowledge, this is the only study in the United States to examine associations between separate SES dimensions and risk factors or disease outcomes. Other studies, however, have examined associations between one measure of SES and one disease risk factor,[6,8,28–32] morbidity,[33] or mortality.[1,33–35] In general, these studies have found that education is more strongly associated with disease than is income or occupation. One of the most complete studies of mortality differentials found that lower SES groups exhibited higher rates of all-cause mortality than did higher SES groups, irrespective of whether education, income, or occupation was used as the measure of SES.[1] Other studies have documented strong inverse associations between education and all-cause mortality[31,34,36] and life expectancy.[37] Framingham study data shows that, of 23 potential contributors to morbidity, only education and age at study enrollment were related in both sexes to "survival with good function."[38] Cardiovascular disease studies have shown that lower levels of education are associated with hypertension,[6,28–29,31,39] cigarette smoking,[6,31,32,40–41] and high cholesterol,[6,32] as well as with cardiovascular morbidity[33] and mortality.[31,33,35]

Why Education May Be the Strongest Predictor of Good Health

Several different mechanisms through which education may positively influence health have been proposed. Fuchs has suggested that both education and health are markers for willingness to delay gratification in order to "invest in human capital."[15] Others have argued that education may simply serve as a marker for intelligence; however, studies showing that environmental factors are the strongest predictors of school dropout lend little support to this hypothesis.[42] Some have suggested that higher education may improve health by conferring economic advantages, but our low correlation coefficients between education and income, as well as the lack of significant income effects on risk factors, argue against this hypothesis. Neither does the health knowledge acquisition that accompanies higher education appear to explain the relationship between education and health, given that provision of information alone appears to be a weak stimulus to human behavior change.[16,37]

One hypothesis we find most plausible is that education may protect against disease by influencing life-style behaviors, problem-solving abilities, and values.[17] Moreover, education may facilitate the acquisition of positive social, psychological, and economic skills and assets, and may provide insulation from adverse influences.[7] Such skills and assets that may accompany higher educational attainment include positive attitudes about health, access to preventive health services,[15] membership in peer groups that promote the adoption or continuation of positive health behaviors, and higher self-esteem and self-efficacy.[43,44]

Summary

There can be no SES measure that is universally valid and suitable for all populations. However, if economics and time dictate that a single parameter be chosen and if the research hypothesis does not dictate otherwise, this study suggests that higher education, rather than income or occupation, may be the strongest and most consistent predictor of good health. □

Acknowledgments

This research was supported by Public Health Service Grant 1RO1–HL–21906 from the National Heart, Lung, and Blood Institute to Dr. John W. Farquhar.

The authors thank Drs. Lawrence Green and David Ragland for comments on an earlier draft, Dr. Helena Kraemer and Ms. Beverly Rockhill for statistical advice, and Ms. Cindy German-Kung for the preparation of tables.

References

1. Ki•gawa EM, Hauser PM. *Differential Mortality in the United States: A Study in Socioeconomic Epidemiology*. Cambridge, Mass: Harvard University Press; 1973.
2. Blaxter M. Evidence on inequality in health from a national survey. *Lancet* 1987;ii:30–33.
3. Black D. *Inequalities in Health: Report of a Research Working Group*. London, England: Department of Health and Social Security; 1980.
4. Haan M, Kaplan G, Camacho T. Poverty and health: prospective evidence from the Alameda County Study. *Am J Epidemiol.* 1987;125:989–998.
5. Marmot MG, Kogevinas M, Elston MA. Social/economic status and disease. *Ann Rev Public Health.* 1987;8:111–135.
6. Matthews KA, Kelsey SF, Meilahn EN, Kuller LH, Wing RR. Educational attainment and behavioral and biological risk factors for coronary heart disease in middle-aged women. *Am J Epidemiol.* 1989;129: 1132–1144.
7. Winkleby MA, Fortmann SP, Barrett DC. Social class disparities in risk factors for disease: eight-year prevalence patterns by level of education. *Prev Med.* 1990;19:1–12.
8. Helmert U, Herman B, Joeckel KH, Greiser E, Madans J. Social class and risk factors for coronary heart disease in the Federal Republic of Germany: results of the baseline survey of the German Cardiovascular Prevention Study. *J Epidemiol Community Health.* 1989;43:37–42.
9. Antonovsky A. Social class, life expectancy and overall mortality. *Milbank Mem Fund Q.* 1967;45:31–73.
10. Mueller CW, Parcel TL. Measures of socioeconomic status: alternatives and recommendations. *Child Dev.* 1981;52:13–30.
11. Hollingshead AB. The indiscriminate state of social class measurement. *Soc Forces.* 1971;49:563–567.
12. Duncan OD. A socioeconomic index for all occupations. In: Reiss AJ Jr, Duncan OD, Hatt PK, North CC, eds. *Occupation and Social Status.* New York: The Free Press of Glencoe; 1961:109–138.
13. Green L. Manual for scoring socioeconomic status for research on health behavior. *Public Health Rep.* 1970;85:815–827.
14. Susser MW, Watson W, Hopper K. *Soci-*

ology in Medicine. New York, NY: Oxford University Press; 1985.
15. Fuchs VR. Economics, health, and post-industrial society. *Milbank Mem Fund Q/Health and Society*. 1979;57:153–182.
16. Williams DR. Socioeconomic differentials in health: a review and redirection. *Soc Psych Q*. 1990;53:81–99.
17. Liberatos P, Link BG, Kelsey JL. The measurement of social class in epidemiology. *Epidemiol Rev*. 1988;10:87–121.
18. Morgenstern H. Socioeconomic factors: concepts, measurement and health effects. NHLBI Workshop on "Measuring Psychosocial Variables in Epidemiological Studies of Cardiovascular Disease." December 1983; Galveston, TX.
19. Farquhar JW, Fortmann SP, Maccoby N, et al. The Stanford Five-City Project: design and methods. *Am J Epidemiol*. 1985; 122:323–334.
20. Farquhar JW, Fortmann SP, Flora JA, et al. Effects of communitywide education on cardiovascular disease risk factors. *JAMA*. 1990;264:359–365.
21. US Bureau of the Census. *1980 Census of Population: Alphabetical Index of Industries and Occupations*. Washington, DG: US Government Printing Office; 1982.
22. Fortmann SP, Rogers T, Haskell WL, Solomon DS, Vranizan K, Farquhar JW. Indirect measures of cigarette use: expired air carbon monoxide vs plasma thiocyanate. *Prev Med*. 1984;13:127–135.
23. US Department of Health, Education, and Welfare. *Lipid Research Clinics Manual of Laboratory Operations*. Vol 1: *Lipid and Lipoprotein Analysis*. Washington, DC: US Government Printing Office; 1974.
24. Fortmann SP, Marcuson R, Bitter PH, Haskell WL. A comparison of the Sphygmetrics SR-2 automatic blood pressure recorder to the mercury sphygmomanometer in population studies. *Am J Epidemiol*. 1981; 114:836–844.
25. Socioeconomic factors: working group summary. In: Ostfeld AM, Eaker ED, eds. *Measuring Psychosocial Variables in Epidemiologic Studies of Cardiovascular Disease: Proceedings of a Workshop*. Washington, DC: US Government Printing Office; March 1985. NIH publication 85–2270.
26. Morgan M. Measuring social inequality: occupational classifications and their alternatives. *Community Med*. 1983;5:116–124.
27. Faia MA. Selection by certification: a neglected variable in stratification research. *Am J Sociol*. 1981;86:1093–1111.
28. Hypertension Detection and Follow-Up Program Cooperative Group. Race, education and prevalence of hypertension. *Am J Epidemiol*. 1977;106:351–361.
29. Dyer AR, Stamler J, Shekelle RB, Schoenberger J. The relationship of education to blood pressure: findings on 40 000 employed Chicagoans. *Circulation*. 1976;54: 987–992.
30. Abramson JH, Gofin R, Habib J, Pridan H, Gofin J. A comparative appraisal of measures for use in epidemiological studies. *Soc Sci Med*. 1982;16:1739–1746.
31. Liu K, Cedres LB, Stamler J, et al. Relationship of education to major risk factors and death from coronary heart disease, cardiovascular diseases, and all causes. *Circulation*. 1982;66:1308–1314.
32. Jacobsen BK, Thelle DS. Risk factors for coronary heart disease and level of education. *Am J Epidemiol*. 1988;127:923–932.
33. Hinkle LE, Whitney LH, Lehman EW, et al. Occupation, education, and coronary heart disease. *Science*. 1968;161:238–246.
34. Snowdon DA, Ostwald SK, Kane RL. Education, survival and independence in elderly Catholic sisters, 1936–1988. *Am J Epidemiol*. 1989;130:999–1012.
35. Hypertension Detection and Follow-Up Program Cooperative Group. Educational level and 5-year all-cause mortality in the Hypertension Detection and Follow-Up Program. *Hypertension*. 1987;9:641–646.
36. Feldman JJ, Makuc DM, Kleinman JC, Cornoni-Huntley J. National trends in educational differentials in mortality. *Am J Epidemiol*. 1989;129:919–933.
37. Sagan LA. *The Health of Nations*. New York, NY: Basic Books, Inc; 1987.
38. Pinsky JL, Leaverton PE, Stokes J. Predictors of good function: the Framingham study. *J Chronic Dis*. 1987;40:159S–167S.
39. Berger MC, Leigh JP. Schooling, self-selection, and health. *J Hum Res*. 1989;24: 433–455.
40. Millar WJ, Wigle DT. Socioeconomic disparities in risk factors for cardiovascular disease. *Can Med Assoc J*. 1986;134:127–132.
41. Wagenknecht LE, Perkins LL, Cutler GR, et al. Cigarette smoking is strongly related to educational status: the CARDIA study. *Prev Med*. 1990;19:158–169.
42. Howard MA, Anderson RJ. Early identification of potential school dropouts: a literature review. *Child Welfare*. 1978;57:221–231.
43. Bunker JP, Gomby DS. Preface. In: Bunker JP, Gomby DS, Kehrer BH, ed. *Pathways to Health: The Role of Social Factors*. Menlo Park, Calif: Henry J. Kaiser Foundation; 1989:15.
44. Cohen S, Syme SL. *Social Support and Health*. New York, NY: Academic Press; 1985.

[6]

Soc. Sci. Med. Vol. 36, No. 9, pp. 1169–1180, 1993
Printed in Great Britain.

0277-9536/93 $6.00 + 0.00

ACCULTURATION AND SYMPTOMS: A COMPARATIVE STUDY OF REPORTED HEALTH SYMPTOMS IN THREE SAMOAN COMMUNITIES

Joel M. Hanna and Maureen H. Fitzgerald

Departments of Physiology and Pacific Basin Rehabilitation Research and Training Center, John A. Burns School of Medicine, University of Hawaii, Honolulu, HI 96822, U.S.A.

Abstract—A health questionnaire, which included a 91 item list of symptoms was administered to three groups of young Samoan adults. These young adults resided in a traditional Samoan village in Western Samoa ($n = 50$), several villages in modernizing American Samoa ($n = 50$) and in urban Honolulu, Hawaii ($n = 52$). Each yes response to a symptom was followed by an expanded interview providing details. The yes answer frequency and the contents of the expanded answers were examined with respect to site of residence. Western Samoan responses differed from the other sites in a number of areas suggesting possible differences related to the process of modernization. These response differences suggest four areas in which the stressors of modernization may have health influences: (1) wage employment outside of the family, (2) increased size of support networks by including non-family members and non-Samoans (3) the greater availability of alcohol, and (4) changes in the perceptions of food.

Key words—acculturation, stress, Samoans

Modernization, with its accompanying changes in life style and stresses of daily living, often results in an 'epidemiological transition' of morbidity and mortality patterns [1, 2]. In a very short period of time, even within a single generation, illnesses of modernization come to rival infectious diseases as primary health concerns. Rapid increases in major health problems such as diabetes [3], cardiovascular disease, high blood pressure [4, 5], minor health problems such as allergy, dental caries, backache [1] and psychosocial problems, including alcohol abuse, drug abuse and suicide [6–9] have been documented in populations undergoing change. While epidemiologists and biologists have tried to identify pertinent biological factors, social scientists have focused upon the changing psychosocial environment. They have usually employed a Selye-derived model in which environmental change precipitates adaptation and maladaptation. According to this model, changes in the psychosocial environment become stressful and lead to a greater morbidity through increased individual adaptive demands. These demands tax the adaptive capacity and lead to increased susceptibility to illness [10, 12]. Identification of the specific psychosocial stressors is difficult because they interact with other variables such as coping mechanisms, buffers, social supports, individual personality characteristics and perceptions which modify their expression [11, 13]. Because of the nature of these confounding variables and the complexity of links, the relationship between stressors and outcome often remains unclear.

Prospective studies to clarify psychosocial relations are difficult in humans, so investigators often take advantage of 'natural experiments' [12] to unravel their complex interactions. These experiments incorporate human populations which have been divided by *in situ* acculturation or by migration, thus permitting contrasts between those who modernize and the 'traditional', who are less modernized. This has provided a useful tool for investigators such as Scotch [14] and Henry and Cassel [15] who demonstrated the potential importance of psychosocial stressors in the regulation of blood pressure, which is a major risk factor for heart disease. They reported that an urban migration or a change in life style by rural peoples is related to subsequent elevations in blood pressure. Later work has verified these observations but has usually employed 'modernization', 'westernization' or 'migration' as state (category) variables. The specific aspects of the environment which contribute to the stressful experience remain undefined, although many examples of stress buffers or social supporting factors have been identified [16–19]. Without a more precise definition of these psychosocial variables as stressors we cannot understand their contributions to the epidemiological transition and thus reduce their role in morbidity and mortality.

There is ample evidence that an epidemiological transition in health patterns is taking place among Samoans. The 'natural experiment' includes populations living in traditional Western Samoa, populations exposed to pressures of American culture in American Samoa, and migrants to American cities [20]. The major health changes include a greater level of obesity [21], higher blood pressure [4], less favorable blood lipid profile [22], reduced physical fitness [23, 24] and elevations in urinary catecholamine output in more modernized men [25]. Most work has focused upon the categorical, 'modernized' environment but some efforts have identified specific stressors in specific communities. Hanna and Baker [26] in Hawaii have presented data suggesting that within migrant communities, individuals with higher blood pressures may be more closely associated with Samoan organizations. DuBois [27] also reported increased family obligations were associated with elevated blood pressure in elderly Samoans living in San Diego. Based upon his study of migrants, Janes [28] has hypothesized that in some cases the social demands from the migrant communities may exceed the benefits received and result in some degree of subjective stress. In another study on the island of Upolu in Western Samoa, James *et al.* [25] have studied adult men exposed to differing degrees of modern influence. They found that college students and sedentary workers excreted higher levels of stress hormones than laborers or villagers. This higher rate of excretion was correlated to a 'modernization work level complex' including mental effort and a lesser degree of life satisfaction. Martz *et al.* [29] examined the effects of other psychosocial stressors in American Samoa. Also employing hormone excretion as a measure of stress they found self-reliant behavior, social support and community participation as significant correlates. Self reliance in particular is not a Samoan virtue, and may represent an acculturation effect. Janes [28] studying a migrant congregation living in the San Francisco Area, has also identified a number of potential stressors ranging from network obligations to low socioeconomic status.

It is clear that some aspects of the psychosocial environment are stressful for Samoans and some have been related to acculturation and modernization. However, because each of these investigations has focused upon a specific location we cannot determine whether the potential stressors are unique to that particular location or if they represent points along a continuum ranging from traditional to modern. The aim of this study was to attempt to identify some stressful aspects of the modernization process by employing a comparative approach. We hope that by taking advantage of the natural experiment experienced by Samoans we can identify some aspects of the change in the psychosocial environment which are perceived as stressful.

METHODS

In 1986 and 1987 we conducted a health survey among young adult Samoans (18–37 years of age) in three communities. These communities—located in rural Western Samoa, rapidly modernizing American Samoa, and urban Honolulu, Hawaii—represent a rough continuum of increasing 'modernization' reflecting *in situ* changes as well as migration to a western urban center. We believed that through a comparative study of young adults we could identify some specific aspects of psychosocial environment which were differentially affected by modernization processes.

Populations

The Western Samoan village is located on the southwest coast of the island of Savai'i and is recognized as one of the most traditional in modern Samoa. The economy is based upon horticulture, family cooperation and remittances from overseas, although some elements of a new market oriented economic system are beginning to emerge similar to those observed elsewhere on the island [30]. The traditional Samoan chiefly hierarchy functions as do many community organizations. There is some wage labor employment by the national government, but this is largely plantation-like. There is no electricity, running water or other hallmarks of a late-twentieth century life style.

The American Samoan sample was taken from seven small villages on the southern coast of the Island of Tutuila from an area which has experienced intensive *in situ* modernization since the end of the Second World War. Electricity, running water, automobiles, imported foods, television and radio are generally available. Although traditional Samoan social organization remains, it has been greatly modified and reduced in importance [31, 32]. The sample itself is composed of individuals who were restudied 5 years after an earlier survey. Their biological and social characteristics have been described elsewhere [23, 32]. The Hawaiian sample resides in urban Honolulu, mostly in high rise public housing developments. This was a convenience sample with age range and a greater than three years of residence in Hawaii as the major criteria. Most men and women are employed and participate in the local economy. Most work at entry-level positions and some are also on welfare [33]. There is a chiefly hierarchy, but its functioning is somewhat reduced and mostly limited to Samoan affairs [32]. Although this was a convenience sample, the socio-demographic characteristics are similar to those for Samoans living in Hawaii taken from the 1980 census. They seem fairly typical in terms of place of birth, education and employment [23, 33]. This community is clearly at the lower end of the socioeconomic spectrum, but seems substantially more affluent than the one in San Francisco described by Janes [28]. The three communities have been described in greater detail by Fitzgerald [34] and by Pearson [23].

Some of the characteristics of our samples are shown in Table 1. The samples are divided between men and women and are relatively young. While stature is similar in all sites, weight shows significant variation among sites with American Samoans heavier than Western Samoans and migrants to Hawaii the heaviest of all. Body Mass Index and skin folds suggest obesity is involved. This type of weight variation has been observed in Samoans and in other

Table 1. Mean characteristics of the samples

	Western Samoa	American Samoa	Hawaii
Men	$N = 25$	$N = 26$	$N = 23$
Age (years)	23.6	24.2	26.0
Height (cm)[a]	173.4	174.2	175.8
Weight (kg)[a]	73.4	84.4	93.7
Systolic pressure(mm)[a]	128.9	127	130.4
Diastolic pressure(mm)[a]	76.6	83.3	76.5
Total yes responses	16.3	27.2	23.7
Drinkers	9	20	12
Employed	7	19	13
Network size[b]	12	28	29
Women	$N = 25$[a]	$N = 24$	$N = 29$
Age (years)	23.6	23.3	24.4
Height (cm)[a]	161.3	162.9	163.7
Weight (kg)[a]	65.0	77.6	86.7
Systolic pressure (mm)[a]	121	113	118.2
Diastolic pressure (mm)[a]	74	74	75.5
Total yes responses	24	36.3	36.4
Drink	1	8	14
Employed	8	12	13
Network size	14	21	25

[a]Some individuals did not provide anthropometric data hence the physical measurements are based upon fewer individuals. These are WS men (24), WS women (25), AS men (26), AS women (22), HI men (22) and HI women (26).

[b]See text for explanation.

migrant and modernizing populations [21]. The blood pressure variation in our three samples is small not conforming with an acculturation model. This probably reflects the relative youth of the samples.

Instruments

As part of a comprehensive survey we administered a health questionnaire which included questions on individual and family health status. Part of that questionnaire was a series of 91 yes–no health items which consisted mostly of symptoms. Although a few items were not actually symptoms this term will be employed for simplicity. The item list is an expanded and modified version of one proposed by Woods [35]. Each person was asked if they had ever experienced any of the health symptoms and for each yes answer, follow-up questions determined the specific details. These expanded answers uncovered details of the symptom and, when appropriate, an example of when it might occur. Analyses of the expanded responses provided us with a greater understanding of the answers and of the specific problems occurring at each site. Examples of some of the items are: Have you ever experienced...? anger, anemia, anxiety, awakening at night, arthritis, asthma, automobile accident and so on. Questions were asked in either English or Samoan depending upon subject preference and the subject was able to follow on a bilingual printed sheet should they wish to do so. Each time a yes answer was given the additional, expanded information was requested.

At the completion of data collection the Item List was reviewed and reduced from 91 to 80 items by eliminating those having no affirmative responses. For example, there were no reported heart attacks and none of the subjects reported cancer so these were dropped from further analysis. For the remaining items the number of yes answers was then computed for each item. An analysis of the expanded answers for each yes was undertaken by listing all given answers for all of the respondents at a given site and then categorizing them into several domains through content analysis [36]. This procedure revealed that many of the yes responses were really normal conditions and did not reflect health problems. Feeling tired, for example, was often answered yes, but during the subsequent follow-up the respondent would suggest this only followed hard work. These normal, non-pathological responses were considered to be 'no' responses, Similarly, many of the yes answers were associated with reproduction (menstruation, pregnancy or lactation) and had little to do with general health. Fitzgerald [34] has described the reproduction-related responses elsewhere. In this paper we will use the answer set with 'normal' yes answers deleted, that is we will discuss only those yes responses which are not expected of healthy people in normal situations.

The frequency of yes responses was averaged for each of the three populations (Table 1). In tabulating the average number of items checked, an analysis of variance revealed that there were significant differences between the sites ($F = 10.9$, $df\,2{,}137$, $P < 0.01$) and the genders ($F = 19.7$, $df\,1{,}137$, $P < 0.01$). The average rate of yes responses of men were less than those of women and those of Western Samoans less frequent than American Samoans and Hawaiian migrants.

To further examine this variation we considered two contrasts based upon models from earlier investigations [20]. First, we followed earlier Samoan research which suggested that for many social and biological characteristics the residents of American Samoa more closely resemble the migrants to Hawaii than they do to Western Samoans. This is a simple acculturation model and was apparent in studies of

Table 2. Western Samoa contrasts with other sites—acculturation effects

Item	W. Samoa	A. Samoa	Hawaii
N	50	50	52
Depression	22	38	40
Nervousness	6	25	27
Awakening in the night	8	21	23
Decreased desire to talk	10	22	21
Dental problems	6	22	29
Desire to be alone	12	31	39
Difficulty in concentrating	9	21	24
Difficulty in making decisions	8	21	20
Feelings of guilt	4	19	25
Headaches	17	38	32
Impatience	8	23	27
Impulsiveness	7	15	17
Increased appetite	6	15	17
Feeling weight gain	2	16	14
Decreased appetite	15	25	24
Decreased food intake	11	23	22
Muscle weakness	7	17	19
Feeling in control	22	36	32
Feelings of well being	28	44	44
Swelling of joints	2	10	9
Restlessness	5	14	16

One way analysis of variance show these items differ at $P < 0.05$ level of significance.

blood pressure, body size, growth [20] and some social characteristics [34]. The general similarity is not only the result of acculturation, but also reflects the fact that many of the migrants to Hawaii are from American Samoa. Items following this pattern are listed in Table 2.

As a second approach we contrasted the three sites by looking for items which differed among them in a regular manner such that Western Samoa was at one extreme and Hawaii was at the other with American Samoa intermediate. This pattern most closely approximates the rough continuum of modernization in which Western Samoa represents a traditional population, American Samoa is experiencing *in situ* acculturative pressures and migrants to Hawaii are exposed to both acculturation and migration pressures. The mode is additive for acculturation and migration. Items following this pattern are listed in Table 3.

After grouping items according to frequency of yes responses some items showed significant variation but did not fall into either of the above categories. These were mostly items in which the number of yes responses in American Samoa was higher than in the other two sites (Table 4).

After each grouping there were some items which showed small differences that were clearly not significant. These were not further analyzed. Other items which showed larger differences were tested with a one way analysis of variance to establish statistical significance and Duncan's New Multiple Range was employed to determine site differences. Items showing statistically significant variation are listed in Tables 2–4.

RESULTS

Acculturative pressures—American Somoa and Hawaii grouping

In much of our earlier research we found that American Samoa and Hawaii were often more similar to each other than either was to Western Samoa. Twenty-one of the items which follow this pattern, and show statistically significant differences are listed in Table 2.

'Feelings of depression' was common at all sites, but the sources of depression, named in the expanded remarks, were quite different. Western Samoans associated depression only with death, illness or separation from family. These themes were also present in American Samoa and Hawaii, but depression additionally resulted from friends' misfortunes (AS) or from problems in the workplace or with love interests (HI). Western Samoan depression is largely

Table 3. Three site contrasts—additive effects of acculturation and migration

Item	W. Samoa	A. Samoa	Hawaii
N	50	50	52
Feelings of anger[a]	40	45	51
Increased food intake[a]	2	11	19
Frequent crying[a]	5	12	22
Feeling lonely[a]	8	23	31
Craving certain foods[a]	20	27	37
Feelings of confusion[a]	13	19	25
Bloating[a]	0	4	10
Muscle cramps[b]	4	18	32

[a]Significant difference between W. Samoa and Hawaii $P < 0.05$.
[b]Three sites differ significantly from each other $P < 0.05$.

Table 4. Items showing other differences

Item	W. Samoa	A. Samoa	Hawaii
N	50	50	52
Parasites	1	1	6
Increased sleeping	0	13	8
Hearing problems	6	14	2
Feeling out of control	3	13	6
Digestive problems	3	9	3
Aches and pains	4	17	8

occassioned by family matters, while elsewhere there are more inclusive causes—friends and work. A similar expanded spectrum is evident in response to other items such as nervousness. In Western Samoa nervousness is infrequent ($n = 6$) and limited to cases of sick children, but in American Samoa ($n = 25$) and in Hawaii ($n = 27$), individual performance becomes the prominent factor. Performance before groups, in school or on the job surpasses family problems as causes for nervousness. Again the causality extends beyond the immediate family and into non-family and work settings. Modernization may thus provide more opportunities for depression and nervousness through expanding the circle of potential causes, beyond the immediate family and into the broader community.

Life in American Samoa and Hawaii also occasions increased difficulty in concentration and in making decisions (Table 2). Expanded explanations for the few occurrences in the village seem trivial—difficulty arises from minor events such as speculation about the future or being distracted in Sunday School. The higher frequency of concentration and decision making problems in the modernized sites is accompanied by some degree of preoccupation. Most prevalent is 'having too much to do', or 'having too many things on my mind', usually with a reference to work or to some social obligation. Once more there seems to be a spectrum of stressors arising from beyond the family and home environment extending to the workplace and the community.

Increased impatience and impulsiveness reflect the differences between the traditional and a more acculturated lifestyle. In Western Samoa, impatience is linked to being angry and impulsiveness to 'all of the time', that is, these are viewed mainly as personality characteristics. In the other sites impatience is closely related to work and to waiting in lines, while impulsiveness is also linked to work and non-desired family social obligations. The underlying difference seems to be an individual personality perspective in Western Samoa as opposed to a situational perspective in the more modernized sites. This is also evident in the item 'feelings of guilt or shame' which is attributed to similar causes in all sites—usually to doing something 'wrong', but the somewhat higher frequencies in Hawaii are further attributed to 'making mistakes on the job' and to behavior associated with drinking which are largely situational.

A desire to be alone was frequently answered affirmative. In Western Samoa 12 individuals reported a desire to be alone, the reasons being to think, to escape family problems or 'to be alone at night'. The 31 American Samoans and 39 Hawaiian residents who wanted to be alone listed similar reasons but were more likely to want to be alone on a regular basis. That is, they clearly wanted to be able to be alone when they chose to do so. Both sites are crowded as compared to the Western Samoan village so this probably reflects a problem common to many urban situations.

Another item 'awakening in the night' is lowest in Western Samoa, and almost exclusively attributed to events surrounding child care which is an activity appropriate for this age group. In the other locations there are additional causes. People in both sites describe noises in the night and nightmares as primary reasons for awakening. Neither is mentioned in Western Samoa. Noise can be a product of living in a more crowded, electronic environment such as Tutuila or Honolulu, but the high frequency of dream-related awakening suggests a psychological component may exist.

The decreased desire to talk also has a common origin at all locations—being tired or angry is the most frequent response. In American Samoa additional reasons were being drunk ($n = 2$) and feeling lonely ($n = 2$). In Hawaii similar causes were given—angry, tired and lonely—but additional causes were being interrupted from some task ($n = 3$) or while watching television ($n = 3$).

In light of the number of studies which have described the obesity of modernized Samoans [21] the 'feeling sensations of weight gain' item is of some interest. Western Samoans do not report feeling weight gain, but American Samoans and Hawaii residents do. They report that they are aware of it most of the time, but especially when they try on clothing. Among women in American Samoa and Hawaii, but not among Western Samoan women, pregnancy is related to weight gain.

There were also two items related to food consumption—decreased appetite and decreased food intake. The expanded answers at all sites indicated sickness or unavailability of specific foods lead to decreases, but in the two modernized locations there were also psychological links. Answers such as 'when I worry' or 'when I'm depressed' were common in American Samoa and Hawaii. Likewise dieting was never given as a reason for reduced food intake in Western Samoa, but was frequently mentioned elsewhere. Drinking alcohol was also a cause for decreased appetite and food intake, but less frequently in Western Samoa than at the other sites. Coincidentally, in Hawaii, of the 24 expanded answers to the difficulty of concentration item, 15 were linked to food. That is, difficulty in concentration was linked to some general preoccupation with or the consumption of specific foods—Samoan foods, milk, oil, raw food—or, eating too much food or too much good food. The significance is not clear but this linkage seems strong in the Hawaii population.

In American Samoa and in Hawaii food seems to have a stronger psychological character than in the Western Samoan villages. In the expanded answers to food related questions villagers focused upon nutrition and taste, while in the more modernized populations there were additional strong linkages to what are often negative affective symptoms—preoccupation, depression, worry and difficulty in concentrating. Modernization may modify the psychological links to foods for these young Samoans.

Two positive items, 'feeling in control' and 'feelings of well being' were also more frequently answered affirmative in the modernized sites. At all locations the most common explanation was 'everyday' or 'all of the time,' thus describing a self perceived personality attribute. In Western Samoa a recent improvement in health was given as the cause of well being ($n = 4$) while in Hawaii a big paycheck was involved ($n = 2$). Such responses were not given in other locations. Feeling in control was also a personality attribute at all locations, but in Hawaii was often associated with anger. We investigated the possibility that the same individuals were answering yes to these two items. This could result in a few individuals skewing the population response. A sign test was performed to determine concordance on the two answers; of the 150 individuals, 46 differed in response with 35 changing in one direction 11 in the other. This was statistically significant ($P < 0.0005$) and a hypothesis of concordance on these two questions was not supported.

Minor physical problems often associated with modernization [1] and the reported physical symptoms support this for the present sample. Among physical items, muscle weakness was reported at all sites and was usually associated with over-exertion on the job. Additional causes in American Samoa and Hawaii were physical workout and drinking. Joint swelling, another physical problem, also differed across the sites but explanations were similar in all locations. The reported swelling included knee and shoulder joints and the causes were hard work. The frequency in joint swelling in American Samoa and Hawaii was simply higher.

Reported dental problems significantly increase from Western Samoa to Hawaii. In the villages few dental problems were reported and these were tooth or gum pain. In American Samoa there are additional reports of pain, a large number of caries and 13 extractions. In Hawaii there are numerous reported fillings with only 6 extractions, probably representing a different type of dentistry. Significantly in Hawaii there are also a number of individuals recognizing dental problems and wanting to see a dentist, but there are also a number ($n = 5$) who admit having cavities and fear seeing the dentist. Even though more extractions are recalled in American Samoa this fear of the dentist is not reported. The more frequent complaints about minor physical problems is probably related to acculturation pressures [1].

Headaches were also more common in the two more modernized locations and were related to aspects of the modern lifestyle. Western Samoa attributed practically all headaches to 'too much sun' ($n = 11$), while lack of sleep and no rest was listed in American Samoa ($n = 4$) and Hawaii ($n = 8$) as principal causes. Hawaii residents listed hangover as the second major cause ($n = 6$). Specific physical and traumatic causes for headaches were equal ($n = 3$) at all sites.

Additive effects of migration and acculturation—three sites contrasts

There were eight questions whose frequencies differed significantly among the three sites in such a manner that the frequency was lowest in Western Samoa, intermediate in American Samoa and highest in Hawaii (Table 3). This may reflect a migration effect superimposed upon modernization. In all cases there were statistically significant differences between Western Samoa and Hawaii, but only for muscle cramps did the three sites differ significantly. In most cases American Samoa and Hawaii did not differ in the statistical sense, but the former was clearly in an intermediate position.

Muscle cramps show significant elevations from Western Samoa to American Samoan to Hawaii. The four reports of cramps in Western Samoa describe excess physical activity associated with chores—carrying wet laundry or long walks. In American Samoa cramps are equally associated with physical work or exercise workouts, while in Hawaii cramps are mostly from workouts with recalled employment-related cramps minimal ($n = 1$). Also included in the expanded answers are descriptions of nighttime cramps: they were absent in Western Samoa, reported twice in American Samoa and seven times in Hawaii. Other studies [23, 24] have discussed apparent parallel differences in levels of physical fitness between the sites. According to those observations the Western Samoan sample is relatively fit, hence they experience the least cramping. In the other locations physically working out, which leads to cramps, may be an attempt to maintain some degree of fitness. It is further noteworthy that 'working out' has become important in American culture and the behavior of these young Samoans reflects that trend.

Of the food related items, a craving for special foods varies across the sites. In Western Samoa the craving is universally for fish or seafood, a normal, but not always available, component of the diet. In American Samoa there are a similar cravings but also for fast foods. The brands specifically mentioned are not found in American Samoa but are probably seen in television commercials imported from the Mainland. In Hawaii the cravings are for fast foods, which are readily available, and Samoan foods, which are not. The variety of foods named also increases in the latter two sites. The item 'increased food intake' has common aspects across the sites. In general, seeing or smelling good food is associated with increased consumption and social events are also closely linked. But, in American Samoa and Hawaii being pregnant is associated with increased food intake. Similarly, at the latter sites drinking alcohol and food consumption are more frequently associated. A response unique to Hawaii is boredom—three individuals say they eat when bored. Thus, in the latter two sites there is a pregnancy association and more frequent linking with alcohol as well as a link to boredom in Hawaii. These are not characteristic of Western Samoan responses. Abdominal bloating is absent in Western Samoa, but is closely linked to eating too much at the other two locations. In Hawaii there is an additional explanation—it accompanies meals, that is bloating is apparently a normal consequence of eating.

In the psychological realm, feelings of loneliness are least frequently reported in Western Samoa with only 16% answering yes and a variety of reasons are given. The levels are much higher in American Samoa (46%) and in Hawaii (62%). In the latter two sites the absence of friends and relatives is reported as the major cause of loneliness. This is a particularly interesting contrast because we have extensive data on genealogical and network relationships for each respondent. Western Samoans report about half of the number of friends and relatives as do the other two sites, yet less frequently feel lonely. This suggests that the quality of the larger networks in Hawaii and American Samoa is in some way inferior to that of networks in the villages. Quantity and quality are clearly not the same.

Two other psychological items, 'anger' and 'feeling confusion' are also shown in Table 3. They follow the trend of increasing frequency but display statistical significance only between the extremes of the Western Samoa and Hawaii sites. Anger was the most frequent affirmative response (WS $n = 40$, AS $n = 45$, HI $n = 51$). The numbers were high and there was little difference between the sites in reported causes. Anger was occasioned by children and spouse in that order. There seemed to be nothing unique to any environment which occasioned anger, except an anger-work association, which was fairly strong in the modernized sites, and not reported in Western Samoa.

Feelings of confusion, while less frequent than anger also increase across the sites becoming greatest in Hawaii. This supports a hypothesis that expectations are more clearly defined in more traditional locations [18, 28] and that acculturative pressures lead to some ambiguity with respect to expectations. As one is further removed from cultural tradition, daily behavior becomes less predictable.

The item 'tearfulness or crying easily' is related to family conflicts in Western Samoa, due to anger or "being beat by my father". In American Samoa and in Hawaii the causes are generally similar—family problems—but an additional cause is provided. Movie and television generated sadness is responsible, especially in Hawaii where 7 of the responses were due to entertainment. Also more prevalent in the modernized sites was empathy with friends or acquaintance's misfortunes.

Other patterns of responses

There were a small number of items which showed statistically significant differences but did not fit into one of the above patterns (Table 4). The item 'have you ever had parasites?' was highest in Hawaii ($n = 6$) and equal in the other sites ($n = 1$). All recalled parasite incidents were pinworms experienced as children, so there seems to be little relevance for the present time. It should be noted that other investigations have suggested the parasite load in Western Samoa is considerable [39] so a 'no' answer to this question from some Western Samoans may be more perception than reality.

The remaining six items were highest in American Samoa with the other sites showing variable relationships. These were: 'increased sleep', 'hearing problems', 'aches and pains', 'digestive problems' and 'feeling out of control'. Increased sleeping was associated with drinking, sickness and pregnancy. It was reported most often in American Samoa and totally absent in Western Samoa. Hearing problems were site specific. In Hawaii working conditions were linked to hearing problems ($n = 2$), while in American Samoa ear infections ($n = 6$) were the cause and in Western Samoa water in the ear ($n = 4$) was the cause. In both Samoas diving for fish on the reef is part of daily subsistence for many individuals in this age group. The responses suggest that water in the ear and ear infections may result from this normal activity. On the Island of Oahu, where all of the Hawaii residents live, reef fishing is not a common undertaking for most Samoans. The reduced number of ear complaints probably reflects the absence of fishing from daily activities.

American Samoans reported feeling 'out of control'—usually as a result of anger ($n = 8$). In Hawaii 3 cases were due to anger and as was one in Western Samoa. Various other causes were given, including drinking at the two more modernized sites (1 each). Digestive problems were also highest in American Samoa and were attributed to either food ($n = 4$) or to some sickness ($n = 3$). In Hawaii all were due to physical pathology and in Western Samoa all were due to food. Finally, in terms of aches and pains American Samoa is highest ($n = 17$). These are attributed to sickness, arthritis and work. The causes are similar in the other sites, just less frequent.

DISCUSSION

In this study we have tried to expand upon the approach of social epidemiology by adding depth. Extending the questionnaire from a simple yes/no format to include an opportunity for expanding upon the answers added a richness to the data that would have otherwise been lost. Analysis of the expanded answers has allowed us to address a broader range of issues than were apparent from the symptom check list. In this discussion we have focused on aspects of symptom reports which seem to reflect a modernization or acculturation effect; an effect which might be related to increased health risk.

There were substantial differences among the three sites in terms of the frequency of yes responses to the eighty items and in the underlying explanations for those responses. The most profound differences were in the contrast between Western Samoa and the other sites. Responses in American Samoa and Hawaii were similar, and even when the reported frequencies differed, the underlying causes tended to be analogous. In many respects American Samoa is both American and Samoan. As noted earlier [32, p. 47] "When compared with Western Samoa, American Samoa appears to have undergone some rather profound changes in response to commercialization of its economy, to urbanization, and to Americanization." We can now extend to the psychosocial sphere a conclusion derived from biological, epidemiological [20] and demographic [32] observations. In addition the present study has defined four areas in which acculturation and migration may prove stressful. These are in the work environment, extension of social networks, increased availability of alcohol and changes in food perceptions.

Occupational stress

Problems in the workplace is a recurrent theme which contributes substantially to individual stress levels and is most evident in American Samoa and Hawaii. An acculturation model is appropriate. Western Samoan men were mostly horticulturists, working on a family plantation and exploiting the reef. Women tended to household chores as well as plantation activities, but occasionally participated in fishing and collecting. Everyday work is carried out with close family members and is not formally supervised. In American Samoa and in Hawaii employment was more varied with clerical, blue collar positions and housekeeping predominating. The element of family participation is more removed so that there is a clear differentiation between employment and family obligations. These populations seem more fully engaged in a modern-style work complex.

Expanded answers illustrate the contrast and provide details of the differences. In Western Samoa the only references to work were in physical terms relating to ear problems, muscle weakness, and swelling of the joints, symptoms which can result from over exertion. Working did not appear in the expanded answers as a factor contributing to other symptoms. On the other hand, in Hawaii and American Samoa, working and the workplace were often discussed and frequently named as contributing factors in other contexts. This was most evident in the items dealing with depression, nervousness, decision making, confusion, impulsiveness, feelings of guilt, and anger; but passing references to occupational problems often appeared in other items as well. Job related stress seems to permeate the lives of many respondents in these two communities.

Perhaps the nature of their employment was a major factor. Clerical and bluecollar workers are especially subject to organizational stresses which are tied to the social character of the unskilled job. These include little chance for advancement, a lack of job security, ambiguity in expectations and role conflicts [12, 40]—aspects of the work situation which characterize many in the present sample of American Samoans and migrants in Hawaii. But there are some other aspects of this type of employment which also have special significance for Samoans. Working is separated from family activity, a situation seldom experienced in traditional Samoa. There is also constant exposure to non-Samoan values [41, 42], and a requirement for a degree of self reliance, which has been associated with elevations in stress hormones for American Samoans [29]. Finally, clerical and office jobs tend to involve some degree of mental effort, a characteristic which has been shown to be more stressful than traditional plantation occupations for Western Samoans [24]. There are many opportunities for occupational stressors in the more modernized sites.

For American blue-collar and clerical workers the consequences of such organizational stresses are often displaced into other, non-work settings where they contribute to violence and family discord [12, 40]. This kind of displacement may contribute to the violence, substance abuse and family problems which seem to characterize migrant communities in Hawaii [43]. In a similar manner the higher levels of physical symptoms in American Samoa and in Hawaii follow a tendency toward somatization of more general complaints by Polynesians [28, 44] and may also represent a displacement. Stressful events on the job become somatisized into headaches, muscle weakness and joint swelling complaints.

It seems clear that in the acculturated communities the existence of occupational stress is greater than in traditional Samoa. For villagers the reported job-related symptoms are largely physical, while in the more modernized communities job-related stress seems to be more frequent, more variable and displaced into other aspects of life. In American Samoa and in Hawaii, work-induced stress may be one of the key psychosocial factors contributing to development of a modern disease profile.

In his study of a Samoan congregation living in the San Francisco area, Janes [28] concluded that participation in a market economy and the concomitant economic deprivation was a major stressor. The workplace itself was also important, but mostly in terms of " social inconsistency" [28, p. 118] wherein a worker held a position above their level of training. As noted earlier the socioeconomic status of the present samples from Hawaii and American Samoa appears somewhat higher than that described in San Francisco. Unemployment at the time of this study was also less of a problem, so economic worries were less important than those related directly to the workplace. In these communities the symptoms were linked to the workplace and the working environment, not to wages or money. We cannot discuss status inconsistency because this was not a focus of our study, but Janes also reported a substantial number of psychosomatic complaints, which is compatible with the displacement phenomenon which we describe.

Social networks

Another apparent stressor accompanying acculturation is an increase in the size of social networks. We estimated individual social networks by requesting each individual to name all of their friends and relatives and to describe interactions with them [32]. The average number of named individuals who were available for support in Western Samoa (mean = 12) was significantly smaller than in American Samoa (mean = 24) and in Hawaii (mean = 27) (Table 1). The major difference was that the larger networks include greater numbers of non-kin social groups, friends, and work mates as well as greater numbers of non-Samoans. These larger networks were not entirely supportive because expanded answers to the items relating to depression, nervousness, feeling angry, difficulty in concentrating, and difficulty in decision making contained negative references to them. The main stressful element seems to be increased social obligations. Other studies among migrant Samoans have suggested how these obligations may evolve. Initially immigrants are heavily dependent upon other Samoans to find employment and to find a place to live as well as assistance with language and cultural problems [41, 42, 45]. In Samoa the immediate family is usually helpful with these concerns, but in Hawaii they can be solved only through developing a larger network of varying composition. While this expanded (and largely ethnic) network continues to be an asset in time of need [46], it can become burdensome in time. Helping other arrivals, support of church and civic activities and remittances to Samoa continue to tax resources and in the long term may have adverse health effects. This may appear as higher blood pressure in Hawaii [26], where those Samoans living in rural and more ethnically Samoan communities show higher blood pressures than those Samoans living in urban and more ethnically mixed areas. Similar suggestions have been forwarded by observers in California where larger networks are also correlated with higher overall health risk [27, 28].

Among non-migrant American Samoans the structural aspects of network demands are less clear, although many of the same features probably exist. American Samoa has been under strong acculturative pressures for a generation with substantial changes in family and traditional social organization [32]. Participation in the local wage economy as a clerk probably has much of the same effect as in Hawaii. Working in the cannery or in government offices extends social networks beyond the traditional family units and will also include non-Samoans with regular exposure to non-Samoan values. The problems of helping new arrivals are not present, but many of the other aspects of migrant networks are present.

In a general way these observations are in conflict with studies stressing the value of ethnic networks and social support in terms of their buffering and stress alleviating capacity [16–19, 47, 48]. While these functions are also characteristic of Samoan networks [27, 45], the evidence shows that this is not invariable. For Samoans in American Samoa, Hawaii and California non-family networking can clearly become a stressor. While some of the negative aspects can arise from acculturation and from non-Samoans, there also appears to be an element which is Samoan, but non-family. We suggest that other investigators also examine ethnic networks from that perspective, since we doubt that Samoans are unique in this respect.

Drinking alcohol

Access to alcohol was a major factor differentiating Western Samoa from the other sites. The number of yes answers for the craving for alcohol item does not significantly differ among the research locations, yet alcohol was a contributing factor to a variety of other symptoms. This was especially true in American Samoa and Hawaii where reported alcohol use was more frequent. Alcohol was related to depression, decreased food intake, decreased talking, muscle weakness, and numerous other items. It was a cause of anger at all sites, but most particularly in Hawaii and American Samoa. There thus appears to be a link of alcohol, anger and aggression with adverse effects on relations with family and friends. This relationship has been established in laboratory and in epidemiological studies [43, 49–52]. In the present study many indirect attributes of alcohol use were described by women who listed a husband or boyfriend's drinking as a cause for anger, depression or other psychological symptoms similar to experiences of Native American women [53]. Men volunteered headaches, anger, decreased appetite and muscle weakness associated with excessive drinking. Alcohol abuse is more prevalent in Hawaii and American Samoa because of easy access to alcohol. The Western Samoan village did not permit alcohol within its limits and strong social pressure was exerted to keep it out. In American Samoa and Hawaii alcohol and the cash to buy it were readily available.

Food

References to food also follow an acculturation model paralleling that described in earlier studies. Bindon [54] and Brown *et al.* [55] have documented an increase in the variety of foods which are consumed in modernized communities as well as a decrease in the consumption of traditional foods such as taro and breadfruit. The food references in the present study depict such a pattern. In the Western Samoan village 'craving special foods' was the least frequent and there were no reported linkages with affect or other psychological parameters. The villagers simply responded that they wanted more of their normal foods. Although they were not totally happy with their diet, western foods did not appear as a craved item. In the modernized sites more complex relationships were described with food related to affect. This was true especially in Hawaii where there was a psychological link between difficulty in concentration, boredom and food. The kinds of food named were also different in acculturated locations with advertised foods most evident. In American Samoa even foods never sold there were craved. The modernization effect of electronic advertising was clearly in evidence.

It might be hypothesized that the differential view of food results from economic considerations. Western Samoans are food producers while the other populations are more dependent upon a paycheck whose future may be uncertain. While we cannot rule out economics, save for complaints surrounding social obligations, financial distress was not closely linked to symptoms and did not seem a major theme in this protocol. Money never appeared in the same context as food.

CONCLUSIONS

In terms of responses to reported health symptoms the acculturated communities in American Samoa and Hawaii more closely resemble each other than does either resemble Western Samoa. There are four main areas of contrast.

(1) The transition from a traditional, family based employment to a modern style occupation is probably a source of stress for acculturated and migrant Samoans. In acculturated communities stresses arising from events surrounding the workplace seem substantial and responses to them may be displaced into other aspects of life.

(2) Migration and acculturation have resulted in larger social networks. The greater size is due to inclusion of more distant relatives, non-kin Samoans and non-Samoans. These larger extra familial networks seem to produce a degree of stress as well as offering social support.

(3) Problems associated with alcohol are more frequent and widespread in the acculturated communities. Drinking is associated with negative health items in all locations, but because of limited accessibility in Western Samoa, alcoholic problems do not seem so prominent. In American Samoa and Hawaii, where alcohol is readily available, both physical and psychological symptoms are associated with its use.

(4) There seem to be changes in perceptions of food and, perhaps, the addition of some psychological elements in the more acculturated communities. The origin and significance of these new elements is not clear.

An aim of this study was to identify some elements which cause a change in morbidity patterns in Samoans as they become modernized and as they migrate from Samoa. This comparative study has suggested there are four areas of difference which may be involved. Reported changes in occupational relations, social networking, alcohol and food consumption can be stressful and in the long run unhealthy. Further investigation of these changes is suggested. We hesitate to extend these conclusions to other non-Samoan populations, but the basic findings may also characterize other groups exposed to pressures of modernization.

Acknowledgements—We would like to express our appreciation to all the people who aided in the work, especially Jay Pearson, Christina Pearson, our Samoan research assistants, and most especially the Samoan respondents. Also to one of the reviewers whose thoughtful comments were most constructive To all of them we say: *faafetai tele lava mo le fesoasoani.* Supported by NIMH grant MH40675.

REFERENCES

1. Corruccini R. and Kaul S. The epidemiological transition and anthropology of minor chronic noninfectious diseases. *Med. Anthropol.* **7**, 36, 1983.
2. Hull D. Migration, adaptation and illness: A review. *Soc. Sci. Med.* **13**, 25, 1979.
3. Zimmett P. The epidemiology of diabetes in Micronesia and Polynesia. In *Epidemiology of Diabetes in Developing Countries* (Edited by Ahuja M.), p. 88. Interprint, New Delhi, 1979.
4. McGarvey S. and Schendel D. Blood pressure in Samoans. In *The Changing Samoans: Behavior and Health in Transition* (Edited by Baker P., Hanna J. and Baker J.), p. 351. Oxford University Press, New York, 1986.
5. Ward R. and Prior I. Genetic and sociocultural factors in the response of blood pressure to migration of the Tokelau population. *Med. Anthropol.* **4**, 339, 1980.
6. Kirby D. G. Immigration, stress and prescription drug use among Cuban women in South Florida. *Med. Anthropol.* **10**, 287, 1989.
7. Rubinstein D. A survey of adolescent suicide in Micronesia. *Pac. Hlth* **15**, 2, 1982.

8. Marshall M. *Weekend Warriors: Alcohol in a Micronesian Culture*. Mayfield, Palo Alto, 1979.
9. Graves T. D. Acculturation, access and alcohol in a triethnic community. *Am. Anthropol.* **69**, 306, 1967.
10. Scott R. and Howard A. Models of stress. In *Social Stress* (Edited by Levine S. and Scotch N.). Aldine Press, Chicago, 1970.
11. Lazarus R. S. The concepts of stress and disease. In *Society, Stress and Disease* (Edited by Levi L.), p. 112. Oxford University Press, New York, 1973.
12. Kasl S. V. Stress and health. *Ann. Rev. Publ. Hlth* **5**, 319, 1984.
13. Maes S., Vingerhoets A. and VanHeck G. The study of stress and disease: some developments and requirements. *Soc. Sci. Med.* **25**, 567, 1987.
14. Scotch N. A. Sociocultural factors in the epidemiology of Zulu hypertension. *Am. J. Publ. Hlth* **53**, 1205, 1963.
15. Henry J. P. and Cassel J. Psychosocial factors in essential hypertension. *Am. J. Epidemiol.* **90**, 171, 1969.
16. Wheeler R. J. and Frank M. A. Identification of stress buffers. *Behav. Med.* **11**, 78, 1988.
17. Marmot M. G. and Syme L. Acculturation and coronary heart disease in Japanese-Americans. *Am. J. Epidemiol.* **104**, 225, 1976.
18. Dressler W., Dos Santos J. E. and Viteri F. E. Blood pressure, ethnicity and psychosocial resources. *Psychosom. Med.* **48**, 509, 1986.
19. Cohen S. and Hoberman H. Positive events and social support as buffers of life change stress. *J. appl. Soc. Psychol.* **13**, 99, 1983.
20. Baker P., Hanna J. and Baker T. (Eds) *The Changing Samoans: Behavior and Health in Transition*. Oxford University Press, New York, 1986.
21. Pawson I. The Morphological Characteristics of Samoan Adults. In *The Changing Samoans: Behavior and Health in Transition* (Edited by Baker P., Hanna J. and Baker T.), p. 254. Oxford University Press, New York, 1986.
22. Pelletier D. L. and Hornick C. A. Blood lipid studies. In *The Changing Samoans: Behavior and Health in Transition* (Edited by Baker P., Hanna J. and Baker T.), p. 327. Oxford University Press, New York, 1986.
23. Pearson J. D. Stress and daily activities in three Samoan groups. Ph.D. Dissertation. Penn State University, 1989.
24. Greska L., Pelletier D. and Gage T. Work in contemporary and traditional Samoa. In *The Challenging Samoans: Behavior and Health in Transition* (Edited by Baker P., Hanna J. and Baker T.), p. 297. Oxford University Press, New York, 1986.
25. James G., Jenner D., Harrison G. and Baker P. Differences in *Catecholamine excretion rates in* Western Samoan men. *Hum. Biol.* **57**, 635, 1985.
26. Hanna J. and Baker P. Biocultural correlates of blood pressure of Samoan migrants to Hawaii. *Hum. Biol.* **51**, 481, 1979.
27. DuBois B. Hypertension and social support: the medical anthropology of older, urban Samoans. Ph.D. Dissertation, University of Hawaii, Honolulu, 1989.
28. Janes C. R. *Migration, Social Change and Health*. Stanford University Press, Stanford, 1990.
29. Hanna J. M., James G. D. and Martz J. M. Hormonal measures of stress. In *The Changing Samoans: Behavior and Health in Transition* (Edited by Baker P., Hanna J. and Baker T.), p. 203. Oxford University Press, New York, 1986.
30. O'Meara T. *Samoan Planters: Tradition and Economic Development in Polynesia*. Holt, Rinehart and Winston, Fort Worth, TX, 1990.
31. Hecht J., Orans M. and Janes C. Social settings of contemporary Samoans. In *The Changing Samoans: Behavior and Health in Transition* (Edited by Baker P., Hanna J. and Baker T.), p. 39. Oxford University Press, New York, 1986.
32. Fitzgerald M. and Howard A. Aspects of social organization in three Samoan communities. *Pacific. Stud.* **14**, 31, 1990.
33. Franco R. *A Demographic Assessment of The Samoan Employment Situation in Hawii*. East-West Center Population Institute, Honolulu, 1984.
34. Fitzgerald M. Modernization and the menstrual experience among Samoans. Ph.D. Dissertation, University of Hawaii, Honolulu, 1989.
35. Woods N. Premenstrual symptoms: model and method. Paper presented at the *Sixth Conference of the Society for Menstrual Cycle Research*, University of Texas, Medical Branch, Galveston, 1985.
36. Rosenthal R. and Rosnow R. *Essentials of Behavioral Research*, p. 124. McGraw-Hill, New York, 1984.
37. Baker P. and Hanna J. Modernization and the biological fitness of Samoans. In *Migration, Adaptation and Health in the Pacific* (Edited by Fleming C. and Prior I.), p. 14. Epidemiology Unit, Wellington Hospital, Wellington, 1981.
38. Hanna J., Fitzgerald M., Pearson J., Howard A. and Martz-Hanna J. Selective migration from Samoa. *Soc. Biol.* **37**, 204, 1990.
39. Wood C. and Gens L. Hematological status of reproductive women in Western Samoa. *Hum. Biol.* **53**, 269, 1981.
40. Baker D. The study of stress at work. *Ann. Rev. Publ. Hlth* **6**, 367, 1985.
41. Graves T. Polynesians in New Zealand industry. In *New Neighbors: Islanders in Adaptation* (Edited by Macpherson C., Shore B. and Franco R.), p. 136. Center S. Pacific Studies, University of California, Santa Cruz, 1978.
42. MacDonald F. New Zealand's multicultural work force. In *New Neighbors: Islanders in Adaptation* (Edited by Macpherson C., Shore B. and Franco R.), p. 131. Center S. Pacific Studies, University of California, Santa Cruz, 1978.
43. Kincaid D. and Yum J. A comparative study of Korean, Filipino and Samoan immigrants to Hawaii: Socioeconomic consequences. *Hum. Org.* **46**, 70, 1982.
44. Gerber E. The cultural patterning of emotions in Samoa. Ph.D. Dissertation, University of California, San Diego, 1975.
45. Macpherson C. Samoan migration to New Zealand & Polynesian migration and settlement. In *New Neighbors: Islanders in Adaptation* (Edited by Macpherson C., Shore B. and Franco R.), p. 11. Center S. Pacific Studies, University of California, Santa Cruz, 1978.
46. Ablon J. Reactions of Samoan burn patients and families to severe burns. *Soc. Sci. Med.* **7**, 167, 1973.
47. Kaplin B., Casse J. and Gore S. Social support and health. *Med. Care* **15**, suppl. 47, 1977.
48. Pilisuk M. and Forland C. Kinship, social networks, social support and health. *Soc. Sci. Med.* **12B**, 273, 1978.
49. Jaffe J., Babor T. and Fishbein D. Alcoholics, aggression and antisocial personality. *J. Stud. Alc.* **49**, 211, 1988.
50. Walker R. and Kivlahan D. Definitions, models and methods in research on sociocultural factors in American Indian alcohol use. *Subs. Alcohol Actions Misuse* **5**, 9, 1984.
51. Kelly T., Cherek D. and Steinberg J. Concurrent reinforcement and alcohol interactions: effects on human aggressive behavior. *J. Stud. Alc.* **50**, 399, 1989.
52. Cherek D., Steinberg J. and Manno B. Effects of alcohol on human aggressive behavior. *J. Stud. Alc.* **46**, 321, 1985.

53. Leland J. Women and alcohol in an Indian settlement. *Med. Anthropol.* **2**, 85, 1978.
54. Bindon J. Breadfruit, bananas, beef and beer: Modernization in the Samoan diet. *Ecol. Food Nutrit.* **12**, 49, 1982.
55. Hanna J., Pelletier D. and Brown V. Dietary changes. In *The Changing Samoans: Behavior and Health in Transition* (Edited by Baker P., Hanna J. and Baker T.), p. 39. Oxford University Press, New York, 1986.

[7]

Depression among the Homeless*

MARK LA GORY
FERRIS J. RITCHEY
JEFF MULLIS
University of Alabama at Birmingham

Journal of Health and Social Behavior 1990, Vol. 31 (March):87–101

Very little is known about one of the most common mental health problems facing the homeless: high levels of depressive symptomatology. This paper explains variation in the prevalence of depressive symptoms (CES-D) for a random sample of 150 shelter- and street-based homeless persons in the Birmingham metropolitan area. Fifty-nine percent of the sample show the signs of "probable clinical caseness"; yet there is significant variation in the level of symptomatology. A modified version of the social resources model explains 31 percent of the variation in CES-D scores. Although psychological resources play an important role in the distress outcome, as predicted, social supports are found to have limited impact on depression. Life circumstances have significant direct effects on depression. Persons with previous histories of mental illness and with extensive life event histories are more susceptible to distress. Younger persons, the chronically homeless, the street-based homeless, the sick, and the less educated are also more likely to experience depression. This study suggests the importance of understanding homelessness both as a psychological condition and as a complex set of life circumstances and physical deprivations.

Social and behavioral scientists writing in the 1980s demonstrated disproportionately high rates of mental illness among the homeless, which indicated the extreme vulnerability of this impoverished population. Indeed, some forms of homelessness may be attributed directly or indirectly to mental illness (Morrisey and Dennis 1986). The homeless condition itself, however, poses potentially grave psychological and physical health risks which result in higher prevalence rates of mental illness (Fischer, Shapiro, Breakey, Anthony, and Kramer 1987; Morrisey and Dennis, 1986; Snow, Baker, Anderson, and Martin 1986). It represents a highly stressful life circumstance, with significant daily struggles, that tends to be preceded or accompanied by multiple life crises (La Gory, Ritchey, O'Donoghue, and Mullis 1989; Lee 1988; Rossi, Fisher, and Willis 1986). In addition, social support systems for the homeless are not likely to function in a manner similar to those for the general population (Caplow, Bahr, and Sternberg 1968; Lee 1987; Rossi et al. 1986).

Although a significant body of literature on homelessness and mental health has accumulated, very little is known about one of the most common mental health problems faced by the homeless: high levels of distress or depressive symptomatology (La Gory et al. 1989; Rossi et al. 1986). Indeed, only two studies focus on depression (Koegel and Burnham forthcoming; Rossi et al. 1986), but neither attempts to explain variation in the prevalence of depressive symptomatology among homeless individuals. In short, we know little about why some homeless people appear less distressed than others.

The purpose of this paper is to explain

* This research was supported by a grant from Birmingham Healthcare for the Homeless Program. The authors are grateful to Walter Ensel, Kevin Fitzpatrick, William Haley, Nan Lin, and several anonymous *JHSB* reviewers for their comments and suggestions on earlier versions of this paper. Address all correspondence to Mark La Gory, Department of Sociology, University of Alabama at Birmingham, Birmingham, AL 35294.

variation in the prevalence of depressive symptomatology in a random probability cluster sample of 150 shelter- and street-based homeless persons in the Birmingham metropolitan statistical area. A modified form of the social resources model (Cassel 1974; Kaplan 1975; Lin, Dean, and Ensel 1986; Nuckolls, Cassel, and Kaplan 1972; Thoits 1982) is employed to explain why some homeless persons experience severe depressive symptomatology while others do not. This model focuses on how personal resources (both social and psychological) help people to cope with external stressors. In statistical terms these resources are mediating factors or intervening variables between 1) demographic variables and life circumstances and 2) health/illness outcomes. The social resources model can be useful in answering several related questions: 1) What role do social supports (Cobb 1976; Lin et al. 1986; Thoits 1982) and psychological resources (Kessler and Cleary 1980; Lin et al. 1986) play in mediating the stress of homelessness? 2) Is the homeless life circumstance so distressful that traditional social science explanations of stress and depression fail to apply? 3) More specifically, is the homeless state such an impoverished condition that informal social supports (i.e., social resources) become irrelevant to the mediation of stressors? In turn, how important are psychological resources, as compared to social resources, for determining depressive symptomatology?

These questions have critical policy implications for the care and treatment of the homeless because the symptoms of depression can aggravate an already life-threatening social and physical condition. They also are important for scholars interested in social psychological models of distress. Whereas studies of distress in the general population typically involve life events affecting "higher-order" needs such as affiliation, esteem, actualization, or learning, the chronic stressor "homelessness" demands resolution of "lower-order" or basic needs related to survival La Gory and Pipkin, 1981; Maslow 1954). The severity of the life circumstance makes it difficult to assess *a priori* the relevance of additional social psychological explanations to the homeless experience. General population models might not be as useful in understanding mental health among the spatially dispossessed.

EXPLANATIONS OF DEPRESSION IN THE GENERAL POPULATION

To understand the etiology of depression among the homeless it is necessary first to consider explanations of distress in the general population. Depression appears to be distributed systematically in the population. Persons under age 50, blacks, women, the poor, the poorly educated, persons with physical illness, and those not currently married have higher rates of depression than persons not in these groups (Aneshensel, Frerichs, and Clark 1981; Eaton and Kessler 1981; Radloff 1975; Seligman 1975; Tausig 1986; Warheit, Holzer, and Schwab 1973). Some scholars have attempted to explain these differences in biological or psychological terms. There is growing support in the social epidemiological literature, however, for an explanation that links social stressors (undesirable life events and situational stressors) and personal resources (psychological and social resources) with illness outcomes such as depression (Lin et al. 1986; Paykel 1982). In this view, undesirable life events (such as death of a loved one, a financial setback, divorce, or a move) disrupt the individual's life and challenge personal coping skills and social resources. Situational stressors—the daily hassles presented by life circumstances—take an equal or even greater toll on personal health (Lazarus and Folkman 1984), whereas the individual's social and psychological resources modify the effects of these hassles and life events on depression (Dohrenwend and Dohrenwend 1978; Kessler and Cleary 1980; Lin et al. 1986). The most widely accepted contemporary version of this modification process is expressed in the mediation model (Lin et al. 1986). The broad outlines of this explanation can be expressed by the following propositions:

- The frequency of undesirable life events and daily hassles experienced by individuals is related directly to the extent of depressive symptomatology.
- The extent of an individual's social supports and coping skills is related inversely to the extent of depressive symptomatology.
- Social support serves as a mediating factor between undesirable life events and depressive symptomatology.
- Coping skills serve as a mediating factor

between undesirable life events and depressive symptomatology.

THE HOMELESS AND DEPRESSION

It is significant that life events, daily hassles, social supports, and individual coping skills are essential ingredients in determining depressive symptoms because each of these factors distinguishes the homeless from other subpopulations. Homelessness itself represents one of the least desirable life circumstances one could imagine, presenting significant daily difficulties for the individual. It involves the coincidence of multiple life crises such as health problems, physical abuse, and job loss (La Gory et al. 1989; Lee 1988; Rossi et al. 1986).

Homelessness also is a state of deprivation in which existing social supports fail to provide essential resources in a crisis. Indeed, some observers describe the homeless as "disaffiliated" or retreatist (Bahr and Caplow 1973; Blumberg, Hoffman, LoCicero, Niebuhr, Rooney, and Shipley 1960; Bogue 1963; Rossi et al. 1986). This traditional view is captured most accurately by Caplow et al.'s (1968, p. 494) definition of disaffiliation as a "detachment from society characterized by the absence or attenuation of the affiliative bonds that link settled persons to a network of interconnected social structures." Affiliation stresses the formal links, particularly the statuses that persons hold with the major institutions of the community and the society, such as family status, employment, voluntary association membership, or political and religious affiliation (Lee 1987). This view is too restrictive, however, and does not fit current conceptions of "social support," which emphasize the importance of informal ties (Kaplan 1975; Lowenthal and Haven 1968; Wellman 1981). The presence of informal ties, friendships, and confidant relationships is documented easily in studies of the "new homeless" (La Gory et al. 1989; Lee 1988). Nonetheless, although the homeless are reasonably well connected socially, these supports often are not adequate for the level of need.

In addition to these problems, some scholars suggest that impoverished groups generally are more vulnerable to feelings of distress (Kessler and Cleary 1980) because they lack adequate psychological coping skills. According to this argument, variation in internal coping skills, particularly mastery and self-esteem, makes some people more likely to be upwardly or downwardly mobile than others and results in class differentials in the ability to deal with stress. Although these differences are by no means well demonstrated in the literature, variation in psychological resources should be addressed in the analysis of homelessness and mental stress. It is certainly likely that in view of the severity of the life crisis, "homelessness," self-esteem, and mastery will be affected at least in the short term (Snow and Anderson 1987). Hence the social and psychological resources for coping will be constrained severely among the homeless and the extent of undesirable life events and daily hassles will be abnormally high, leading us to expect significant prevalence levels of depression.

A MEDIATION MODEL FOR HOMELESS DEPRESSION

This paper attempts to clarify the varied psychological responses to homelessness by testing the mediation model depicted in Figure 1. Before discussing the operational definition of variables, we will review the hypothetical relationships in the model. The model contains several hypothesized direct and indirect effects of predisposing variables. These variables include individuals' sociodemographic characteristics as well as their life circumstances.

Predisposing Variables: Sociodemographic Characteristics

Several personal background factors have been mentioned as significant exogenous variables in the depression outcome. Older persons, whites, men, married people, people in good physical health, the better educated, and those with higher incomes generally have been found to have lower prevalences of depression (Aneshensel et al. 1981; Eaton and Kessler 1981; Radloff 1975; Seligman 1975; Tausig 1986; Warheit et al. 1973). Because the homeless have uniformly low incomes (median monthly income is $122 for the sample) and are unlikely to be currently married (only 7% in the sample), income and marital status are not included in the model of

FIGURE 1. Mediation Model for Depression among the Homeless

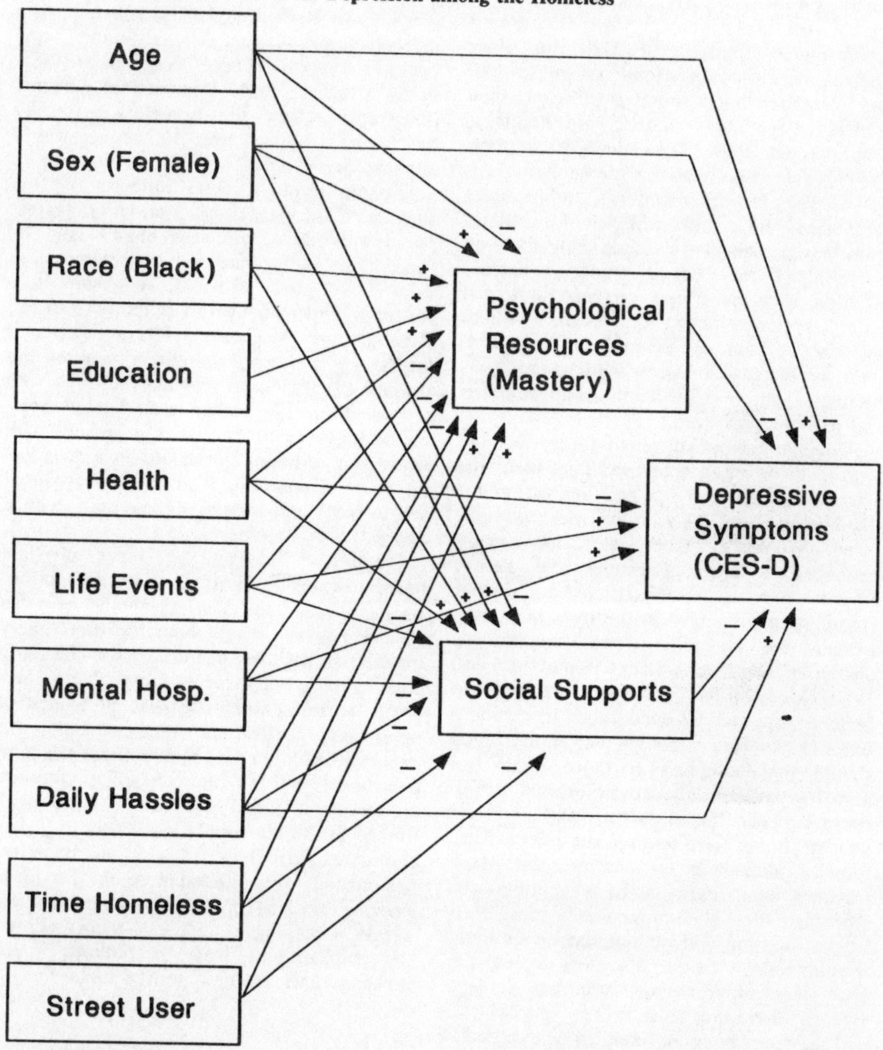

homeless depression. Age, sex, race, education, and health, however, are hypothesized to be significant for depression outcomes. We will consider in turn each variable's relationship to depression.

Age is expected to have a direct effect on depressive symptomatology as well as indirect effects through psychological resources and social supports. Previous research suggests that depression in the general population is reduced with age (Lin et al. 1986) because of cohort effects. Persons who grew up during the economic depression of the 1930s, a period when homelessness and transience were commonplace, learned to expect less of their environment. There is no reason to believe that this relationship would diminish among the homeless.

Aging also affects social support systems and psychological resources. Because of role losses associated with age and because of some reduction in the activities of daily living, mastery tends to diminish with age. Older homeless persons, like the general population of the elderly, thus should experience higher levels of depression because of their reduced mastery. Further, in older populations, close family (children and spouse) and neighbors are more significant than friends for everyday support (Ward, La Gory, and Sherman 1988). These everyday support systems are virtually absent for the homeless; they literally have no neighbors, and most are unmarried. It is also difficult for elderly homeless persons to maintain long-standing friendships because normal modes of communication such as phone conversations and letters are unreliable for people without residences. Thus age should be associated with an increase in depression through its indirect negative effects on social supports and psychological resources.

Although general studies of depression find women to be more depressed than men, the relationship between sex and depression for the homeless is likely to be more complicated. Women's higher rates are usually explained in terms of gender role theory. Because they are socialized to have deeper emotional involvement in the lives of others, women are generally more sensitive to disruptive life events (Kessler and McLeod 1984). Men, on the other hand, are taught to be in control and are encouraged to exhibit a sense of mastery. Although such socialization should make depression more likely for homeless women, the environmental differences between homeless men and homeless women should have an opposite effect. Most females' shelters in our sample are 24-hour facilities that house women continuously, whereas males' shelters generally close early in the morning and do not reopen until the evening. As a result, homeless males may have less support than homeless females (whose environment is more "sociopetal") and they may be more likely to be exposed to the many environmental stressors associated with homelessness. Ultimately the males' advantage regarding symptomatology should be reduced.

Race also should exhibit mixed relationships with depression. Although race should have no direct relationship with depressive symptomatology, general population studies show that blacks are more likely to experience certain stressful life events (Dohrenwend and Dohrenwend 1969), but that their social supports and sense of mastery are higher. Blacks benefit more than whites from the presence of extended families (Hill and Shackleford 1975; Lee 1987), which in turn increase opportunities for emotional and material support. These benefits are less likely to accrue to black homeless persons, however, because the homeless generally have fewer familial ties. Hence we would expect only a weak indirect relationship to depression through social supports. At the same time, in view of discrimination against racial minorities, homeless blacks may be more likely to attribute their homelessness to racism and less likely to consider it a reflection of personal worth or ability (Yancey, Rigsby, and McCarthy 1972); the result would be a stronger indirect relationship through psychological resources.

Education, like other class-related variables, tends to be correlated inversely with depression. Although it should have no direct effect on depression, it provides a sense of self-esteem and mastery that may reduce depressive symptoms.

Finally, as Tausig (1986) notes, physical health has special significance for depression. Its impact on the homeless should be even greater: not only are the homeless more likely to characterize their health as poor (La Gory et al. 1989), but these health problems also are more burdensome because of a lack of predictable shelter and medical care. We expect health to exhibit both a direct effect on depression and an indirect effect through mastery and social support. Persons with limited health are simply less likely to feel in control of their lives. In addition, homeless persons in poor health are more likely to place extreme burdens on their support systems, which, according to exchange theory (Emerson 1962), will lead to reduced social exchange and fewer supportive social ties.

Predisposing Variables: Life Circumstances

Four aspects of life circumstances are believed to have important symptom outcomes for the homeless: life events, daily hassles, the type of environment occupied, and how long the person has been homeless. The effects of life events and daily hassles on depression should be mediated by social supports. We believe, however, that homelessness represents such extreme poverty that as events and hassles accumulate, support systems become less capable and less willing to respond. According to exchange theory, such one-sided social relationships are extremely fragile (Emerson 1962). Thus the mediating capacity of social support will be significantly lower than that found in general populations.

Regarding psychological resources, persons experiencing stressful life events and multiple daily hassles are more likely to have a sense of being out of control; this feeling contributes to greater distress. Furthermore, the greater the number of stressors, the more energy and effort must be devoted to identity work (Snow and Anderson 1987). At the same time, the chance of success is less because the homeless state requires that the greatest effort be expended on satisfying more basic needs (La Gory and Pipkin 1981).

The type of environment occupied by a homeless individual also should be important. Although the homeless generally lack spatial control, not all homeless environments are the same. Street environments (sidewalks, alleyways, bridge underpasses, parks, or other public places and buildings) are certainly different living and sleeping environments from shelters and missions. Although neither environment offers the privacy, security, or predictability of a traditional home, each type of living arrangement yields a different set of choices. Shelters are sociopetal (spaces that bring people together), while street environments are sociofugal (spaces that separate people). At the same time, shelters encourage and reward dependent behaviors (Hoch and Slayton 1989), whereas the street provides minimal, albeit superficial, autonomy. These differences are likely to have consequences for depression outcomes. Persons who use street environments live in a setting where the probability of social contact is reduced. In such environments stressors are less likely to be mediated by social supports. On the other hand, persons using that type of environment may be slightly more likely to experience an increased sense of mastery or control over their environment.

Finally, length of time homeless should have indirect effects on depressive symptoms. The longer a person remains homeless, the less responsive social networks are likely to be, as resources become overtaxed. The recency of homelessness also is hypothesized to affect the individual's psychological resources. Snow and Anderson (1987) point out that the homeless engage actively in identity work, attempting to reestablish a positive self-image. Being cast into or labeled with a new identity such as "homeless person" involves an initial period of social and psychological disruption. Eventually, however, individual identities and psychological resources become capable of being repaired (Snow and Anderson 1987). Hence the longer a person remains homeless, the greater the probability of psychological adjustment to that condition and the less the likelihood of experiencing the symptoms of depression.[1]

METHOD OF STUDY

Sampling and Survey Procedures

One serious obstacle to the study of the homeless is the lack of an agreed-on definition of homelessness. To be homeless literally means to be without home, or, as described more precisely by Rossi, Wright, Fisher, and Willis (1987), "without customary access to a conventional dwelling or residence." The literature on homelessness, however, offers many interpretations of the terms "customary and regular access" and "conventional dwellings." In some studies, for example, persons who are housed marginally are defined as homeless, as are persons residing in single-room occupancy hotels. We adopted a more conservative approach and included only what might be termed the "literally homeless."

Our data on the homeless were taken from the survey phase of the Homeless Enumeration and Survey Project conducted in early 1987 (La Gory et al. 1989). We used an earlier enumeration to establish sample parameters for that survey. The enumeration involved a census of homeless persons in the 22 shelters serving homeless clients in the Birmingham metropolitan statistical area as well as persons without residence sleeping in public places in a 368-square-block area of downtown. Building on the research strategies of Lee (reported in Cuoto, Lawrence, and Lee 1985), we conducted the enumeration in the early morning hours (3:30–5:30 a.m.) in order to reduce the possibility of mistaking "homed" persons for homeless. The enumeration established a conservative count of homeless by sex, race, estimated age, and geographic site (shelter versus street). We found 103 people on the streets and counted 498 in the shelters.

We followed this census two months later

with an interview survey of 150 homeless adults. Data for the present paper are derived from that survey. The survey population was a random probability sample with quotas for the variables of race, sex, and geographic site based on the enumeration figures. For convenience and security, we conducted interviews during the day at the 22 shelters as well as in public places and soup kitchens. We used screening questionnaires for street interviews in order to distinguish the homeless from the homed and the unsheltered from the sheltered homeless.

The interview was about an hour in length and involved an array of topics including basic demographics, housing and employment histories, the circumstances that led to homelessness, life event histories, self-reported physical and mental health symptoms, and the extent of family and friendship networks as well as instrumental and expressive supports. Interviews were conducted in private by trained, experienced interviewers. Of 155 people asked for interviews, only one refused, for a response rate of 99.3 percent. Three interviews were discarded because of incomplete data; one was a duplicate.

Table 1 addresses the representativeness of the survey sample relative to the demographic makeup of the homeless population as established by the enumeration. Generally speaking, the survey sample reflected the enumerated population fairly well.

This population is unique, however. Because of their special nature, these data differ from those used to predict depression symptoms in general populations: the data are cross-sectional rather than longitudinal. Although this is a drawback, a longitudinal design was not feasible in view of our limited resources and the special difficulties encountered with such a mobile group.

Measurement of Variables

Depression. Depressive symptomatology is measured by the Center for Epidemiological Studies Depression (CES-D) scale (Radloff 1975; Weissman, Scholomskes, Pollenger, Prusoff, and Locke 1977), a scale used widely for assessing self-reported depressive symptoms. The scale consists of 20 items, each of which is scored from 0 to 3 depending on the frequency of the symptoms during the week before the interview. It has been shown to have high internal consistency (Radloff 1977) and strong test-retest reliability (Ensel, Lin, and Dean 1986). Its "sensitivity" (ability to predict a diagnosis of depression) is

TABLE 1. Sample Representation Relative to the Birmingham Enumeration

Respondent Characteristic	Enumeration Population[a]		Survey Sample		Significance[b]
	%	(N)	%	(N)	
Age					
20–39	53.8%	(269)	54.0%	(81)[c]	N.S.
40–59	39.6	(198)	40.0	(60)	N.S.
60+	6.6	(33)	6.0	(9)	N.S.
Totals	100.0	(500)[d]	100.0	(150)	
Sex					
Male	78.8%	(462)	76.7%	(115)	N.S.
Female	21.2	(124)	23.3	(35)	N.S.
Totals	100.0	(586)[e]	100.0	(150)	
Race					
White	60.9%	(354)	68.7%	(103)	$p < .05$
Nonwhite	39.1	(227)	31.3	(47)	$p < .05$
Totals	100.0	(581)[f]	100.0	(150)	
Site					
Sheltered	82.8%	(495)	80.7%	(121)	N.S.
Street	17.2	(103)	19.3	(29)	N.S.
Totals	100.0	(598)	100.0	(150)	

[a] Enumeration figures are based on observations; age is estimated.
[b] One-tailed tests.
[c] Includes two between 18 and 20 years of age.
[d] Excludes 76 under 20 years old (children) and 22 individuals for whom age was not discernible.
[e] Excludes 12 for whom sex was not discernible.
[f] Excludes 17 for whom race was not discernible.

reasonably good. Boyd, Weissman, Thompson, and Myers (1982), for example, show that the CES-D scale is a highly sensitive predictor of diagnosed depression (using SADS/RDC criteria), with more than 80 percent of those above the cut-off for "possible clinical caseness" (16+) diagnosed as depressed. Specificity (the capacity to predict who is not depressed) is also quite favorable; more than 91 percent of the respondents were predicted correctly to have a nondepressive diagnosis (using the Diagnostic Interview Schedule) when the 21+ cutoff was used for the CES-D (Ensel et al. 1986). In the current study, reliability is quite high, with a Cronbach's alpha of .887 and item-to-total correlations ranging from .24 to .74.

Predisposing variables: sociodemographic. Sex and race are scored as dichotomous variables, with whites and males assigned a score of 0. Age is treated as an interval-level measure and education as an ordinal-level measure (0–4 years, 5–7 years, grade school education, 9–11 years, high school degree, post high school-trade, some college, college degree, postgraduate education). Finally, the individual's health status is assessed by the use of a subjective health scale ranging from 4 for excellent health to 1 for poor health.

Predisposing variables: life circumstances. Two life event variables are built into the model. One is a scale designed to detect the occurrence of 11 life crises similar to those listed in the life events scales developed by Holmes and Rahe (1967) and by Lin et al. (1986). These events include job loss, marital problems, eviction, jail or imprisonment, trouble getting along with friends and relatives, expulsion from school, sexual abuse, physical abuse, crime victimization, hospitalization for drug abuse, and hospitalization for alcohol abuse. All scale items are correlated significantly with the total score, but the scale displays only moderate reliability, with a Kuder-Richardson score of .61.

We separated out previous hospitalization or mental illness from other life events to test its independent effect on the depression outcome. This event serves as a rough control for any preexisting psychological conditions.[2]

We also employ several additional life circumstance measures. Homelessness is conceptualized more properly as a life circumstance than as a life event because it is a condition that extends over time. Homelessness as circumstance can be assessed by the time elapsed since the event of becoming homeless occurred. The time interval used here is weeks; the variable is logged because of its skewed distribution (median = 20 weeks).

Another measure of life circumstance is the daily hassles that a homeless person experiences. For our purposes we use a scale of daily environmental hassles, which asks questions about the person's current dissatisfaction with his or her living arrangements. The scale consists of nine potential problems ranging from physical factors (e.g., crowding, dirt, noise) to social factors (e.g., rules, the way people act, lack of privacy). Because the distribution was skewed (mean = 1.86, standard deviation = 2.12), the variable was logged. A high score indicates greater dissatisfaction with the environment. The scale is reliable (Cronbach's alpha .775, item-to-total correlations from .29 to .58).

A final measure of the homeless life circumstance is the respondent's use of the environment. This measure is delineated by a dummy variable distinguishing those who used the street (abandoned buildings, public places, outdoor settings, construction sites, automobiles) during the two weeks before the survey from those who used only more controlled, sociopetal settings (such as shelters, SROs, motels, or friend's or relative's housing). A score of 1 indicates a "street user."

Psychological resources. Lin and associates (1986) suggest that several types of psychological resources are relevant to the depression outcome, including sense of personal competence and self-esteem. In view of the high likelihood of intercorrelation between these two elements, our conceptualization of psychological resources is limited to personal competence—more specifically, to one aspect of self-perceived competence, namely mastery. Mastery is defined as "the extent to which one regards one's life chances as being under one's own control" (Pearlin and Schooler 1978). This study uses the scale developed in 1978 by Pearlin and Schooler. Higher mastery scores designate greater psychological resources. Reliability is adequate, with a Cronbach's alpha equal to .689.

Social supports. Social support can be defined as the perceived or actual instrumental and expressive functions provided by social networks and confidants (Lin et al. 1986). We developed a social support scale that indicates the presence or absence of an array of instrumental and expressive ties. The presence of seven types of instrumental assistance (money, advice, food, clothing, shelter, ride, help when sick) and the source of each type of action (friends, relatives, or both) are included. Additional items show whether respondents had visited or communicated with family or other close relatives during the last three months and whether they had friends in Birmingham and/or elsewhere; another item tapped perceived support ("On the whole, do you feel you have enough people and places to turn to when you need help?"). Each item was assigned a 0 or a 1 on the basis of the presence or absence of the characteristic; the items were summed to produce a measure of the extent of social support. Thus higher scale scores indicate more extensive support. Scale scores range between 0 and 19. Items are all correlated significantly (r = .23 to .58) with the total scale score; the scale displays high reliability, with a Kuder-Richardson score of .84.

RESULTS

Our sample shows a striking prevalence of depressive symptomatology. In many studies (Comstock and Helsing 1976; Lin et al. 1986; Weissman et al. 1977) a score of 16 or above on the CES-D is used as the threshold for "possible depression," and 20 or more as an indicator of "probable depression." Whereas less than 20 percent of the general population usually scores 16 or above (Comstock and Helsing 1976; Eaton and Kessler 1981; Ensel et al. 1986; Frerichs, Aneshensel, and Clark 1981), nearly 75 percent of our sample report this significant level of symptomatology. In addition, approximately 59 percent have a score of 20 or more. In general populations, the mean CES-D scores typically fall below 10, with a strong positive skew. In contrast, our sample mean was 23.5, with a standard deviation of 12.45; the deviation was normal. These facts lead us to suspect that a highly significant mental health issue has gone unnoticed in the recent barrage of research on the homeless. Such deep sadness and distress as evidenced by these scores indicate pervasive mental strain. It is essential to understand why some people in our sample were more subject to this strain than others.

Tables 2, 3, and 4 yield such an understanding. Table 2 presents zero-order correlations between variables in the original model, along with their means, standard deviations and ranges. Table 3 reports significant standardized regression coefficients for the modeled depression outcome; Table 4 presents decomposed zero-order correlations for the mediation model. The model explains 31 percent of the variation in depressive symptomatology for the homeless sample. It appears, however, that the dynamics of depression in this sample do not match those observed previously in the general population. Although both social support and mastery have significant direct effects on depressive symptomatology, their ability to mediate the life circumstances of homeless persons is quite limited.

Mastery has the most significant direct effect on depressive symptomatology. It mediates the impact of mental hospitalization and health on depression as hypothesized. Healthier people and those without a history of mental hospitalization exhibit greater psychological resources and thus fewer depressive symptoms. One demographic variable, education, also has a significant indirect effect on depression through mastery; better-educated people exhibit more mastery. Mastery does not, however, mediate the effect of their life circumstance variables such as life event histories, daily hassles, street use, or the length of time a person has been homeless; nor does it have the hypothesized significant relationship with age, sex, or race. Despite this fact, significant differentials exist in coping skills. Such differences, even more than variation in other life circumstances, are especially important for explaining differences in depression among the homeless poor. To cope even modestly with this uniquely stressful life situation requires a great deal of inner strength. Good health and better education are critical factors in determining such strength among the homeless.

The number of life events, previous mental hospitalization, the extent of social supports, and age also have significant direct influence on depression as hypothesized. Younger persons, persons with a previous record of mental hospitalization, persons with limited social resources, and persons who have experienced many undesirable life events are

TABLE 2. Zero-Order Correlations between Variables in the Original Model

	Age	Sex	Race	Education	Health	Life events	Mental hospital	Time homeless	Daily hassles	Street user	Psychological resources (mastery)	Social support	CES-D
Sex (female)	−.297***												
Race (black)	−.170**	−.033											
Education	−.045	.237***	−.011										
Health	−.131*	−.088	.051	.213**									
Life events	−.178**	.048	−.146*	−.216**	−.059								
Mental hospital	−.157*	.164*	−.082	.086	−.102	.375***							
Time homeless (log)	−.198**	−.112*	−.006	−.231***	−.100	.151*	.060						
Daily hassles (log)	−.264***	−.158*	.035	−.085	−.101	.035	.028	.078					
Street user	.001	−.345***	−.046	−.254***	−.069	.032	−.106*	−.018	.334***				
Psychological resources (mastery)	−.073	.023	.014	.241***	.292***	−.141*	−.195**	−.110*	−.013	−.007			
Social support	−.445***	.239***	.033	.186**	.204**	.141*	.069	−.270***	−.023	−.185**	.193**		
CES-D	−.185**	.107*	−.104*	−.145*	−.221**	.338***	.314***	.121*	.167*	.008	−.413***	−.076	
Mean	39.7	.23	.31	5.0	2.6	3.5	.17	3.2	.79	.43	16.9	8.1	23.5
Standard deviation	11.7	.42	.47	1.8	1.0	1.9	.38	1.6	.73	.50	3.8	4.9	12.4
Minimum	18.0	0 = Male	0 = White	1 = 4 years	1 = Poor	0	0 = No	0.0	0.0	0 = No	7	0	0
Maximum	74.0	1 = Female	1 = Black	9 = Post grad.	4 = Excel.	7 = 7+	1 = Yes	6.9	2.2	1 = Yes	24	19	52

* $p<.05$; ** $p<.01$; *** $p<.001$; one-tailed tests.
N = 150.

TABLE 3. Regression Coefficients for Mediation Model Predicting Depression (CES-D)

	Dependent Variables					
	Psychological Resources (Mastery)		Social Support		CES-D	
Independent Variables	*Beta*	b (S.E. b)	*Beta*	b (S.E. b)	*Beta*	b (S.E. b)
Age	−.062	−.020 (.032)	−.367	−.153*** (.037)	−.165	−.176* (.091)
Sex (female)	.023	.208 (.861)	.060	.690 (.983)	.074	2.176 (2.260)
Race (black)	−.023	−.189 (.689)	−.026	−.276 (.798)	—	—
Education	.205	.434* (.194)	—	—	—	—
Health	.225	.855** (.328)	.133	.645* (.369)	−.079	−.978 (.926)
Life events	−.028	−.057 (.188)	.127	.328 (.212)	.221**	1.456** (.499)
Mental hospital	−.190	−1.917* (.907)	−.038	−.491 (1.037)	.128	4.186* (2.508)
Time homeless	−.009	−.021 (.206)	−.195	−.592** (.234)	—	—
Daily hassles	.007	.039 (.484)	−.031	−.212 (.560)	.109	1.857 (1.293)
Street user	.046	.352 (.712)	−.157	−1.540* (.813)	—	—
Psychological resources (mastery)	—	—	—	—	−.322	−1.043*** (.242)
Social supports	—	—	—	—	−.128	−.335* (.203)
Constant		13.715*** (2.388)		14.082*** (2.551)		45.565*** (7.112)
R^2 (Significant variables)	.154		.282		.310	

* p<.05; ** p<.01; *** p<.001; one-tailed test.
N = 150.

more susceptible to high symptom levels. Apparently no matter how psychologically resourceful or how well supported some homeless individuals are, the number of undesirable life events, previous mental health problems, and age have important, independent effects on feelings of distress. This finding suggests that there are qualitatively different experiences of homelessness which go beyond the constructed realities of the homeless individual. In addition, it points to the inability of informal social supports to mediate meaningfully the stressful circumstances of a homeless existence.

Although social support does have a modest, statistically significant direct effect on depressive symptomatology, its mediating function is at best weak. Specifically, four variables (age, health, time homeless, and street use) display small but significant indirect effects on depression through social support. As predicted, older people have less extensive support systems; nonetheless, elders are less distressed. In addition, people using street environments, the physically less healthy, and the longer-term homeless have fewer supports. As hypothesized, street residence is sociofugal. Such "nonplace" residential environments exacerbate an already debilitating condition. Although in some cases this type of residence is chosen (by approximately 50 percent in this sample), it is apparent that it does not contribute to a sense of well-being. According to an exchange perspective, persons whose homelessness is recent rather than chronic and persons who are healthier are more likely to have supportive social ties.

Despite the statistical significance of the

TABLE 4. Decomposed Zero-Order Correlations between Predictor Variables and CES-D: Mediation Model

		Indirect Effects			
Predictor Variable	Direct Effects	Via Psychological Resources (Mastery)	Via Social Support	Joint Effects	r
Age	−.165*	.020	.047***	−.087	−.185**
Sex (female)	.074	−.007	−.008	.048	.107*
Race (black)	0	.007	.003	−.114	−.104*
Education	0	−.066*	0	−.079	−.145*
Health	−.079	−.072**	−.017*	−.053	−.221**
Life events	.221**	.009	−.016	.124	.338***
Mental hospital	.128*	.061*	.005	.120	.314***
Time homeless	0	.003	.023**	.095	.121*
Daily hassles	.109	−.002	.004	.056	.167*
Street user	0	−.015	.020*	.003	.008
Psychological resources (mastery)	−.322***	—	—	−.091	−.413**
Social supports	−.127*	—	—	.051	−.076

* p<.05; ** p<.01; *** p<.001; one-tailed test.
N = 150.

indirect effects, the total impact of these variables through social support is quite small (.077); social support is correlated so highly with age (−.445) that it obfuscates the already modest mediating role. In addition, the mediation model's key proposition concerning the intervention of social support in the relationship between life events and depression fails to hold for the homeless; thus the rather nonconsequential intervening effect is emphasized further.

DISCUSSION

Although recent work shows that the prevalence of mental illness among the homeless is much lower than originally thought (Fischer et al. 1987; Morrisey and Dennis 1986; Snow et al. 1986; Stark 1987), that is not to say that the homeless are psychologically healthy or that the homeless condition itself does not pose grave mental health risks. Perhaps one of the most prevalent mental health problems facing the homeless is the rather silent problem of depression. This paper demonstrates how potentially serious the problem is. Nearly three out of four homeless persons in this study exhibit the symptomatology of "possible clinical caseness," and 59 percent show the signs of "probable clinical caseness."

The correlates of depression for this sample exhibit both similarities to and differences from the general population. The differences found here, of course, must be tempered with the understanding that these findings are not based on longitudinal data, nor are they the result of comparisons with a matched sample of homed individuals. Although social supports and mastery play a statistically significant role in mediating symptom outcomes, their importance for the homeless population is different from that for the general population. As hypothesized, social supports have a more modest effect on depressive symptoms, whereas psychological resources in the form of mastery play a more important role. The most dramatic aspect of these findings is the small size of both the direct and the mediation effects of supports. Although many homeless persons are affiliated, their social supports cannot play the effective role in mediating stressful events that they play for the average person, not only because of the multiple undesirable life events that the homeless experience but also because of the relatively limited economic resources of their support systems. This point is underscored by our surprising finding concerning the positive relationship between life events and social supports (although it is not statistically significant when other variables are controlled). The homeless have support systems, and these systems respond to need, but we expected that in view of the crisis-laden lives of the homeless, such supports would stop responding as demands on them increased. The problem for the homeless is not one of unresponsive networks; rather, social supports cannot reduce distress as effectively in this very needy population as in other groups. Such a finding indicates the potential importance of service providers in the intervention process. Homelessness represents a condition so devastating that personal ties are almost ineffectual. A significant question for future research is "How effective can secondary ties be in reducing distress levels in this population under siege?"

Perhaps the most interesting finding is the extent to which psychological resources, in the form of mastery, influence the level of depressive symptomatology. Even though Kessler and Cleary (1980) see psychological resources as critical in explaining depression outcomes among the poor, it is difficult to anticipate the extent of their importance. Homelessness is a devastating life event, one that interferes with the satisfaction of basic physical needs. Despite the challenge to "lower-order needs," psychological resourcefulness has a much stronger influence on distress levels than does any objective condition (social support, life events, health, environmental use, sex, or age). One needs remarkable inner strength to be homeless and yet to maintain one's psychological equilibrium. This distress, of course, cannot be resolved by the individual alone; yet apparently no objective resources currently available to the homeless can substitute for this internal asset in moderating depression. This fact suggests the importance of developing new intervention strategies. As Hoch and Slayton (1989) argued recently, current strategies are not working in moderating the harmful effects of homelessness.

Another important finding is the tremendous variation in the experience of homelessness. Perhaps the most consistent theme in the homelessness research of the 1980s has been the demographic diversity of the homeless population. Our research suggests that this objective diversity is paralleled by significant variation in the level of distress. Younger persons, persons who have experienced greater numbers of undesirable life events, persons previously hospitalized for mental problems, persons with a limited sense of their own resourcefulness, and persons with less extensive social supports are much more vulnerable than others to the debilitating effects of the homeless condition. Similarly, the street-based homeless, the chronically homeless, the physically ill, and the less educated are more susceptible to depression because of their limited social or psychological resources. "Homelessness" is a convenient label for a variety of objective and subjective conditions of impoverishment. Thus the array of mental health outcomes is equally varied, although depression symptoms generally are elevated in this population.

Future research should determine the significance of high prevalence levels of depressive symptoms among the homeless. Some researchers may find nothing alarming in the fact that nearly 60 percent of the homeless show the symptoms of probable depression. Indeed, such levels could be seen as a natural, even healthy reaction to a severely impoverished condition. Although high levels of depression are not surprising, we must understand that they are potentially serious. The consequences of depression for the homeless have been overlooked. Homelessness is not merely a devastating physical condition; it also has quite significant psychological consequences that may intensify physical deprivations (Radloff 1977). The sadness and apathy associated with depression may interfere with normal social relations and with the motivation necessary to solve life problems. Such a cycle could be extremely debilitating to homeless individuals, worsening an already severe objective condition. In short, the presence of depression may isolate individuals further from the psychological and social resources necessary to solve their problem; thus the depressed homeless may be less likely to leave the streets quickly. It is imperative that further research be conducted to examine this potential cycle.

NOTES

1. Because of the absence of longitudinal information on the homeless, neither this research nor earlier work can establish causal direction. In fact, it could be the case that psychological adjustment decreases with time homeless.
2. Because we lack information concerning previous dates for mental hospitalization, it is possible that the first episode of homelessness may have occurred before institutionalization. Because this is not a longitudinal design, it is also plausible in some cases that depression predated homelessness and hospitalization.

REFERENCES

Aneshensel, Carol S., Ralph R. Frerichs, and Virginia A. Clark. 1981. "Family Roles and Sex Differences in Depression." *Journal of Health and Social Behavior* 22:379–93.

Bahr, Howard M. and Theodore Caplow. 1973. *Old Men Drunk and Sober*. New York: New York University Press.

Blumberg, Leonard U., F.H. Hoffman, V. LoCicero, H. Niebuhr, James F. Rooney, and Thomas E. Shipley. 1960. *The Men on Skid Row: A Study of Philadelphia's Homeless Man Population*. Philadelphia: Department of Psychiatry, Temple University.

Bogue, Donald. 1963. *Skid Row in American Cities*. Chicago: Community and Family Study Center, University of Chicago.

Boyd, Jeffery, Myrna M. Weissman, Douglas Thompson, and Jerome K. Myers. 1982. "Screening for Depression in a Community Sample." *Archives of General Psychiatry* 39: 1195–1200.

Caplow, Theodore, Howard M. Bahr, and David Sternberg. 1968. "Homelessness." Pp. 494–99 in *International Encyclopedia of the Social Sciences*, vol. 6, edited by D. Stills. New York: Macmillan.

Cassel, John. 1974. "An Epidemiological Perspective of Psychosocial Factors in Disease Etiology." *American Journal of Public Health* 64: 1040–43.

Cobb, Sidney. 1976. "Social Support as a Moderator of Life Stress." *Psychosomatic Medicine* 38:300–14.

Comstock, George W. and Knud Helsing. 1976. "Symptoms of Depression in Two Communities." *Psychological Medicine* 6:551–63.

Cuoto, Richard, Risley Lawrence, and Barrett Lee. 1985. "Healthcare and the Homeless of Nashville: Dealing with a Problem without a Definition." *Urban Resources* 2:17–23.

Dean, Alfred. 1986. "Measuring Psychological Resources." Pp. 97–111 in *Social Support, Life Events, and Depression*, edited by N. Lin, A. Dean, and W. Ensel. New York: Academic Press.

Dean, Alfred and Nan Lin. 1977. "The Stress Buffering Role of Social Support." *Journal of Nervous and Mental Disease* 165:403–13.

Dohrenwend, Barbara S. and Bruce P. Dohrenwend. 1978. "Some Issues in Research on Stressful Life Events." *Journal of Nervous and Mental Disease* 166:7–15.

———. 1981. "Life Stress and Illness: Formulation of the Issues." Pp. 1–28 in *Stressful Life Events and Their Contexts*, edited by B.S. Dohrenwend and B.F. Dohrenwend. New York: Prodist.

Durkheim, Emile. 1897. *Suicide*, translated by J. Spaulding and G. Simpson. New York: Free Press.

Eaton, William and Larry G. Kessler. 1981. "Rates of Symptoms of Depression in a National Sample." *American Journal of Epidemiology* 114:528–38.

———. 1985. *Epidemiology Field Methods in Psychiatry: The NIMH Epidemiologic Catchment Area Program*. New York: Academic Press.

Emerson, Richard. 1962. "Power Dependence Relations." *American Sociological Review* 27(1): 31–41.

Ensel, Walter, Nan Lin, and Alfred Dean. 1986. "Correlates of Depressive Symptoms (CES-D) and Major Depressive Episodes (DIS)." Paper presented at the annual meetings of the American Public Health Association, Washington, D.C.

Fischer, Pamela, Sam Shapiro, William Breakey, James Anthony, and Morton Kramer. 1987. "Characteristics of the Homeless: Findings of the Baltimore Epidemiologic Catchment Area Study." *DIS Newsletter* 4:6–7.

Frerichs, Ralph R., Carol S. Aneshensel, and Virginia A. Clark. 1981. "Prevalence of Depression in Los Angeles County." *American Journal of Epidemiology* 113:691–9.

Hill, Robert and Lawrence Shackleford. 1975. "The Black Extended Family Revisited." *Urban League Review* 1:18–24.

Hoch, Charles and Robert Slayton. 1989. *New Homeless and Old*. Philadelphia: Temple University Press.

Holmes, Thomas and Richard Rahe. 1967. "The Social Readjustment Rating Scale." *Journal of Psychosomatic Research* 11:213–18.

Jeffrey, C.R. 1971. *Crime Prevention through Environmental Design*. Beverly Hills: Sage.

Kaplan, Burton. 1975. "Toward Further Research on Family and Health." Pp. 89–106 in *Family and Health: An Epidemiological Approach*, edited by B. Kaplan and J. Cassel. Chapel Hill: Institute for Research in Social Science, University of North Carolina.

Kessler, Ronald C. and Paul Cleary. 1980. "Social Class and Psychological Distress." *American Sociological Review* 45:463–78.

Kessler, Ronald C. and Jane D. McLeod. 1984. "Sex Differences in Vulnerability to Undesirable Life Events." *American Sociological Review* 49:620–31.

Koegel, Paul and M.A. Burnham. Forthcoming. "Problems in the Assessment of Mental Illness among the Homeless: An Empirical Approach." In *Homelessness: The National Perspective*, edited by M. J. Robertson and M. Greenblatt. New York: Plenum.

La Gory, Mark and John Pipkin. 1981. *Urban Social Space*. Belmont, CA: Wadsworth.

La Gory, Mark, Ferris Ritchey, Timothy O'Donoghue, and Jeff Mullis. 1989. "The Homeless of Alabama: A Diversity of People and Experiences." Pp. 1–20 in *Homelessness in America*, edited by J. Momeni. Westport, CT: Greenwood.

Lazarus, Richard S. and Susan Folkman. 1984. *Stress, Appraisal and Coping*. New York: Springer.

Lee, Barrett, 1987. "Homelessness and Community." Paper presented at the annual meeting of the American Sociological Association, Chicago, IL.

______. 1988. "Homelessness in Tennessee." Pp. 181–204 in *Homelessness in the United States*, edited by J. Momeni. Westport, CT: Greenwood.

Lin, Nan, Alfred Dean, and Walter Ensel (eds.). 1986. *Social Support, Life Events, and Depression*. New York: Academic Press.

Lowenthal, Margaret F. and C. Haven. 1968. "Interaction and Adaptation: Intimacy as a Cultural Variable." *American Sociological Review* 33:20–30.

Maslow, Abraham. 1954. *Motivation and Personality*. New York: Harper & Row.

Myers, Jerome K., J.J. Lindenthal, and Max P. Pepper. 1975. "Life Events, Social Integration and Psychiatric Symptomatology." *Journal of Health and Social Behavior* 16:421–27.

Myers, Jerome K., J.J. Lindenthal, Max P. Pepper, and D. Ostrander. 1972. "Life Events and Mental Status." *Journal of Health and Social Behavior* 33:398–406.

Morrisey, Joseph P. and Deborah Dennis. 1986. "NIMH-Funded Research Concerning Homeless Mentally Ill Persons: Implications for Policy and Practice." In *Proceedings of Third Annual Meeting of NIMH-Funded Researchers Studying Homeless Mentally Ill Persons*. Washington, DC: Division of Education and Service Systems Liaison, NIMH.

Newman, Oscar. 1973. "Defensible Space: Crime Prevention through Urban Design." *Ekistics* 36:325–32.

Nuckolls, Katherine G., John Cassel, and Burton Kaplan. 1972. "Psycho-Social Assets, Life Crises and the Prognosis of Pregnancy." *American Journal of Epidemiology* 95:431–41.

Paykel, Eugene S. (ed.). 1982. *Handbook of Affective Disorders*. New York: Guilford.

Pearlin, Leonard I., Morton A. Lieberman, Elizabeth Menaghan, and Joseph Mullan. 1981. "The Stress Process." *Journal of Health and Social Behavior* 22:337–56.

Pearlin, Leonard I. and Carmi Schooler. 1978. "The Structure of Coping." *Journal of Health and Social Behavior* 19:2–21.

Rabkin, Judith G. and Elmer Struening. 1976. "Life Events, Stress, and Illness." *Science* 194:1013–20.

Radloff, Lerore S. 1975. "Sex Differences in Depression: The Effects of Occupation and Marital Status." *Sex Roles* 1:249–265.

______. 1977. "The CES-D Scale: A Self-Report Depression Scale for Research in the General Population." *Applied Psychological Measurement* 1:385–401.

Rossi, Peter H., Gene Fisher, and Georgianna Willis. 1986. *The Condition of the Homeless of Chicago*. Amherst: Social and Demographic Research Institute.

Rossi, Peter, James Wright, G. Fisher and G. Willis. 1987. "The Urban Homeless: Estimating Composition and Size." *Science* 235:1336–41.

Seligman, Martin E.P. 1975. *Helplessness: On Depression, Development and Death*. San Francisco: Freeman.

Selye, Hans. 1956. *The Stress of Life*. New York: McGraw-Hill.

Snow, David and Leon Anderson. 1987. "Identity Work among the Homeless: The Verbal Construction and Avowal of Personal Identities." *American Journal of Sociology* 92:1336–71.

Snow, David, Susan G. Baker, Leon Anderson, and Michael Martin. 1986. "The Myth of Pervasive Mental Illness among the Homeless." *Social Problems* 33:407–23.

Stark, Louisa. 1987. "Blame the System, Not Its Victims." Pp. 7–12 in *Homelessness: Critical Issues for Policy and Practice*, edited by J. Kneerim. Boston: Boston Foundation.

Tausig, Mark. 1986. "Prior History of Illness in the Basic Model." Pp. 267–80 in *Social Support, Life Events, and Depression*, edited by N. Lin, A. Dean, and W. Ensel. New York: Academic Press.

Thoits, Peggy. 1982. "Conceptual, Methodological, and Theoretical Problems in Studying Social Support as a Buffer against Life Stress." *Journal of Health and Social Behavior* 23: 145–59.

Ward, Russell A., Mark La Gory, and Susan Sherman. 1988. *The Environment for Aging*. Tuscaloosa: University of Alabama Press.

Warheit, George, Charles E. Holzer, and J.J. Schwab. 1973. "An Analysis of Social Class and Racial Differences in Depressive Symptomatology: A Community Study." *Journal of Health and Social Behavior* 14:291–99.

Weissman, Myrna M., D. Scholomskes, M. Pollenger, B.A. Prusoff, and Ben Z. Locke. 1977. "Assessing Depressive Symptoms in Five Psychiatric Populations: A Validation Study." *American Journal of Epidemiology* 106:203–14.

Wellman, Barry. 1981. "Applying Network Analysis to the Study of Social Support." Pp. 171–200 in *Social Networks and Social Support*, edited by B.H. Gottlieb. Beverly Hills: Sage.

Yancey, William, L. Rigby, and J.D. McCarthy. 1972. "Social Position and Self-Evaluation: The Relative Importance of Race." *American Journal of Sociology* 78:338–59.

[8]

Uncertainty and the Lives of Persons with AIDS

ROSE WEITZ
Arizona State University

Journal of Health and Social Behavior 1989, Vol. 30 (September):270–281

This article uses interview data to explore how 23 gay and bisexual men who had AIDS were affected by and managed uncertainty. Before diagnosis these individuals had to find ways to cope with uncertainty about their risk of contracting AIDS and about their initial symptoms. After diagnosis they had to find answers to their questions about why they contracted this disease, whether they would be able to function in the short run, whether their illness would kill them, and whether they would be allowed to live and (if death was unavoidable) to die with dignity. The data suggest that persons with AIDS respond to the uncertainties of their illness by attempting to assert as much control as possible over their lives, through such divergent strategies as seeking and avoiding knowledge about their illness.

Uncertainty exists whenever people lack a cognitive framework for understanding their situations and thus feel that they cannot predict the outcomes of their behaviors. At least as far back as Malinowski ([1926] 1948), researchers have recognized that few people tolerate uncertainty well; therefore most people seek ways to reduce it or, if that is not possible, to cope with it. Researchers have identified means of dealing with uncertainty as disparate as developing magical rituals (Felson and Gmelch 1979) and gathering scientific information about the consequences of various possible actions (Janis and Mann 1977). Most recently, scholarly interest in uncertainty has produced a vast literature on how persons perceive and respond to the risks of natural and technological disasters (e.g., Douglas and Wildavsky 1982; National Research Council 1982; Slovic, Fischhoff, and Lichtenstein 1977).

Medical sociologists have long recognized that uncertainty is a critical issue for chronically and terminally ill persons (Conrad 1987, pp. 7–9; Glaser and Strauss 1968) and a major source of stress in their lives (Mishel 1984; Mishel, Hostetter, King, and Graham 1984; Molleman, Krabbendom, Annyas, Koops, Sleijfer, and Vermey 1984). To cope with this uncertainty, such persons, like others in stressful situations, can use two basic strategies: vigilance and avoidance.

In vigilance, persons attempt to reduce uncertainty by seeking knowledge and acting on that knowledge. For example, ill persons whose physicians prove unable to diagnose their problems can research possible diagnoses themselves (Schneider and Conrad 1983; Stewart and Sullivan 1982). Once their illnesses are identified, they can reduce uncertainty about why disease has struck them and about what they can expect in the future by searching for similarities between their cases and those of fellow sufferers (Comaroff and Maguire 1981; Cowie 1976; Roth 1963; Schneider and Conrad 1983; Wiener 1975).

In avoidance, people cope with uncertainty by protecting themselves against unpleasant knowledge. For example, many ill persons deal with uncertainty about the meaning of their initial symptoms by attributing those symptoms to less serious ailments or to preexisting illnesses and by avoiding any contact with physicians (Cowie 1976; Schnei-

* Direct all correspondence to Rose Weitz, Department of Sociology, Arizona State University, Tempe, AZ 85287-2101. This research was made possible by a grant from the Arizona Disease Control Research Commission and by a small grant from the Arizona State University College of Liberal Arts and Sciences. The comments of Peter Conrad, Rochelle Kern, Karolynn Siegel, and the anonymous reviewers were much appreciated, as was the research assistance of Kathleen Abbott, Melissa Bolyard, and Shirley Philp.

der and Conrad 1983). Even after they seek medical care, they may prefer not to know their diagnoses or prognoses and may ignore persons who propose pessimistic definitions of their situations (Comaroff and Maguire 1981; McIntosh 1976).

Although these two strategies may appear antithetical, they are linked in fact by a common goal: the construction of normative frameworks that enable individuals to explain their situations to themselves. These frameworks give people the sense that they understand what has happened and will happen to them. By making the world seem predictable, these frameworks help individuals to choose (albeit sometimes from among limited options) how they will live their lives. Thus even when normative frameworks are factually inaccurate and when the resulting actions seem short-sighted or self-destructive, I would hypothesize that these frameworks reduce the stresses of uncertainty, for they enable people to feel that they are at least minimally in control of their lives. In this paper I suggest that in the final analysis, it is this sense of control which enables people to tolerate uncertainty.

AIDS and Uncertainty

This paper describes how uncertainty affects persons with AIDS (or PWAs, as they call themselves), and how they cope with that uncertainty. Few published research studies have analyzed the experiences of PWAs; none has looked specifically at the issue of uncertainty. Instead the social science literature on AIDS consists largely of quantitative studies regarding why people do or do not change their sexual behavior to protect themselves against infection (reviewed in Becker and Joseph 1988).

Because most medical authorities believe that AIDS eventually kills all its victims, it may seem that uncertainty is not an issue for PWAs. As this paper will show, however, uncertainty affects PWAs in several ways.[1] Even before health problems appear, persons who are at risk for AIDS must wonder whether they will develop the disease. Once symptoms become evident, PWAs are uncertain how to interpret and respond to those symptoms. After they receive their diagnoses, PWAs must question why this calamity has befallen them. Because AIDS causes unpredictable flare-ups and remissions, PWAs face uncertainty each morning about how ill they will be that day. As their illness progresses, they also experience anxiety about whether they will be able to live with dignity even though they are ill, and about whether AIDS eventually will kill them. Finally, those who conclude that death is inevitable must wonder whether they will be allowed to die with dignity.[2] This paper will describe how PWAs seek control over these uncertainties and how their illness impairs their ability to do so.

METHODS AND SAMPLE

Between July 1986 and March 1987, I interviewed 25 Arizona residents who had either AIDS or AIDS-related complex (ARC).[3] Four to six months after the initial interviews, I reinterviewed 13 respondents. (Two respondents declined to participate in the follow-up interviews, two moved without leaving addresses, and eight died or suffered brain damage in the interim). Two of the 25 respondents were heterosexual women who had used intravenous drugs. The rest were men, all of whom described themselves as gay or bisexual (although none mentioned any recent relationships with women). Three of these men also had used drugs. The data presented in this paper come from the 23 initial and 11 follow-up interviews with gay and bisexual men, except where noted otherwise.

At the time I began the study, the Arizona Department of Health Services had confirmed 110 reports of AIDS cases. State officials believed that approximately 40 of these persons were still living, as well as an unknown number of persons with ARC. Because AIDS is still rare in Arizona, the situation of PWAs there is very different from that in places like New York or California, where most of the previous research on PWAs has taken place. Research conducted in Arizona can help us to understand what it is like to have AIDS in an area which lacks a politically powerful gay community and in which AIDS is just beginning to have an impact. Therefore this study can help us to predict what the lives of PWAs will be like in the future, as the disease spreads from the current centers of infection to more conservative and more typical areas of the country.

Most respondents learned of this study

through letters mailed to them by the Arizona AIDS Project (N=15) or the Tucson AIDS Project (N=4), two nonprofit groups that offer emotional and financial support to PWAs. To increase sample size and diversity I posted signs in gay bars, placed announcements in gay newspapers and in the mainstream press, and announced the study in AIDS political action groups. I also asked several physicians and AIDS support group counselors to inform their clients of the study. Finally, I asked my respondents to give my name to any other PWAs they knew. No names were given to me by any source; instead, PWAs were invited to contact me if they wanted to participate.

The sample is comparable to the state population in regard to religion and is comparable to the population of reported Arizona AIDS cases in regard to sex, geographical location (overwhelmingly urban), and mode of transmission (Arizona Department of Health Services 1987). Because participation in the interviews required both mental competence and some physical stamina, the sample undoubtedly underrepresents the more seriously ill PWAs. It also underrepresents persons with Kaposi's sarcoma (8% of the sample but 21% of reported cases), perhaps because these individuals did not want a stranger to see their disfigurement. In addition, the sample underrepresents nonwhites (0% of the sample but 13% of reported cases), who typically are less well integrated into the AIDS support networks and therefore were less likely to have heard of the study. Finally, the sample overrepresents persons in their thirties (60% of the sample but 42% of reported cases) and underrepresents older persons. Unfortunately, there is no way of knowing how well the state's statistics on reported AIDS cases reflect the actual distribution of AIDS cases.

The data for this paper were obtained through semistructured interviews. I entered each interview with a preset list of questions, but also probed any new topics that arose during the interview. Initial interviews ranged from two to five hours in length and averaged about three hours; follow-up interviews were considerably shorter. All interviews were audiotaped and transcribed, and took place at respondents' homes unless they preferred another location (usually my home). I attempted to ask all questions and to respond to all answers in an unbiased and nonjudgmental manner, whether my respondent was describing sadomasochistic homosexual behavior or fundamentalist Christian theology. I believe that I was successful in that no respondents acted hostilely, broke off the interviews (except from physical exhaustion), or suggested in any other way that they felt uncomfortable in discussing these issues with me.

Following the suggestions of Glaser and Strauss (1967), I analyzed the data using categories that I developed from the respondents' descriptions of their situations. After each interview I revised the interview schedule to focus it more closely on these emerging themes. When the themes were collapsed and reorganized, they formed the structure of this paper.

FINDINGS

Uncertainty affects PWAs at many levels. From the time when they realize that they are at risk, they must question whether they will contract AIDS. Once they start to have symptoms, they must wonder what those symptoms signify. And once they are diagnosed, they must question why they have contracted AIDS and whether they will be able to function tomorrow, to live with dignity, to "beat" AIDS, or to die with dignity. The following sections show how these uncertainties affect PWAs and how they cope with their situations.

"Will I get AIDS?"

Fear of contracting AIDS permeates the lives of many gay and bisexual men. Finding this uncertainty too much to endure, several respondents dealt with their fear by assuming that they were infected long before they were diagnosed. The rest, however, had lived through long months of anxiety about whether they would become ill; although they could change their behavior to protect themselves against future infection, they could not stop the disease's development if they were infected already.

Unable truly to control their health prospects, these men coped with uncertainty about whether they would contract AIDS by finding ways at least to *feel* that they were in control of their lives. They did so by developing theories that explained why they were not really at risk, despite their behaviors. Typically these theories suggested that AIDS attacks only physically weak, "promiscuous" persons, who choose their partners unwisely. The theories also emphasized that AIDS occurs only elsewhere. One Phoenix resident explained that he and his friends had not followed safe sex guidelines because they had convinced themselves that "there's only nine people in Arizona who have it and four of them are dead and two of them live in Tucson. So what are your chances? Even though we knew about it and we knew how awful it was, it was like, no, that's something that happens someplace else, not in Phoenix."

As more cases of AIDS appeared, however, these theories provided less comfort (especially for the nine respondents who had seen friends or lovers die). As a result, most found themselves alternately denying and brooding on the risks they had taken. Emotionally they were unable to accept the fact that they might die from a dread disease; yet intellectually they could not reject the possibility. One man shifted in a matter of moments from describing how his fear of contacting AIDS had kept him awake nights to describing how he "thought it would never happen to me."

Beginning in mid-1985, Arizonans could eliminate some uncertainty by having their blood tested to learn whether they had been exposed to the AIDS virus. The test could reduce uncertainty significantly for those who tested negative. For those who tested positive, however, the test merely replaced one form of uncertainty with another because it could not show whether they would develop AIDS. Moreover, a positive test result could increase stigma and anxiety significantly (Beeson, Zones, and Nye 1986; Moulton 1985). As a result, all but two of the men decided that they would feel more in control of their destinies if they refused to obtain such potentially ambiguous knowledge. As one said, "I figured if I was tested and tested positive, I'd worry myself into coming down with it, . . . so I decided against it. . . . If I came down with it, I came down with it, and I'd have to worry about it then."

"What do my symptoms mean?"

People who have been infected with AIDS may remain asymptomatic, and therefore ignorant that they are infected, for several years. Once symptoms start to appear, however, these individuals must decide what the symptoms mean and how or whether they should react.

Because symptoms generally build gradually, PWAs at first can accommodate to the difficulties they cause. As a result, like persons who develop other chronic illnesses (Bury 1982, p. 170; Cowie 1976, p. 88; Schneider and Conrad 1983; Stewart and Sullivan 1982), they may explain their symptoms initially using preexisting cognitive frameworks which minimize the symptoms' importance. Several men blamed their night sweats and exhaustion on the Arizona heat. Others confused the symptoms of AIDS with the side effects of drug use; both can cause weight loss, sweating, and diarrhea. Although these theories eventually proved wrong, in the interim they allowed the men to feel that they understood their situations and thus helped them to reduce stress.

Although in some cases the men minimized their symptoms out of ignorance, in other cases they appeared to have chosen consciously or unconsciously to downplay their symptoms because they preferred uncertainty to the certainty of the AIDS diagnosis. One individual explained that he did not go to a physician despite a variety of symptoms because "I didn't want to find out I had AIDS. Even though I kind of figured I did, I didn't want to know. I wanted to live a normal life for as long as I could." By avoiding the physicians he was able to assert control over his emotional well-being despite his lack of control over his physical well-being.

Those who minimize their symptoms for whatever reason may defer seeing a physician for some time. As the disease progresses, however, they find eventually that they can neither control their bodies nor maintain their everyday living patterns. Once they reach this point, PWAs can no longer maintain their cognitive frameworks and are motivated to seek diagnosis and treatment.

As they discover soon, however, seeing a physician does not necessarily end their uncertainty. Many physicians simply lack the knowledge needed to diagnose AIDS (Lewis, Freeman, and Corey 1987). Others may not consider diagnoses of AIDS unless they know that their clients are at risk, even if their clients' symptoms fit the classic patterns for AIDS. Yet clients may not disclose that they are at risk for fear of the social consequences.

Even if physicians have the intellectual knowledge to diagnose AIDS, they may lack the emotional ability to do so. Several respondents complained that physicians neither tested them for AIDS nor diagnosed them with AIDS, even though the respondents had multiple, classic symptoms, stated that they were gay, and requested AIDS testing. One man described how his physician refused several requests for AIDS testing, even though the physician knew that he was gay and that something was wrong with his immune system:

> I was concerned. The symptoms were there, and I was not getting any better, not feeling any better, still getting weaker and weaker, losing more weight, and I kept mentioning all these things and I said, "Look, I've been reading more articles about AIDS." And he said, "Oh, people are just panic-stricken. You don't have AIDS. I'm not doing a test on you."

Stories like this suggest that even in obvious cases some physicians consciously or unconsciously avoid diagnosing AIDS.

For all these reasons, then, PWAs may not receive accurate diagnoses until several months after they seek care. Initially, some of my respondents accepted or even welcomed the alternative diagnoses that their physicians proposed. When symptoms continued, however, these men found themselves in what Stewart and Sullivan (1982, p. 1402) described (with regard to multiple sclerosis) as "an ambiguous and uncertain limbo," in which they suffered anxiety about the meaning of their symptoms and could not function normally, but lacked social support for adopting the sick role (cf. Bury 1982, p. 172; Schneider and Conrad 1983; Stewart and Sullivan 1982; Waddell 1982). Consequently they could not maintain these positions indefinitely. To cope with this situation, some respondents went from doctor to doctor to obtain a diagnosis. Others researched their symptoms, diagnosed themselves, and then pressed their physicians to test them for AIDS. Only then did their uncertainty about the nature of their illnesses end.

"Why have I become ill?"

A diagnosis of AIDS ends individuals' uncertainty about what is wrong with them, but it raises new questions about why this terrible thing has happened to them. Only by answering these questions can PWAs make their illness comprehensible.

Despite the price exacted by AIDS, two of my subjects developed positive explanations for their illnesses. One, a fundamentalist Christian, felt that God had given him AIDS to enable him to share his religious faith with others. He had accepted several invitations to speak about having AIDS at schools and churches, and had used these opportunities to share his belief "that you can be a homosexual and still go to heaven." Another, whose disastrous choice of lovers had left him suicidal on several occasions, considered his diagnosis literally an "answer to a prayer." He believed that God had given him AIDS as a way of providing the extra incentive he needed to avoid any further romantic entanglements.

The rest, however, had no such comforting explanations. Their search for meaning was painful, set as it was in the context of popular belief that AIDS is punishment for sin.

At least on the surface, the majority rejected the idea that AIDS was divine punishment. Instead they argued that AIDS results from the same biological forces that cause other illnesses. Consequently they dismissed the idea that they or anyone else deserved AIDS. As one man said:

> Nobody deserves it. I have friends that say, "Well, hey, if we weren't gay, we wouldn't get this disease." That's bullshit. I mean, I don't want to hear that from anybody. Because no germ has mercy on anybody, no matter who they are—gay, straight, babies, adults.

Yet other statements by some of these men suggested that at a less conscious level they did feel that they were to blame for their illnesses (cf. Moulton 1985). One man denied that he deserved AIDS but suggested later that AIDS might have been God's way of punishing him for being gay or "for not being a good person. . . . I should have helped people more, or not have yelled at somebody, or been better to my dad even though we have never gotten along. . . . Maybe if I had tried to get along better with him, maybe this wouldn't be happening."

Others maintained that they did not deserve AIDS, but used language which suggested considerable ambivalence. Several attributed their illness not to their "nonmonogamy" or "multiple sexual partners" but rather to their "promiscuity." One man said he contracted AIDS "probably because I was a royal whore for about four years." Their use of such morally loaded terms suggests that they were not describing their behavior objectively but were condemning it on moral grounds. Thus it seems that they believed emotionally, if not intellectually, that they deserved punishment, although perhaps less severe punishment than AIDS.

Still other respondents had no doubts that they deserved AIDS. Some felt that they deserved AIDS simply because of their lack of forethought in engaging in high-risk behaviors. One man stated, "I knew better. I mean, it's like, you deserve it. You knew what was going on and yet you slipped and this is the consequence." Others stated explicitly that they deserved AIDS as punishment for their immoral activities. Among these men a diagnosis of AIDS seemed to unleash preexisting guilt about being gay or bisexual (or, in one case, about using drugs). Such guilt seemed particularly prevalent among the nine respondents from fundamentalist Christian or Mormon families; more than half of these men expressed regret about being gay and two-thirds believed at least partially that they deserved AIDS. One fundamentalist Christian who had engaged in homosexual behavior for several years said, "I reaped what I sowed: I sowed sin, I reaped death. I believe, biblically, I received AIDS as a result of my sexual sin practices."

Regardless of how an individual explained why he developed AIDS, simply having an explanation made it easier to tolerate having the illness. For this reason the persons who showed the most distress were those who believed that others deserved to get AIDS but that they themselves did not. Consequently they raged at the unfairness of their situation. As one respondent stated:

> I get real angry. I don't know how to explain why I got it and somebody else didn't because I don't consider myself that I was that promiscuous. When I go out I see other guys out in the bars and they're hopping around, two and three guys a night basically, and it's like why aren't they getting it? Why is it me?

Similarly, some persons who believed that they were born gay considered it unfair that their innate orientation put them at risk for AIDS. Therefore they had to cope not only with the physical trauma of illness but also with the emotional trauma of losing their faith that this is a just world.

"Will I be able to function tomorrow?"

Like many chronic illnesses, AIDS causes unpredictable flare-ups and remissions. As a result, PWAs can never know from one day to the next how sick they will be. As one man said:

> Probably the hardest thing is not knowing when you're well what's going to happen tomorrow because when you're well all you're thinking about is, "What am I going to get? What's the next infection I'm going to have to put up with?" Of course, when you're sick it's like, "Well, I hope they can make me well. I wonder if they can or not."

Because PWAs can become incapacitated without warning, they expose themselves to possible disappointment whenever they make long- or even short-range plans. One man said that he feared going "for a little trip tomorrow even though I am capable of doing that, but I may have diarrhea and who wants to be driving down the highway with shit in your pants?" He and others like him accepted that they had lost control over their physical health. As one man said, "AIDS has become my life. I live for AIDS. I don't live for me anymore, I live for AIDS. I'm at its beck and call and I'll do what it tells me when it tells me." Therefore they chose to avoid making plans as a way to protect themselves against disappointment (cf. Charmaz 1983). By acknowledging their lack of control over their physical health they could assert control over their emotional health.

This strategy was not without cost, however; although it protected PWAs against disappointment, it increased their frustration. As one man explained, "I may have a day where I feel great, where I have plenty of energy and everything is fine, and then you have nothing going, you're just sitting there in the house rotting. So that is really frustrating." Consequently PWAs must walk a tightrope—making the plans they need in order to lead a meaningful life without setting themselves up for disappointment when those plans collapse. For this reason several respondents compared themselves to recovering alcoholics, who must learn to live "one day at a time."

"Will I be able to live with dignity?"

AIDS takes its toll on the human body in many ways, some of which leave individuals with little dignity during either their living or their dying. Consequently PWAs face tremendous uncertainty about the nature of their remaining days.

Fear of death is minimal compared to fear of what their lives may become. In the words of a man who had already suffered one agonizingly debilitating episode, "Death doesn't bother me. Being ill as I was terrifies me." In particular, PWAs fear that they will be among the 70 percent who suffer neurological impairment or the 10 percent who become disfigured by the lesions of Kaposi's sarcoma. They especially fear esoteric illnesses whose effects they cannot predict. As one respondent said:

> I'm not [as] afraid of getting infections from people as I am from inanimate objects, like fruits and moldy tile. . . . I know what a cold is like. . . . [It's] something that I have experienced. I've never experienced a mold infection.

PWAs have little control over whether they will develop such infections. To cope with the uncertainty that this lack of control creates, some PWAs try to develop a realistic picture of what they can expect in the future. To learn about the consequences and treatments of various infections (as well as to obtain emotional support), PWAs may attend support groups offered by community organizations. Others research their illnesses on their own, in some cases developing extensive libraries on AIDS. The knowledge that they gain allows them to feel that they can respond appropriately if some problem should arise, and thus that they can exert some control over their situations.

Other PWAs cope with anxiety about what their lives will be like by attempting to maintain unrealistic images of their futures. One man had not joined an AIDS support group because he did not "want to see what other people [with AIDS] look like." This sentiment was especially common among the healthier respondents, who feared that gaining knowledge would lead to depression and that choosing to maintain ignorance was therefore the more sensible approach.

"Will I be able to 'beat' AIDS?"

All PWAs must grapple with questions about the likelihood of an early death. These questions seem least answerable to those who initially receive diagnoses of ARC. Faced with conflicting, probabilistic estimates of when and whether they will contact AIDS, persons with ARC experience enormous stress. In the words of one respondent whose diagnosis changed from ARC to AIDS between the initial and the follow-up interviews:

> The worst feeling was when I was ARC, waiting for a bomb to explode. Not knowing when or if ever it would do it. There was always that tentative (sic) in my life that it may or may not—beware! Now that the diagnosis has come in, it's like "Okay. I can relax now. The worst is over."

Even persons diagnosed with AIDS, however, may continue to wonder whether God or medicine will cure them. To cope with this uncertainty and to gain a sense of control over their lives, they search for and adopt any courses of action that might preserve or improve their health. A few respondents relied primarily on prayer. The rest ate more balanced meals, took vitamins, limited their use of caffeine, tobacco, and illegal drugs, and exercised, if possible. They tried to limit their exposure to germs by (for example) avoiding animals and swimming pools and by scanning public buses for passengers who looked unhealthy before choosing a seat. They also sought any treatments, including the experimental, the illegal, or the toxic, which might increase their chances for survival.

Faced with the prospects of an early death, some PWAs are willing to go to extraordinary lengths to obtain promising treatments. The drug most in demand by my respondents was zidovudine (formerly called azidothymidine or AZT). Zidovudine is now available by prescription (although it costs about $12,000 per year). During most of the study period, however, PWAs could obtain zidovudine legally only if they were among the few chosen to participate in pharmaceutical experiments. The rest had to rely on various subterfuges. Some convinced their physicians to diagnose them inaccurately so they would meet the experimenters' criteria. Others received zidovudine from physicians who continued to collect pills from the researchers for clients who had died. Still others obtained unused pills from friends who were research subjects. These friends gave away pills that the experimenters had instructed them to destroy when they had forgotten to take their pills on schedule or had skipped them because of unpleasant side effects. Friends also could obtain an extra set of pills to give away by registering as research subjects under two names with two physicians.

Finally, PWAs also tried to increase their chances for survival and their sense of control over their lives by maintaining a positive attitude. As one man explained, "The main killer with having AIDS is that mental psyche, because your mind controls your body. . . . There are so many people that can't get past that 'I'm sick and going to die.' And therefore, they don't even start—they die." He and others like him simply refused to believe that they would die or to make plans for their deaths. One man said that he had not written a will because of "that whole will to live bit. Once I get that done, that means one less thing I have to do. As long as I don't have it done, it seems like, well, I can't die yet." He went on to explain his belief in the importance of

> . . . being active about this disease, whether it involves drinking a certain kind of tea or standing on your head twice a day or doing something, something that gives the patient a feeling of control over his own life that if you do these things, this might help you a little bit. . . . It's a sense of being in control, of being actively involved in your own health, which in itself produces health.

"Will I be able to die with dignity?"

Despite the lengths to which PWAs will go to survive, their greatest fear is not death but being kept alive against their will and beyond the point of meaningful life. As one respondent said, "I'm not afraid to die. I can truthfully say I'm not. I'm a Christian, I'm saved, and I'm going to heaven. It's getting from here to there that worries me. That's the rough spot."

To alleviate uncertainty and to maintain a sense of control over the nature of their dying, several respondents had made plans to commit suicide if that seemed to be warranted. As one man explained, "If I'm going to die, I would rather it be my business. I guess it's a lack of control. I want to reassert as much control as I can." Others had decided to let the disease take its natural course. They had signed living wills to prohibit physicians from keeping them alive by extraordinary means and had decided to stop taking their medications as soon as life no longer seemed worthwhile: One man had thrown away all his medications without informing his physician. As he explained, "I don't want to die, but I don't have a choice. I have to—period. I mean, no question. So if I have to die, why not tackle the chore and get it over with?"

Learning to Live with AIDS

By the time of the follow-up interviews (four to six months after the initial interviews), AIDS had become far more comprehensible to my respondents. They now had cognitive frameworks that enabled them to understand the changes in their bodies. One man said:

> I remember, a little over a year ago when I was first told what I had, it was very frightening. . . . You didn't know what the future held. A lot of that has been, at least, resolved. I don't worry about it so much, as I did in that respect. It's still not something I want, but I guess you learn to live with it a little better. Then, when you get a case of pneumonia, you know what it is and you don't really think anything of it, other than the fact that "Well, we know what's caused this."

Not only had uncertainty been reduced; it also had become an accepted part of life. Stress had decreased because the men had learned both to assert control over some aspects of their lives and to accept that they could not control other aspects. One man, comparing his feelings at the initial and the follow-up interviews, said, "All I think I've done is adjust to it. I'm not so afraid. I guess

I have realized that there's nothing that I can do about it."

Although more respondents still hoped for a cure, their frenetic search had abated. As one respondent said:

> At first, I got on the bandwagon of vitamins and getting nutrition and proper meals and eating my spinach and everything. One day I finally said, "What for?" It's not going to save me. I don't know of anybody that has not died from AIDS just because they ate spinach."

Those who accepted that death was inevitable now focused on living for the present—doing whatever they could do to give pleasure to themselves and their loved ones. By doing so they could feel that they controlled their present circumstances at least partially, even if they could not control their futures.

DISCUSSION

Previous studies showed that uncertainty is a central concern for all seriously ill persons. This study suggests that uncertainty and its ramifications may have an even greater impact on PWAs than on those who suffer from most other illnesses, for several reasons. First, PWAs are more likely than most to know before diagnosis that they are at risk. As a result they suffer difficulties that other ill persons do not experience, because uncertainty and anxiety often sap their emotional energy and physical resources months or even years before they become ill.

Second, PWAs are more likely to feel guilt about the behaviors that led to their becoming ill. Thus, when faced with uncertainty about why they became ill, they are more likely to conclude that it was a deserved punishment. Moreover, PWAs are far more likely to find that their friends, families, and the general public also believe that PWAs cause and deserve their own illness. As a result, these others often reinforce the guilt that PWAs feel.

Third, PWAs are more likely to face difficulties in obtaining an accurate diagnosis. Like other illnesses, AIDS can be difficult to diagnose because it is rare and causes multiple symptoms. These problems are exacerbated because physicians often deliberately (although sometimes unconsciously) avoid questions or actions that would lead to diagnosis.

Fourth, PWAs face greater uncertainty than other ill persons in predicting how their illness will affect their lives; AIDS causes more extensive and less predictable physical and mental damage than most other illnesses.

Fifth, because AIDS is such a new disease, PWAs are more likely to lack answers to their questions about treatment and prognosis. Moreover, because physicians' knowledge about AIDS is developing rapidly and changing constantly, PWAs often are reluctant to trust the answers they do receive.

Uncertainty can be even more troublesome for PWAs who (unlike those described in this paper) are not gay men. Such PWAs face additional problems in obtaining diagnoses because they may not know that they are at risk. Some women, for example, do not know that their male partners are bisexual. Some bisexual men (as well as many heterosexuals, including those who use drugs) may believe that only gays are at risk. Moreover, their physicians may be less alert for and knowledgeable about AIDS than the physicians of gay men, who often specialize in gay health care.

After diagnosis, PWAs who are not gay and who cannot argue that God-given biological needs forced them to put themselves at risk for AIDS may experience more guilt and more loss of self-esteem than gay men. (In fact, all three gay drug users in the sample exhibited more guilt about their drug use than about their sexuality.) Nongay PWAs (especially women) also experience more difficulty in predicting their futures because so many studies have examined only how AIDS affects the health of gay men. Moreover, they are far less likely to have networks of fellow sufferers to whom they can turn for advice and information. Some live on the margins of society and lack either access to or knowledge of community resources. Others either are unwilling to accept help from groups dominated by gay men because of their own homophobia or are unable to obtain help because their problems are too different from those of gay men. Finally, other PWAs may suffer greater uncertainty than gay men about whether they might transmit AIDS to others. Many gay men function in social circles where everyone is presumed to be at risk, but other PWAs may be overwhelmed by the belief that they are the sole potential source of infection for their loved ones.

Yet despite all the difficulties faced by PWAs because of uncertainty, they are not completely helpless. As this paper has described, they find ways to reduce or (if necessary) to live with uncertainty.

These data on how PWAs cope with uncertainty have significant implications for the study of uncertainty in general: they highlight the role of control in making uncertainty tolerable. Previous research on uncertainty hinted that loss of control might make uncertainty stressful; studies on helplessness demonstrated that loss of control causes stress and depression (Lazarus 1966; Peterson and Seligman 1984). This study specifies further the links among uncertainty, loss of control, and stress. As this paper has shown, individuals can cope with uncertainty by developing normative frameworks that make their situations comprehensible. These frameworks, combined with other tactics (such as deciding not to make plans, in the case of PWAs), help individuals to gain control or at least the sense of control over their lives. Thus in some situations they enable people to reduce uncertainty. In other situations, where uncertainty is either unavoidable or preferable to certainty, such frameworks enable people to reduce the stresses of living with uncertainty.

POLICY IMPLICATIONS

According to Janis (1983), people can handle stressful situations most effectively if they feel that they are in control of their lives. To achieve this goal he proposes "stress inoculation," in which people 1) are given information about what to expect, which is realistic but which still allows them to maintain optimism; 2) are encouraged to identify possible actions that can help them to survive and to find internal and external resources that would allow them to take those actions; and 3) are helped to develop their own plan for responding to their situation.

The results of this study support Janis's model; they, too, suggest that the key to coping with the uncertainty of having AIDS is achieving a sense of control. Thus if we are to improve PWAs' lives, doctors, counselors, relatives, and others who care for or about PWAs must learn both how uncertainty affects PWAs and how they can help PWAs to feel that they are in control. Paradoxically, in some cases this process will mean learning to recognize when PWAs would prefer to maintain uncertainty rather than to learn the truth about their situation. As Janis suggests, knowledge is counterproductive if it makes persons feel that their situations are hopeless. In most cases, however, help will entail involving PWAs in their own care—making sure that they understand what is happening to them and believe that decisions (including decisions about when to terminate care) are left to them. In addition, caregivers must learn to go beyond simply providing information; they also must learn to help PWAs identify their internal and external resources and decide on their own plan of action—even if the resulting steps seem useless or even harmful (cf. Cohen and Lazarus 1983). Health care workers need to understand that both trust and therapeutic effectiveness will suffer unless they learn to convince PWAs that they can discuss safely and honestly any nonmedically approved actions they are taking.

Finally, those who care for or about PWAs must recognize that PWAs have a strong need to find a logical explanation for their illness. Physicians, counselors, and AIDS activists must learn that although talking in terms of "risk behaviors" can be useful in discussing the possibility of AIDS with persons not yet infected, it can reinforce guilt feelings among those who have AIDS and thus can increase their emotional difficulties. Family members and friends, as well as health care workers, must learn to ascertain whether PWAs are blaming themselves and to intervene in such instances, or at least to refer them for counseling. In sum, those who work with PWAs need to learn how psychosocial factors affect PWAs and to develop ways of responding to PWAs' emotional as well as physical problems.

NOTES

1. Although uncertainty about contagion is a major cause of social rejection, this paper does not address how uncertainty affects PWAs' social relationships. I have chosen to address that subject in a separate paper both because of its complexity and because stigma rather than uncertainty seems to be the more crucial factor affecting PWAs' social lives.

2. These various aspects of uncertainty need not be sequential. For example, individuals may question whether they will be well enough to work tomorrow even before they obtain names for their illnesses.
3. For this analysis I combined persons with AIDS and persons with ARC because I could not separate the two categories adequately. Some individuals said that they had ARC when they clearly had AIDS, some said that they had AIDS when they seemed to have ARC, and some vacillated in their statements about which disease they had. Since these interviews were conducted, the Centers for Disease Control have broadened their definition of AIDS to include most cases considered previously as ARC.

REFERENCES

Arizona Department of Health Services. Feb. 2, 1987. *Definitive and Presumptive AIDS Cases in Arizona and AIDS Related Complex (ARC): Surveillance Report for Arizona*.

Becker, Marshall H. and Jill G. Joseph. 1988. "AIDS and Behavioral Change to Reduce Risk: A Review." *American Journal of Public Health* 78:394–410.

Beeson, Diane, Jane S. Zones, and John Nye. 1986. "The Social Consequences of AIDS Antibody Testing: Coping with Stigma." Paper presented at the annual meeting of the Society for the Study of Social Problems, New York.

Bury, Michael. 1982. "Chronic Illness as Biographical Disruption." *Sociology of Health and Illness* 4:167–82.

Charmaz, Kathy. 1983. "Loss of Self: A Fundamental Form of Suffering in the Chronically Ill." *Sociology of Health and Illness* 5:168–95.

Cohen, Frances and Richard S. Lazarus. 1983. "Coping and Adaptation in Health and Illness." Pp. 608–35 in *Handbook of Health, Health Care, and the Health Professions*, edited by David Mechanic. New York: Free Press.

Comaroff, Jean and Peter Maguire. 1981. "Ambiguity and the Search for Meaning: Childhood Leukemia in the Modern Clinical Context." *Social Science and Medicine* 15B:115–23.

Conrad, Peter. 1987. "The Experience of Illness: Recent and New Directions." *Research in the Sociology of Health Care* 6:1–31.

Cowie, Bill. 1976. "The Cardiac Patient's Perception of His Heart Attack." *Social Science and Medicine* 10:87–96.

Douglas, Mary and Aaron Wildavsky. 1982. *Risk and Culture*. Berkeley: University of California Press.

Felson, Richard B. and George Gmelch. 1979. "Uncertainty and the Use of Magic." *Current Anthropology* 20:587–89.

Glaser, Barney G. and Anselm L. Strauss. 1967. *The Discovery of Grounded Theory: Strategies for Qualitative Research*. New York: Aldine.

———. 1968. *Time for Dying*. Chicago: Aldine.

Janis, Irving L. 1983. "Stress Inoculation in Health Care: Theory and Research." Pp. 67–99 in *Stress Reduction and Prevention*, edited by David Meichenbaum and Matt E. Jaremko. New York: Plenum.

Janis, Irving L. and Leon Mann. 1977. *Decision Making: A Psychological Analysis of Conflict, Choice, and Commitment*. New York: Free Press.

Lazarus, Richard S. 1966. *Psychological Stress and the Coping Process*. New York: McGraw-Hill.

Lewis, Charles E., Howard E. Freeman, and Christopher R. Corey. 1987. "AIDS-Related Competence of California's Primary Care Physicians." *American Journal of Public Health* 77:795–800.

Malinowski, Bronislaw. (1926) 1948. *Magic, Science, and Religion and Other Essays*. Boston: Beacon.

McIntosh, Jim. 1976. "Patients' Awareness and Desire for Information about Diagnosed but Undisclosed Malignant Disease." *Lancet* 2: 300–303.

Mishel, Merle H. 1984. "Perceived Uncertainty and Stress in Illness." *Research in Nursing and Health* 7:163–71.

Mishel, Merle H., Thelma Hostetter, Barbara King, and Vivian Graham. 1984. "Predictors of Psychosocial Adjustment in Patients Newly Diagnosed with Gynecological Cancer." *Cancer Nursing* 7:291–99.

Molleman, Eric, Pieter J. Krabbendam, Albertus A. Annyas, Heimen S. Koops, Dirk T. Sleijfer, and Albert Vermey. 1984. "The Significance of the Doctor-Patient Relationship in Coping with Cancer." *Social Science and Medicine* 18:475–80.

Moulton, J. M. 1985. "Adjustment to a Diagnosis of AIDS or ARC in Gay Men." Ph.D. dissertation, California School of Professional Psychology, Berkeley.

National Research Council. 1982. *Risk and Decision Making*. Washington, DC: National Academy Press.

Peterson, Christopher and Martin E.P. Seligman. 1984. "Causal Explanations as a Risk Factor for Depression: Theory and Evidence." *Psychological Review* 91:347–74.

Roth, Julius A. 1963. *Timetables*. Indianapolis: Bobbs-Merrill.

Schneider, Joseph W. and Peter Conrad. 1983. *Having Epilepsy: The Experience and Control of Illness*. Philadelphia: Temple University Press.

Slovic, P., B. Fischhoff, and S. Lichtenstein. 1977. "Behavioral Decision Theory." *Annual Review of Psychology* 28:1–39.

Stewart, David C. and Thomas J. Sullivan. 1982. "Illness Behavior and the Sick Role in Chronic Disease: The Case of Multiple Sclerosis." *Social Science and Medicine* 16:1397–1404.

Waddell, Charles, 1982. "The Process of Neutralisation and the Uncertainties of Cystic Fibrosis." *Sociology of Health and Illness* 4:210–20.

Wiener, Carolyn L. 1975. "The Burden of Rheumatoid Arthritis." Pp. 1–88 in *Chronic Illness and the Quality of Life*, edited by Anselm L. Strauss. St. Louis: Mosby.

***ROSE WEITZ** is an associate professor at Arizona State University. She is currently working on a book on* Living with AIDS, *to be published next year by Rutgers University Press. She is the author, with Deborah A. Sullivan, of* Labor Pains: Modern Midwives and Home Birth.

[9]

Migrant Labor and Sexually Transmitted Disease: AIDS in Africa*

CHARLES W. HUNT

University of Oregon

Journal of Health and Social Behavior 1989, Vol. 30 (December):353–373

Acquired immune deficiency syndrome (AIDS) is worldwide, but the clinical and epidemiological pattern of the disease in Africa is different from that in developed areas. "Type 1 AIDS" occurs in industrialized North America and Europe; it has a distinctive sex ratio (16:1) and risk pattern of IV drug use and sexual practices. "Type 2 AIDS" occurs in Third World countries, particularly in eastern, southern, and central Africa. It is characterized by an entirely different sex ratio (1:1) and by distinctively different risk patterns. Both epidemics are caused by the HIV-1 virus. The key concept for understanding the origins of the differences between Type 1 and Type 2 AIDS is the migratory labor system in eastern, central, and southern Africa. This system causes long absences, increased family breakdown, and increased numbers of sexual partners. Historically the organization of this labor market has created a population which suffers from epidemics of sexually transmitted diseases. These historical patterns are presented as evidence for the contemporary transmission of AIDS. When contemporary AIDS and HIV-1 seropositivity prevalence data are examined, a systematic temporal and geographic pattern emerges for the AIDS epidemic in Africa. Despite a paucity of good data, the prevalence data from eastern, central, and southern Africa support the thesis of migrant labor's role in the transmission of AIDS.

The following paper integrates four areas of history, research, methodology, and theory. First, it incorporates a scientific understanding of the HIV-1 virus and the action of this virus in the creation of acquired immune deficiency syndrome (AIDS). The modes and methods of transmission in both Africa and the United States are the basis of understanding in the following discussion.

Second, in combination with an understanding of the biology of the HIV-1 virus and of the AIDS that results, this paper uses an analysis of epidemiology known as "historical materialist epidemiology." Accordingly it assumes the primacy of economic life, economic patterns, and economic development. This economic foundation sets the basic parameters of health and illness in society. This method of approach is derived from work done by such early thinkers as Frederick Engels, Rudolf Virchow, and Salvador Allende (Waitzkin 1983, pp. 65–85). This early work was followed in the 1970s and 1980s by a great deal of research and writing on disease and health. The historical materialist approach was taken in a series of articles concerning coronary heart disease and hypertension (Eyer 1975; Eyer and Sterling 1977; Schall and Kern 1986), cancer (S. Epstein 1976, 1978), suicide (Hopper and Guttmacher 1979; Waldron and Eyer 1975), occupational health and safety (Chavkin 1984; Navarro 1982; Navarro and Berman 1983; B. Smith 1981), women's longer life span as compared with men's (Waldron 1986), and the expansion and contraction of economic cycles and mortality rates (Eyer 1977; Waldron and Eyer 1975). This approach may be described as a method that "relates patterns of death and disease to the political, economic, and social structures of society" (Waitzkin 1978, p. 272). Special applications have been made to Third World

* Direct correspondence to Charles W. Hunt, Department of Sociology, University of Oregon, Eugene, OR 97403.

societies, relating underdevelopment, dependency theory, and health (Doyal 1981; Navarro 1974; Turshen 1977).

Third, this paper's assertions are based on a study of the historic, social, and economic development of eastern, central, and southern Africa, the Africa of migrant labor and the labor reserve. The development process has been described by dependency theory; therefore this paper is grounded in dependency theory (Amin 1976; Foster 1986; Frank 1967; Leys 1975; Rodney 1982; Saul and Arrighi 1973). World systems theory has elaborated on dependency theory; the work in this paper also complements the studies in world systems theory on the household in the world economy (Friedman 1984; Martin 1984; J. Smith 1984; Wallerstein 1984; Wallerstein and Martin 1979). The structure of the household, its size, and its varying composition, as well as degree of proletarianization, wage and nonwage work, and migrancy, are integrated into the following analysis with considerations of health, well-being, and disease. These household structures are defined by their place in the world system; consequently, it is argued in the subsequent presentation, health and disease are defined by place—core or periphery—in that system.

Finally, an understanding of the medical and population geography of central, eastern, and southern Africa is integrated into the thesis advanced in this paper (see Hall and Langlands 1975; Kabera 1982; Langlands 1975; Meyer 1988; Prothero 1977, 1983; White 1978). The population's geographical movements in these regions of Africa, often termed oscillations rather than migrations, give rise to the characteristic concentrations of labor around plantations, mines, and other capital investments. These movements, interacting with historical development patterns, give rise to the labor reserve, the rural farming area which often is in decline because of the patterns established by dependency and migrant labor (P. Epstein and Packard 1987). This pattern of movement and labor market affects Africans' family and sexual patterns (see Murray 1977, 1980, 1981); as I argue here, it creates a population that is susceptible to sexually transmitted disease (STD), AIDS in particular. A study of past spatial patterns—the medical geography of STDs—will reveal the historical relationship of STDs to migrant labor. This pattern, it is argued, has been repeated in the AIDS epidemic of the 1970s and 1980s.

AFRICA AND AIDS

Acquired immune deficiency syndrome is epidemic in the United States, but it is more than an epidemic. AIDS is a pandemic: it is *worldwide* in distribution and began almost simultaneously in a number of areas in the world. World Health Organization (WHO) officials estimate that "over 250,000 cases of AIDS have already occurred, that between five and 10 million people worldwide are infected with the AIDS virus and that within the next five years about one million new AIDS cases can be expected" (Mann, Chin, Piot, and Quinn 1988, p. 82). By March 1, 1988, there were 81,433 reported AIDS cases in 133 countries (WHO 1988).

AIDS has appeared in the Pacific Oceania complex of islands and Australia, in South and Central America, and, although delayed, in Asia. Nowhere, however, was its appearance more ominous than in Africa (Andersen, May, and McLean 1988).

It is extremely difficult to judge the exact extent of AIDS in Africa, either geographically or in the population (Konotey-Ahulu 1987, pp. 206–207). Rwanda, Burundi, the Congo, Zimbabwe, Botswana, Zaire, Zambia, Kenya, and Uganda seem to be particularly afflicted (Mann and Chin 1988; Mann et al. 1988). These countries form what has been called "the AIDS belt" across eastern, central, and southern Africa.

AIDS was first discovered to be present in Africa when it was diagnosed in upper-class Africans seeking treatment in European hospitals. The first African cases were diagnosed in Europe shortly after the first diagnosis of AIDS occurred in the United States (Quinn, Mann, Curran, and Piot 1986). African AIDS, however, has two distinctive aspects in relation to the AIDS epidemic in the United States.

First, the sex ratio of those who have AIDS in Africa is approximately 1:1, an equal number of females and males (Biggar 1986; Brunet and Ancelle 1985; Curran, Morgan, Hardy, Jaffe, Darrow, and Dowdle 1985; Mann and Chin 1988; Mann et al. 1988; Mann, Francis, Davachi, et al. 1986; Mann, Francis, Quinn, et al. 1986; Quinn 1987; Quinn et al. 1986). This ratio is in sharp contrast to the 16:1 ratio of males to females in Europe and the United States (Quinn et al. 1986). The disparity is related to the different risk patterns associated with African and with North American AIDS cases. In Africa neither homosexuality, homosexual sexual patterns, nor IV drug use are associated with AIDS or found as a means of transmission for the AIDS virus (Biggar 1987; Brunet and Ancelle 1985; Carswell 1987; Clumeck et al. 1985; Kreiss 1986; Moodie 1988; Quinn 1987).

When the illness is studied epidemiologically, primarily *sexually active heterosexuals* are seen to evidence the highest incidence of AIDS in Africa. Females who have AIDS in Africa tend to be younger than males, and often are single. There appears to be a higher incidence of AIDS among prostitutes than among African women generally (Biggar 1986; Brunet and Ancelle 1985; Quinn 1987; Quinn et al. 1986). Because women contract AIDS in Africa much more often than in North America, and because it appears that AIDS can be transmitted across the placenta from the infected mother to the fetus, there are many more children with AIDS in Africa than in the United States (Mann, Francis, Davachi, et al. 1986); in fact, children constitute almost one-third of all AIDS cases in Africa (Hilts 1987). As in the United States, AIDS in Africa appears to occur much more frequently in large cities than in the rural areas, at least at the present (although this may be a reporting bias, as we will discuss later). As in Europe and the United States, those who are discovered to have the AIDS virus frequently have a medical history of previous venereal diseases and appear to be more sexually active than those without AIDS (Quinn 1987; Quinn et al. 1986). The patterns of AIDS infection in the industrialized countries of North America and Europe is so distinctive in relation to the pattern in Africa, Haiti, and parts of Central and South America that the former is often termed "Pattern 1 AIDS" and the latter "Pattern 2 AIDS" (Mann and Chin 1988; Mann et al. 1988; Piot, Plummer, Mhalu, Lamboray, Chin, and Mann 1988).

AIDS in Africa has a second distinctive aspect. In the United States and in Europe a definite series of "opportunistic" infections occurs with AIDS, such as Kaposi's sarcoma (a skin cancer), toxoplasmosis (a parasitic disease spread by cats and chickens, which is usually harmless for those not suffering from AIDS), or a type of pneumonia. In Africa, in contrast, the opportunistic infections usually do not include any of these. Generally the infections suffered by AIDS patients in Africa involve the stomach or the digestive system, some skin diseases (in some cases Kaposi's sarcoma), tuberculosis, herpes zoster, and meningitis (Quinn et al. 1986). Thus in Uganda, AIDS is termed "slim disease" because of the wasting that occurs as a result of these infections. AIDS in Africa is epidemiologically and clinically quite distinct from AIDS in Europe or in North America. In fact, "the definition of AIDS used in the West needs to be broadened for use in Africa" (Norman 1985).

If the biological agent of the disease is the same in North America and Europe as in Africa—and research has proved that this is the case (Biggar 1986)—why do AIDS in Africa and AIDS in the United States look and act so different? Why is the same biological cause linked to such different demographic and clinical results? In short, why are there Pattern 1 and Pattern 2 AIDS epidemics? The answer lies in the social/historical environment in which the biological cause, the HIV virus, acts.

When AIDS is viewed in this way, one can advance a strong thesis that the main historical fact of African social, political, and economic reality is the situation of underdevelopment and the position of dependency in which many African nations find themselves with respect to the core capitalist countries. This relationship of underdevelopment and dependency, particularly as it affects African health, labor market organization, and rural agricultural development, has largely determined the pattern of the disease in Africa.

DEPENDENCY AND AIDS

First we will examine African historical and economic development in terms of industrialization and the development of a labor market. Then we will discuss the effect of this development on rural and agricultural areas. This background will help us to understand how these factors interact with the AIDS virus.

The pattern of industrial development in southern, eastern, and central Africa, which was followed by colonization of this area by the European powers and has continued to the present, was based largely on a migrant labor system (Crush 1984; Davidson 1983; Doyal 1981, pp. 11–119; Freund 1984, 1988; Gugler, 1968; Gutkind and Wallerstein 1976; Karugire 1980; C. Leys 1975; R. Leys 1974; Mamdani 1976; Parpart 1983; Roberts 1979; Sathyamurthy 1986; Stichter 1985; Turshen, 1977, 1984; Wallerstein and Martin 1979). Mining, railroad work, plantation work, and primary production facilities absorbed capital investment and became enclaves of development in an immense, underdeveloped continent. Just as these industries absorbed capital, they absorbed large quantities of labor from the rural areas, concentrating great numbers of male workers. The effect on these men and on their families is described well by Lesley Doyal (1981) in *The Political Economy of Health:*

> The migrant labor system affected Africans' lives in many fundamental ways. Whatever the miseries of industrialization in Britain, it was usually possible for workers to keep their families together, but this has not been the case in third world countries. In Tanganyika, for example, male workers were typically recruited from designated labour supply areas great distances from the centres of economic activity. This entailed prolonged family separations which had serious physical and psychological repercussions for all concerned. The populations of African towns 'recruited by migration' were characterized by a heavy preponderance of men living in intolerably insecure and depressing conditions and lacking the benefits of family life or other customary supports (p. 114).

Through the migrant labor process and the enclave development system, the African workers, largely male, concentrated at the site of industry, agriculture, or extraction. In many cases the resulting depletion of males from the rural villages and farms caused a marked deterioration in women's ability to carry on alone and to provide for their families. A reduction in labor available to do farm work resulted from the men's employment-related migration (Stichter 1985). The dependency ratio (the number of very young and very old) increased in the rural areas and in the labor reserves (Murray 1981). In many cases, women began to change crops; although these crops were prolific and could feed many mouths, with the added benefit of requiring less labor input, they were largely carbohydrates rather than protein. Cassava is such a crop (Stichter 1985). This change in cropping patterns led to protein deficiencies and compromised the immune systems of persons living in the labor reserves (McCance and Rutishauser 1975). In fact, some studies show that simply the increased labor demand on women, with the reduction in time to attend to their children's nutritional concerns, leads to declines in children's nutritional status whether or not cropping patterns and crops have changed (Vaughn and Moore 1988).

Lack of labor to assist in land clearing produced overcropping of already-cleared areas, deterioration of the land, and loss of fertility. The loss of fertility also contributed to a reduction in yield, which further encouraged the growing of higher-yield crops on poorer soils, although these crops were less nutritious than in the past (Stichter 1985). A "bachelor wage" system usually produced little money income for migrant laborers to send back to a family on the labor reserve; thus the labor reserve subsidized other sectors of the economy to its own detriment (Stichter 1985). This cycle continues in a process of declining agriculture.

In addition, and particularly in recent decades, many unmarried rural women saw no means of adequate support for a family and thus emigrated to the city at a young age (see Murray 1981; Stichter 1985). Family conflict and separation also have caused many young women to migrate to the cities and to concentrations of male labor. Unfortunately, however, very few women have found wage labor or work of any kind (Doyal 1981, p. 116; Stichter 1985); there is little wage employment for women in the developing African economy (Stichter 1985, pp. 144–78). Some—perhaps many—of these women become prostitutes and enter the marginal or secondary labor market in the areas surrounding the large concentrations of men and development (Doyal 1981; Stichter 1985).

The combination of the migrant labor system with a heavy prepondernance of male laboring jobs and long familial separations caused a breakdown in family and sexual patterns in central and southern Africa (Murray 1981). An explosion of both prostitution and sexually transmitted diseases (STDs) in these populations occurred well before the

AIDS virus made an appearance (Bennett 1975; Brown, Zacarias, and Aral 1985; Rampen 1978; Sajiwandani and Babbo 1987; Sathyamurthy 1986). As Doyal 1981 states:

> . . . venereal disease became—and still remains—a major health problem in many parts of the third world where it was previously unknown. It is hardly surprising that the disruption of the economic and personal foundations of family life led to the disintegration of long-established marital and sexual patterns. In this context, the growth of prostitution represented one form of adaptation to the intolerable strains faced by men and women alike. In the case of male migrants, the absence of their wives was compounded by the fact that their new environment was almost exclusively masculine. This unequal sex ratio made it difficult for men to establish stable sexual liaisons with women, and encouraged prostitution. For the women involved, prostitution was usually a matter of sheer economic necessity . . . The structure of the colonial economy made it virtually impossible for women to sell their labour . . . most were compelled to live off the low wages of male workers. Often this involved either formal or informal prostitution (p. 115–16).

The development of the migrant labor and industrial pattern led to serious health consequences, particularly to an epidemic of sexually transmitted diseases in central and southern Africa. This pattern was clear even in 1981, when Doyal wrote the above (Osoba 1981).

In addition to the "pull" effect of industrialization and the migrant labor markets and the "push" effect of declining agriculture with reduced labor inputs, a "push" effect was produced by capital's takeover of African agriculture (Loewenson 1988; Sanders and Davies 1988). As in many Third World countries, the best and most fertile lands are used by capital to produce agricultural goods for export. Local food production is marginalized on poor land; rural labor needs become seasonal; as a result of large-scale monoculture and mechanization, rural "overpopulation" is "pushed" into urban slum areas. In these areas poor health, disease, and malnutrition abound. Employment is difficult, especially for women; family life may become difficult (Stichter 1985). The result, as with the "pull" effect of large capital developments, is the social creation of a population especially vulnerable to venereal disease and particularly to AIDS (P. Epstein and Packard 1987, pp. 10–17).

As a consequence of the migrant labor pattern and the capitalist takeover of rural African agriculture, AIDS had a ready population that suffered from an unusually high level of sexually transmitted diseases. Because of residual lesions and injury, the higher incidence of previous venereal disease (especially if untreated) increases the likelihood of contracting AIDS (Quinn et al. 1986, pp. 957–58; Stamm, Handsfield, Rompalo, Ashley, Roberts, and Corey 1988).

The manner in which labor is handled in migrant labor situations makes the resulting epidemics much worse. Such a labor system, in which migrants recruited from rural areas surround industrial and extractive developments, does not require care for the health or the safety of the working population. As long as labor power is in surplus in the rural and urban areas because of the expansion of capitalist agriculture and the existence of the labor reserve, injured or incapacitated workers can be replaced easily by subsequent migrants. Workers who no longer can work under such conditions simply return to their villages (Doyal 1981, p. 119). Further, workers' ability to combat poor working conditions and to demand health benefits from employment is severely compromised because migrant laborers are historically difficult to unionize or to organize for resistance to employers (Stichter 1985).

Urban slum dwellers, who lack medical care because of unemployment, also return home regularly when ill, carrying urban disease back to their rural villages (Doyal 1981). Thus a woman who is a prostitute and who becomes ill is very likely to return to her home village to be cared for by relatives.

In the case of sexually transmitted diseases and many other illnesses, this return home has tragic consequences. Tuberculosis and STDs are carried back to the village, infecting areas where they have not been seen before and striking populations that lack resistance or previous exposure. "Whether or not these migrants survived their diseases, the diseases invariably survived them, often spreading rapidly among an increasingly susceptible population" (Doyal 1981, p. 119).

Therefore there is little question that AIDS

strikes a population which is not only susceptible to sexually transmitted diseases but which is also structured socially to hasten the transmission of the HIV-1 virus. Such structuring of a population to make it vulnerable to STDs is an integral part of the peripheral status of eastern, central, and southern Africa. As argued above, the social structuring of the family unit and labor migrancy are related closely to partial proletarianization and incomplete separation from the land, characteristics of a peripheral labor force (Friedman 1984; Martin 1984; J. Smith 1984; Wallerstein 1984; Wallerstein and Martin 1979).

Past data on prevalence of sexually transmitted diseases show clearly that the pattern of STD spread described above has occurred. For instance, in studies completed in the 1960s and early 1970s, the primary risk factor for gonorrhea in eastern Africa was male labor migrancy, with a pool of infection in the female prostitute population (Bennett 1962; Verhagen and Gemert 1972). The pattern of spread from urban and labor concentrations to rural areas also was confirmed for gonorrhea (Bennett 1964). Prevalence data also establish that higher rates of STDs are present around labor concentrations.

An especially well-documented example in west Africa may suffice to show this relationship. In Cameroon, migrant workers "were and are considered to be a major cause of a high incidence of venereal disease among the population in the plantation environs" (DeLancey 1978, p. 172). This is the area of labor concentration in Cameroon; DeLancey regards the return of migrant laborers to rural areas as a problem in this area. Further, a 1949 health survey showed a 4.2 percent rate of gonorrhea infection in rural areas far from these labor concentrations, in contrast to 13.1 percent and 10.4 percent rates in areas directly surrounding the concentrations. In 1948 a 21 percent rate of gonorrhea infection was found in the heart of the migrant labor district in Cameroon (DeLancey 1978, p. 179). Labor migrancy in west Africa has declined since the 1940s, however, so this pattern may no longer be in evidence in that area.

Urethral stricture is a common long-term result of STD, particularly of gonorrhea. A spatial mapping of this condition for Zambia, in east central Africa, shows that it is most prevalent in the copper belt of Zambia, the primary labor concentration area. The second highest area of prevalence is in the northeast of Zambia, a labor reserve area (Kibukamusoke 1975). Further, the condition is much more prevalent in Uganda in the labor concentration area: it forms a half moon around Kampala and Lake Victoria, and shows secondary concentrations in the West Nile district and in Kigezi and Ankole. Migrant labor is drawn from these areas into the Kampala area (Kibukamusoke 1975).

Thus the pattern of the eastern and central African labor market—a migrant labor system based on labor reserves, surpluses of laborers, and a laboring population separated only partially from the land—may account for many of the differences between the AIDS epidemic in the United States in the African population. In Africa as in North America, AIDS required a population that was vulnerable to sexually transmitted diseases. In each case the virus first made its inroads into these populations. In Africa, a population structured socially by capitalist agriculture and a labor market created in its present form by dependency development gave AIDS the foothold it required. The prevalence of malnutrition, malaria, measles, and other diseases that resulted from the collapse of local food production and from Africa's dependency development pattern has resulted in a population whose health is continually compromised. Large numbers of persons have immune systems weakened not only by diseases but also by malnutrition, a condition which also may help to set the stage for AIDS infection (P. Epstein and Packard 1987; Hall and Langlands 1975; McCance and Rutishauser 1975). In North America, a gay population that had had a sexually transmitted disease problem for at least a decade was the foothold for the HIV virus (Altman 1986; Shilts 1987). In each case the initial stages of the epidemic were determined by the population in which the virus was able to establish itself. In both cases it appears that although these populations affect profoundly the perceptions of AIDS, the HIV-1 virus will not confine itself to these sites. They are simply the populations that were most vulnerable at the outset.

This model for the spread of the AIDS epidemic relies on the scientific understanding of the HIV-1 virus and of its transmission capabilities. We know that this virus is spread in much the same way as hepatitis B, by body fluids and particularly during sexual activity. We also know that previously untreated STDs, especially when they may cause breaks in the skin or ulcers, increase the likelihood of infection on exposure to HIV-1 (Schoub et al. 1988; Simonsen 1988; Stamm et al. 1988). Both in Africa and in the United States, large numbers of sexual partners increase the possibility of infection with HIV-1 and the resulting development of AIDS (Carswell 1987; Curran 1985).

This model of the AIDS epidemic in eastern and central Africa also relies on an understanding of historic patterns of development in this area. The context of dependency development, combined with studies of medical and population geography for the region, gives an outline of the probable high-prevalence areas in countries in east Africa and indicates which groups in the population will have high prevalence and high incidence rates of HIV-1 infection. The following section will discuss in greater detail the implications of this model in medical and population geography and in population subgroups by presenting a series of hypotheses regarding the prevalence rates of HIV-1 infection, primarily in Uganda and in neighboring Burundi and Rwanda in eastern Africa.

AIDS: THE PATTERN OF AN EPIDEMIC IN AFRICA

If the model that was presented above its valid for the AIDS epidemic in eastern and central Africa, the pattern in which the epidemic appears should show some evidence of the expected modes of transmission. In other words, if the epidemic occurs geographically in areas with high concentrations of male migrant labor, and particularly among males and females who have high levels of heterosexual activity, then high prevalence or incidence rates should appear first geographically in areas where labor is concentrated. Further, two population groups in these areas should be affected: the male migrant laborers themselves and their partners, usually female prostitutes living near the enclave of development. Thus a high rate of infection in these two groups would fit the model.

Further, if the spread of the HIV-1 virus occurs through the return of male migrant laborers and female prostitutes to their villages due to illness, the second geographic sites that should begin to show high rates of infection are those areas in eastern and central Africa known as labor reserves. If we assume that the rural areas are infected with HIV-1 after the labor concentration areas are infected, these rural areas should show lower prevalence rates than the labor concentration areas. Yet the labor reserves—the migrant labor pool areas—should show higher rates of infection than surrounding rural areas which do not provide migrant labor. Thus prevalence of HIV-1 in the areas from which migrants are drawn by contract in order to provide the workers necessary for production should lag somewhat behind the areas where these workers labor. When the workers return home carrying HIV-1, it is assumed in this model that they will pass the infection on to their partners and to others after their return.

The prostitutes from these areas of male migrant labor concentration also tend to return home when illness prevents them from continuing their work. This trend may be less definite because prostitutes are not dismissed formally. They may continue prostitution activities and delay returning home, even though they are quite ill. They may be able to continue working and generating some income, although their capacity may be reduced considerably.

The brief discussion in this paper concerning the historical, social, and economic development of eastern, central, and southern Africa points in a number of directions for further research and study. As a start, available data concerning HIV-1 seropositivity and AIDS prevalences can be used to test the pattern of the epidemic. Do the available data on seropositivity and AIDS prevalence fit the pattern that would result from the description presented above? We can use this description to generate the following 14 hypotheses based on the above argument:

1. Geographically, areas of migrant labor concentration should show high prevalence rates of HIV-1 infection. These sites include mining areas, commercial plantations, and some large cities.
2. Geographic areas from which migrant laborers are drawn should show high rates of prevalence for HIV-1 infection.
3. The prevalence of HIV-1 infection in labor reserves should be higher than in

rural areas that do not form labor reserves.

4. Geographic areas from which young women migrate to become prostitutes should show high prevalence levels of HIV-1 infection. These rates should be higher than for other rural areas. Again, the rate of HIV infection in rural labor reserves should be higher than in areas of stable commodity production by peasants.
5. Because of earliest transmission by migrant labor to the rural labor reserves, HIV-1 seropositivity should appear earlier in these areas than in surrounding rural areas or in areas of stable peasant agricultural commodity production. This difference may be due to temporal differences in transmission as well as to reduction in the number of sexual partners once a migrant laborer returns home.
6. The prevalence rates for areas where migrant labor is concentrated should be somewhat higher than for the rural labor reserves, the areas from which migrant labor is drawn.
7. HIV-1 seropositivity should appear earliest in the areas where migrant labor is concentrated, such as mining areas, plantations, and cities.
8. Migrant laborers themselves should show higher rates of infection than other groups in the population.
9. For male migrant workers, the rate of HIV-1 seropositivity may increase with length of labor contract or time away from the family.
10. There should be a lower rate of prevalence among permanent migrant laborers who are allowed to take their families to the job site.
11. Prostitutes concentrated in areas where male migrant labor is located should show higher rates of infection than other women in the population. Further, prostitutes located in areas of migrant labor concentration should show higher levels of HIV-1 seropositivity and AIDS than prostitutes in areas migrant labor does not concentrate. These rates should bias the age and marital status data concerning women who are infected with HIV-1. Therefore infected women should be younger and more often single than infected men.
12. Higher prevalences and earlier occurrences should appear among those who previously suffered sexually transmitted diseases (STDs). This population is constructed socially and biologically to transmit these diseases.
13. There should be lower prevalences among persons on the rural labor reserves who have not migrated for laboring contracts, and among their families.
14. HIV-1 seropositivity should evidence a complex pattern of spread. The epidemic will not spread from rural areas to the city, as would be posited by a disease which is endemic for long periods of time in rural areas and which breaks out into the larger population because of social disruption. Such a pattern should appear earlier and in higher prevalences in rural areas. Rather, HIV-1 seropositivity should evidence a movement from areas of labor concentration to rural labor reserves and outward from these latter foci of infection to the general rural community. The degree of movement of HIV-1 seropositivity and AIDS into a labor reserve should depend on the quantity of migrant labor employed from that reserve, the length of time of contracts or absences, the age of laborers who migrate, the type of employment to which migrants are moving, the number of women leaving for the city and the work they obtain, and the rate of return of ill women and migrant laborers. The direction of movement should depend on where most of the migrant labor originates, where recruiting occurs, and from what areas women are leaving. In other words, numerous factors that influence the sexual and migratory patterns in eastern, central, and southern Africa will affect the spread and transmission of HIV-1 seropositivity and AIDS. The principal organizing factor, however, is the fact of labor migrancy and the labor reserve. From this central point one can begin to investigate the variations and the complex movement of the epidemic.

DATA AND PREVALENCE SURVEYS

Do the available data support the 14 hypotheses presented above? Do the actual AIDS prevalence and seropositivity studies conducted in eastern, central, and southern Africa conform to these hypotheses? Caution is advised because, as already mentioned, data are sometimes unreliable and fragmentary. In addition, as mentioned earlier, the ELISA test for HIV-1 immune response may be much less reliable in Africa than elsewhere (Biggar et al. 1985). Of course, in Uganda the use of the WHO case definition (Berkeley, Okware, and Naamara 1989), which does not rely on laboratory work, makes this unreliability less of a problem.

Further, the process of HIV-1 transmission, which was outlined above, is dynamic. Much of the data concerns prevalence, which can be examined spatially or geographically; incidence data are relatively scarce. Prevalence data are inherently static, not dynamic, and we can only infer the dynamic process from the static data. It is rare, however, to find truly adequate data in social science; therefore let us pursue the available data to see if they agree with the above model and with the hypotheses that the model has generated. In the discussion that follows refer to Figure 1, a map of Uganda, including district names. See also Figure 2 which shows the labor concentration areas and the labor reserve areas in Uganda. This map is derived from historical accounts and migration data from the Ugandan census (Kabera 1982; Mamdani 1976; Gimui 1982).

FIGURE 1. Map of Uganda

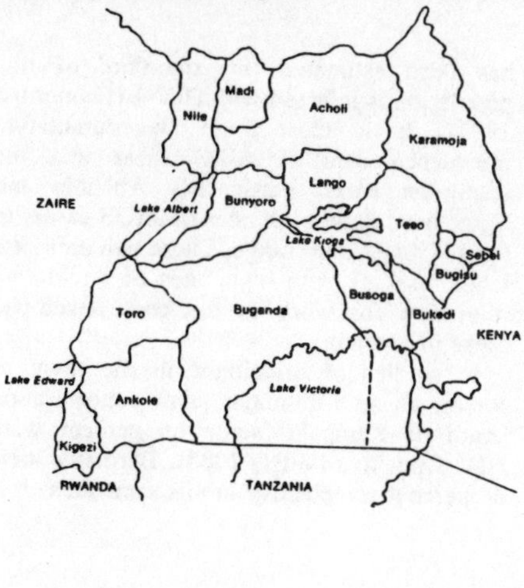

Hypotheses 1, 2, 3, 4, 5, 6 & 7

These hypotheses concern the geographical and temporal distributional evidence for the pattern of HIV-1 transmission outlined above. Geographical distribution is capable of eliciting transmission patterns in some diseases (Hall and Langlands 1975; Hunter 1974; McGlashan 1972; Meade 1980; Pyle 1979).

It is clear that AIDS cases and HIV infection generally have been most serious in cities in Uganda and in much of eastern Africa (Berkley et al. 1989; Biggar 1986; Economist 1987; Georges et al. 1987; Harden 1986; Harden 1987; Mann, Francis, Quinn, et al. 1986; Mugerwa and Giraldo 1987; Mugerwa, Widy-Wirski, and Okwake 1987; Van de Perre 1984). These are areas of labor concentration. This conclusion is also confirmed by cumulative prevalence data from Uganda (see Figure 3), which establish that the highest prevalence rate of AIDS in Uganda is contained in the half-moon area along the lakeshore of Lake Victoria, particularly in the Masaka and Kampala-Entebbe areas (Berkley et al. 1989, p. 83).

The problem with these data is that they reflect not only the possible reality of the epidemic but also the availability of medical facilities in these regions of Africa. Most medical facilities that are capable of recognizing and diagnosing AIDS in central and eastern Africa are concentrated almost exclusively in cities (Hall and Langlands 1975; Navarro 1974). Thus these areas will show a predominant number of diagnosed cases. Individuals from rural areas may not even be able to travel to the cities for diagnosis and may be either misdiagnosed or not treated at all. It has been noted frequently that AIDS patients in eastern Africa are more well-to-do than the average population (Georges et al., 1987; Harden 1987; Van de Perre 1984). This finding also may reflect the comparative ease with which the most affluent classes are able to enter the medical system in contrast to poorer or rural individuals.

In Uganda, however, it has been claimed that the prevalence of HIV-1 seropositivity does not seem as high in Kampala as elsewhere (Economist 1987), and that the southwest areas of the country have higher HIV-1 prevalence rates. This conclusion seems to be refuted by recent, more comprehensive studies and cumulative prevalence data (Carswell 1987; Berkley et al. 1989) (see

FIGURE 2. Labor Concentrations and Labor Reserves in Uganda

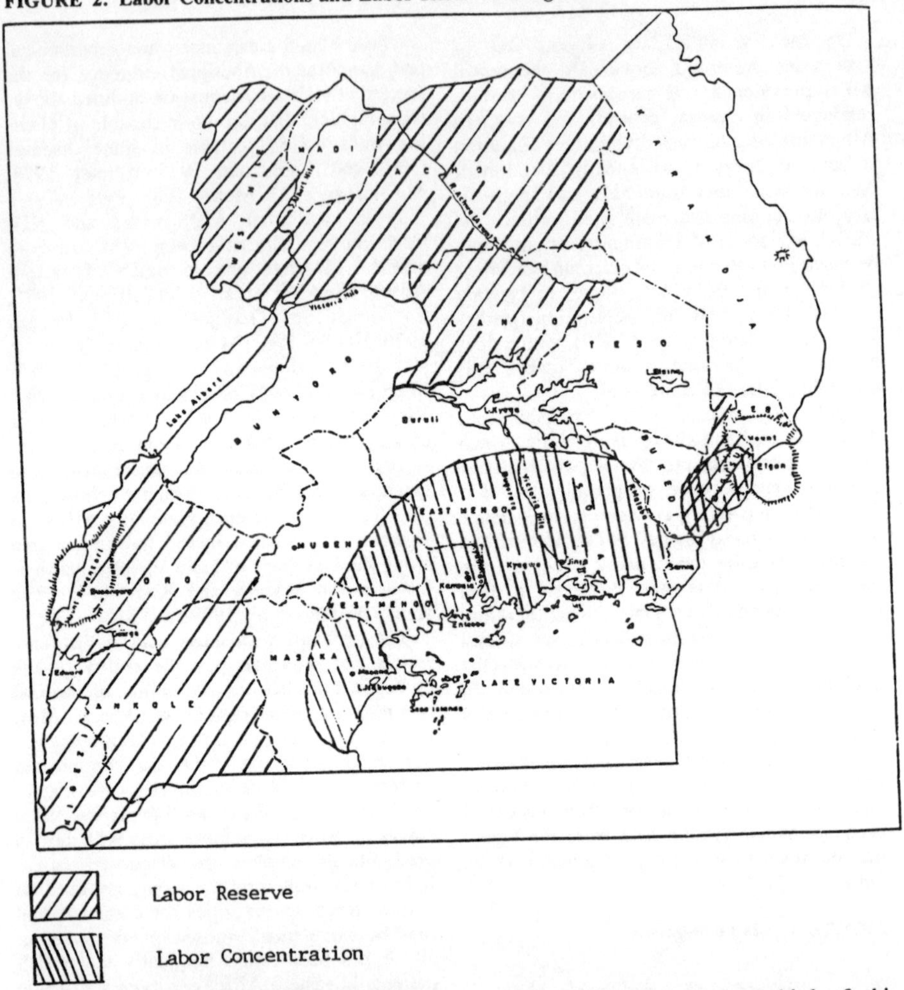

Figure 3). In general, rural residents, particularly in the peasant farming areas of central Uganda, seem to have a rather low rate of HIV-1 seropositivity and AIDS (Berkley et al., 1989; Carswell 1987; Harden 1987; Van de Perre 1984). In Rwanda and Zaire the infection rate in the country is far lower than the very high rate in the cities (Specter 1986). We can say, however, that rural southwestern Uganda appears to have very high prevalences of AIDS cases and HIV-1 infection (Berkley et al. 1989; Economist 1987; Serwadda, Seqankambo, Carswell, Bayley, Tedder, Weiss, Mugerwa, Lwegaba, Kirya, Downing, Clayden, and Dalgleish 1985). It has been estimated that one-third of this population is infected with HIV-1 (Economist 1987). It is clear from the cumulative prevalence data of AIDS cases that the southwest areas, particularly Anchole and Toro, have quite high rates of AIDS cases, in the 11-50/100,000 range. These two areas are labor reserves with high rates of circulating migration for work in the core developed areas in Uganda.

In studies of prostitutes in the town of Rakai, an area of major labor concentration south of Kampala, some 86 percent were HIV-1 positive (WHO 1988). Barmaids were 80 percent seropositive in this same area. It is

FIGURE 3. AIDS Cumulative Prevalence by District in Uganda

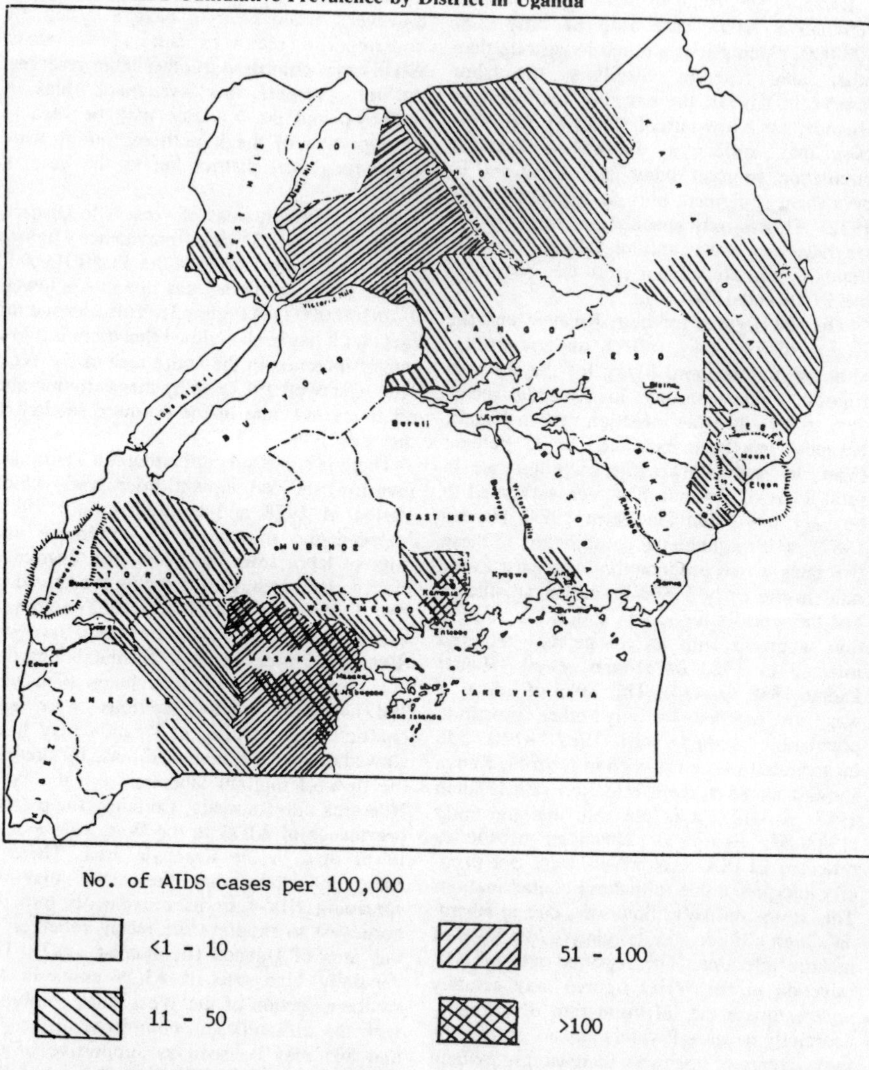

easy to see the high cumulative rates of AIDS cases in this area on the map of Uganda (see figure 3). In fact, this area south of Kampala has one of the highest rates of AIDS in Uganda, comparable to the Kampala-Entebbe area (see Figure 3).

The countries of Burundi and Rwanda have not established an AIDS surveillance system such as the one in place in Uganda. However, the WHO has collected some cumulative figures for AIDS cases in these two countries. These figures were accumulated until 31 December 1988 and they establish that Burundi's prevalence rate of AIDS cases is 13/100,000, with a total of 1408 cases of AIDS (WHO 1989, p. 113). This rate is comparable to the high rate found in Ugandan labor reserves such as the West Nile, Lango, Acholi, Bugisu, Toro, and eastern Ankole. Further, the data show that Burundi has the second highest national cumulative prevalence rate of AIDS cases in Africa, higher than the overall rate for Uganda (WHO 1989, p. 113).

Rwanda, according to these figures, has a cumulative AIDS case rate of only 2.8/100,000, placing it at a much lower rate than other labor reserves. Similarly, the labor reserve in Kigezi, the extreme southwest of Uganda, has a low rate of 1-10/100,000. This case may reflect a diminished rate of circulating migrant labor and increases in permanent settlement outside Kigezi (Kabera 1982). This is only speculation, however, as we have no really accurate figures for the trends in migratory labor from this district in the 1970s and 1980s.

The low figures for both Rwanda and the Kigezi district may reflect underreporting, although this is more likely for the Rwanda figures. Underreporting in Rwanda seems very likely since the infection rate in Kigali, Rwanda, has been estimated at 25 percent (Van De Perre 1984). The infection rate in rural areas of Rwanda has been estimated to be very low (Van De Perre 1984; Harden 1987), so it might be the combination of these two rates which produce the somewhat lower rate. In the early 1980s Rwandan prostitutes had the world's highest infection rate among this subgroup with an 80 percent reported infected in 1983–84 (Mann, et al. 1986a; Padian 1988, p. 414). This level of infection was not reached by any other prostitute population studied until 1987 when 535 incarcerated women studied in Nairobi, Kenya showed an 85 percent infection rate (Padian 1988, p. 414). It is possible that the early (1983–84) figure for Rwandan prostitutes reflected ELISA tests which were not properly interpreted due to malaria contamination. This seems unlikely, however, due to Rwanda's high altitude and its relative low level of malaria infection. The reported rate of HIV infection in the WHO figures may actually underestimate the infection rate in Rwanda, especially because Rwanda has not shown the same degree of openness increasingly evident among other Eastern African nations with regard to AIDS.

Underreporting seems less likely in the Kigezi district, since the area has been served (at least in the 1960s, the most recent report) by two government hospitals, two mission hospitals, two health centers and a number of dispensary/maternity units (Hall and Langlands 1975, p. viii). This might be an area for further research. However, the surveillance system in Uganda is passive, not legally required, and may underreport cases (Berkeley et al. 1989, p. 82). The Kigezi District, however, would have to have a systematic underreporting bias to explain its lower rate of AIDS cases compared to other labor reserves. At the present, this systematic bias is unknown and the low rate may be seen as unsupportive of the hypotheses put forward on geographical distribution in the case of Kigezi.

In the southern areas of West Nile District, cumulative AIDS case prevalence figures establish that the rate is in the 11-50/100,000 range. In the northern areas, the rate is lower, 1-10/100,000 (see Figure 3). This, despite the fact that it has been claimed that there is a low rate of infection in the entire area of the West Nile (Carswell 1987). Why this variation and relatively low rate in the northern section of the West Nile?

There is some indication that the Tanzanian invasion and subsequent civil war, which started in 1978 and continued until 1985, impeded the movement of commerce and migrant labor from the West Nile district to the Kampala area, thus delaying the spread of HIV-1 (Avirgan and Honey 1982; Carswell 1987; Mamdani 1988). Further, the Nile River itself often forms a "formidable barrier to communication" and interchange (Carswell 1987). Unlike many previous wars and conflicts, the fighting in Uganda may have slowed down the spread of disease by slowing the flow of migrant laborers from the West Nile area into Kampala. Certainly the present prevalence of AIDS in the West Nile area is lower than in the Kampala area. There is some indication that the army may be spreading HIV-1 in its movements into the northwest to suppress the recent rebellion in this area of Uganda (Economist 1987). The generally high rate of AIDS cases in the southern section of the West Nile, combined with the difficulties in commerce in the 70s and 80s may be seen as supportive of the hypotheses which we have advanced for temporal and spatial distribution of the AIDS epidemic.

Many cite Acholi in central-northern Uganda as the leading area of migratory labor (Kabera 1982; Mamdani 1976). Acholi's cumulative rate of AIDS cases is second only to that of the labor concentrations around Kampala-Entebbe and Masaka (see Figure 1), with a 51-100/100,000 rate in the western sections of Acholi. The western section of Lango and the eastern section of Acholi also contain unusually high cumulative rates of AIDS at 11-50/100,000. Both of these findings support the hypotheses on spatial and temporal distribution of AIDS.

In eastern sections of Uganda, a high rate of cumulative AIDS case prevalence, 11-50/100,000, occurs in Bugisu area, also a major labor reserve and a source of migrant labor. This high rate extends northward into the Karamoja District which is not a major labor reserve area. In general, however, these results are supportive of hypotheses one through seven.

It is difficult to determine if the syndrome occurred earlier in the urban labor concentrations than in the labor reserves, but one can argue that the higher cumulative prevalence rates in the Kampala-Entebbe and Masaka labor concentrations are consistent with an earlier appearance. Certainly, it can be argued that AIDS seems to have had a longer time to reach high epidemic levels in these labor concentrations.

When considering countries other than Uganda, Burundi, and Rwanda, in areas of labor concentration such as the copper mines of Zambia and Zaire, the evidence is consistent with a higher rate of spread of HIV-1 (Harden 1987). In Lusaka, the capital of Zambia, the rate for blood donors was 15 percent in 1986. In the northern copper belt areas, the rate of HIV-1 seropositivity among blood donors was 13 percent (Harden 1987; Melbye, Mads, Bayley, Manuwele, Clayden, Blattner, Tedder, Njelesani, Mukelabai, Bowa, Levin, Weiss, and Biggar 1986). Zambia has always had a clearer pattern of labor concentrations and labor reserves than Uganda, because the copper belt has dominated the economic development of that country (Kay 1967; Mamdani 1976; Parpart 1983; Roberts 1979). Unfortunately, we have little data from labor reserve areas in Zambia to compare with the data from the copper belt. In Zaire it is clear that the rural prevalence of HIV-1 is low (Nzilambi et al., 1988) and that urban prevalence, at least in Kinshasa, is quite high (Mann et al., 1986a). Hardly any data exist in Zaire, however, to allow comparison of these results with those in labor reserve areas.

Hypotheses 8, 9, and 10

Migrant laborers themselves should show higher rates of HIV-1 infection than others in the population; these data should correlate with family factors and with length of contracts. As with the other hypotheses, data on this point are scarce. There are only two studies that concentrate on migrant laborers in eastern, southern, and central Africa; we may use national data to draw some conclusions concerning this group.

In 1986, 74 truck drivers for a large freight company in Kampala (Uganda) were tested for HIV-1. Some 55.9 percent of the drivers were seropositive (Carswell 1987; Economist 1987). The overall HIV-1 infection rate for Kampala was estimated in 1986 to be approximately 10 percent (Harden 1986). Thus, we can say that in Uganda truck drivers have a much higher rate of infection than others in the population. These drivers and their mates, known as "turnboys," were either Ugandan or Kenyan nationals and had large numbers of sexual partners, particularly prostitutes (Carswell 1987).

In South Africa, the country with the most highly "developed" system of migrant labor, we might expect clearer findings in regard to HIV-1 seropositivity. South Africa has a very systematic labor reserve policy, termed a "homelands" policy; workers usually are banned from living with their families near where they contract to work. Thus the familial separation is enforced more strictly in South Africa, particularly in the mining regions.

In a study of South African migrant miners, 30,000 miners were selected randomly for HIV-1 testing. Some labor reserve areas and some countries showed a seropositive rate in the migrant labor group as high as four percent. In 1987, however, South Africa reported an overall infection rate of 0.1 per cent, with only 46 cases of full-blown AIDS. Therefore it would appear that the AIDS epidemic is concentrated in the migrant labor population in South Africa. This pattern is recognized by South African medical authorities (Ijsselmuiden et al. 1988; Sher 1986).

Finally, with regard to migrant laborers, the countries of Rwanda and Burundi, particularly the former, seem to have a serious problem with AIDS infection (Biggar 1987; Brunet and Ancelle 1985; Harden 1987; Mann et al. 1988a and b; Quinn et al. 1986; WHO 1989). It is noteworthy that these two mountainous countries send massive numbers of migrant laborers to the labor concentration areas of Uganda. In fact, they constitute labor reserves for Uganda; some 380,000 Rwandans and 140,000 Rundi have lived in Uganda. These individuals come to Uganda as migrant laborers and usually are only temporary residents. A large proportion of the migrant laborers in the areas around Kampala come from these two countries (Hall and Langlands 1975, pp. 7–8). The high cumulative prevalence of AIDS cases in Burundi and the likelihood of high prevalences in Rwanda argue strongly for the hypothesis that AIDS prevalence will be high among these migrant laborers.

It is impossible to determine from these data whether the earliest cases of AIDS in South Africa or in central or eastern Africa occurred among migrant laborers. If we assume, however, that the AIDS epidemic is new in many of these areas (see Carswell, Sewankambo, Lloyd, and Downing 1986), we may say that the prevalence data indicate where the epidemic began. Thus although cases may show up earlier in isolated groups in South Africa, the prevalence among migrant laborers argues for an early appearance in this group. Unfortunately, there are hardly any data on other migrant laborers or on their family and sexual patterns; nor are these data correlated with length of contract, working conditions, and other factors. This lack of data militates against truly definitive conclusions.

Hypothesis 11

One of the best-documented facts about the AIDS epidemic in Africa is its incredibly high prevalence rate among prostitutes in all countries. Prostitutes are at high risk for HIV-1 infection (Mann et al. 1988b) and are recognized world-wide as transmitters of HIV-1 (Carael, Van de Perre, Lepage, Allen, Nsengumuremyui, Van Goethem, Ntahorutaba, Nzaramba and Clumeck 1988; Day 1988; Hudson, Hennis, Kataaha, Lloyd, Moore, Sutehall, Whetstone, Wreghitt and Karpas 1988; Padian 1988). In different areas of the world the practice of prostitution varies from the United States where prostitutes develop a professionalization associated with "marked distance between their working and private lives (Day 1988, p. 421)," to the much more informal situation in Sub-Saharan Africa, where prostitution is difficult to define (Day 1988, p. 424).

Rates of infection among some prostitute groups range from 27 percent in Kinshasa, Zaire to 66 percent in Nairobi, Kenya and 88 percent in Butare, Rwanda (Mann, Francis, Quinn, et al. 1986). Overall infection rates in Rwanda are approximately 25 percent in Kigali, although rural infection rates are almost zero (Harden 1987; Van de Peere 1984). In a survey of 327 persons concluded in 1986 in the Central Africa Republic, 19 percent of prostitutes were seropositive, compared to a 4 percent overall infection rate for prostitutes in the Central Africa Republic (Specter 1986). In Tanzania a 1986 study of 225 prostitutes established a 29 percent seropositivity rate (Padian 1988, p. 414).

A study in Kenya showed a 4 percent rate of HIV-1 infection in Nairobi prostitutes in 1980 (Kreiss 1986). In 1987 the prevalence among 115 prostitutes in Nairobi was 65 percent. None of these women had been infected by HIV-1 only one year before. More than one-half of the new cases were attributed to the presence of genital ulcers and to the use of birth control pills, which apparently increase the probability of HIV-1 infection (Specter 1986).

The infection rate for women overall is consistently much lower than for prostitutes, as would be expected. The rate for sexually active persons of both sexes is approximately 20 percent (Mann et al. 1988, p. 85). In fact, women of childbearing age evidenced approximately a 10 to 15 percent infection rate in 1986 in Kampala, Uganda (Harden 1987). In one hospital in Kampala, 13 percent of 1,000 pregnant women were found to be HIV-1 seropositive in 1986. The same hospital showed a prevalence of 24 percent one year later among 170 pregnant women (Blaine 1987; Carswell 1987).

In all of the countries of this region, the mean age of men with seropositivity was greater than the mean age of seropositive women (Quinn 1987; Quinn et al. 1986; Mann, Francis, Quinn, et al. 1986a). Women account for most of the AIDS cases in the 20–29 age group in Kinshasa, Zaire. Most of the cases in the 40–49 and 50–59 age groups are male, although both of these groups generally contain smaller cohorts of AIDS cases than the 20–29 group (Mann, Francis, Quinn et al. 1986). Among those suffering from AIDS, women are more likely to be unmarried than men (Mann, Francis, Quinn, et al. 1986; Quinn 1987; Quinn et al. 1986).

All of this evidence points to a sexually transmitted disease in which the number of partners increases the risk of exposure to the infection (Carswell 1987; Clumeck et al. 1985; Kreiss 1986; Serwadda et al. 1985; Van de Perre 1984). Prostitutes, having large numbers of partners, are particularly at risk, but the pattern also fits the larger social model which has been advanced. Young women migrating to concentrations of male migrant labor become prostitutes in order to earn a living in an environment in which women are rarely employed in wage labor or other "legitimate" jobs.

Hypothesis 12

There is little question that persons who were previously infected by sexually transmitted diseases are at higher risk for HIV-1 infection because of the continued high number of sexual partners. (Pepin, Plummer, Brunham, Piot, Cameron, and Ronald 1989). This pattern may be evidence of a life situation, such as migrant laboring, which gives rise to an unstable sexual life. Further, as mentioned earlier, this group also increases its risk if sexually transmitted diseases are untreated or if lesions and ulcerations are present to allow infection more easily.

Hypothesis 13

Unfortunately, it is not possible to compare migrant workers with persons from the same labor reserve area who do not migrate because there seems to be little information reflecting tests of migrant workers themselves. Thus at present we have little ability to compare prevalence rates in this way.

Hypothesis 14

There is little question of the complex nature of the AIDS epidemic in central, eastern, and southern Africa (Biggar 1987; Carswell 1987). This complexity may blind observers to the existing patterns and without geographic, historic, and economic information about the region observers cannot understand the map of cumulative prevalences of AIDS.

Yet on the basis of much of the data dealing with urban and rural prevalences of HIV-1 seropositivity and AIDS cases, it is quite clear that a rural-to-urban spread pattern is not present. Urban infection rates are considerably higher than rural (Berkley et al. 1989; Carswell 1987; Carswell et al. 1986; Clumeck et al. 1985; Nzilambi et al. 1988; Peterson et al. 1987; Recene et al. 1987; Van de Perre 1984; Wender, Schneider, Gras, Fleming, Hunsmann, and Schmitz 1986). Therefore these data provide additional refutation of the argument that the HIV-1 virus was somehow endemic in rural Africa and then broke out into the broader community because of war and social disruption. Such an argument is not supported by the prevalence patterns we have seen here. It is much more logical to argue that this disease spread as a result of the complex migratory labor patterns in the eastern, central, and southern African economy. This would explain the complex pattern of cumulative AIDS prevalences seen in Uganda. The effects of these patterns on sexual practices and on the stability of the Africa family in these regions help to set up the pattern of AIDS epidemic, whose outline we can see from the scanty evidence available.

There seems to be substantial evidence, particularly in geographical cumulative prevalence data, as well as in HIV-1 seropositivity prevalence data among some specific population groups and geographical areas, that would support the model which we presented for the AIDS epidemic in Eastern Africa. In a rather striking manner, this evidence supports the concept that the HIV-1 virus, and the resulting AIDS, first struck the labor concentrations in Uganda and then moved outward to the labor reserves, carried by migrant laborers and prostitutes as they return to their birthplaces for care and assistance with illnesses consequent to infection with this virus.

CONCLUSION AND SUMMARY

The Western press and (to some extent) the Western scientific establishment have attempted to locate the origins of the HIV-1 virus, the biologically causative agent for AIDS, in Africa. In my opinion this attempt is based on a "victim-blaming" mentality and is fundamentally racist (Hunt 1988). The desire to see serious disease as coming from somewhere else, as an invasion, as a foreigner, is widespread (Sontag 1978, 1989; Brandt 1985). The "African origins" theory is based on many weak arguments; almost all have been disproved, including the genetic relationship of the HIV-1 virus to the simian variety of retrovirus found in the green monkey of equatorial Africa (see Gallo 1987; Mulder 1988). The "African origins" myth also arose because cases of AIDS were discovered earlier in Africa than in Europe or in North America. This argument, too, has been refuted decisively (see Carswell et al. 1986; Garry et al. 1988; Huminer, Rosenfeld, and Pitlik 1987; Hunt 1988).

One of the remaining props of the "African origins" myth is the pattern of spread of the disease in eastern, central, and southern Africa. The thesis of this paper provides an alternative explanation to the myth insofar as the myth is supported by the rapid or early spread of HIV-1 seropositivity in Africa. The historical pattern of sexually transmitted disease in eastern, central, and southern Africa is related intimately to dependency development and to migrant labor. It provides a much more adequate explanation for the rapidity and the complexities of the spread of HIV-1 seropositivity in Africa than do any assumptions about the origins of HIV-1. "African origins" theories contradict the evidence not only genetically and clinically, but also epidemiologically.

In the foregoing discussion an alternative epidemic pattern has been presented for AIDS in eastern, central, and southern Africa. This pattern has appeared in other areas where migrant labor markets were combined with dependency development and where workers were separated incompletely from the land; it has occurred, for instance, in western Africa. This pattern is rooted in migratory labor markets and is based in systematic economic, historic, and social development. Previous epidemics of STDs occurred in eastern, central, and southern Africa, resulting from the conjunction of the same historic, economic, and social factors. Those epidemics demonstrate medical/geographic and temporal patterns that are based in the movements of labor between concentrations of work and industry and the labor reserve.

The data on HIV-1 seropositivity and AIDS prevalence in Africa are sparse, scattered, small in scale, and often inaccurate. Yet even in view of these limitations, the available data on HIV-1 seropositivity and AIDS surveillance and testing in eastern, southern, and central Africa support the historical pattern and the labor market relationship in the AIDS epidemic now ravaging Africa. The highest prevalence rates of AIDS and HIV-1 seropositivity occur in the concentrations of industry and development in Uganda. In the rural labor reserves, particularly in Burundi, Rwanda, and southwestern Uganda, very high prevalence rates of HIV-1 seropositivity and AIDS also occur, but those rates are not as high as in the industrial and developed areas. Labor reserves in parts of Uganda where prevalence rates of seropositivity and AIDS are low show isolation from traditional labor migration because of war and social disruption over the last decade. The general rate of rural infection in eastern, southern, and central Africa is quite low.

There is some evidence of high rates of HIV-1 seropositivity among migrant laborers themselves. Certainly, prostitutes have very high rates of seropositivity and AIDS, as would be expected by most social theories of STDs. Further, those who suffered from previous STDs appear more likely to contract HIV-1 seropositivity and therefore AIDS. This interaction in the AIDS epidemic reinforces the historic patterns of STDs already occurring in this region in Africa.

In conclusion, the epidemic of HIV-1 seropositivity in Uganda and in other countries of the area is a social event, not simply a biological occurrence (see Stark 1977). Although a biological understanding of HIV-1 is necessary, it is inadequate. The epidemic of HIV-1 seropositivity and AIDS in Africa must be understood socially, in its historically specific context, or not at all.

REFERENCES

Altman, Dennis. 1986. *AIDS in the Mind of America*. Garden City, NY: Anchor/Doubleday.

Amin, Samir. 1976. *Unequal Development: An Essay on the Social Formations of Peripheral Capitalism*. New York: Monthly Review Press.

Anderson, R.M., R.M. May, and A.R. McLean. 1988. "Possible Demographic Consequences of AIDS in Developing Countries." *Nature*, March: 228.

Avirgan, Tony and Martha Honey. 1982. *War in Uganda: The Legacy of Idi Amin*. Westport, CT: Lawrence Hill.

Becker, W.B. 1986. "HTLV-III Infection in the RSA." *South African Medical Journal* Supplement, October 11:26–27.

Bennett, F.J. 1962. "The Social Determinants of Gonorrhea in an East African Town." *East African Medicine* 39(6):332–42.

———. 1964. "Gonorrhea: A Rural Pattern of Transmission." *East African Medical Journal* 41(4):163–67.

———. 1975. "Venereal Disease and Other Spirochaetal Diseases." Pp. 64–65 in *Uganda Atlas of Disease Distribution*, edited by S.A. Hall and B.W. Langlands. Nairobi: East African Publishing House.

Berkley, Seth, Samuel Okware, and Warren Naamara. 1989. "Surveillance for AIDS in Uganda." *AIDS*. 3:79–85.

Biggar, Robert J. 1986. "The AIDS Problem in Africa." *Lancet*, January 11:79–83.

———. 1987. "AIDS in Subsaharan Africa." *Cancer Detection and Prevention* Supplement 1:487–91.

Biggar, Robert J., Mads Melbye, Prem S. Sarin, Paul Demedts, Charles Delacollette, Wim J. Stevens, Paul L. Gigase, Luc Kestens, Anne J. Bodner, Leopold Paluku, and William A. Blattner. 1985. "ELISA HTLV Retrovirus Antibody Reactivity Associated with Malaria and Immune Complexes in Healthy Africans." *Lancet*, September 7:520–23.

Brandt, Allan M. 1985. *No Magic Bullet: A Social History of Venereal Disease in the United States since 1880*. New York: Oxford University Press.

Brown, Stuart T., Fernando R.K. Zacarias, and Sevgi O Aral. 1985. "STD Control in Less Developed Countries: The Time Is Now." *International Journal of Epidemiology* 14(4): 505–509.

Brunet, J.B. and R.A. Ancelle. 1985. "The International Occurrence of the Acquired Immunodeficiency Syndrome." *Annals of Internal Medicine* 103(5):670–74.

Carael, Michel, Philippe H. Van de Perre, Philippe H. Lepage, Susan Allen, Francois Nsenquimuremyi, Christian Van Goethem, Melanie Ntahorutaba, Didace Nzaramba and Nathan Clumeck. 1988. "Human Immunodeficiency Virus Transmission Among Heterosexual Couples in Central Africa." *AIDS*. 2:201–205.

Carswell, J. Wilson, 1987. "HIV Infection in Healthy Persons in Uganda." *AIDS* 1(4): 223–27.

Carswell, J. Wilson, N. Sewankambo, G. Lloyd, and R.G. Downing. 1986. "How Long Has the AIDS Virus Been in Uganda?" *Lancet*, May 24:1217.

Chavkin, Wendy (ed.). 1984. *Double Exposure: Women's Health Hazards on the Job and at Home*. New York: Monthly Review Press.

Clumeck, Nathan, Marjorie Robert-Guroff, Philippe Van de Perre, Andrea Jennings, Jean Sibomana, Patrick Demol, Sophie Cran, and Robert C. Gallo. 1985. "Seroepidemiological Studies of HTLV-III Antibody Prevalence among Selected Groups of Heterosexual Africans." *Journal of the American Medical Association* 254(18):2599–2602.

Crush, Jonathan. 1984. "Uneven Labour Migration in Southern Africa: Conceptions and Misconceptions." *South African Geographical Journal* 66(2):115–32.

Curran, James W. 1985. "The Epidemiology and Prevention of the Acquired Immunodeficiency Syndrome." *Annals of Internal Medicine* 103(5): 657–62.

Curran, James W., Meade Morgan, A.M. Hardy, H.W. Jaffe, W.M. Darrow, and W.R. Dowdle. 1985. "The Epidemiology of AIDS: Current Status and Future Prospects." *Science* 229: 1352–57.

Davidson, Basil. 1983. *Modern Africa*. New York: Longmans.

Day, Sophie. 1988. "Prostitute Women and AIDS: Anthropology." *AIDS*. 2:421–28.

DeLancey, Mark W. 1978. "Health and Disease on the Plantations of Cameroon, 1884–1939." Pp. 151–79 in *Disease in African History: An Introductory Survey and Case Studies*, edited by Gerald W. Hartwig and K. David Patterson. Durham: Duke University Press.

Doyal, Lesley, with Immogen Pennell. 1981. *The Political Economy of Health*. Boston: South End Press.

Economist. 1987. "In the Heart of the Plague." *The Economist*, March 21–27:45.

Epstein, Paul, and Randall Packard. 1987. "Ecology & Immunity." *Science for the People*, Jan/Feb:10–17.

Epstein, Samuel S. 1976. "The Political and Economic Basis of Cancer." *Technology Review* 78:1–7.

———. 1978. *The Politics of Cancer*. San Francisco: Sierra Club Books.

Eyer, Joseph. 1975. "Hypertension as a Disease of Modern Society." *International Journal of Health Services* 5(4):539–58.

———1977. "Prosperity as a Cause of Death." *International Journal of Health Services* 7: 125–50.

Eyer, Joseph and Peter Sterling. 1977. "Stress-Related Mortality and Social Organization." *Review of Radical Political Economy* 8(1):1–44.

Foster, John Bellamy. 1986. *The Theory of Monopoly Capitalism: An Elaboration of Marxian Political Economy*. New York: Monthly Review Press.

Frank, Andre G. 1967. *Capitalism and Underdevelopment in Latin America*. New York: Monthly Review Press.

Freund, William. 1984. *The Making of Contemporary Africa: The Development of African Society since 1800*. Bloomington: University of Indiana Press.

______. 1988. *The African Worker*. New York: Cambridge University Press.

Friedman, Kathie. 1984. "Households as Income-Pooling Units." Pp. 37–55 in *Households and the World Economy*, edited by Joan Smith, Immanuel Wallerstein, and Hans-Dieter Evers. Beverly Hills: Sage.

Gallo, Robert C. 1987. "The AIDS Virus." *Scientific American* 256(1):46–56.

Garry, Robert F., Marlys H. Witte, A. Arthur Gottlieb, Memory Elvin-Lewis, Marise S. Gottlieb, Charles L. Witte, Steve S. Alexander, William R. Cole, and William L. Drake. 1988. "Documentation of an AIDS Virus Infection in the United States in 1968." *Journal of the American Medical Association* 260(14): 2085–87.

Georges, Alain J., Paul M.V. Martin, Jean-Paul Gonzalez, Daniele Salaun, Christian C. Mathiot, Gerard Grezenguet, and Marie-Claude Georges-Courbot. 1987. "HIV-1 Seroprevalence and AIDS Diagnostic Criteria in Central African Republic." *Lancet*, December 5:1732–33.

Gimui, Kiboma. 1982. "Spatial Inequalities and Population Redistribution with Reference to Uganda." Pp. 146–49 in *Redistribution of Population in Africa*, edited by John I. Clarke and Laszek A. Kosinski. London: Heinemann.

Gugler, Josef. 1968. "The Impact of Labor Migration on Society and Economy in Sub-Saharan Africa: Empirical Findings and Theoretical Considerations." *African Social Research*, December 6:463–86.

Gutkind, Peter C.W. and Immanuel Wallerstein. 1976. *The Political Economy of Contemporary Africa*. Beverly Hills: Sage.

Hall, S.A. and B.W. Langlands. 1975. *Uganda Atlas of Disease Distribution*. Nairobi: East African Publishing House.

Harden, Blaine. 1986. "Uganda Battles AIDS Epidemic." *Washington Post*, June 2:A1, A18.

______. 1987. "AIDS Seen as Threat to Africa's Future." *Washington Post*, May 31:A1, A18.

Hilts, Philip J. 1987. *Washington Post*, "AIDS Takes Heavy Toll of African Children." October 10:A6

Hooper, Ed. 1987. "AIDS in Uganda." *African Affairs* 86(345):469–77.

Hopper, K. and Sally Guttmacher. 1979. "Rethinking Suicide: Notes toward a Critical Epidemiology." *International Journal of Health Services* 9:417–38.

Hudson, Christopher P., Anselm J.M. Hennis, Peter Kataaha, Graham Lloyd, A. Timothy Moore, Gordon M. Sutehall, Rod Whetstone, Tim Wreghitt and Abraham Karpas. 1988. "Risk Factors for the Spread of AIDS in Rural Africa: Evidence from a Comparative Seroepidemiological Survey of AIDS, Hepatitis B and Syphilis in Southwestern Uganda." *AIDS*. 2: 255–60.

Huminer, David, Joseph B. Rosenfeld, and Silvio D. Pitlik. 1987. "AIDS in the Pre-AIDS Era." *Reviews of Infectious Diseases* 9(6):1102–1108.

Hunt, Charles W. 1988. "Africa and AIDS: Dependent Development, Sexism and Racism." *Monthly Review* 39(9):10–22.

Hunter, John M. (ed.). 1974. *The Geography of Health and Disease*. Chapel Hill: University of North Carolina, Department of Geography.

Ijsselmuiden, C.B., M.H. Steinberg, G.N. Padayachee, B.D. Schoub, S.A. Strauss, E. Buch, J.C.A. Davies, C. DeBeer, J.S.S. Gear, and H.S. Hurwitz, 1988. "AIDS and South Africa—Towards a Comprehensive Strategy. Part I, Part II, and Part III." *South African Medical Journal* (73):461–64.

Kabera, John B. 1982. "Rural Population Redistribution in Uganda since 1900." Pp. 192–201 in *Redistribution of Population in Africa*, edited by John I. Clarke and Leszek A. Kosinski. London: Heinemann.

Karugire, S.R. 1980. *A Political History of Uganda*. Nairobi: Heinemann.

Kay, George. 1967. *A Social Geography of Zambia*. London: University of London Press.

Kibukamusoke, J.W. 1975. "Diseases of the Genito-Urinary System." Pp. 121–24 in *Uganda Atlas of Disease Distribution*, edited by S.A. Hall and B.W. Langlands. Nairobi: East African Publishing House.

Konotey-Ahulu, Felix I.D. 1987. "AIDS in Africa: Misinformation and Disinformation." *Lancet*, July 25:206–207.

Kreiss, Joan K. 1986. "AIDS Virus Infection in Nairobi Prostitutes: Spread of the Epidemic to East Africa." *New England Journal of Medicine* 314(7):414–18.

Langlands, B.W. 1975. "Introduction: The Geographic Basis to the Pattern of Disease in Uganda." Pp. 1–10 in *Uganda Atlas of Disease Distribution*, edited by S.A. Hall and B.W. Langlands. Nairobi: East African Publishing House.

Leys, Colin. 1975. *Underdevelopment in Kenya: The Political Economy of Neo-Colonialism*. Los Angeles: University of California Press.

Leys, R. 1974. "South African Gold Mining in 1974: 'The Gold of Migrant Labour.'" *African Affairs* 74 (295):196–208.

Loewenson, Rene. 1988. "Labour Insecurity and Health: An Epidemiological Study in Zimbabwe." *Social Science and Medicine* 27(7): 733–41.

Mamdani, Mahmood. 1976. *Politics and Class Formation in Uganda*. New York: Monthly Review Press.

______. 1988. "Uganda in Transition: Two Years of the NRA/NRM." *Third World Quarterly* 10(3):1155–81.

Mann, Jonathan and James Chin. 1988. "AIDS: A Global Perspective." *New England Journal of Medicine* 319(5):302–303.

Mann, Jonathan M., James Chin, Peter Piot, and Thomas Quinn. 1988. "The International Epidemiology of AIDS." *Scientific American* 259(4): 82–89.

Mann, Johathan M., Henry Francis, Farzin Davachi, Paola Baudoux, Thomas C. Quinn, Nzila Nzilambi, Ngaly Bosenge, Robert L. Colebunders, Peter Piot, Ndoko Kabote, Pangu Kaza Asila, Miatudila Malonga, and James W. Curran. 1986. "Risk Factors for Human Immunodeficiency Virus Seropositivity among Children 1–24 Months Old in Kinshasa, Zaire." *Lancet*, September 20:654–56.

Mann, Jonathan M., Henry Francis, Thomas Quinn, Pangu Kaza Asila, Ngaly Bosenge, Nzila Nzilambi, Kapita Bila, Muyembe Tamfum, Kalisa Ruti, Peter Piot, Joseph McCormick, and James W. Curran. 1986. "Surveillance for AIDS in a Central African City." *Journal of the American Medical Association* 255(23):3255–59.

Martin, William G. 1984. "Beyond the Peasant and Proletarian Debate: African Household Formation in South Africa." Pp. 151–67 in *Households and the World Economy*, edited by Joan Smith, Immanuel Wallerstein, and Hans-Dieter Evers. Beverly Hills: Sage.

Mayer, Jonathan D. 1988. "Migrant Studies and Medical Geography: Conceptual Problems and Methodological Issues." Pp. 136–54 in *Conceptual and Methodological Issues in Medical Geography*, edited by Melinda S. Meade. Chapel Hill: University of North Carolina, Department of Geography.

McCance, R.A. and I.H.E. Rutishauser. 1975. "Childhood Malnutrition." Pp. 89–92 in *Uganda Atlas of Disease Distribution*, edited by S.A. Hall and B.W. Langlands. Nairobi: East African Publishing Huse.

McGlashan, N.D. (ed.). 1972. *Medical Geography: Techniques and Field Studies*. New York: Harper and Row.

Meade, Melinda S. (ed.). 1980. *Conceptual and Methodological Issues in Medical Geography*. Chapel Hill: University of North Carolina, Department of Geography.

Melbye, Mads, Anne Bayley, J.K. Manuwele, Susan A. Clayden, William A. Blattner, Richard Tedder, E.K. Njelesani, K. Mukelabai, F.J. Bowa, Arthur Levin, Robin A. Weiss, and Robert J. Biggar. 1986. "Evidence for Heterosexual Transmission and Clinical Manifestations of Human Immunodeficiency Virus Infection and Related Conditions in Lusaka, Zambia." *Lancet*, November 15:1113–15.

Moodie, T. Dunbar. 1988. "Migrancy and Male Sexuality in the South African Gold Mines." *Journal of Southern African Studies* 14(2): 228–56.

Mugerwa, R. and G. Giraldo. 1987. "Some Clinical Aspects of AIDS in Uganda." Paper presented at Second International Symposium on AIDS and Associated Cancers in Africa, Naples. Abstract S.3.2.

Mugerwa, R., R. Widy-Wirski, and S. Okwake. 1987. "Assessment of a Provisional WHO Clinical Case—Definition of HIV Related Illness in the Referral Hospital of Uganda." Paper presented at Second International Symposium on AIDS and Associated Cancers in Africa, Naples. Abstract TH-89.

Mulder, Carel. 1988. "Human AIDS Virus Not from Monkeys." *Nature* (333):396.

Murray, Colin. 1977. "High Bridewealth, Migrant Labour and the Position of Women in Lesotho." *Journal of African Law* 21 (1):79–96.

———. 1980. "Migrant Labour and the Changing Family Structure in the Rural Periphery of South Africa." *Journal of Southern African Studies* 6(2):139–56.

———. 1981. *Families Divided: The Impact of Migrant Labour in Lesotho*. Cambridge: Cambridge University Press.

Navarro, Vincente. 1974. "The Underdevelopment of Health or the Health of Underdevelopment." *Politics and Society*, Winter:267–93.

———. 1982. "The Labor Process and Health: A Historical Materialist Interpretation." *International Journal of Health Services* 12(1):5–29.

Navarro, Vincente and Daniel M. Berman (eds.). 1983. *Health and Work under Capitalism: An International Perspective*. Farmingdale, NY: Baywood.

Norman, Colin. 1985. "Politics and Science Clash on African AIDS." *Science* 230:1140–42.

Nzilambi, Nzila, Kevin M. DeCock, Donald N. Forthal, Henry Francis, Robert W. Ryder, Ismey Malebe, Jane Getchell, Marie Laga, Peter Piot, and Joseph B. McCormick. 1988. "The Prevalence of Infection with Human Immunodeficiency Virus over a 10-year Period in Rural Zaire." *New England Journal of Medicine* 318(5):276–79.

Osoba, A.O. 1981. "Sexually Transmitted Diseases in Tropical Africa." *British Journal of Venereal Disease* 57:89–94.

Padian, Nancy S. 1988. "Prostitute Women and AIDS: Epidemiology." *AIDS*. 2:413–419.

Parker, Richard. "Acquired Immunodeficiency Syndrome in Urban Brazil." *Medical Anthropology Quarterly* 1(2):155–75.

Parpart, Jane L. 1983. *Labor and Capital on the African Copperbelt*. Philadelphia: Temple University Press.

Pepin, Jacques, Francis A. Plummer, Robert C. Brunham, Peter Piot, D. William Cameron, and Allan R. Ronald. 1989. "The Interaction of HIV Infection and Other Sexually Transmitted Diseases: An Opportunity for Intervention." *AIDS*. 3:3–9.

Peterson, Hans D., Bjarne O. Lindhardt, Peter M. Nyarango, Tula R. Bowry, Alex K. Chemtal, Kim Krogsgaard, and Albert Bunyasi. 1987. "A Prevalence Study of HIV Antibodies in Rural Kenya." *Scandinavian Journal of Infectious Diseases* 19:395–401.

Piot, Peter, Francis A. Plummer, Fred S. Mhalu, Jean-Louis Lamboray, James Chin, and Jonathan Mann. 1988. "AIDS: An International Perspective." *Science* 239:573–79.

Prothero, R. Mansell. 1977. "Disease and Mobility: A Neglected Factor in Epidemiology." *International Journal of Epidemiology* 3(6):259–67.

______. 1983. "Medical Geography of Tropical Africa." Pp. 137–53 in *Geographical Aspects of Health*, edited by N.D. McGlashan and J.R. Blunden. San Francisco: Academic Press.

Pyle, Gerald F. 1979. *Applied Medical Geography*. New York: Wiley.

Quinn, Thomas C. 1987. "AIDS in Africa: Evidence for Heterosexual Transmission of the Human Immunodeficiency Virus." *New York State Journal of Medicine* (May):286–89.

Quinn, Thomas C., Jonathan M. Mann, James W. Curran, and Peter Piot. 1986. "AIDS in Africa: An Epidemiological Paradigm." *Science* 234: 955–63.

Rampen, F., 1978. "Venereal Syphilis in Tropical Africa." *British Journal of Venereal Disease* (54):364–68.

Ratnam, Attili V., Shahida N. Din, Subhash K. Hira, Ganapati J. Bhat, D.S.O. Wacha, A. Rukmini, and Raphael C. Mulenga. 1982. "Syphilis in Pregnant Women in Zambia." *British Journal of Venereal Disease* 58:355–58.

Recene, U., S. Orach, and A. Petti. 1987. "HTLV III-TB Association in Northern Uganda (Gulu District)." Paper presented at Second International Conference on AIDS and Associated Cancers in Africa, Naples. Abstract TH-80.

Roberts. A. 1979. *A History of Zambia*. New York: Africana.

Rodney, Walter. 1982. *How Europe Underdeveloped Africa*. Washington, DC: Howard University Press.

Sajiwandani, Jonathan and K.S. Babbo. "Sexually Transmitted Diseases in Zambia." 1987. *Journal of the Royal Society of Health* 5:183–86.

Sanders, David and Rob Davies. 1988. "The Economy, the Health Sector and Child Health in Zimbabwe since Independence." *Social Science and Medicine* 27(7):723–31.

Sathyamurthy, T.V. 1986. *The Political Development of Uganda: 1900–1986*. Brookfield, VT: Gower.

Saul, John S. and Giovanni Arrighi. 1973. *Essays on the Political Economy of Africa*. New York: Monthly Review Press.

Schall, Peter L. and Rochelle Kern. 1986. "Hypertension in American Society: An Introduction to Historical Materialist Epidemiology." Pp. 73–89 in *The Sociology of Health and Illness: Critical Perspectives*. 2nd ed., edited by Peter Conrad and Rochelle Kern. New York: St. Martin's.

Schoub, B.D., A.N. Smith, S.F. Lyons, S. Johnson, D.J. Martin, G. McGillivray, G.N. Padayachee, S. Naidoo, E.L. Fisher, and H.S. Hurwitz. 1988. "Epidemiological Considerations of the Present Status and Future Growth of the Acquired Immunodeficiency Syndrome Epidemic in South Africa." *South African Medical Journal* 74:153–57.

Serwadda, D., N.K. Sewankambo, J.W. Carswell, A.C. Bayley, R.S. Tedder, R.A. Weiss, R.D. Mugerwa, A. Lwegaba, G.B. Kirya, R.G. Downing, S.A. Clayden, and A.G. Dalgleish. 1985. "Slim Disease: A New Disease in Uganda and Its Association with HTLV-III Infection." *Lancet*, October 19:849–52.

Sher, R. 1986. "Acquired Immune Deficiency Syndrome (AIDS) in the RSA." *South African Medical Journal* Supplement, October 11: 23–26.

Shilts, Randy. 1987. *And the Band Played On: Politics, People, and the AIDS Epidemic*. New York: Penguin.

Simonsen, J. Neil. 1988. "Human Immunodeficiency Virus Infection among Men with Sexually Transmitted Diseases: Experience from a Center in Africa." *New England Journal of Medicine* 319(5):1274–78.

Smith, Barbara E. 1981. "Black Lung: The Social Production of Disease." *International Journal of Health Services* 11(3):343–59.

Smith, Joan. 1984. "Nonwage Labor and Subsistence." Pp. 64–89 in *Households and the World Economy*, edited by Joan Smith, Immanuel Wallerstein, and Hans-Dieter Evers. Beverly Hills: Sage.

Sontag, Susan. 1978. *Illness as Metaphor*. New York. Farrar, Straus, and Giroux.

______. 1988. *AIDS and Its Metaphors*. New York: Farrar, Struas, and Giroux.

Specter, Michael. 1986. "AIDS Infection and Birth Control Pills." *The Washington Post*, May 31:A18.

Stamm, Walter E., H. Hunter Handsfield, Anne M. Rompalo, Rhoda L. Ashley, Pacita L. Roberts, and Lawrence Corey. 1988. "The Association between Genital Ulcer Disease and Acquisition of HIV Infection in Homosexual Men." *Journal of the American Medical Association* 260(10):1429–33.

Stark, Evan. 1977. "The Epidemic as a Social Event." *International Journal of Health Services* 7(4):681–705.

Stichter, Sharon. 1985. *Migrant Laborers*. New York: Cambridge University Press.

Turshen, Meredeth. 1977. "The Impact of Colonialism on Heath and Health Services in Tanzania." *International Journal of Health Services* 7:7–35.

———. 1984. *The Political Ecology of Disease in Tanzania*. New Brunswick: Rutgers University Press.

Van de Perre, Philippe. 1984. "Acquired Immunodeficiency Syndrome in Rwanda." *Lancet*, July 14:62–69.

Vaughn, Megan and Henrietta Moore. 1988. "Health, Nutrition and Agricultural Development in Northern Zambia." *Social Science and Medicine* 27(7):743–45.

Verhagen, A.R. and W. Gemert. 1972. "Social and Epidemiological Determinants of Gonorrhea in an East African Country." *British Review of Venereal Disease* 277(48):277–86.

Waitzkin, Howard. 1978. "A Marxist View of Medical Care." *Annals of Internal Medicine* (89):264–78.

———. 1983. *The Second Sickness: Contradictions of Capitalist Health Care*. New York: Free Press.

Waldron, Ingrid. 1986. "Why Do Women Live Longer than Men?" Pp. 34–44 in *The Sociology of Health and Illness*, edited by Peter Conrad and Rochelle Kern. New York: St. Martin's.

Waldron, Ingrid and J. Eyer. 1975. "Socioeconomic Causes of the Recent Rise in Death Rates for 15–24 Year Olds." *Social Science and Medicine* (9):383–96.

Wallerstein, Immanuel. 1984. "Household Structures and Labor-Force Formation in the Capitalist World-Economy." Pp. 17–22 in *Households and the World Economy*, edited by Joan Smith, Immanuel Wallerstein, and Hans-Dieter Evers. Beverly Hills: Sage.

Wallerstein, Immanuel and William G. Martin. 1979. "Peripheralization of Southern Africa: Changes in Household Structure and Labor-Force Formation." *Review* III(2):325–71.

Wender, I., J. Schneider, B. Gras, A.F. Fleming, G. Hunsmann, and H. Schmitz. 1986. "Seroepidemiology of Human Immunodeficiency Virus in Africa." *British Medical Journal* 293: 782–85.

White, Richard. 1978. *Africa: Geographic Studies*. London: Heinemann.

World Health Organization (WHO). 1988. "A Global Response to AIDS." *Africa Report*, November–December:13–16.

World Health Organization (WHO). 1989. "Statistics from the World Health Organization and the Centers for Disease Control." *AIDS*. 3:113–17.

***CHARLES W. HUNT** is a graduate student and graduate teaching fellow at the University of Oregon, Eugene. His current research is in Medical Sociology and AIDS Epidemiology. He also works in the areas of political economy, sociology of developing countries, and social movements.*

[10]

Soc. Sci. Med. Vol 36, No. 7, pp. 949–955, 1993
Printed in Great Britain

0277-9536/93 $6.00 + 0.00
Pergamon Press Ltd

HIV TRANSMISSION THROUGH SOCIAL AND GEOGRAPHICAL NETWORKS IN UGANDA

CHRISTINE OBBO

Chateau de la Mothe, St Private des Prés, 24410 St Aulaye, France

Abstract—Long distance drivers and prostitutes at trading centres and towns have been targeted as groups that engage in risky sexual behaviours that promote HIV transmission. While towns and stops along highways have been linked to HIV transmission, the role of small urban and rural centres have been overlooked. There is need to study socio-geographical mating networks because situations not deemed to be risky may be an important aspect of HIV transmission.

Key words—HIV, mating networks, socio-geographical proximity, Uganda

GENERAL INTRODUCTION

The main purpose of this paper is to suggest that high AIDS casualties in some communities require that research priorities be focused equally upon risky behaviour as well as risky situations. Furthermore, it is a proposal that researchers be open to new issues that may lead to new insights.

The pattern of AIDS incidence in Uganda is complex. However, population movement dominates the picture. The HIV infections and the AIDS disease are related to rural–urban and regional migration, the black market economy of the 1970s, and the political unrest which caused unprecedented movements of both civilian and military populations in the last two decennia. This paper focuses upon the geographical and social networks that have contributed to the spread of HIV. The emphasis here is not so much on risky behaviour as on risk situations. In a few years it will be possible to map out the intensity of HIV infections and AIDS death in all districts. Figure 1 is a modest attempt to indicate national transmission patterns resulting from the movement of traders, migrant labourers and soldiers. Figure 2 shows the distinctive transmission patterns in Rakai, the worst hit district, as distance from the fishing villages on Lake Victoria, location of rural centre and townships along the main roads leading to the capital Kampala. These patterns are reflected in numbers of orphans, abandoned homes and numbers of afflicted people in villages.

The most obvious and often commented upon population movements involve truck drivers (and their assistants, the turn boys) and the prostitutes in urban centres along the highways. While this would account for the spread of HIV to the areas that commonly supply truck drivers, it does not explain the spread to other areas. A much more promising model relates the HIV spread to the labour importing and exporting areas. The idea is that the HIV virus and the resulting AIDS first struck the labour concentrations in Uganda and then moved outward to the labor reserves, carried by migrant labourers and prostitutes as they returned to their birth places for care and assistance after being infected and falling ill in the urban areas [1]. In Uganda, AIDS is generally regarded as an urban problem. This is because the earliest deaths were of urban dwelling professionals and business people. Estimates of the epidemiology of infection so far support this view. The rates of urban infections are substantially higher than rural rates. However, rural and urban areas are not either or situations, they are interdependent. The majority of Ugandans live in rural areas. However, ruralites and urbanites exchange visits regularly as personal and family demands dictate. During the 1970s, periodic levels of state violence and generalized anarchy in different areas forced people to escape alternately to the villages when the towns became too dangerous, and to rural centers and urban areas when the villages were deemed unsafe. Normally, men and women migrate to towns primarily to escape rural poverty and secondly for many social and personal reasons. Returnees from high migrant labour concentrations, male migrant labourers and their female sexual worker partners (local as well as a few migrants), were the first known AIDS cases in most villages.

One study has associated high HIV prevalence and high incidence of AIDS deaths with the patterns of labour migrations [1]. This model applies to the rural areas that export labourers to the towns as well as to the regional rural areas that supplied workers to other rural areas which had demands for extra labour in cash crop production. Studies during the 1960s associated the high incidence of sexually transmitted diseases (STDS) in Teso District with male labour migration to Buganda (Central district) [2]. Returning migrants infected their girlfriends and wives. Currently, high rates of HIV infections in both Teso and Gulu districts are attributable to the presence of troops dealing with political unrest. The military is increasingly recognized as important in HIV trans-

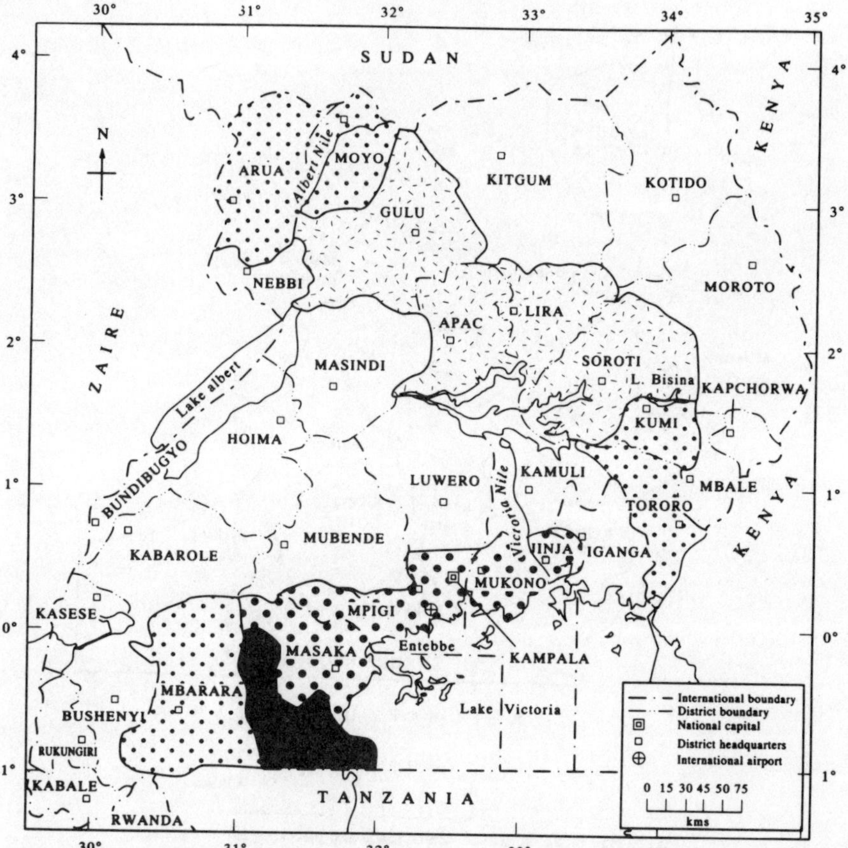

Fig. 1. Map of Uganda districts showing differing patterns of HIV transmission. Labour exporting ▣; Labour importing ▣; Soldiers ◫; Illicit trade ■.

mission [3]. The traditional labour exporting areas of West Nile have low HIV prevalence because the district has been isolated geographically and development policies in the last 20 years. The West Nile population can be divided into those in the rural areas who merely hear of AIDS deaths at funerals and the Kampala urban population (who rarely visit their home areas) who exhibit high incidence of AIDS deaths. Kampala (as well as Rakai and Masaka) is one of the worst affected districts [4].

Lake Victoria was the scene of intense smuggling during the 1970s because it connects Uganda, Kenya and Tanzania. During the day traders and porters waited in fishing villages and neighbouring towns. Every night fleets of fishing canoes converged on the fishing villages along the shores in Rakai. Young men were employed to row and unload the canoes. Some young men worked as porters to quickly whisk away the goods to hideaway places in neighbouring villages. Traders who were well off would have the trucks to take the goods to the capital, but middling traders used bicycles to move their goods to townships and urban centres. In the fishing villages, the rural centres services developed to cater to the traders. Rental rooms, eating places and drinking places attracted women who supplemented their meagre bar waitressing income or worked solely to entertain the traders. As expected, the traders acquired multiple wives as well as girlfriends. Inflation created such an ambiance of prosperity that even porters were considered rich by poor women with no other access to money than through sex work. All these men paid periodic visits to their villages where they had wives as well as girlfriends. The personal stories of the AIDS epidemic show that different populations were affected in waves. The first wave of

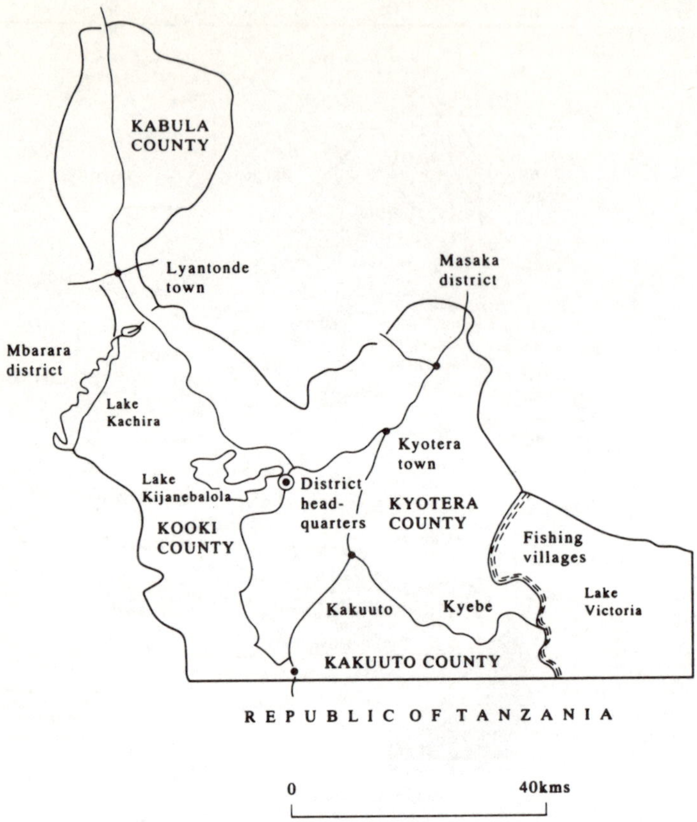

Fig. 2. Map of Rakai district. Major roads and places named in the article.

afflictions and deaths was in trading and polygamous households. Usually the women outlived their husbands for periods varying from 6 months to a year. The earliest orphans inherited houses built of permanent materials, despite the fact that the construction on some was incomplete. Some orphans had money available to continue their education. The areas most affected in this first wave were in Kakuuto county, particularly the sub-counties of Kakuuto, Kyebe and Kasasa situated adjacent to the fishing villages and where most of the smuggling networks were pervasive. The personal stories of the second wave of the AIDS epidemic was concentrated in Kooki county, which had the highest number of educated people working in professions all over the district towns and the capital city, Kampala. The AIDS death involved businessmen (bankers, hotels and lodge owners) and professionals employed in the civil service as magistrates, district educational officers, school teachers, veterinary and agricultural extension officers. Again, this wave involved people with money and power to put them in risky situations. The inheritance of these orphans was similar to that of the first wave.

The third wave of AIDS death was manifested among residents of rural and urban centres along the Kampala road. It has been observed that AIDS is a disease of development [5], and that small urban centres play an important role in economic development [6]. The services in these centres were responses to the travelling populations, and marketing activities attracted increased concentrations of people at periodic intervals. Kyotera town is such a service centre with lodges, restaurants, a bank, petrol stations, etc. Kyotera is the largest town in Rakai district because all the main roads dissecting the district pass through it, including the main Tanzania–Kampala road running through the district and the international road from Rwanda via Mbarara district (both areas have reported high AIDS deaths). Lyantonde rivals Kyotera not only in the number of AIDS deaths, but also that they have lost up to three distinctive waves of business and commercial elites since 1987. A footnote must be added that, since 1990 many people from these towns have migrated to the border town of Tororo and Busia in the East where there are extensive economic opportunities. AIDS deaths are on the rise in these AIDS refuge towns.

GEOGRAPHICAL PROXIMITY AND SOCIAL MATING NETWORKS

Ever since HIV transmission became associated with sex, research and intervention programmes have been focused on persuading people to change risky behaviours that are likely to expose them to infection. There has been no discussion of risky situations other than discos, truck stops and bars. The argument here is that there are many apparently normal practices that are, in fact, risky situations. In this section, two such situations are examined: the urban mating networks based on common school background and work place, and the rural mating networks based on residential proximity. The networks were constructed by interviewing the actors. Altogether 20 urban and 15 rural people were interviewed through open ended instructional questions about their present and past close friends. Although these were supposed to be personal narratives, people were much more likely to talk about other people's relations than their own because of the nature of the subject. The rural networks were unstructured by interviewing the actors, the neighbours and friends in 1989. The connections in each case were confirmed by at least four respondents in an attempt to avoid unsubstantiated gossip. In addition, the participant observer researcher stayed long enough in the area to be able to evaluate the relative accuracy of solicited and unsolicited information.

URBAN ELITE MATING NETWORKS

"We are all dying" was a refrain I heard at every funeral. For a long time it seemed to me like a remark anyone surrounded by morbidity and mortality would make. It was made by urbanites and ruralites alike to refer to the AIDS epidemic. The predominant heterosexual mode of HIV transmission and the nonexistence of a cure were common knowledge. The tattered appearance of 'sex workers' at bar lodges in Masaka and Rakai towns suggested that many men were avoiding risky behaviours. However, one day after a funeral of a bank executive, people divided into groups as they hung around. In one group there was animated discussion which seemed not to refer to the epidemic in general, but was focused upon those present. Remarks that were repeated several times included: "AIDS is a death sentence." "This is a calamity, we are all going to perish." "It is a pity we are all going to die." But a remark that was made by a woman who had been silent throughout the discussion provided a significant lead to the researcher. She said, "It is our mating patterns that are finishing us off." In the following months, the people in the group were interviewed regarding the meaning of the remark. The catastrophe envisaged and feared was based on the common knowledge of the widespread endogamous mating among friends and co-workers. The interviews further revealed that friendship networks formed on the basis of school attendance, social, ethnic and religious backgrounds, and work place associations became the basis of social, practical and emotional support. Within these networks, some relationships occasionally became sexual. A common occurrence, cases where members of the network would quarrel and break up with their lovers or wives after a misunderstanding and turn to their friends in the networks for consolation or replacement. Members of the networks were secure and familiar with each other and usually ready to do anything for each other. Most of the mating was within this context involving both married and unmarried members.

Network X (Scheme 1) was ethnically homogeneous and consisted of people aged between 30–45 who had attended the same secondary school, some of whom were related to each other. The network consisted of two unmarried people, a divorcee, and the rest were married. A had died of AIDS and it was at his funeral that the network members were first discovered. But, as one woman suggested, "We are in shock. There is reluctance to acknowledge any sexual association with him." The survivors worried because the deputy head of the department was rumored to be afflicted with HIV (he died of AIDS 5 months after the research was completed). He had been married for 2 years before he died, but his wife shows no signs of affliction. The women in the network expressed anxiety and the unmarried male civil servants showed hostility to any reference to AIDS.

Network Y was based on networks formed when at University and it was ethnically heterogeneous. However, the world of elites seems small indeed, and networks X and Y were connected (see Scheme 1). In 1990, network Y had two AIDS deaths and there was one affliction. Members of the networks worried about AIDS. However, some members were sexually active inside and outside the networks. Members felt that it was safer to confine the relationships within the network, and men said that they avoided sex workers. The women said that they could not ask their male network friends to wear condoms under any circumstances, although some had experiences of contracting sexually transmitted diseases from network lovers. The illusion that there was no need to use condoms because the sexual relationships within the network were occasional and were with people who were known and presumed safe was being exposed by the deaths of close friends. As of June 1992, only C in network Y and B in network X remain unafflicted.

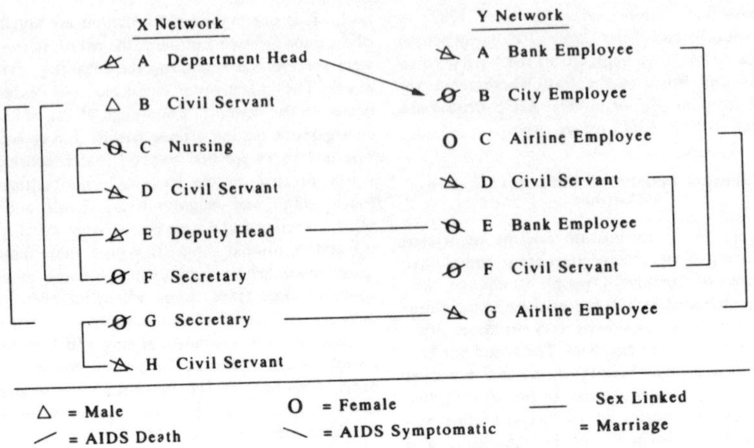

Scheme 1. Urban elite mating networks.

Most couples in Uganda had faith in 'Zero grazing', men increasingly stayed at home, confided in their wives and some even apologized to their wives for staying out late and missing family happenings. However, on the subject of condoms, the discussion centered around what men might do. For example, an official who was in charge of health education (including AIDS) in schools in 1989 had never seen condoms and when one was shown to her, she was flabbergasted. She intimated that her husband, a medical doctor, would kill her if he saw her with a condom. There might be some exaggeration about supposed men's reactions, but the important thing is that negative reactions are anticipated. There is an increase in condom use and this must be among the urban elites.

RURAL MATING NETWORKS

Rural areas are divided into administrative units varying in size from counties, sub-counties and villages (Resistance Council Area). The smallest units are villages, and each has a traditional name. After being in the field for only 6 months, the differing patterns of deaths in the sub-county emerged. Some villages had no deaths of locally residing people. Other villages seemed to have clusters of local affliction and deaths in some neighbourhoods. This seemed puzzling. In some cases, as many as five neighbouring houses would have had AIDS death and affliction, in others every other second house would be so affected. When neighbours were asked about the patterns, men made statements like, "Women are the greatest spreaders of AIDS." Or, both men and women said, "Some people are so wicked that they will quietly wipe out the village with AIDS." The answers seem to suggest that clandestine sexual activities were suspected and that the vectors had a hidden agenda to wipe out everyone. Interviews with the surviving family members and neighbors revealed close friendship between the homesteads. The couples tended to visit each others homes for lunch or tea on Sundays. During the week, the women occasionally visited each other in late afternoons; the men visited in the evenings while the wives prepared the evening meals. But in a neighborhood, neighbors would also visit different neighbors at different times. Informants insisted that these evening visits provided ample opportunities for clandestine sexual activities. However, one rarely heard of fights because, in the words of one informant, "A cuckolded man who discovers the goings-on usually revenges by counter cuckolding, even if it takes him a lifetime to do so." These men do not always succeed because some women either have no wish to be unfaithful to their husbands or may have wind of their husband's carrying on which they do not consider as solved by sleeping with the other women's husbands. In these cases, hatred and avoidance usually develop between the families. There are other opportunities that provide occasional or prolonged sexual relations. For example, the practice of young women returning to be with their mothers for the last weeks of their pregnancy and following childbirth, was aimed at providing the woman rest from tiring chores so as to conserve energy for birth and also for recovery afterwards. This, however, apparently offered some men 'opportunities to sneak women friends into the house when other household members were preoccupied with work'. Silence was considered good manners (buntu bulamu) on the part of household members to see, hear or say nothing to the absent wife. Other examples that encouraged adultery are: the practice of installing women in separate homesteads by polygamous men; and the common occurrence of women deserting (Kunoba) their

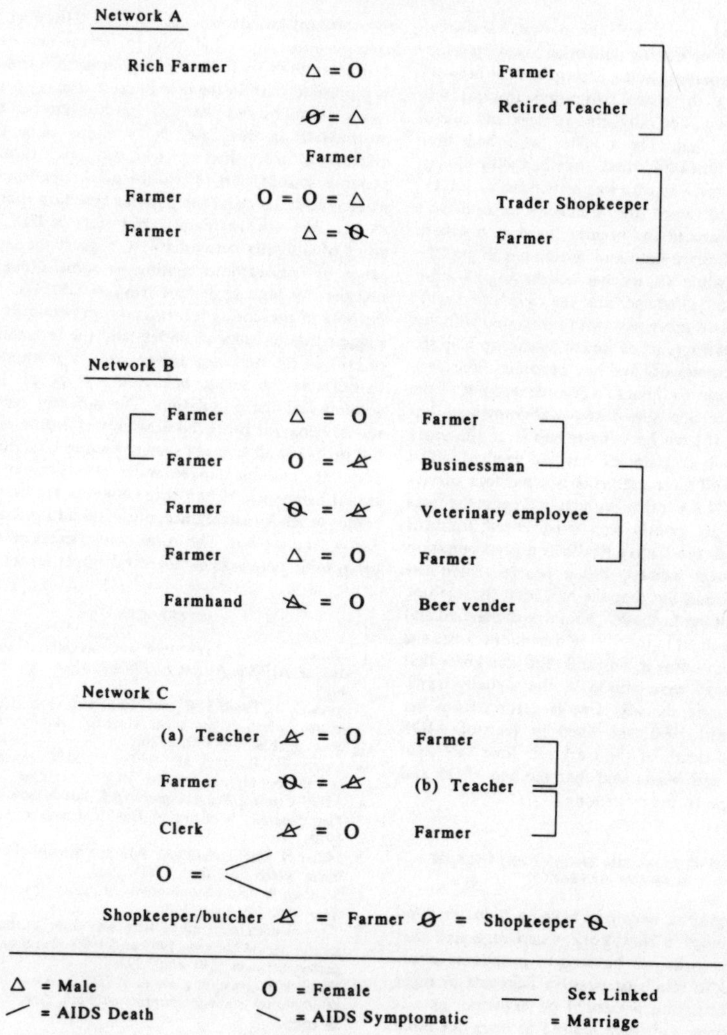

Scheme 2. Rural mating networks.

husbands because of marital discord, neglect or maltreatment. These separations were supposed to be temporary until a man came to explain himself and claim his wife. In cases of beatings, he was required to pay a fine and to promise not to repeat his actions. Both husbands and wives in the situation regard liaisons with other people as justified. Most marriages usually end by these separations where a woman deserts permanently and hides or when a reconciliation fails. However, the failure of marriage may follow several such separations. During the interim, pregnancies occurred and it was common knowledge that some families had children among them who resembled men among their friends and neighbours.

These practices were identified by informants as contributing to the high AIDS casualty rates observed in sections of some villages. Following is a brief representation of sexual networks in a village with high AIDS casualties.

The women in networks A, B and C were all full-time cultivators and men predominantly weekend cultivators. However, the predominant mode of employment for both men and women was full-time subsistence farming. Some men in the networks were involved in non-agricultural occupations. Shown in Scheme 2 are three mating networks based on socio-geographical proximity and a description for network C. In Network C there were two monogamous teachers, one had died. The polygamous clerk and one of his wives had died. The butcher who had been married three times had died, together with his last wife, and the surviving wife was bedridden with HIV.

It all started when the butcher's second wife deserted her husband and became the second wife of the clerk. He bought land and settled her in another county. Meanwhile. (b) teacher was having an affair with the wife of (a) teacher and the clerk's first wife. As the clerk spent more time with his second wife, his first wife increasingly relied on (b) teacher to help the children with homework and book supplies. The clerk and his wife were Catholics so divorce was out of the question for her. She viewed what was going on as her cross. Maria, (b) teacher's wife, had over the years endured difficult pregnancies that had resulted in five miscarriages and three stillbirths. She has four surviving children. Like other village women, she was overworked, ate poorly and experienced frequent pregnancies. Reproductive health is a preoccupation for most village women. When Maria visited the diviner, she found out that she had been the last one to know about her husband's affairs with married and unattached women in the village during the times she was away from home in hospital. She also knew that her miscarriages were caused by the sexually transmitted infections she was always getting from her husband. Until 1990, she lived in fear of AIDS following the death of the clerk. In June 1992, (b) teacher died and Maria said that she had AIDS and does not hope to live very long.

CONCLUDING REMARKS: THE IMPORTANCE OF NETWORK RESEARCH

Socio-geographic networks have been documented by recent studies in New York which suggested that the same networks can be used to propagate information, and to reinforce positive behavior changes [8]. The information presented on networks here is limited in scope and there is need to map out more relationships based on large samples. However, the exercise underscores the need for researchers to be flexible enough to follow serendipitous information as it presents itself in the field because it may open up issues, questions and practices that hitherto had been overlooked. In this case, the stimulus came from informants' unsolicited remarks and issues raised in previous studies, particularly the preoccupation with women's adultery and the popular assertion that it is women who are the main transmitters of HIV. The point of studying networks is to suggest the significance of endogamous mating in some groups as revealed by high casualties from AIDS. The main purpose of presenting information on networks is to suggest that in order to understand the transmission of HIV in the rural and urban areas, it is important to examine the sexual behaviours of people in all segments of the population. The different types of sexual behavior practiced now existed before AIDS, but people at all levels of society need to be sensitized about the possible dangers inherent in some of their sexual behaviors. Urban elite networks are based on common school attendance, professional associations and working place. The rural networks show socio-geographic networks of the rural upper strata.

REFERENCES

1. Hunt C. W. Migrant labor and sexually transmitted disease: AIDS in Africa. *J. Hlth soc. Behav.* **30,** 353–373, 1989.
2. Arya O. P., Taber S. R. and Nsanzo H. Gonorrhea and female infertility in rural Uganda. *Am. J. Obstet. Gynecol.* **138,** 929–932, 1980.
3. Lyerly W., Barry S. and Miller N. HIV transmission and the military. *AIDS Soc. Bull.* **1,** (4), 1990.
4. AIDS Control Programme *AIDS Surveillance Report: First Quarter.* Ministry of Health, Entebbe, Uganda, 1990.
5. Miller N. and Carballo M. AIDS: a disease of development. *AIDS Soc. Bull.* **1,** (1), 1989.
6. Southall A. (Ed.) Small towns in Africa revisited. *Afr. Stud. Rev.* **31,** 1–16, 1988.
7. The research referred to here was done during a 10-month period between 1989 and 1990, and a six month period between 1991 and 1992.
8. Wallace R. Travelling waves of HIV infection on a low dimensional 'sociogeographic' network. *Soc. Sci. Med.* In press.

Part III
Social Demography

[11]

Soc. Sci. Med. Vol. 23, No. 4, pp. 393–415, 1986
Printed in Great Britain. All rights reserved

0277-9536/86 $3.00 + 0.00

THE PATTERNING OF HEALTH BY SOCIAL POSITION IN CONTEMPORARY BRITAIN: DIRECTIONS FOR SOCIOLOGICAL RESEARCH

SALLY MACINTYRE

MRC Medical Sociology Unit, 6 Lilybank Gardens, Glasgow G12 8QQ, Scotland

Abstract—Associations are described between health (variously measured) and occupational class, gender, marital status, age, ethnicity and area of residence, using British data. It is argued that when exploring the social patterning of health, illness and death, it would be profitable for sociologists to consider several or all of these social positions, and to develop models of general vulnerability to ill-health rather than of specific etiology. Three main types of explanation, artefact, health selection and social causation, are reviewed, and six general points are made about how sociological research on social patterning in health should proceed.

Key words—social position, physical and mental health, social causation, health selection

INTRODUCTION

In recent years in Britain a great deal of attention has been given, by social epidemiologists and medical sociologists among others, to inequalities in health [1]. The focus has mainly been on differences in mortality, morbidity and service use between groups classified by the British Registrar General's Classification of Occupations, and discussion has centred around the magnitude of these differences, their variation or otherwise over time, and reasons for their existence or continuation.

In this article I wish to place these debates in a broader and perhaps more traditional context: that of interest in observed social regularities in experience of health, illness and death. Health is associated with a number of social positions; exploring why this should be so tells us something about the causes of health and illness, and also something about social systems and social processes. In this paper I do not assume that observed variations in health are necessarily due to social inequalities or other forms of social disadvantage; rather I treat these inequalities as one out of a number of possible explanations for such variations. I therefore chose to use the term 'social patterning', rather than 'inequalities', in health, since the latter term has developed connotations of: (a) referring specifically to class inequalities and (b) referring, as Blaxter put it, to "unacceptable inequalities, or alternatively unjust, disfunctional, unnecessary or preventable inequalities" [2].

In this paper the following social positions have been chosen for particular attention; social (occupational) class, gender, marital status, age, ethnicity and area of residence. These have been selected because of their consistently observed associations with various distributions of health and illness, their relevance for sociological theories of social differentiation, and their pertinence for social and medical policies. Although age, gender and ethnicity may initially be thought of as biological characteristics, it is clear from historical and cross-cultural evidence that in all societies they are attributed with social significance which may shape the consequence of being a particular age, sex or ethnic origin. Area of residence, similarly, may have social or cultural consequences as well as purely topographical ones. These six variables are therefore conceptualized here as positions on dimensions of social differentiation which may be associated with particular patterns of life chances.

The first section of this review summarizes evidence of associations between these social positions and health, and concludes with some general comments about this evidence. The second section reviews explanations for observed associations between social position and health and concludes with suggestions for strategies for further research.

EVIDENCE OF ASSOCIATIONS BETWEEN SOCIAL POSITION AND HEALTH

Associations between people's social position and their health have been observed and commented on for over a century in Britain [3–6]. While great advances have been made since then in our understanding of disease processes, less progress has been made in understanding either the social factors side of the equation or the processes intervening between social position and observed health or ill-health. Thus while it has been observed for some time than a person's social class of origin or achievement, gender, marital status, age, ethnic group and area of residence are all correlated with his or her mental and physical health and likelihood of death (from all causes or specific causes), detailed study of why this should be so is surprisingly sparse. Indeed the existence of the correlations themselves, which would not have surprised observers in the nineteenth century, is often treated as if it were a novel disclosure. (Note, for example, the public attention devoted to the Black Report on inequalities in health [1].) As Blaxter has observed in relation to childhood health:

"A great deal of effort has gone into the task of proving, again and again, that these socially associated differences in the health status of children do exist: almost as if this were something that society did not wish to believe, and had to re-discover at regular intervals. To continue to prove, however, that children's health and development differ according to the occupational social class of their father does little towards explaining why this should be so" [7, p. 219].

This section briefly outlines the main associations between social position and health and illness as they have been reported in Britain. It should be noted that in Britain there is much more evidence available about occupational class in relation to health than there is about the other social positions of interest. Most routinely collected statistics and research studies in Britain gather data on social class, age and sex, and present tables broken down by these variables: fewer present data by marital status, ethnicity, or area of residence.

Where possible the material summarised in this section includes mortality (all-cause and disease-specific); physical and mental illness (self-reported and deriving from screening instruments); selected health-related continuous variables (e.g. height, blood pressure, birth-weight, edentulousness); and self-perceived health. Actual figures are presented so that the magnitude, as well as the direction, of the associations is clear to the reader. Data on health service contacts have been avoided since, given variations in illness behaviour and in availability of services, they are an extremely unreliable indicator of health or illness. For ease of exposition a discussion of the conceptualisation and measurement of the selected social positions, and of health, follows rather than precedes the presentation of these data.

Occupational class

'Class' in this section refers to occupational class as measured by the British Registrar General.

Consistent gradients are observable for both men and women in mortality by occupational class. For example, among people aged between 15 and 64 in England and Wales in 1971, the ratio of social class V to social class I death rates was 2.5 to 1 [8]. The greater risk of death for lower occupational classes exists for virtually all of the 'chapters' for causes of death in the International Classification of Disease, e.g. for congenital anomalies, infective and parasitic diseases, respiratory diseases, diseases of the digestive system, disease of the circulatory system, diseases of the blood and blood-forming organs and most types of cancer [9].

The occupational class of one's father is associated with chances of survival in the perinatal period; there are consistent gradients in stillbirths and neonatal mortality by occupational class, and an excess of deaths in the post neonatal period in classes IV and V compared to classes I–IIIm [10]. Steep gradients in mortality by class of parents are found again towards the end of the first year of life and persist throughout childhood and adolescence (after which own, rather than parental class, is usually measured) [9].

The combination of the occupational class gradients in mortality in childhood with those in adulthood (i.e. up to 64) means that a newborn male, subject to the mortality rates recorded in 1970–2 for social class I aged up to 65 years, would expect to live 5.12 years longer than one subject to the rates for social class V, the expectation of life for the former being 70.91 years and for the latter 65.79 years assuming no class gradient in mortality after age 65. Similar calculations based on the assumption of continued class differences in mortality after 65 would give a figure of 7.17 years (expectation of life 72.19 and 65.02 for social class I and V respectively) [9].

For chronic and acute illness there are gradients by occupational class, these being steeper for the former than for the latter. Between 1971 and 1976 the rate of limiting long-standing illness per 1000 population, self-reported to the General Household Survey (GHS), was three times greater among unskilled manual workers than among professional workers. For men the rate of restricted activity in the 2 weeks prior to interview (the operationalisation of acute illness) was 130% higher among unskilled workers than among professionals [8]. In 1982 men in semi and unskilled manual jobs were over twice as likely as men in professional jobs to have been absent from work in the 4 weeks prior to interview because of their own illness or injury [11].

Mental health and well-being have also been shown to be associated with occupational class. Although different conditions tend to show different patterns by occupational class, screening measures such as the General Health Questionnaire (GHQ) tend to show a higher proportion of caseness and/or a greater number of psychiatric symptoms the lower the social class [12].

Numerous other distributions of health-related variables show similar gradients by occupational class. The heights of children and of adults, for example, vary systematically by class, height being regarded as a good general indicator of health and nutritional status [13]. In 1980 in Britain the average height of both men and women in class I was around 4 cm higher than that of their class V counterparts of similar ages [14]. The Whitehall study of male civil servants reported a difference of 5 cm between the average heights of those in the highest and the lowest employment grades [15], and found that being 6 feet tall or more was less than half as common in the lowest grade as among the administrative grade [16]. Among members of the 1946 birth cohort, studied at the age of 36, there were differences of 3 cm between the mean height for men in social class I and those in social class V, and 4 cm between those in social class I and those currently unemployed. For women there was a height difference of 5 cm between those in classes I and V (measured by their own occupation). Similar gradients in adult height were recorded by the social group of the individual's parents [17].

There is an association between birth-weight and father's occupational class, the incidence of low birth-weight rising with falling family social class. In 1980 the percentage of babies less than 2500 g at birth rose from 5.6 in class I to 8.7 in class V [10]. Among adults the prevalence of obesity is greatest for men among social class III manual, while for women it is greatest among those in households headed by someone in classes IV or V [14].

Several recent studies have shown that men in

lower occupational classes have significantly higher systolic and diastolic blood pressure than those in higher classes. The Whitehall study found that 11% of the administrators, 12% of the professional and executive, 14% of the clerical and 16% of the 'other' grades had a systolic blood pressure of 160 mmHg or greater [16]. Among the 1946 birth cohort studied at age 36, although mean systolic blood pressure in men was highest among the lower occupational classes (125 among social class V men, and 124 among unemployed men, compared with 120 in social class I), there was no significant difference among men or women in the distribution of systolic or diastolic blood pressure by current occupational class. However, men and women of low social group of origin had significantly higher blood pressure than those of higher social group of origin [18].

The prevalence of edentulousness is related to occupational class; among adults in England and Wales in 1978, 11% of those in social class I had no teeth compared with 47% in social class V [19]. Among men, 10% in the professional class reported problems with vision (whether or not they wore glasses) compared with 16% in the unskilled class; among women the comparable figure was 10% compared with 21%, i.e. twice as many in the unskilled as in the professional classes reported difficulty with their eyesight [11]. Finally in this brief account of various health indicators by class, it is worth including a recent finding from the Oxford Family Planning Association Study that among women who stopped using contraception with the intention of conceiving, the lower the occupational class of the husband the lower were the chances of conceiving [20].

Self-perceived health (as distinct from self-reported illness, as measured by the GHS) is also correlated with occupational class. Hunt, McEwan and McKenna have reported significant differences between social classes on the 'energy', 'pain', 'sleep' and 'physical mobility' sections of part I of the Nottingham Health Profile, and on the 'paid employment', 'jobs around the house', 'social life' and 'hobbies' sections of part II of the profile [21]. Blaxter reported that self-perceived 'well-being' and 'fitness' scores were higher among non-manual than among manual class respondents, while scores for 'chronic disease', 'illness' and 'disability' were highest among manual class respondents [22].

Thus occupational class (whether of self, father or husband) has repeatedly been shown to be associated with a diverse collection of health measures, including death from all causes or from specific causes, physical and mental illness, height, weight for height, birth-weight, blood pressure, dental condition, ability to conceive and self-perceived health. These class variations in mortality, morbidity, and other health related variables have been reported extensively during the last decade in Britain and there exist a number of reviews of the evidence [1, 7, 8, 9, 23, 24].

Gender

Differences between the sexes appear to be sufficiently obvious for most social or health data to be presented and analysed separately for each sex. The assumption that there will be distinctive profiles for each sex on any given variable is so taken-for-granted, however, that the data often remain treated separately rather than being subject to systematic comparison or attempts to account for the difference. In this sense, as Morgan has argued: "Gender, as a key variable, is both ubiquitous and hidden" [25].

Male mortality is higher than female mortality in Britain from before birth; from the end of the first trimester of pregnancy there are more male than female foetuses, but male foetuses are more likely to be spontaneously aborted. Stillbirths, neonatal and infant mortality rates are all higher among males than females, although it should be noted that the difference between male and female death rates in early life has been declining in Britain over the last 50 years [10]. Among adults the male excess of deaths persists. In 1971, for example, the ratio of male to female death rates hovered at just under 2 to 1 in all social groups in England and Wales [9]. Male/female mortality differences can also be expressed in terms of expectation of life. For men and women born in Britain in 1979 the expectation of life at birth was 70.2 and 76.2 years respectively. The difference, 6 years, is greater than at the beginning of this century: the expectation of life at birth in 1901 was 48.00 for men and 51.6 for women, a differences of 3 years [26]. The longer life expectancy of women is a relatively recent historical pattern, and one related to the extent of development; in some developing countries, such as India and Papua New Guinea, women have higher death rates and a shorter life span than men, as they did in industrialised societies in earlier historical periods [27, 28].

The causes of death differ between men and women. Among young people proportionately more men than women die of accidents and violence (around 70% male deaths compared with around 35% female deaths). After the age of 35 the most common causes of death are cancer and circulatory disease (the latter comprising heart disease and strokes), with proportionately more men dying of circulatory disease and more women dying of cancer. Between the ages of 50 to 55, for example, over 50% of male deaths are from circulatory disease, compared with less than 30% from cancer; the figures are reversed for women, with less than 30% of deaths being from circulatory disease and more than 50% being from cancer [26].

Although men have higher death rates than women, women tend to report slightly more illness than men. In 1982, for example, among adults aged 16–44, 21% men and 23% women reported long standing illness, 10% men and 12% women reported limiting long standing illness, and 8% men and 12% women reported some restricted activity due to illness in the 14 days before interview. Men reported an average of 19.6 days of restricted activity due to illness in the previous year, while women reported 25.6. Differences of similar magnitude occur at other ages, and within social classes [11].

Evidence about sex differences in mental illness is difficult to interpret and fraught with conceptual problems [29, 30]. However, most studies of the prevalence of psychiatric morbidity or of mental well being (whether based on population screening instruments, surveys in general practice or hospital admission rates) have reported striking gender differences

[12]. Women are considerably more likely than men to be diagnosed as suffering from psychoneurotic conditions (such as depression or anxiety), psychosomatic conditions and manic depressive psychoses. In the most developed countries a ratio of around 2 to 1 of women to men among treated depressives has been reported; but among some developing countries (principally India and Papua New Guinea) there is a male excess of treated depressive illness [29].

Men's average height is greater than that of women; in 1980, men in social classes I and II averaged 175.7 cm while women in the same classes averaged 162.5 cm: men in social classes IV and V averaged 172.3 cm while women in the same classes averaged 159.6 cm [14]. A Body Mass Index ($BMI = H/W^2$) shows that while more men than women were 'over-weight' (39% men compared with 32% women had a BMI of over 25), fewer men than women were 'obese' (6% men compared with 8% women had a BMI of over 30) [14].

In early life blood pressure tends to be higher among men than among women. Among the 1946 birth cohort studied at the age of 36, for example, the mean systolic and diastolic blood pressures for men were 123 and 78 respectively, while for all women they were 114 and 73 and for all non-pregnant women they were 115 and 73 [18]. At around the age of 55, however, there is a cross-over effect in industrial countries, such that women's blood pressure is higher than that of men at later ages [31]. Among the 1946 birth cohort women's peak flow expiration measures were considerably lower (i.e. poorer) than men's within each social class group [32].

Fewer men than women have no teeth; in 1978 in England and Wales 24% men, compared with 32% women, had no teeth [19]. Fewer men than women report having difficulty with eyesight, whether or not they have their eyesight corrected; 12% compared with 15% [11].

For self-reported health, women scored significantly higher (i.e. worse) than men on all sections of part I of the Nottingham Health Profile, and on 'jobs around the home', 'social life' and 'personal relationships' sections on part II [21]. In Blaxter's study, men reported higher scores (i.e. 'better' self-perceptions), for self-reported well being and fitness, and less chronic disease and frequency of illness, than women [22].

There have been a number of recent British and American reviews of gender differences in mortality and in physical and mental health [28–30, 33–39].

Marital status

Although variations in mortality and morbidity by marital status were first noted in the last century [6], marital status is seldom used as an independent variable in studies of health. Although, for example, data on marital status is collected in the General Household Survey, few distributions of health variables have been presented by marital status in recent years.

From the available evidence it appears that married people generally have lower death rates than people who have never been, or who were previously but are no longer, married. The Longitudinal Study (a study of a 1% sample from the 1971 Census, followed up via registerable events such as births, marriages, deaths and cancer-registration) recorded Standardised Mortality Ratios (SMRs) among men aged 45 to 64 varying from 95 for the married to 128 for the divorced and 135 for the single and widowed. For women in the same age group the SMRs ranged from 97 for the married to 149 for the divorced. The difference between being single (i.e. never married) and being married tends to be less for women than for men at all ages [24].

The marital status of a child's parents at the time of its birth is associated with the likelihood of it dying in infancy. Illegitimate children have higher stillbirth, post neonatal mortality, and low birth-weight rates than even social class V legitimate infants, and their neonatal mortality rates are nearly as high as for social class V [10]. In 1982 infant mortality rates in Scotland were 10.4 per thousand for legitimate children and 17.1 per thousand for illegitimate children. In Glasgow the comparative figures for the same year were 10.8 and 15.8 per thousand [40].

There are few national data available on marital status in relation to self-reported or physician-assessed physical morbidity. A preliminary analysis of unpublished data from the 1981 GHS shows that up to 60 years of age married persons are less likely to report long standing chronic illness than single or formerly married persons. For example, at ages 40–49, 30% married men, 36% single men, 36% widowed men, 37% divorced men and 42% separated men reported chronic illness. For women in the same age group the proportions were 30% married, 35% single, 32% widowed, 36% divorced and 54% separated. After the age of 60 the pattern of chronic illness by marital status is less consistent. The proportions reporting acute illness do not show such a regular pattern by marital status, single and married people showing little difference, although the highest rates are always reported in one of the formerly married categories. Married men reported better health in the previous year than single men in all age groups between 30 and 70, but there is no such pattern for women and there is no consistent pattern by the formerly married categories [41].

Rates of psychiatric disorders as detected by community surveys are also higher among the separated and divorced than among the married [12]. It has been suggested that marriage is more stressful for women than for men and that there will therefore be higher rates of mental illness among married women than among married men, and higher rates for married than for unmarried women [38, 42]. Although the former suggestion tends to be borne out (but rates are higher for women than for men in all marital categories), the latter does not [29]. In general, however, the evidence does suggest that in terms of likelihood of death, and physical or mental ill health, being unmarried may be more risky for men than women, as Durkheim originally suggested in his 1897 work on suicide [43].

In the 1946 birth cohort mean blood pressures were highest at age 36 for those not living with a spouse or partner and never previously married (126 systolic for men and 114 systolic for women). Blood pressure values for those cohabiting, and for those divorced, widowed or separated, were intermediate between single and married [17]. Shaper *et al.* reported significantly high blood pressure (systolic and diastolic) for single men as compared with those of all other marital statuses, among those studied as part of the Regional Heart Study [44].

The main British review of marital status and health is by Myfanwy Morgan [45].

Age

As Finch has noted, data on age is almost always collected in social research, but frequently not used as a topic for analysis in its own right [46]. As with gender, one reason for the ubiquity but invisibility of age as a topic for analysis in research on health may be that it is taken-for-granted as a physiological characteristic. However, observed relationships between age and any dependent variables may be due to period or cohort effects as well as to ageing, and even if they are due to ageing they may be attributable to social as well as physiological aspects of growing older. Data on associations between age and other variables therefore have to be approached with care, particularly if they are derived cross sectionally. We also have to be cautious about extrapolating the past or present to the future (current estimates of life expectancy, for example, are based on presently prevailing death rates, i.e. those experienced by previous generations).

The patterns of all-cause and cause-specific mortality alter with age. Death rates are high up to 4 years of age (4210 and 3195 per million for males and females respectively) then decrease up to later childhood. For males the rate rises abruptly in late adolescence, and continues to rise thereafter, while for females there is a more gradual increase (between the ages of 15 and 24 the male/female death ratio is well over 2) [24]. Accidents and violence are important causes of death among young persons from 15 to 24 (though there are relatively few deaths in this age group), cancer is an important cause of death in middle age and early old age, and circulatory and respiratory diseases become increasingly important as causes of death with increasing age [26].

Perinatal and infant mortality rates show a U-shaped relationship with maternal age, being highest for mothers under 16 and lowest for those between 25 and 35. In England and Wales in 1980, for example, perinatal mortality rates were 18.6, 16.5, 12.0, 12.6 and 17.7 per thousand for mothers aged respectively under 16, 16–19, 20–24, 25–29, 30–34 and 35 and over [10].

There is a steady gradient in self-reported chronic illness with age. In 1982 the percentage of males reporting long standing illness rose from 21% among 16–44 year olds to 41% among 45–64 year olds and 58% among 65–74 year olds; comparable figures for women were 23, 42 and 58%. The percentage of males reporting limiting long standing illness rose from 10% among 16–44 year olds to 41% among 65–74 year olds; the comparable figures for women were 12% rising to 39%. For acute illness, that is, restricted activity in the 14 days prior to interview, there is a much less marked increase with age. Among men the percentage rose from 8% among 16–44 year olds to 11% among 45–64 year olds and 14% among 65–74 year olds; for women the increase was even less, the comparable figures being 12, 14 and 15% [11].

Height varies with age among adults as well as children. In 1980 the average height of males fell from a peak of 176.0 cm among 20–24 year olds to 170.0 cm among 60–64 year olds, and the average height of women from a peak of 161.9 cm among 30–34 year olds to 158.5 cm among 60–64 year olds [14]. Birth-weight shows a normal curve with maternal age for first pregnancies, i.e. lighter babies are born to younger and older mothers [47]. Among women the proportion overweight and/or obese rises steadily with age, while for men there is a peak in the late 40s and another in the early 60s [14].

In industrial societies (but not in hunter–gatherer, pastoral or traditional agricultural societies), blood pressure values tend to rise with increasing age, by an average of 0.5 mm Hg per year for men and 0.9 mm Hg per year for women in systolic blood pressure, and 0.2 and 0.4 mm Hg respectively in diastolic blood pressure [48]. The proportion of the population with no teeth rises with age: in 1978 3% of those aged 25–34, 48% among those aged 55–64 and 87% among those aged over 75 were edentulous [19]. The proportion reporting difficulty with eyesight (whether or not glasses were worn) doubles between the ages of 16–44 and 65–74 [11]. Fertility declines with increasing age, as recently demonstrated by the Oxford Family Planning Association study; compared with a standard of 1.0 for a reference group of nulliparous women aged 25–27, the relative fertility rates of nulliparous women fell with age to 0.55 among 36–37 year olds and 0.48 among 38–39 year olds. Among parous women, relative fertility rates declined to 0.49 among those over 40 compared with 1.0 for the reference group of 25–27 year olds [20].

Studies using the Nottingham Health Profile have found that the worst scores for self-perceived health tend to occur in middle age and then in very old age, with a drop in reported problems between [49, 50]. The only significant social class differences on this measure occur in the age group 20–44; after 45 social class differences were found for only a few areas or for none. There were significant age differences on part I of the Profile, scores tending to rise after 45, and on part II on all items except for impact on paid employment and sex life, for which scores tend to fall after 64 [21]. Blaxter found that while self-perceived 'fitness' decreased with age among men and women, and 'well-being' also decreased with age among men, 'well being' showed a more complex relationship to age among women, being highest among those aged 50–59 and lowest at the extremes of age (under 30 and over 70) [22].

It should be reiterated that most of the above findings may reflect period or cohort effects as much as ageing effects. Only prospective designs can disentangle the relative importance of these effects.

Ethnicity

In Britain, unlike countries such as the U.S.A., there is little systematic evidence about mortality or morbidity by ethnic groups since ethnic or racial data are not recorded in census, health service or other routinely collected statistics. National studies therefore have to rely on place of birth which is recorded on death certificates and in the 1971 census, and which refers to immigration rather than ethnic affiliation [24, 51–53] (although several investigators have tried to establish ethnic affiliation for those born in India or Africa by use of the names recorded on death certificates, e.g. Refs [51, 53]). Much of the British work on ethnicity and health thus tends to be based on local or *ad hoc* studies, or to concentrate on specific conditions affecting ethnic minority groups, such as thalassaemia, sickle cell anaemia or rickets [54, 55].

Marmot, Adelstein and Bulusu were able to compare the mortality of immigrants both with that prevailing in their country of birth and with that prevailing in England and Wales. Indian and African born immigrants were allocated to ethnic groups according to the names recorded on the death certificates. Most of the male immigrant groups had lower age standardised mortality than that of their countries of birth and that of all males in England and Wales. The main exception is men migrating from Ireland, who have higher mortality than men in Ireland or in England and Wales. With the exception of immigrants from Europe, immigrant women have higher SMRs than those prevailing in England and Wales, and lower SMRs than those in their countries of origin. Among migrants female death rates are higher than mens within each social class [51].

Irish immigrants display the same social class gradients in death rates as are found in England and Wales, i.e. highest in the lowest social classes. The same relation of mortality with class is not found in other immigrant groups; immigrants from Europe as a whole show no gradient in mortality from social class I to IV, immigrants from the Indian subcontinent show a gradient from class I to III but none in the manual classes, while among immigrants from the Caribbean the highest mortality is in class I, and the non-manual classes have a higher mortality than the manual classes [51].

There are marked differences between immigrant groups in causes of death. For example, there are high rates from hypertension and stroke, and low rates from ischaemic heart disease, among immigrants from the Caribbean; high rates from ischaemic heart disease, infections and diabetes and low rates from cancer among those from the Indian subcontinent; high rates from cirrhosis of the liver, accidents and violence, and TB among those from Ireland; and high rates from cirrhosis and alcohol-related cancers and low rates from ischaemic heart disease and respiratory disease among those from France [51]. Variations in cause of death by ethnic group have also been reported among those born in the Indian sub-continent. Proportional mortality ratios for cancer were lower for Hindus than for Moslems, and were lowest for Punjabis. Mortality due to ischaemic heart disease, high in all groups, was highest among Moslems [53].

While adult mortality in immigrants from the New Commonwealth is generally low compared to Britain as a whole, the same is not true for early mortality in the next generation. Stillbirth, neonatal and post neonatal mortality rates are higher for children of mothers born in Pakistan, India and Bangladesh, African Commonwealth countries and the West Indies, than for children of mothers born in the U.K. Perinatal mortality rates for children whose mothers were born in Australia, Canada, New Zealand, Gibralta, Malta, Cyprus and the rest of Europe were lower than those for U.K. born mothers [52]. Enhanced perinatal risk also applies to the children of mothers classified as Asian in terms of ethnicity rather than place of birth. In 1975–81 in Bradford, for example, the stillbirth rate among Asians was 15.5 per thousand births compared with 8.7 among non-Asians; infant mortality was 21.6 for Asians compared with 14.1 for non-Asians. Although 70% Asian mothers were in social classes IV and V, compared with 23.2% non-Asians, they experienced excessive rates of death from congenital abnormalities compared with non-Asians in the same social class; the rates of death from congenital abnormalities being 12.4 per thousand total births among Asians compared with 4.8 among non-Asians. Similarly, although Asian mothers have different child-bearing patterns from non-Asians, when controls for age and parity were introduced they still had higher perinatal mortality [56].

There are few data on physical or mental illness by country of birth or ethnic affiliation. The General Household Survey, for example, has not published material on ethnicity and health (although it does collect ethnic data). In Britain Asians show lower rates of mental disturbances, suicides and admissions to mental hospitals than either whites or other immigrant groups, and West Indians have lower rates of affective and depressive illnesses than the rest of the population and higher rates for schizophrenia [54]. The incidence of low birth-weight is high among children born to mothers born in India and Bangladesh, Pakistan, the African Commonwealth and the West Indies [10].

Other national data on indicators of health and functioning (height, weight, blood pressure etc) are not available by ethnicity.

Marmot *et al.* [51] and Fox and Goldblatt [24] provide useful evidence and discussions on immigrant mortality, and Donovan [54] and Fitzpatrick and Scambler [55] provide general reviews.

Area of residence

Area of residence has long been observed to be associated with mortality and morbidity. The first national review of area mortality appeared in the 9th Annual Report of the Registrar General, for the years 1838–44 [4], and the first decennial supplement was published in 1864 [5]. It is interesting to note the historical persistence of area variations within the U.K.; Lancashire had the highest mortality rates in England in 1838–44 and still does so today [57].

For men aged 40–69 the worst death rates in the industrial world are found in Finland, its standardised mortality rate being 1707 per 100,000. Scotland ranks second worst, with a rate of 1626, Northern Ireland fifth with a rate of 1519, and England and Wales fourteenth with a rate of 1355. For women aged 40–69 Scotland had the worst rate, 872 per 100,000; Northern Ireland was fourth with 818 and England and Wales twelfth with 720 [58].

Within the U.K. there is a gradient in mortality from low in the South and East of the country to high in the North and West. In 1969–73, for example, all-cause SMRs for men varied between 89 in East Anglia and 112 in the North West, while the SMRs for women varied between 93 in East Anglia and 109 in the North West [57]. Gradients by social class vary between areas, being steeper in the North and North West than in the South and East, but social class standardisation has virtually no effect on the SMRs for the regions; for men aged 15–64 in 1970–72 the social class standardised SMRs varied between 83 in East Anglia and 116 in the North West [9].

These regional gradients are found for most causes of death, and for all of the major causes, i.e. circulatory disease; malignant neoplasms; respiratory disease; and accidents, poisoning and violence; which accounted respectively for 51, 20, 14 and 4% of all deaths in 1969–73 [57]. West, investigating variations in ischaemic heart disease, showed that significant geographical variations in mortality in England and Wales mainly reflected differences in age at death rather than in cause of death [59].

Perinatal and infant mortality follows a similar gradient from the South East to the North West of England and Wales; social class standardised infant mortality rates, as a percentage of England and Wales deaths, varied from 88 in East Anglia to 111 in Yorkshire [9].

There are variations within, as well as between, regions in Britain. Fox, Jones and Goldblatt [60] looked at variations in mortality between areas of the country divided into 36 clusters derived by grouping census wards on the basis of 40 census variables [61, 62]. Areas with significantly high SMRs for men were: inner areas with low quality older housing, overspill estates, urban local authority estates with good job opportunities, mining areas, inner city council estates, and multi-occupied and immigrant inner areas [60]. Those with significantly low SMRs included modern high status areas, established high status suburban areas, residential retirement areas and others classified as high status. In general there was therefore a pattern of high mortality in low status areas and low mortality in high status areas. The Greater Glasgow Health Board (GGHB) reports that within the Glasgow conurbation, some areas experience mortality rates as low as, or lower than, those found in the healthiest countries in the world, while others experience rates as high as the highest found anywhere in the industrialized world. Examination of SMRs for persons under 65 in various neighbourhoods within Glasgow City, and in adjacent areas covered by the GGHB, reveals that SMRs in the worst quintile are 2.3 times those in the best quintile [63]. Similar variations between small areas have been reported for other urban areas such as Bristol [64].

People living in the South West and South East of Britain are taller than those living in the North or North West. The percentage of men above 182.5 cm, for example, varied from 13% in East Anglia and the rest of the South East, to 8% in Scotland and the North West and 4% in Wales. Comparable figures for women above 170 cm were 5% in East Anglia, 8% in the rest of the South East, 6% in Scotland and 2% in Wales and in the North West. Both men and women living in Wales were significantly shorter than the rest of the population, and men and women living in Scotland were marginally shorter than the British average [14].

Shaper *et al.* found a pronounced variation between towns in mean systolic and diastolic blood pressure among males, with low values in the South and East and high values in the North. Mean systolic blood pressure ranged from 136 mm Hg in Guildford and Shrewsbury to 153 mm Hg in Dunfermline, and mean diastolic blood pressure ranged from 77 mm Hg in Lowestoft to 88 mm Hg in Dunfermline; there was thus a substantially bigger difference than that between social classes (the major differences between towns in mean systolic blood pressure remained when age, body mass index, alcohol use, smoking, social class and marital status were taken into account) [44]. Dental health shows similar patterns; 21% adults in London and the South East have no teeth compared with 33% in the North [19].

General remarks on the epidemiological evidence

Before outlining the explanations advanced for the observed associations between social position and health, it is useful to make four main comments about the evidence presented above.

Firstly, few reviews systematically examine all (or even several) of these social positions in connection with health. There has been considerable interest recently in relationships between occupational class and health, and some interest in gender, marital status, ethnicity and area in relationship to health [28, 30, 45, 54, 65], but very little interest in examining health in relation to all of these social positions. Sociologists have of course always been interested in class, gender, marital status, age and ethnicity, but mainstream (or even medical) sociology has seldom studied these axes of social differentiation in relationship to life chances conceptualised in terms of health. Collating the above evidence of social patterning in health proved surprisingly difficult because it involved so many different sources and separate bodies of research literature. Yet if one is to develop a clearer understanding of how any one of these social positions relates to health, it is useful to look at the other positions as well. Exploring the processes connecting one social position with health can produce useful insights about linkages between other social positions and health, and the testing of resulting hypotheses can clarify and refine knowledge about the specificity or generalisability of the processes involved.

Empirically of course any individual simultaneously occupies a position on all of these dimensions, and their interactions may have important consequences; viewing a teenage Pakistani woman living in Bradford and married to a self-employed shopkeeper purely in terms of either her age, ethnicity, gender, area of residence or occupational class of household is to ignore the other dimensions of her social position that may crucially affect her life-chances. Many forms of disadvantage related to ill-health are themselves inter-correlated (for example, being non-white, working in an unskilled occupation or being unemployed, living in the inner city, being the female head of a single parent family) and disaggregating these components may misleadingly mask the effects of these simultaneous and overlapping vulnerabilities [66, 67].

Secondly, occupancy of the social positions described tends to be associated, empirically, with a wide range of sometimes disparate-appearing health experiences. Being male, of unskilled occupation, unmarried, or living in the North or West of Britain, appears to be linked to an increased probability of a diversity of adverse health experiences including death from motor vehicle accidents, pedestrian accidents, homicide, suicide, heart disease, infectious diseases, respiratory diseases, congenital anomalies etc and likelihood of ill health in a variety of forms. Thus for example while much attention has been devoted in the last decade or so to coronary heart disease as a major cause of premature death in Western societies, it is apparent that greater risk of heart disease goes together with greater risk of death from all causes, whether the risk is associated with occupational class, maleness, unmarried status, employment grade or area of residence. This point is made in relation to geographical variations by West, who found that significant geographical variations in mortality in England and Wales mainly reflected differences in age at death, irrespective of cause of death, and who commented that:

"Public health measures should not be directed towards eradicating 'an IHD specific toxin' in the England and Wales environment, since mortality from other causes demonstrates similar associations with socio-economic variables, but should be directed towards alleviating early death from all causes (including IHD) by modifying the environmental micro-climate and improving socio-economic circumstances" [59, p. 250].

Similarly, risk factors for ill health, such as cigarette smoking, obesity, or the occurrance of threatening life events, tend to be associated with a range of adverse health experiences rather than demonstrating etiological specificity.

Rather than starting with a particular health problem and searching for specific etiological processes influencing it, an approach which has proved very successful when applied by biomedical scientists, particularly to infectious diseases, it seems more fruitful for sociologists to explore why particular social positions render their occupants generally vulnerable to a whole range of ill health (or alternatively, generally prone to a range of good health outcomes). From the viewpoint both of increasing our understanding of the processes linking social structure with patterns of health and ill-health, and of assessing the effectiveness of medical and social interventions, it seems sensible to build models of the general vulnerability or resistance of social groups to adverse health, broadly conceived. This is particularly important given the increasing prevalence of chronic (and multiple) disease with multifactorial etiology; an increasing interest in a holistic, rather than reductionistic, view of health [68–70]; and the above-noted tendency for occupancy of a given social position to be empirically associated with a range of health outcomes. This does not imply aggregating all health outcomes together in an undifferentiated manner, as suggested by Brown and Harris, who adduce the different processes involved in the etiology of schizophrenia and depression as grounds for focussing on the specific etiology of only one of these, depression, rather than mental illness in general [71]. Even if the etiological processes are somewhat different, one can still start from the social position and document vulnerability or resistance to a range of specified outcomes.

Thirdly, none of the social positions of interest, or the variables used to represent them, are unproblematic or self-evident in their meaning, measurement or significance.

Occupational class as measured by the Registrar General is clearly something very different from Marxian or Weberian conceptualisations of social class or status. Alternative classificatory schemes for analysing social stratification have been suggested by sociologists [72–74] but the RG scheme has been remarkably persistent despite its (lack of) theoretical base. Recent critiques have largely focussed on Stevenson's purposes in compiling the classification in the way he did, since the precise criteria for allocating an occupation to a class are unclear [75–77].

The ubiquity and persistence of the RG classification in government and health statistics has tended to lead to the reification of occupational class; that is, it is sometimes treated as though it were a fixed and material attribute of individuals that somehow 'causes' certain outcomes, rather than as a convenient system of social classification imposed on a complex social reality by investigators with certain research purposes. As Illsley argued in relation to low birth-weight:

"Social class is an intellectual and social construct, it has no material form and cannot directly affect the development of the foetus in its uterine environment or cause its premature expulsion."

However, as he goes on to point out:

"Yet its relationship with so many aspects of child and adult illness and death . . . shows that it nevertheless has biological significance" [78, p. 74].

Thus despite the conceptual problems which exist with the RG classification, whatever social reality is sorted by this classification does, empirically, seem to have significance for people's life chances and physical and mental health (although there are variations within 'classes' that also need to be explored) [76, 79]. A proper sociological task is therefore to get behind the labels created by this classificatory system and to explore their meaning for the everyday lives and life chances of those on whom the labels are imposed.

Age and sex may be, as Szreter argues, "physiologically determined and relatively indisputable attributes of individuals which have been recognised since long before the emergence of modern sociology as carrying important consequences for those individuals' observable attitudes and behaviour" [75, p. 225]. However, we similarly have to be careful not to reify these as simple and self evident attributes 'causing' patterns of ill-health. Both are based on biological classifications, but biology tells us little about their meaning and significance within any given culture or historical period. In all societies age and sex are recognised as dimensions of social differentiation, with significance for access to material resources, power, status, rights and obligations and interconnections with legal, economic, religious, military and other institutions. The actual significance of occupancy of particular age and sex roles, and its consequences for social life and health, is however culturally and historically variable and cannot be taken for granted [25, 30, 46]. The same applies to marital status, ethnicity and area of residence: their social and health significance is dependent on the historical and cultural context, and what they 'mean' is therefore not self evident.

Although the earlier account of health correlates of these social positions treated these variables as given, and simply summarised selected associations with health, it is evident that even if they are causally implicated in health (see next section), none of them is likely directly to cause health outcomes; rather they are markers for the complex set of social conditions and processes which may be causally implicated. A major concern of medical sociologists should therefore be to unpack these variables in terms of their meaning and significance for patterns of day to day living, and to understand the processes intervening between these measures and health outcomes.

Fourthly, the above account listed a number of health-related outcomes, mainly adverse ones, without defining health. The conceptualisation and measurement of health is bedevilled by a number of conceptual, definitional and practical problems [80]. The WHO definition of health as "a state of complete physical, mental and social well being and not just an absence of disease" has been much criticised for being Utopian and impossible to operationalise, but it is laudable in at least attempting to formulate health in positive terms, rather than in terms of lack of pathology. This is particularly important given the increasing importance of multiple (and multi-caused) chronic illness and disability [81, 82]; the discovery that many people carry supposedly pathogenic substances such as viruses or bacteria without manifest illness [70]; the realisation that persons with high levels on some continuous variables, such as blood pressure or blood sugar, may not shown the symptoms normally associated with high levels; and the findings from screening studies that very few people are without some abnormalities that can be defined as disease, even though many of the affected individuals are unaware of the disorder [83–87].

Sociologists normally distinguish between disease (objective disorder), illness (subjective unwellness) and sickness (the social role of the ill person). For disability, distinctions are made between impairment (biological disorder), disability (functional condition) and handicap (reduced social and economic activity due to impairment or disability) [88]. The distinction between disease and illness is important because there is not necessarily a direct relationship between them. It is quite possible to feel ill without there being any evidence of disease, or to be diseased without feeling ill. It appears to be more common to be 'diseased' without feeling ill than vice versa. Post mortem findings frequently reveal serious organic pathology of which the deceased was unaware and which was not the cause of death [89]. Signs and symptoms may be unnoticed or assumed to be part of ordinary life, as has been found for decayed teeth [83], smoker's cough [90] and for foot problems [91]. The Peckham experiment conducted health overhauls on 4002 individuals and found that no more than 10% were without clinically recognisable disorders of one sort or another, and that of those in whom disorders were detected only around 30% were aware of them [84].

Similarly, people's perceptions of their own health may be relatively unrelated to their perceptions of the presence or absence of either disease or illness. Among a random sample of 2500 adults in Bermondsey and Southwark, less than 5% reported no ailments in the previous 14 days. However, 35% respondents described their state of health as 'perfect', 34% as 'good', 21% as 'fair' and only 10% as 'poor' [87]. Similar findings are consistently reported in the GHS, with high prevalence and incidence of reported illness co-existing with positive self evaluation of general health. Although self ratings of general health are associated with self reported chronic and short term health problems, the associations are very weak; in 1978, for example, while 89% of men who reported neither chronic nor acute ailments described their health as good, so did 46% of those who reported both chronic and acute ailments [92].

Although it is thus useful at an abstract level to formulate health in the manner recommended by WHO, it is probably less useful to attempt to generate a single, global, unidimensional measure of health so defined and more fruitful to use or develop multidimensional models or measures appropriate for the particular purpose at hand. The dimensions to be used might well include physical, mental and 'social' health, and objective and subjective definitions, with various further sub-distinctions. The Alameda County study, for example, looked at what it called objective measures of physical health in terms of recurrent symptoms, chronic conditions, impairments and disability. It then used what the authors called subjective measures of physical health such as whether the respondent felt seriously bothered by the symptoms or conditions; whether the respondent felt in good, fair or poor health for people of the same age; measures of mental health; and measures of social health viewed in terms of occupational, marital and community adjustment [69, 73]. Another set of distinctions is offered by Blaxter, who examined five different dimensions of health: the absence/presence of disease, illness (frequency of symptoms), functional ability/disability, fitness/unfitness and well being/malaise. She also makes a useful distinction between health state (a transitory condition) and health status (the general characteristic of being healthy or unhealthy) [22].

Important tasks for sociologists are to continue to develop subjective measures of health [49, 94]; to pursue work on lay people's conceptualisations of health [22, 95, 96]; to explore the relationship between self-reported and clinically-assessed illness; and to develop the use of continuous objective health measures such as height and birth-weight [13, 77, 78].

EXPLANATIONS FOR ASSOCIATIONS BETWEEN SOCIAL POSITION AND HEALTH

The existence of associations between social position and health and illness is fairly well known and relatively undisputed. There is however more uncertainty and dispute about why the associations should exist. Yet an understanding of the reasons for these observed associations is crucial not only for theoretical reasons, increasing our knowledge of basic social processes, but also for practical reasons, assisting the formulation or evaluation of policies designed to improve the health of the population or of sub-groups within it.

At the most general level there are three possible types of process accounting for observed associations between social position and health and illness:

1. Artefact, e.g. (a) the social position is related to another social or physical characteristic which is the 'true' cause of the health status; that is, the apparent relationship is spurious, or (b) the definition or measurement of either the social position or the health status effects or produces the observed relationship.
2. Health selection, e.g. unhealthy people do poorly in the labour or marriage markets, or healthy people are more likely to move in search of better jobs.
3. Social causation, e.g. being of low occupational class or unmarried is bad for your health.

Although there has recently been some theoretical debate about the relative importance of these three processes in explaining gradients in health by occupational class [1, 97, 98], there has, until recently, been less empirical work testing the relative importance of these processes or exploring in detail how they might actually operate in practice, and little attention has been given to these processes as they might operate for other social positions such as gender, age, marital status, ethnicity and area of residence.

Artefact explanations

(a) A commonly advanced explanation of the artefact type is that an observed relationship between one social position and health is 'really' caused by another social position which is highly intercorrelated with the first and which is the true cause of the health outcome. Area variations in health, for example, are often 'explained' in terms of the social class composition of the areas in question; that is, it is suggested that what appears to be an area effect is really a class effect. One problem with this type of artefact explanation is that it is often implicit and untested; another is that it simply shifts the burden of explanation from one rather crude set of indicators to another equally crude set, without aiding understanding of the processes involved.

The possibility that observed associations between health and marital status, ethnicity, or area are artefactual in this sense have, however, been examined in a number of studies. As hinted earlier, Marmot, Adelstein and Bulusu using national data [51], and Gillies *et al.*, using Bradford data [56], considered the possibility that apparent ethnic variations in adult or perinatal mortality respectively were due to the social class composition of the ethnic groups in question. They found however that the ethnic variations existed within each social class and therefore could not be regarded as social class artefacts. Macintyre looked at the social class of women in Scotland having legitimate and illegitimate babies, and found a difference in perinatal mortality rates by legitimacy within social classes; she concluded that apparent differences in early deaths by marital status of mother were not an artefact of social class [99]. Similar exercises have been conducted on area variations. The Decennial Supplement on Occupational Mortality for 1970–72 found that regional variations in adult and perinatal mortality could not be 'explained away' as artefacts of social class [9]. Shaper *et al.* found that variations in blood pressure between towns in Britain remained when age, marital status, social class and other factors were taken into account [44]. Elbourne and Pritchard have shown that differences in perinatal mortality rates between Aberdeen and Cardiff were due to social class and area effects acting independently [100].

Such evidence suggests that many of the observed variations in health by one social position cannot be explained away in terms of the true cause of the health measure being another, interrelated, social position. More work needs to be done, however, to explore these possibilities and, in particular, to provide empirical evidence to address the response of "it's all due to social class" that so frequently greets findings with other social positions as the independent variable.

(b) Although it has been demonstrated in the epidemiological literature that variations in diagnostic fashion over time, or between places or doctors, may influence apparent variations in disease or mortality rates [16, 101], and in the sociological literature that patients may be diagnosed or treated differently according to their social positions [102], there has been little systematic attempt to explore the extent to which variations in health statistics may be the result of rate-producing processes similar to those which have been described for crime or suicide rates [103, 104].

It is possible that diagnosis, of cause of death, or of mental or physical illness, may be influenced by the diagnostician's knowledge of the social class, age, sex, marital status or ethnicity of the person involved. While the possibility of such a process producing biases in rates of death or illness has often been acknowledged, there has been, as Bloor *et al.* [98] have noted, little systematic empirical research in Britain on the extent and direction of such biases. The few empirical studies that have been conducted have tended to focus on psychiatric disorder (e.g. Ref. [105], rather than on cause of death or on physical illness.

There has been consideration of measurement artefacts affecting apparent all-cause mortality gradients by occupational class. The Registrar General, for example, has suggested that there may be numerator/denominator biases affecting class gradients based on cross-sectional data [9]. Work by Fox, Goldblatt and Jones from the Longitudinal Study suggests that, for men at least, such biases do not in fact distort the gradients too much [106].

There has also been consideration of the possibility that changes in the British occupational structure (and its classification) over time have contributed towards an apparent continuation of mortality gradients by occupational class since the last war. The Black Report for example used the term 'artefact explanation' solely to apply to the suggestion:

"that continuities in the pattern of health inequality in the twentieth century may be more a reflection of changing trends in the occupational structure of society than of a causal link between material welfare and health" [1, p. 154].

The Black working group, though acknowledging that there had been changes in the occupational structure and its classification, dismissed this sort of artefact explanation fairly summarily. The Registrar General, however, noted that reclassifying men by occupational class according to the 1950 classification of occupations reduced the SMRs in social class V from 151 to 134 in 1959–63 and from 139 to 123 in 1970–72 (the reclassification had only minimal effects on the rates for social class I men) [9]. This reclassification suggests that inequalities between social classes may not have been maintained to the extent suggested by the Black committee. Illsley has followed this line of argument even further. He argues that:

"changes in the economic, industrial and technological structure of our society have led over the period covered by our national data (1911 to date) to very substantial shifts in the distribution of occupations which change the meaning of occupational class in relation to equality. In other words the results of a comparison include, and are rendered meaningless by, the measurement tool itself" [107].

This particular debate, about whether there are persisting class gradients in mortality in the face of open access to the welfare state and increasing equalisation of life chances, is bound to continue given its theoretical and political importance.

In general, although artefact explanations are referred to in theoretical discussions of social differentiation in health, or are used to discount the possible causal relevance of one social position by suggesting that it is another one which is causally implicated, little systematic empirical attention has been given to artefact explanations, other than those for all-cause mortality gradients by occupational class among men [98].

Health selection

Although health selection is frequently mentioned in theoretical or general accounts of the social patterning of health and disease, there has been little systematic empirical work on this topic. At one time there was considerable interest in the competing health selection versus social causation hypotheses in accounting for the observed association between rates of mental illness, such as schizophrenia, and low social class or living in a disorganised inner city area [108, 109], but there has been less work recently in this tradition. Most contemporary work on health selection has tended to focus on occupational class [110], or on unemployment and health [111–113].

Stern has argued that in periods with considerable social mobility, comparison of social class mortality rates by achieved social class is insufficient and should be supplemented or replaced by rates calculated according to social class of origin [97]. The national birth cohort studies are able to use both measures. Wadsworth has shown from the 1946 birth cohort how social class and illness may be dynamically related over time. Boys with serious illnesses were more likely to come from lower social class families, and in adult life boys who had been seriously ill as children, even though they were no longer ill, significantly more often than boys who had not been ill experienced a fall in social class relative to that of their family of origin. For boys from manual class families of origin the effect was to double the rate of unemployment among those who had been seriously ill as children (8.0% unemployed at age 26) compared with those who were healthy as children (4.4% unemployed at age 26) [114]. Although Wadsworth found no significant gradient in blood pressure at age 36 by current occupational class, he did find a significant gradient by social class of origin, which suggests that health selection could not account for the difference in adult blood pressure [18]. Illsley has shown that tall women with better physique tend to be upwardly socially mobile at marriage and to have better perinatal outcome, while short women with poorer physique tend to be downwardly socially mobile at marriage and to have poorer perinatal outcome [115]. The finding that tall women are more likely to be upwardly socially mobile has been replicated on the 1946 birth cohort [114] and on a recent national sample [14].

The OPCS Longitudinal Study considered possible health selection explanations for regional variation in mortality and for the observed mortality patterns for immigrants to England and Wales. SMRs for people who had a different address in 1966 from that in 1971 were, for males, 107 for those who moved within a county, 91 for those who moved between counties in a region, 89 for those who moved between regions, and 89 for those who moved from outside England and Wales. For females the equivalent SMRs were 112, 94, 92, 72 [24]. After examining the time elapsing since migration, Fox and Goldblatt suggest that for men there is clear evidence of selection for initial ill-health among migrants within regions, and selection for good health among migrants between regions. For women they found a more complex pattern in that there were both healthy and unhealthy subgroups in those moving between regions. Fox and Goldblatt also explored the possibility that healthy people move from regions of high mortality (the North and West) to areas of low mortality (the South and East). They found that regional gradients in mortality existed among migrants by region of origin and by region of destination, and that the latter were slightly steeper. Migrants from the South and East to the North and West had higher mortality (SMRs of 103 and 113 for men and women respectively) than those moving in the opposite direction (SMRs of 83 and 89 respectively). They concluded that migration was unlikely to explain differences except in areas greatly affected by migration [24]. Analysis of the mortality of those entering England and Wales suggested that these immigrants (other than the Irish) were a select, healthy group, but Fox and Goldblatt caution that low mortality in the years after census may derive from pre-existing socio-economic differences between those who leave a country and those who stay behind, or from various measurement biases [24]. Marmot *et al.*, interpret their findings on male immigrant mortality in terms of selective processes as well as retention of life style [51].

Fox and Goldblatt also explore the possiblity that variations in mortality by marital status were due to selection factors, by examining observed and expected deaths by sex, age, marital status and year of death. Among younger people SMRs for the married rise with length of follow up and those for the single fall, that is, the difference narrows over time. The change in SMRs is, however small, and health-related mobility is unlikely to account for much of the differential. On the other hand, time trends in SMRs for older men suggest that health-selection may play a major role in producing marital status differentials, with relatively healthy men remarrying after widowerhood. There appears to be a health-selection effect operating between the ages of 15 and 44 for married women, but not at other age groups, or for single or widowed women [24].

Fox, Goldblatt and Jones looked at deaths among men in 1971–75 and 1976–81 in relation to their social class in 1971. They found that the mortality gradient by 1971 social class was steeper in 1976–81 than in 1971–75, and suggested that any selection effect that had occurred in the shorter period (i.e. occupation at 1971 census already being influenced by ill health which led to death in 1971–75) had attenuated by the later period, and that the figure for the latter therefore represented the effects of accumulated life chances rather than selection effects [106]. Moser and Goldblatt, on the basis of a similar analysis of women's mortality, showed that the relative mortality for those in the manual occupational classes increased between 1971–75 and 1976–81, while the relative mortality of those in non-manual social classes hardly changed, indicating that differentials by occupation were unlikely to be based on selection effects [116].

Used similar time-based arguments, Berkman and Breslow suggested that if ill health had caused 'social disconnection', rather than vice versa, in the Alameda County study, one would expect that people seriously ill enough to have few social ties would die mostly in the years following the baseline survey; this was found, however, not to be the case. The Alameda County study, unlike the British Longitudinal Study, obtained self-reported physical health measures on their respondents and were thus also able to control for physical health as measured in the baseline survey. They found that their social network index predicted mortality at all levels of physical health, and concluded that the association between social networks and mortality was not merely the reflection of underlying poor health [69]. The Whitehall study, similarly, controlled for health status at entry to the study and found that, although there was a gradient by employment grade at entry, this could not fully account for the steep gradient in deaths from coronary heart disease and other conditions across employment grades [15]. These studies illustrate the importance of a prospective approach to teasing out the relative importance of health selection versus social causation; the Alameda County and Whitehall studies also illustrate the importance of having health measures in any baseline survey.

Other contributions to this debate have been a more theoretical, or at least a less empirical, level. Stern presented a stylised illustrative model of how a systematic health-related selection process can lead to those of lower social class of achievement having a higher mortality rate even though the rates are equal by social class of origin [97]. The Black Report considered what it called "theories of natural and social selection", but suggested that there was little evidence for social drift caused by physical disease, and argued that such theories would not adequately account for the steepness of social class gradients in childhood and early life, since occupational drift caused by ill health could have no opportunity of operating by then [1].

Although there is thus some fascinating work on the possible role of health selection in observed relationships between social position and health, there are still many gaps in the field. Firstly, much of this work applies to specific problems and selected samples; for example, unemployed men [111], working versus non-working women [112], or assortative mating among child-bearing women [115, 117]. Secondly, most of the existing work, apart from the Longitudinal Study's analyses of migration and marriage, deals with social class. Although health selection cannot 'cause' gender, age or ethnicity, it can shape observed gradients in health according to these variables through selective migration and survivorship, so the process is worth exploring in terms of these variables as well as for occupational class, marriage and area of residence.

Thirdly, most of it remains at an associational level, leaving open the question of how such selective processes might actually operate, i.e. how unhealthy men might be extruded from the work-force or move down an occupational hierarchy; how married women chose or are chosen to return to the work-force; how mate selection might in practice be connected with height and vigour; how decisions are made by internal or international migrants to move in search of work and how this relates to their family's or other agencies' views of their health; how health might be implicated in decisions about whether and whom to marry, or in the break-up of marriage; and how social mobility might be affected by health. These processes should interest sociologists, and we need to explore the processes intervening between the health status (or change in health status) and the occupancy of a particular social position (or shift in social position).

Social causation

Theories of social determinants of patterns of health and illness have a long and respectable tradition. Hippocratic writings dating from around 400 B.C. stressed the importance for human health of environmental factors such as the quality of air, food and water, climate and topography, and general living habits and saw health as an expression of harmony between the environment, way of life and human nature [76].

There has been much interest in social determinants of health since the public health movement in the nineteenth century, and the literature on this topic is too voluminous to summarise comprehensively or review in detail. The main points in current ideas about social determinants of health are therefore briefly described with one or two issues highlighted for illustrative purposes, and then some general points are made about the current state of knowledge in this field.

Three broad strands in research and policy formulation can be discerned. There is an interest in the influence on health of, firstly, living conditions and the circumstances of people's lives; secondly, behaviours; and thirdly, knowledge, attitudes and values. The first two strands are sometimes seen as competing explanations for social patterning in health; Doyal *et al.* for example, counterpose what they call 'environmentalist' and 'lifestyle' explanations for cancer incidence [118], and the Black Report compares 'structural/materialistic' and 'cultural/behavioural' explanations of social class inequalities in health [1]. While at the extreme they can be seen as competing explanations (in that they imply different sorts of medical and social interventions), they probably interact and it may be more helpful to find the right balance between them rather than viewing them as mutually exclusive. The third group, knowledge, attitudes and values, is usually conceptualised as mediating between social position and health either by moderating the impact of life circumstances on health, by causing the behaviours that influence health, or by acting directly on health.

Life circumstances

The public health movement in Britain in the mid and late nineteenth century focussed attention on a wide range of environmental and social risks to health, including occupational hazards, adulterated foods, urbanisation, poverty, unclean water supplies, poor sanitation, the employment of women and children, air pollution, overcrowded and poorly ventilated housing and so forth [3]. McKeown and others have argued that public health measures designed to reduce environmental hazards, plus the general rise in living standards over the last century, did more to contribute to the improvement of the health of the population than did specific medical interventions (whether curative or preventive) [119]. Despite these improvements, there are still, however, real differences in living conditions and personal circumstances between social groups that may contribute to differences in their health experiences–differences, for example, in their work settings, housing, access to amenities, command over resources, physical and social threats from the environment and resources to cope with such threats.

Occupation, and its related work settings, has for long been shown to influence health, and since occupation varies by social class by definition, and by gender, age, marital status (at least for women), ethnicity and area of residence, occupational influences on health may mediate between these social positions and health. There has been much discussion in the Registrar General's Decennial Supplements on Occupational Mortality about the direct versus indirect effects of occupation on health, and techniques such as social class standardisation, and the comparison of mortality rates between men working in particular occupations and their wives, have been employed to tease out the relative importance of direct occupational risks as compared with general living conditions. Analysis of cause-specific mortality rates for each occupational order, controlling for social class, shows that some occupations have high death rates from all or most causes (for example, furnace, forge, foundry and rolling mill workers have high death rates from all causes but particularly from cancer of the lung and stomach and from respiratory and circulatory diseases); some have average death rates but seem subject to specific risks (for example, wood-workers have low SMRs but have an excess of deaths from cancers of the nose and sinus); and others have consistently low deaths for all causes (for example, the age, sex and social class standardised death rates for ministers of the crown, MPs and senior Government officials was 61) [9]. Occupations classified as being in the same social class groups can have markedly different mortality rates. Jones and Cameron illustrate this by listing selected occupations within social classes and showing all-cause SMRs among men aged 15–64 varying from 42 to 116 in social class 1, 54 to 175 in social class II, 59 to 104 in social class IIIn, 47 to 156 in social class IIIm, 81 to 171 in social class IV, and 80 to 160 in social class V [76].

The assumption underlying the comparison between men working in particular occupations or industries and their wives, namely that similar mortality patterns represent general conditions of living rather than direct occupational risks, has been challenged. Men may bring home with them hazards from work such as dust or asbestos fibres and these may lead to high rates of related diseases in both spouses [9]. High rates of cervical cancer are found in women married to men in specific occupations (mainly 'dirty' jobs involving mineral oils) [118].

In addition to occupation, employment and unemployment may influence health, and the likelihood of unemployment (and its practical and psychological consequences) may differ between social groups. A considerable amount of work has been conducted recently showing that over and above the 'healthy worker effect', unemployment may have detrimental effects on mental and physical well-being [111, 120, 121].

Occupation and employment are highly correlated with a variety of socio-economic and psycho-social processes influencing health, and in addition to the more obvious direct physical risks of particular occupations there may be many features of occupations that influence health. Many of these are described in the occupational health literature.

Housing has long been regarded as influencing health, and type of housing tends to vary between social groups and areas of the country. The Longitudinal Study showed that for both men and women a simple three-fold classification of housing tenure, owner occupiers, private renters and council house tenants, was strongly associated with mortality (in 1971–75 the SMRs for men so classified were, respectively, 91, 105 and 114, and for women they were 93, 100 and 113). Differences in mortality based on housing characteristics were greatest for respiratory disease, but among males there was a steep gradient for malignant neoplasms, and among females one for circulatory disease [24]. McCarthy *et al.* have recently shown that among council house tenants, those living in 'poor' housing areas reported more respiratory symptoms than those living in 'good' housing areas (having controlled for age, household class, smoking and work experience). Respiratory symptoms were associated with flats rather than houses, and with older accommodation [122].

Access to other amenities has also been implicated in the production of health. Mortality is high among those without access to household amenities such as inside w.c.'s, baths and running hot water. Perhaps less predictably, household car ownership differentiates between people with different mortality risks, in general and within each housing tenure category [24]. For women aged 15–59, for example, SMRs in 1976–81 by housing tenure and access to cars in 1971 were 78 and 108 for owner occupiers with and without cars, 83 and 136 for private tenants with and without cars, and 98 and 139 for local authority tenants with and without cars [116].

Similar evidence has been produced about other features of living conditions, such as income, wealth and the physical environment. Attempting to understand the connections between social position, each aspect of living conditions taken separately, and health, is frustrating for two main reasons. The first is that empirically many features of living conditions cluster (e.g. the unemployed may be poor, live in poor housing, have no car, etc.) and therefore confound each other. The second is that the observed association tells us noting about the processes connecting the living conditions with health. For example, does having a car in the household directly influence health (and if so, how? Do car owners use the car for recreational visits to the country, to speed up commuting time, to shop for more nourishing foods?) or is it that having a car is a marker for other characteristics which influence health (and if so, what are the important ones? Income, priorities for allocating income, desire to be in control of one's life?). These questions cannot easily be addressed from the existing, epidemiological level evidence.

One element of people's life circumstances that might influence health and life expectancy is access to, and treatment by, the health care system and health professionals. There is considerable evidence that some health care resources are unevenly distributed in respect of all the social positions of interest, with those social groups most in need receiving a lower proportion of health care resources than their needs might merit, the 'inverse care law' enunciated by Tudor Hart [123]. In Britain most of the research on this topic has concerned the distribution of health care by social class [1, 124–126] and by region or area [127, 128]. For example, Buchan and Richardson have shown that general practitioners spend longer with middle class than with working class patients [129], and Cartwright has also shown that in some respects the quality of hospital care may be poorer for lower social class patients [130, 131]. There has been less research on the availability and quality of health care according to other axes of social differentiation, and the isssue of the extent to which the National Health Service does offer equality of access to care to all citizens is one that is still disputed [126].

A still more disputed, but under-researched, issue is the extent to which differential access to health care matters for mental or physical health and for survival. McKeown [119] and others have argued that curative (and even preventive) medical interventions may have had less impact on changes over time in life expectancy than have changes in living standards, and it has been shown that medical treatment, such as intensive care for heart attack victims [132], bed rest for women pregnant with twins [133], or routine antenatal care [134] may have little or even deleterious effects compared with less interventionist care. However, we know surprisingly little about the contribution that health care makes to the experience of health or illness, or to the likelihood of death, among different social groups in the population at any one point in time. Rather, it either tends to be assumed that most health care is relatively ineffectual in influencing morbidity or mortality patterns in the community, or that health care is an important contributor to such patterns, without much empirical evidence being offered for either assumption.

Other, more psychological aspects of living conditions have been shown to affect health and to be differentially distributed among social groups. There is a large literature on life events and their impact on physical and mental health [71, 135–137], and it has been shown that the occurrence and nature of threatening life events may differ between social classes and between areas. In a study of pregnant women, for example, it was found that single women and those in social classes IV and V experienced significantly more major life events during pregnancy than those in social classes I and II, and that those major life events were significantly associated with lower birthweight (this effect also occurred independently of social class) [138]. Among women in Camberwell, the rate of severe household life events differed between working and middle class women (though only for those with children at home), with working class women having nearly three times as many severe household events as middle class women, and the occurrence of life events being associated with the onset of depression [71]. In another study it was found that women in Camberwell had a more threatening environment than those living in Walthamstow; they had four times as many 'general crises' (such as burglary, theft of car, accidents, physical attacks on the women or someone close to her, contact with the police or courts, loss of family pets), and more events such as the woman or her husband changing job, than women in Walthamstow [136]. In another comparison it was found that women in Camberwell had 1.8 times more 'regular' life events, 1.34 times more 'irregular' life events and eight times as many 'disruptive' life events, than women living in Lewis, in the outer Hebrides [139].

Within the tradition of life events research, socio-environmental stress is often conceptualised as being acute, and consisting of specific changes or events which appear stressful and disease-producing (or resistance-reducing). However, events such as the death of a spouse or being laid off work, in addition to constituting acute and threatening life events, also create states such as widowhood or unemployment which may represent sources of chronic difficulties and stress. Lazarus and Cohen have suggested that 'chronic hassles', which involve dealing with difficult situations on a day to day basis, may be more taxing of adaptive energy than short term situations [140]. Such chronic hassles may have to do with either living conditions (problems over housing, income, etc.) or social relations (unpleasant neighbours, an unhappy marriage, etc.).

Social networks and social support (usually distinguished as referring respectively to the structure and to the nature of social ties), have also been shown to influence health and to be differentially distributed between social groups and types of area. In the Alameda County study four kinds of social contact were investigated: marriage, contact with extended family and close friends, church membership, and other group affiliation. Each of these was independently associated with subsequent mortality, from a wide variety of diseases, even when physical health at baseline interview was controlled. A social network index combining these four showed a consistent pattern of higher mortality among the least socially connected (except for women aged 50–59), the age-adjusted relative risks being 2.3 for men and 2.8 for women [69]. The same study showed that the extent of social networks was associated with socio-economic status (the higher the SES the more social contacts), geographical mobility (the greater the mobility the fewer the contacts), occupational mobility (the greater the mobility the fewer the contacts), and ethnicity (for every age and sex group, except women aged 60–69, whites scored higher on the social network index than either blacks or others). At younger ages rural dwellers had stronger social ties but at older ages urban dwellers, especially those in 'non-poverty' areas, had stronger social ties. Low social ties and low socio-economic status, living in an urban poverty area, and being non-white, were independently associated with high mortality [69].

Other studies have shown a number of effects on health of social support or social networks. For example, close ties may buffer the effect of threatening life events [71], improve recovery time for heart attack victims [141] decrease rates of pregnancy complications [142] and influence help-seeking behaviour [143].

From the above brief and selected review it is clear that various aspects of people's circumstances from the most material (living in poor housing) to the least material (having close social ties), have been shown both to influence health and to be differentially distributed among social groups. Although to a certain extent some of these life circumstances can be seen as resulting from people's own choices, they can also be seen as constraints or opportunities provided by the physical and social environment, and changes in them may require social, economic or political intervention rather than the reform of individuals.

Behaviours

Remedies for the second main group of possible social influences on health do tend to be seen as very much involving the reform of individuals. Increasing attention has been paid over the last decade or two to the contribution of behaviours to health, and it has indeed been argued that: "the greatest potential, and perhaps the greatest problem for preventative medicine, now lies in changing behaviour and attitudes to health" [144]. Many of the major health problems of today, such as heart disease and cancer, are seen as attributable to individual behaviour patterns and therefore more appropriately attacked by attempting to change these behaviour patterns rather than by focussing on curative procedures [144–146]. The Royal Commission on the Health Service summarised this view as follows:

"The most obvious preventable conditions are those which can be attributed directly to the way we live. Smoking is an important contributory factor in lung cancer, bronchitis and coronary heart disease, but in 1976, 49% of adult men and 39% of adult women smoked cigarettes. Road accidents account for about 6500 deaths in Britain each year.... Excess blood alcohol contributes massively to road accidents, and alcoholism to other accidents and to social problems. The wrong kind of food encourages obesity and dental decay ... Reduction in smoking and alcohol related illness, the prevention of road accidents and mitigating their results, improved nutritional policies, should be the prime targets for prevention ... " [147, p. 42].

Cigarette smoking and alcohol consumption can be used to illustrate the contribution of behaviour to health, and the distribution of behaviour among social groups.

Cigarette smoking has been unequivocally demonstrated to be a major cause of premature death, from heart disease, chronic bronchitis, lung cancer and other conditions, and to produce much ill health and disability [118]. Cigarette smoking is highly class-related. In 1982 in Britain 20% of men in professional occupations smoked cigarettes compared with 49% of men in unskilled manual occupations; the equivalent gradient for women was 21 to 41%. More men than women smoke (38% compared with 33%), and male smokers smoke more heavily than female ones. Among men aged 35–49 the prevalence of smoking among the widowed, divorced and separated was 59% compared to 44% among the single and 39% among the married; for women aged 35–49 the prevalence of smoking was 49% for the widowed, divorced and separated, 34% for the single and 37% for the married. The prevalence of smoking was lowest in East Anglia and highest in the North West [11].

Alcohol consumption shows a more complex relation to health, good health being associated with light to moderate consumption and poor health being associated with both abstinence and moderate or heavy consumption [69, 148]. In 1982 8% of men in professional occupations compared with 33% of men in unskilled manual occupations were 'heavier' drinkers. Men were more likely to be heavier drinkers than women. Drinking patterns were associated with types of industry (with heavier drinking in the construction, coal mining, mineral extraction and metal and chemical manufacturing industries) and with employment (there were more abstainers among the economically inactive, and more heavier drinkers among the unemployed). Alcohol consumption was related to stage of family life-cycle (i.e. whether there were children and how old they were) and to marital status (for example, 47% of formerly married men aged 25–44 were heavy or moderate drinkers, compared with 30% single men and 28% married men of the same age). There were regional gradients in drinking patterns, there being a higher prevalence of heavy drinking in the North and West than in the South and East [11]. For more detailed accounts see Dight [149] for Scottish patterns and Wilson [150] for England and Wales.

Epidemiological studies have shown that smoking and drinking, and a range of other behaviours such as taking recreational physical exercise, diet, engaging in high risk activities, sexual and contraceptive practices, and so forth, are associated with health and risk of ill health or death (involving not only the individual concerned but also their offspring), and are differentially engaged in by different social groups. However, these correlations with social group do not explain all the variations between these groups in their health. For example, in the Whitehall study both cigarette smoking and physically active leisure pursuits were associated with employment grade (men in the lowest grade were twice as likely as those in the highest grade to smoke cigarettes and only half as likely to take physically active recreation), and were correlated with the risk of coronary heart disease (and other) mortality; but these behaviours and the other risk factors examined explained only a small part of the variance in mortality between employment grades [16]. The Aladema County findings that five common health related 'behaviours' (cigarette smoking, physical activity, alcohol consumption, obesity and sleeping patterns) were significantly associated, separately and jointly, with mortality risks, has been widely reported. The association between these health practices and mortality was found to be independent of a wide range of factors including self reported physical health at the time of the baseline survey, year of death, socio-economic status, race, preventive practices and psychological factors. Less widely known is their finding that people of low socio-economic status, males, and black or other non-white ethnic groups had higher mortality than their higher socio-economic status, female, or white counterparts even when controlling for these health behaviours [69]. This accords with other findings that relationships between, for example, social class and health are not simply reducible to differences in specified risk factors; a working class smoker is more likely than a middle class smoker to be adversely affected by smoking, for example [47]. Nevertheless these behaviours are seen as important targets for intervention because they make a major contribution to health and are seen as being amenable to change.

There have been numerous criticisms of the DHSS view of the contribution to the promotion of health that would be made by changing behaviours. One, relating to the point just made, is that other factors, known or unknown and acting singly or in combination, influence health and produce social differentials, and that these also need attention [147]. Another is that behaviours may not be as subject to individual choice and control as some of the health education literature implies. As Pill and Stott suggest of the DHSS view:

"It assumes that everyone has the resources and the autonomy to effect the necessary changes in behaviour and lead healthier lives" [151, p. 49].

Antonovsky has put this point more forcibly when he suggests:

"Over and above the misplaced ideological implications of blaming the victims, the changes in lifestyle are often forced on us by the social organisation within which we live and in which individual choice plays only a minor role" [152, p. 102].

This point is returned to at the end of this section.

Another type of behaviour often mentioned in discussions of variations in health is use of health services. In Britain there is evidence that the use of most types of health care, whether general practitioner or hospital based, and preventive or curative, varies systematically with the social positions reviewed here [1, 30, 45, 54, 126]. There is indeed a large literature on illness behaviour, use of services and compliance with treatment among various social groups. However, there is much less evidence than there is about behaviours such as smoking and alcohol consumption that use of health services actually contributes much to patterns of morbidity and mortality (see the discussion of this point on p. 406). It is thus not clear how much of the variation between social groups in their health or likelihood of survival can validly be attributed to the well-documented variations in illness behaviour or differential use of services. Much health promotional literature, or work directed towards reducing differentials in health, tends however to ignore this lacuna and uncritically to treat the provision and use of health services as a major contributor to health or to differentials in health [153, 154].

Knowledge, attitudes and values

A third (and interconnected) group of types of explanation for variations in health consists of knowledge, attitudes and values. Such cognitive and emotional factors are seen to influence health either indirectly, by shaping behaviours which are the more proximate causes of health, or more directly, by having some more diffuse and general impact on health independently of behaviour.

Examples of the first type include knowledge of, for example, the nutritional value of various foodstuffs [155], the immunological, nutritional and emotional advantages of breast feeding [156], the risks of smoking [157] or the benefits and hazards of oral contraception [158]. It is these sorts of knowledge and beliefs towards which many health educational programmes are directed. Attitudes often seen as relevant include those pertaining to the extent to which health is under the individual's control [151, 159, 160], the evaluation of the risks of behaviours [157], orientation towards preventive health measures [161, 162], and attitudes towards food, smoking, drinking and contraception. Cultural or subcultural norms relating to health behaviour include expectations of appropriate age, marital and sex-role behaviours; for example, that adult men in certain social groups should drink alcohol [149, 150], that women should no longer engage in physical recreation outside the home once they are married

[163], that Asian women should stay indoors [164, 165], and a whole set of values relating to food (who prepares it, in what form, and for whom) [166]. Other values include the importance of health as opposed to other aspects of life. (Type A personality, thought by some to be implicated in the genesis of coronary heart disease [168], might also be included in this list of emotional or value orientations influencing health, although there is dispute about whether the type A behaviour patterns stem from characteristics of the individual or from features of his or her environment [169].) These cognitive or emotional characteristics are differentially distributed among social groups and are seen to influence health via behaviours. The literature on the relationship between knowledge, attitudes and behaviour is too extensive to summarise here; a good review is given in Marsh and Matheson's "Smoking Attitudes and Behaviour" [158].

The second type of emotional or cognitive factor is seen to have a direct effect on health, without behaviour necessarily intervening, by influencing the way people respond to their lives and environments. Brown and Harris, for example, emphasise the traditional sociological view that what is significant for social action (or in this case, reaction) is the subjective meanings people attribute to the world about them. They suggest that the impact of life events is mediated by the meanings given to these events, and stress that they are concerned:

"not just with the fact that as a result of rehousing a housewife walks further to the shops or sees few friends *but with how she perceives and reacts emotionally to these changes*" [72, p. 5: emphasis in original].

Other authors have stressed the importance of various psychosocial 'sets' that may influence people's capacity to deal with the world, such as coping styles [138, 141, 170], locus of control [171], learned helplessness [172], or sense of coherence [153]. There is a large literature on coping strategies, locus of control etc and there is much research underway in this and the stress fields; too much to review in detail here. It should be noted, however, that coping styles or other 'sets' are not necessarily seen as randomly distributed in the population, but are often viewed as resources differentially distributed by social group. Antonovsky puts this in his typically forthright way when he states:

"Of course, it matters very much where one is located in the social structure. Social classes, ethnic and racial groups, men and women do not all share the same set of life experiences. To generalize about national societies without awareness of the great difference it makes whether one is an Appalachian coal miner, a suburban upper-middle-class housewife, or a university professor is to obscure any possible understanding of differences in the sense of coherence" [153, p. 227.

General points

To summarise, three broad types of possible social causes of health have been identified and studied, life circumstances, behaviours and beliefs/attitudes. The distinction between these three types of explanation for social patterning of health is important because each has rather different implications for the likely effectiveness of various medical and social policies. Depending on the preferred or fashionable explanatory model, interventions may be directed at life circumstances (for example, by improving housing standards, up-grading welfare benefits, improving employment opportunities), at behaviours (for example, legislating for compulsory seat-belt use, encouraging physical recreation, banning smoking in public places), or at knowledge, attitudes and values (for example, by teaching proper nutritional skills, encouraging people to believe that giving up smoking could be possible and beneficial, or changing ideas about the domestic division of labour).

Six general points can be made about the current state of research into social factors or processes influencing health. Firstly, in studying the social determinants of health sociologists should not restrict themselves to chains of causation each link of which can somehow be regarded as 'psychosocial'. Physiological processes or the material environment may be the immediate 'cause' of health states or statuses, but the person's exposure or vulnerability to these physical causes may be socially shaped, and therefore a proper topic for sociologists. In this regard I differ from those who suggest that sociologists have most to contribute by concentrating on the direct involvement of the social environment in the production of disorder, for example, by cognitive or emotional responses directly producing physical or psychiatric disorder [72]. While this approach may usefully emphasise the role of interpretations and evaluations of events or experiences, it is unduly restrictive and tends to lead both to an under-emphasis on socio-economic and material factors, and to a division into 'social illnesses' (mainly psychiatric or functional disorders) and 'non social illnesses' (mainly organic ones of interest to bio-medical scientists), a division which seems unrealistic given the associations observed between social position and a whole range of adverse health outcomes including 'organic' ones such as cancer, heart disease, stroke etc.

Secondly, as noted earlier, much of the recent work tends to concentrate on psycho-social factors, such as life events or social support. This sometimes creates or reinforces an assumption that the only contribution social position may make to health is via stress or exposure to life events, thereby leading to neglect of more mundane and practical features of people's everyday lives. Being out of work, or widowed, can affect disposable income, wealth, access to other material resources (for example, telephone or a car), eating patterns, use of time, housing etc, and these changes can influence health either separately from or in interaction with stress, stigma or alterations in self esteem. These mundane features of daily life are, however, rarely examined. Brown and Harris's point that what is important about rehousing a woman is her interpretation of the event [72], may be valid when dealing with the etiology of depression, but other aspects of the rehoused woman's health may be affected independently of social meanings: she may, for example, become fitter if she has to walk further to the shops, or more tired if she can no longer share transporting the children to school with her friends.

Thirdly, much recent work has focussed on the effect on health of lifestyle, viewed as voluntarily chosen behaviours such as smoking, alcohol consumption or recreational exercise. This emphasis on voluntarily chosen behaviours may deflect attention from external constraints or chance factors in influencing people's everyday lives. 'Diet' for example, tends to be conceived rather narrowly in terms of choice of wholemeal bread or consumption of refined sugar and animal fats, and health education efforts are directed at inculcating conventional nutritional wisdom [172]. But what someone eats may depend less on their ideas about the value of fibre or the dangers of cholesterol, and more on the accessibility, opening hours and buying policies of food shops in the locality; the division of domestic labour in the home; the time and money available for food shopping and preparation; or whether his/her employer supplies a canteen and what it supplies. Similarly, an individual's energy expenditure may depend on local housing and transport policies; the number and age of his/her children; the distance of their school from home; the nature of his/her employment; and the domestic division of labour, at least as much as upon whether he/she goes jogging or does aerobics. However, one consequence of the contemporary interest in voluntarily chosen life-styles is that only very narrowly conceived 'health behaviours' tend to be considered, and large areas of people's lives that could be equally significant to health are ignored [173]. As noted earlier, the environmentalist/materialist/structuralist type of explanation is often seen as competing with the behavioural/cultural/lifestyle type of explanation [1, 8, 119, 174]. This polarisation is unfortunate because it means that protagonists tend only to look within their own preferred paradigm rather than taking elements from both and seeing how they might interact.

Fourthly, many studies (particularly the more intensive, sociological ones) have used relatively restricted population samples, consisting, for example, of one social class [96, 152], one sex [15, 72, 161], one ethnic group (most British studies exclude non-whites) or a single age group [97, 152]. The restrictions are usually imposed in order to simplify the analysis by reducing variability in the population under scrutiny, or for convenience of fieldwork (or both), and as such are perfectly understandable. While many of these studies are individually excellent, there is however often a failure subsequently to make systematic comparisons with other groups in the population to assess the generalisability of the findings. This can lead to the possibility either of fallaciously over-generalising from the group studied, or of fallaciously assuming that the process in question is unique to the group studied, because we do not have population values for the phenomenon of interest.

Fifthly, much research focusses on deviant or problematic groups (or ones considered anthropologically strange by policy-makers or researchers) such as the working classes or ethnic minorities. This is understandable in terms of researchers wishing to study policy-relevant issues of topical public concern, but it can result in invalid implicit comparisons with the 'normal'. For example, we may tend to think we know what it is like to be married, employed, a two-parent family, heterosexual, middle class or middle aged, and therefore fail to study people so circumstanced. Not only may this lead to lack of knowledge about such people, but it may also lead to fallacious assumptions about how the groups that are studied differ from these 'normal' groups. A related point is that there is a tendency to focus on transitional states (becoming a parent, getting divorced, being made unemployed) and to neglect long-term stable states (being a parent, a divorcee or unemployed). These two tendencies together lead to a concentration on the suddenly problematic, which, though understandable in terms of policy relevance, leaves considerable gaps in our knowledge.

Sixthly, there is occasionally a tendency to look in detail at some phenomenon, behaviour or process implicitly involved in a model of the social production of health (for example, health beliefs, illness behaviour, use of health services, or doctor/patient interaction), without explicating their supposed role in the production of health or testing whether they are actually related to health outcomes. Thus there is for example a lot of work on differential use of health services by class, gender, etc which appears to be based on the assumption that use of health services is consequential for health outcomes, but which never actually examines or tests this assumption (see p. 406).

Taken together these features of much existing work on social determinants of health mean that we know quite a lot about some behaviours (e.g. smoking, alcohol consumption, use of health services etc), some social circumstances (e.g. life events, social support), some population groups (e.g. male civil servants, children and their mothers, working class groups, elderly people), some transitions (to motherhood, unemployment, widowhood), and some settings in which health beliefs may be transmitted or expressed (mother–daughter transmission, doctor/patient interaction). However, there are other behaviours, circumstances and population groups about which we know less (for example, we know little about diet, life events or health beliefs among men, or among middle class or middle-aged people; and surprisingly little is known about the health of adult women) and it is difficult to gain an overview of various processes and their influence on health, either because they tend to be treated separately or because they are not linked to health outcomes. This is not to decry the value or validity of individual pieces of research, but to suggest that the focus on individual issues may detract from our ability to view the processes linking social structure and health from a broader perspective.

Finally, there have been two major shifts during the last century in ideas about the social patterning of health and illness. One has been away from looking at material conditions of life (such as overcrowding, poverty, bad ventilation, polluted water supplies, occupational hazards) to looking at psychosocial aspects of living (such as social support, stress, life satisfaction, life events), as etiological factors in disease. The other has been away from viewing the processes intervening between social position and health outcomes as being largely outwith the control of the individual concerned (for example, the availability of clean air and water, provision of proper sewerage arrangements, or the design of working class housing), towards viewing these processes as being largely within the individual's own control (for example, by modifying behaviours such as smoking, alcohol consumption, sexual activity, amounts of exercise or by introducing new coping strategies). These perspectives need to be integrated by studying the relative importance of, and interactions between, material and psycho-social, and constrained and voluntaristic, determinants of patterns of health and illness. This integration is important because a focus on one of these poles at the expense of the other may lead to misdirected and unsuccessful attempts at intervention.

Artefact, health selection and/or social causation

The three types of explanatory model described here, artefact, health selection and social causation, are sometimes treated as though they are competitive and mutually exclusive [1, 98, 107]. There is, however, no *a priori* reason to suppose that they could not operate independently, consecutively or interactively to produce observed patterns of social differentiation in health. For example, starting life with a health disadvantage such as low birth-weight seems to produce greater vulnerability to further health and social disadvantage among those born into poor social circumstances than among those born into good social circumstances [79]. If we wish to elucidate the processes underlying observed associations between social position and health and illness it is, therefore, necessary to take all three processes, artefact, selection and causation, into account. Sorting out their relative importance is not just of idle or academic interest; the effectiveness of medical or social interventions depends on the validity of our theories about the contribution of these three types of process to any given health field. Whether or not action is taken to improve the health of certain groups perceived to be disadvantaged (whether middle aged men at risk of heart disease, Asians with tuberculosis, or single parents and their children), and what actions are taken, will be based on beliefs about the reasons for the apparent health disadvantage, and the efficacy of these actions will then depend on the accuracy of these beliefs.

CONCLUSIONS

In this article I have collated and presented British material demonstrating associations between social position and health, using a variety of indicators of health and avoiding those relating to service use. I have shown that each of the selected positions, occupational class, gender, marital status, age, ethnicity and area of residence, is apparently related empirically to a wide range of health outcomes. I have argued that it would be profitable to attempt to pull together the currently rather separate strands of research on these social positions, and to attempt to develop models of social regularities in general vulnerability to, or protection from, ill-health. I have also suggested that we need to 'unpack' categories such as class, gender etc and to explore the everyday lives of those categorised along these dimensions.

I have reviewed three main types of explanation for observed social regularities in health, artefact, health selection, and social causation. Under the social causation heading I have outlined research in three major areas implicated in models of the social production of health: life circumstances; beliefs, attitudes and values; and behaviour. I argued that the three broad types of explanation need not be seen as competing or mutually exclusive, and that we need more prospective sociological research on unselected populations to explore, empirically, the processes linking social position and health.

Acknowledgements—The author is supported financially by the Medical Research Council of Great Britain. She would like to thank Mildred Blaxter, Mick Bloor, Iain Chalmers, Sarah Cunningham-Burley, John Fox, Raymond Illsley, Rex Taylor, Mike Wadsworth and Rory Williams, and the two anonymous referees for Social Science and Medicine, for their helpful comments on an earlier draft of this paper. She would also like to thank Nicky Britten, Ken Mullen and Mike Wadsworth for allowing hitherto unpublished data to be presented.

REFERENCES

1. Black D. *Inequalities in Health: Report of a Working Group*. DHSS, HMSO, London, 1980.
2. Blaxter M. *A Comparison of Measures of Inequality in Morbidity*. Paper presented at European Science Foundation Workshop on Inequalities in Health, City University, September 1985.
3. Poor Law Commissioners. *Report of an Inquiry into the Sanitary Condition of the Labouring Population of Great Britain*. HMSO, London, 1842.
4. Registrar General. *Ninth Annual Report of the Registrar General of Births, Deaths and Marriages in England*. HMSO, London, 1849.
5. Registrar General. *Supplement to the Twenty Fifth Annual Report of the Registrar General of Births, Deaths and Marriages in England*. HMSO, London, 1864.
6. Farr W. The influence of marriage on the mortality of the French people. *Trans. natn. Ass. Promot. Soc. Sci.* 504, 1858.
7. Blaxter M. *The Health of the Children*. Heinemann, London, 1981.
8. Townsend P. and Davidson N. *Inequalities in Health: the Black Report*. Penguin, Harmondsworth, 1982.
9. Office of Population Censuses and Surveys. *Occupational Mortality*. Decennial Supplement for 1970–72, England and Wales, HMSO, London, 1978.
10. Macfarlane A. and Mugford M. *Birth Counts: Statistics of Pregnancy and Childbirth*. National Perinatal Epidemiology Unit (in collaboration with OPCS), HMSO, London, 1984.
11. Office of Population Censuses and Surveys. *General Household Survey 1982*. HMSO, London, 1984.
12. Goldberg D. and Huxley P. *Mental Illness in the Community*. Tavistock, London, 1980.
13. Floud R. Measuring the transformation of the European economies: income, health and welfare. *Discussion Paper 33*. Centre for Economic Policy Research, London, 1984.
14. Knight I. *The Height and Weight of Adults in Great Britain*. OPCS, HMSO, London, 1984.
15. Marmot M. G., Rose G., Shipley M. and Hamilton P. J. S. Employment grade and coronary heart disease in British Civil Servants. *J. Epidem. Commun. Hlth* **32**, 244, 1978.

16. Rose G. A. and Marmot M. G. Social class and coronary heart disease. *Br. Heart J.* **45,** 13, 1981.
17. Wadsworth M. E. J. MRC National Survey of Health and Development, Bristol, personal communication.
18. Wadsworth M. E. J., Cripps H. A., Midwinter R. E. T. and Colley J. R. T. Blood pressure at age 36 and social and familial factors, cigarette smoking and body mass in a national birth cohort. *Br. med. J.* In press.
19. Office of Population Censuses and Surveys. *Adult Dental Health in England and Wales in 1978.* HMSO, London, 1982.
20. Howe G., Westhoff C., Vessey M. and Yeates D. Effects of age, cigarette smoking and other factors on fertility: findings in a large study. *Br. med. J.* **290,** 1697, 1985.
21. Hunt S., McEwan J. and McKenna S. P. Social inequalities and perceived health. *Effect. Hlth Care* **2,** 151, 1985.
22. Blaxter M. Self-definition of health status and consulting rates in primary care. *Q. J. Soc. Affairs* **1,** 131, 1985.
23. Carter C. and Peel J. (Eds) *Equalities and Inequalities in Health.* Academic Press, London, 1976.
24. Fox A. J. and Goldblatt P. O. *Longitudinal Study: Socio-Demographic Mortality Differentials 1971–75,* Series LS No. 1. HMSO, London, 1982.
25. Morgan D. Gender. In *Key Variables in Social Investigation* (Edited by Burgess R.). Routledge and Kegan Paul, London, 1986.
26. Central Statistical Office. *Social Trends 14,* 1984 edn. HMSO, London, 1985.
27. United Nations. *Demographic Yearbook.* UN, New York, 1981.
28. Waldron I. Sex differences in illness incidence, prognosis and mortality. *Soc. Sci. Med.* **17,** 1107, 1983.
29. Briscoe M. Sex differences in psychological well-being. In *Psychological Medicine,* Monograph supplement 1. Cambridge University Press, Cambridge, 1982.
30. Clarke J. Sexism, feminism and medicalisation—a decade review of literature on gender and illness. *Sociol. Hlth Illness* **5,** 62, 1983.
31. MacQueen D. and Celantano D. Social factors in the etiology of multiple outcomes: the case of blood pressure and alcohol consumption patterns. *Soc. Sci. Med.* **16,** 397, 1982.
32. Britten N. MRC National Survey of Health and Development, Bristol, personal communication.
33. Waldron I. Why do women live longer than men? *Soc. Sci. Med.* **10,** 349, 1976.
34. Waldron I. An analysis of causes of sex differences in mortality and morbidity. In *The Fundamental Connection Between Nature and Nurture* (Edited by Gove W. and Carpenter G. R.). Lexington Books, Lexington, Mass. 1982.
35. Verbrugge L. M. Females and illness. Recent trends in sex differences in the US. *J. Hlth Soc. Behav.* **17,** 387, 1976.
36. Verbrugge L. M. Sex and gender in health and medicine. *Soc. Sci. Med.* **12,** 329, 1978.
37. Verbrugge L. M. Multiple roles and physical health of women and men. *J. Hlth Soc. Behav.* **24,** 16, 1983.
38. Gove W. R. Sex differences in the epidemiology of mental disorder: evidence and explanations. In *Gender and Disordered Behaviour; Sex Differences in Psychopathology* (Edited by Gomberg E. S. and Franks C.). Brunner/Mazel, New York, 1979.
39. Gove W. R. and Hughes M. Possible causes of the apparent sex difference in physical health: an empirical investigation. *Am. sociol. Rev.* **44,** 126, 1979.
40. Greater Glasgow Health Board. *Maternity and Child Health Statistics 1982,* 1982.
41. Mullen K. MRC Medical Sociology Unit, Glasgow, personal communication.
42. Gove W. R. and Tudor J. F. Adult sex roles and mental illness. *Am. J. Sci.* **78,** 812, 1973.
43. Durkheim E. *Suicide.* Free Press, New York, 1951.
44. Shaper A. G., Pocock S. J., Walker M., Cohen N. M., Wale C. J. and Thomson A. G. British Regional Heart Study: cardiovascular risk factors in middle aged men in 24 towns. *Br. med. J.* **283,** 179, 1981.
45. Morgan M. Marital status, health, illness and service use. *Soc. Sci. Med.* **14A,** 633, 1980.
46. Finch J. Age. In *Key Variables in Social Investigation* (Edited by Burgess R.) Routledge and Kegan Paul, London, 1986.
47. Carr-Hill R. and Pritchard C. *The Development and Exploitation of Empirical Birthweight Standards.* Macmillan, London, 1985.
48. Waldron I., Nowotenski M., Freimer M., Henry J. P., Post N. and Witten C. Cross-cultural variation in blood pressure: a quantitative analysis of the relationships of blood pressure to cultural characteristics, salt consumption and body weight. *Soc. Sci. Med.* **16,** 419, 1982.
49. Hunt S. and McEwan J. The development of a subjective health indicator. *Soc. Hlth Illness* **2,** 231, 1980.
50. Hunt S., McKenna S. P., McEwan J., Williams J. and Papp E. The Nottingham health profile: subjective health status and medical consultation. *Soc. Sci. Med.* **15A,** 221, 1981.
51. Marmot M. G., Adelstein A. M. and Bulusu L. *Immigrant Mortality in England and Wales, 1970–78. Studies on Medical and Population Subjects,* Vol. 47, OPCS, HMSO, London, 1984.
52. Adelstein A. M., MacDonald Davis I. and Weatherall J. *Perinatal and Infant Mortality: Social and Biological Factors, 1975–77. Studies on Medical and Population Subjects,* No. 41. OPCS, London, HMSO, 1980.
53. Balarajan R., Bulusu L., Adelstein A. M. and Shukla V. Patterns of mortality among migrants to England and Wales from the Indian sub-continent. *Br. med. J.* **289,** 1185, 1984.
54. Donovan J. Ethnicity and health: a research review. *Soc. Sci. Med.* **19,** 663, 1984.
55. Fitzpatrick R. and Scambler G. Social class, ethnicity and illness. In *The Experience of Illness* (Edited by Fitzpatrick R., Hinton J., Newman S., Scambler G. and Thompson J.). Tavistock, London, 1984.
56. Gillies D. R. N., Lealman G. T., Lumb K. M. and Congdon P. Analysis of ethnic influence on stillbirths and infant mortality in Bradford 1975–81. *J. Epidem. Commun. Hlth* **38,** 214, 1984.
57. Office of Population Censuses and Surveys. *Area Mortality.* Decennial Supplement, 1969–73, England and Wales, HMSO, London, 1981.
58. World Health Organization. *World Health Statistics Quarterly,* Vol. 35. WHO, Geneva, 1982.
59. West R. Geographical variations in mortality from heart disease in England and Wales. *Br. J. Prev. Soc. Med.* **31,** 245, 1977.
60. Fox A. J., Jones D. R. and Goldblatt P. O. Approaches to studying the effects of socio-economic circumstances on geographic differences in mortality in England and Wales. *Br. med. Bull.* **40,** 309, 1984.
61. Webber J. and Craig J. Which local authorities are alike? *Popul. Trends* **5,** 13, 1976.
62. Webber R. The classification of residential neighbourhoods: an introduction to the classification of wards and parishes. *PRAG Technical Report TP23,* Centre for Environmental Studies, 1977.
63. Greater Glasgow Health Board. *10 Year Report 1974–1983,* 1984.
64. Townsend P., Simpson D. and Tibbs N. *Inequalities of Health in the City of Bristol*: a preliminary review of statistical evidence, Department of Social Administration, University of Bristol, England, 1984.

65. Howe G. *National Atlas of Disease Mortality in the United Kingdom.* Nelson, London, 1970.
66. Illsley R. and Mullen K. The health needs of disadvantaged client groups. In *Oxford Textbook of Public Health* (Edited by Holland W. W.), Chap. 12, Vol. 4. Oxford University Press, Oxford, 1985.
67. Scottish Office. *A Study of Multiply Deprived Households in Scotland.* Central Research Unit, Edinburgh, 1980.
68. Cassel J. Psychosocial processes and 'stress': theoretical formulation. *Int. J. Hlth Serv.* **4,** 471, 1974.
69. Berkman L. and Breslow L. *Health and Ways of Living: the Alameda County Study.* Oxford University Press, Oxford, 1983.
70. Open University. *The Health of Nations.* Open University Press, Milton Keynes, 1985.
71. Brown G. and Harris T. *The Social Origins of Depression.* Tavistock, London, 1978.
72. Hall J. and Jones D. Social grading of occupations. *Br. J. Sociol.* **1,** 31, 1950.
73. Goldthorpe J. and Hope K. *The Social Classification of Occupations; a New Approach and Scale.* Clarendon Press, Oxford, 1974.
74. Coxon A. J. and Jones C. L. *Class and Hierarchy: the Social Meaning of Occupations.* Macmillan, London, 1979.
75. Szreter S. The Registrar General's social classification of occupations. *Br. J. Sociol.* **xxxv,** 552, 1985.
76. Jones I. G. and Cameron D. Social class—an embarrassment to epidemiology. *Commun. Med.* **6,** 37, 1984.
77. Pritchard C. and Carr-Hill R. *The Empirical Problem of Female Social Class.* Macmillan, London, 1987.
78. Illsley R. and Mitchell R. G. (Eds) *Low Birthweight: a Medical, Psychological and Social Study.* Wiley, Chichester, 1984.
79. Askham J. Delineation of the lowest social class. *J. Biosocial Sci.* **1,** 327, 1969.
80. Macintyre S. Health and Illness. In *Key Variables in Social Investigation* (Edited by Burgess R.). Routledge and Kegan Paul, London, 1986.
81. Morris J. N. *The Uses of Epidemiology.* Livingstone, Edinburgh, 1967.
82. Dubos R. *Man, Medicine and Environment.* Penguin, Harmondsworth, 1968.
83. Morris J. N. A medical examination of 1592 workers. *Lancet* **1,** 51, 1941.
84. Pearse I. H. and Crocker L. H. *The Peckham Experiment: a study of the Living Structure of Society.* Allen & Unwin, London, 1943.
85. Koos E. *The Health of Regionville: What the People Thought and Did About It.* Hefner, New York, 1954.
86. Epson J. *The Mobile Health Clinic*: an interim report on a preliminary analysis of the first 1,000 patients to attend, mimeo. London Borough of Southwark, 1969.
87. Wadsworth M. E. J., Butterfield W. J. H. and Blaney R. *Health and Sickness: the Choice of Treatment.* Tavistock, London, 1971.
88. World Health Organization. *International Classification of Impairments, Disability and Handicap.* WHO, Geneva, 1980.
89. Tuckett D. Becoming a patient. In *Introduction to Medical Sociology* (Edited by Tuckett D.). Tavistock, London, 1976.
90. Holland W. W. and Waller J. Population studies in the London Borough of Lambeth. *Commun. Med.* **126,** 153, 1971.
91. Clarke J. Trouble with feet. In *Occasional Papers on Social Administration,* No. 29. Bell, London, 1969.
92. Office of Population Censuses and Surveys. *General Household Survey 1978.* HMSO, London, 1980.
93. Kessler I. I. and Levin M. L. *The Community as an Epidemiological Laboratory.* Johns Hopkins University Press, Baltimore, 1970.
94. Wright S. Subjective evaluation of health: a theoretical review. *Soc. Indicat. Res.* **16,** 169, 1984.
95. Blaxter M. and Paterson E. *Mothers and Daughters: a Three-Generational Study of Health Attitudes and Behaviour.* Heinemann, London, 1982.
96. Williams R. Concepts of health: an analysis of lay logic. *Sociology* **17,** 185, 1983.
97. Stern J. Social mobility and the interpretation of social class mortality differentials. *J. Social Policy* **12,** 27, 1983.
98. Bloor M., Samphier M. and Prior L. Artefact explanations of inequalities in health: an assessment of the evidence. *Sociol. Hlth Illness.* In press.
99. Macintyre S. *Marital Status and Pregnancy Outcome: a Research Proposal.* Mimeo, MRC Medical Sociology Unit, Glasgow, 1984.
100. Elbourne D. and Pritchard C. *Perinatal Outcome and Related Factors: Social Class Differences Within and Between Geographical Areas.* Paper presented at European Society for Aspects of Reproduction, Aberdeen, September 1985 (mimeo NPEU, Oxford).
101. Reid D. and Rose G. Assessing the comparability of mortality statistics. *Br. med. J.* **251,** 1437, 1964.
102. Aitken Swan J. The epidemiological background. In *Experience with Abortion: A Case Study of North-East Scotland* (Edited by Horobin G.), Chap. 1. Cambridge University Press, Cambridge, 1973.
103. Kitsuse J. and Cicourel A. A note on the use of official statistics. *Social Probl.* **11,** 131, 1963.
104. Douglas J. D. *The Social Meanings of Suicide.* Princeton University Press, Princeton, 1967.
105. Marks J., Goldberg D. and Hillier V. Determinants of the ability of general practitioners to detect psychiatric illness. *Psychol. Med.* **9,** 337, 1979.
106. Fox A. J., Goldblatt P. O. and Jones D. R. Social class mortality differentials: Artefact, selection or life circumstances. *J. Epidem. Commun. Hlth* **39,** 1, 1985.
107. Illsley R. Occupational class, selection, and the production of inequalities. In *Generating Inequalities: Health and Social Mobility* (Edited by Wilkinson R.), Tavistock, London, 1986.
108. Hollingshead A. G. and Redlich F. C. *Social Class and Mental Illness.* Wiley, New York, 1958.
109. Goldberg E. M. and Morrison S. L. Schizophrenia and social class. *Br. J. Psychiat.* **109,** 785, 1963.
110. Wilkinson R. *Generating Inequalities; Health and Social Mobility.* Tavistock, London, 1986.
111. Moser K. A., Fox A. J. and Jones D. R. Unemployment and mortality in the OPCS Longitudinal Study. *Lancet* **8,** 1324, 1984.
112. Arber S., Gilbert N. and Dale A. Paid employment and women's health: a benefit or a source of role strain? *Sociol. Hlth Illness.* **7,** 375, 1985.
113. Stern J. The relationship between unemployment, morbidity and mortality in Britain. *Populatn Stud.* **37,** 61, 1983.
114. Wadsworth M. E. J. Serious illness in children and its association with later life achievement. In *Generating Inequalities: Health and Social Mobility* (Edited by Wilkinson R.). Tavistock, London, 1986.
115. Illsley R. Social class selection and class differences in relation to stillbirths and infant deaths. *Br. med. J.* **233,** 1520, 1955.
116. Moser K. and Goldblatt P. Mortality of women in the OPCS Longitudinal Study; differentials by own occupation and household housing characteristics; *Working Paper Number 28,* Social Statistics Research Unit, City University, 1985.
117. Illsley R. *Professional or Public Health? Sociology in Health and Medicine.* Nuffield Provincial Hospital Trust, London, 1980.
118. Doyal L., Green K., Irwin A., Russell D., Stewart F., Williams R., Gee D. and Epstein S. *Cancer in Britain,*

The Politics of Prevention. Pluto Press, London, 1983.
119. Mackeown T. *The Role of Medicine: Dream, Mirage or Nemesis.* Nuffield Provincial Hospitals Trust, London, 1976.
120. Mullen K. The social context of unemployment and health: a review of the literature. *Occasional Paper Number 8,* Institute of Medical Sociology, University of Aberdeen, 1985.
121. Warr P. B. and Jackson P. R. Men without jobs; some correlates of age and length of unemployment. *J. occup. Psychol.* **57,** 77, 1983.
122. McCarthy P., Byrne D., Harrison S. and Keithley J. Respiratory conditions: effects of housing and other factors. *J. Epidem. Commun. Hlth* **39,** 15, 1985.
123. Tudor Hart J. The inverse care law. *Lancet* **1,** 405, 1971.
124. Brotherston J. Inequality: is it inevitable? In *Equalities and Inequalities in Health* (Edited by Carter C. and Peel J.). Academic Press, London, 1976.
125. Cartwright A. and O'Brien M. Social class variations in health care. In *Sociology in the NHS, Sociological Review Monograph 22* (Edited by Stacey M.). University of Keele, Keele, 1976.
126. Walters V. *Class Equality and Health Care.* Croom Helm, London, 1980.
127. West R. R. and Lowe C. R. Regional variations in need for and provision and use of child health services in England and Wales. *Br. med. J.* **2,** 843, 1976.
128. Skrimshire A. *Area Disadvantage, Social Class, and the Health Service.* Department of Social and Administrative Studies, University of Oxford, Oxford, 1978.
129. Buchan I. C. and Richardson M. E. *Time Study of Consultations in General Practice.* Scottish Home and Health Department, 1973.
130. Cartwright A. *Human Relations and Hospital Care.* Routledge and Kegan Paul, London, 1964.
131. Cartwright A. *The Dignity of Labour.* Tavistock, London, 1979.
132. Cochrane A. *Effectiveness and Efficiency.* Nuffield Provincial Hospital Trust, London, 1972.
133. Saunders M. S., Dick J. S., Brown I. McL., McPherson K. and Chalmers I. The effects of hospital admission for bed rest on the duration of twin pregnancy: a randomised trial. *Lancet* **ii,** 793, 1985.
134. Hall M., Macintyre S. and Porter M. *Antenatal Care Assessed.* Aberdeen University Press, Aberdeen, 1985.
135. Dohrenwend B. P. and Dohrenwend B. S. *Stressful Life Events: Their Nature and Effects.* Wiley, New York, 1974.
136. Murphy E. and Brown G. Life events, psychiatric disturbance and physical illness. *Br. J. Psychiat.* **136,** 326, 1980.
137. Lazarus R. S. *Psychological Stress and the Coping Process.* McGraw–Hill, New York, 1966.
138. Newton R. and Hunt L. Psychosocial stress in pregnancy and its relation to low birthweight. *Br. med. J.* **288,** 1191, 1984.
139. Prudo R., Harris T. and Brown G. W. Psychiatric disorder in a rural and an urban population: 3. Social integration and the morphology of affective disorder. *Psychol. Med.* **14,** 327, 1984.
140. Lazarus R. S. and Cohen J. B. Environmental stress. In *Human Behaviours and Environment, Advances in Theory and Research* (Edited by Altman I. and Wohlwill J. F.), Vol. 2, p. 89. Plenum Press, New York, 1977.
141. Finlayson A. Social networks as coping resources. *Soc. Sci. Med.* **10,** 97, 1976.
142. Nuckolls C. B., Cassel J. C. and Kaplan G. H. Psychosocial assets, life crisis and prognosis of pregnancy. *Am. J. Epidem.* **95,** 431, 1972.
143. McKinlay J. B. Social networks, lay consultation and help-seeking behaviours. *Soc. Forces* **51,** 275, 1973.
144. Department of Health and Social Security. *Prevention and Health: Everybody's Business.* A re-assessment of public and personal health, HMSO, London, 1976.
145. Lalonde M. *A New Perspective on the Health of Canadians.* Ministry of National Health and Welfare, Ottawa, 1974.
146. Sutcliffe P. *Health and Behavioural Change.* Report by a Working Party of Health Services Research Committee, Scottish Home and Health Department, 1981.
147. Merrison A. *Report of the Royal Commission on the National Health Service.* Cmnd 7615, HMSO, London, 1979.
148. Marmot M. R., Rose G., Shipley M. J. and Thomas B. J. Alcohol and mortality: a U-shaped curve. *Lancet* **1,** 580, 1981.
149. Dight S. E. *Scottish Drinking Habits.* OPCS, HMSO, London, 1976.
150. Wilson P. *Drinking in England and Wales.* OPCS, HMSO, London, 1980.
151. Pill R. and Stott N. Concepts of illness causation and responsibility: some preliminary data from a sample of working class mothers. *Soc. Sci. Med.* **16,** 43, 1982.
152. Antonovsky A. *Health, Stress and Coping.* Jossey-Bass, London, 1979.
153. Department of Health and Social Security. *Prevention and Health: Reducing the Risk, Safer Pregnancy and Childbirth.* HMSO, London, 1977.
154. Short Report. Second Report from the Social Services Committee, Session 1979–80. *Perinatal and Neonatal Mortality,* Vol. 1. HMSO, London, 1980.
155. Blaxter M. and Paterson E. The goodness is out of it: the meaning of food to two generations. In *The Sociology of Food and Eating* (Edited by Murcott A.). Gower, London, 1983.
156. Macintyre S. Rhetoric and Reality: mothers' breast feeding intentions and experiences. In *Research and the Midwife, Conference Proceedings, 1982 and 1983* (Edited by Robinson S.). Chelsea College of Nursing Research Unit, 1983.
157. Marsh A. and Matheson J. *Smoking Attitudes and Behaviour.* Office of Population Censuses and Surveys, HMSO, London, 1983.
158. Cartwright A. *How Many Children?* Routledge and Kegan Paul, London, 1976.
159. Blaxter M. The causes of disease: Women talking. *Soc. Sci. Med.* **2,** 59, 1983.
160. Calnan M. *Health, Health Risks and Inequalities: an Exploratory Study of Women's Perceptions.* Paper presented at BSA Annual Medical Sociology Conference, Sheffield. Health Services Research Unit, University of Kent, Canterbury, Kent, 1984.
161. Rosenstock I. M. What research in motivation suggests for public health. *Am. J. publ. Hlth* **50,** 295, 1960.
162. Rosenstock I. M. Why people use health services. *Milbank Mem. Fund Quart.* **3,** 94, 1966.
163. Porter M. Willing deviants? A study of childlessness. Unpublished PhD thesis, University of Aberdeen, 1980.
164. Ford J. A., Colhoun E. M. and Dunnigan M. G. Rickets and osteomalacia in the Glasgow Pakistani community. *Br. med. J.* **226,** 677, 1972.
165. Goel K. M., Sweet E. M., Logan R. W., Warren J. M., Arneil G. C. and Shanks R. A. Florid and sub-clinical rickets among immigrant children in Glasgow. *Lancet* **1,** 1141, 1976.
166. Murcott A. *The Sociology of Food and Eating.* Gower, London, 1983.
167. Rosenman R. H. and Friedman M. Type A behaviour. In *Coronary Prone Behaviour* (Edited by Dembroski T. M. *et al.*). Springer, Berlin, 1978.
168. MacQueen D. and Siegrist J. Social factors in the etiology of chronic disease: an overview. *Soc. Sci. Med.* **16,** 353, 1982.

169. Rahe, R. H. The pathway between subjects' recent life changes and their near-future illness reports. In *Stressful Life Events: Their Nature and Effects* (Edited by Dohrenwend B. and Dohrenwend B.). Wiley, New York, 1974.
170. Rotter J. B. *Generalised Expectancies for Internal Versus External Control Re-inforcement*. Psychological monographs No. 80, 1966.
171. Seligman M. E. D. *Helplessness: On Depression, Development and Death*. Freeman, San Francisco, Calif., 1975.
172. Health Education Council. *Food for Thought*. HEC, London, 1985.
173. Health Education Council. *Looking After Yourself?* HEC, London, 1979.
174. Doyal L. and Pennell I. *The Political Economy of Health*. Pluto Press, London, 1979.

[12]

Sara Arber

Chronic Illness over the Life Course: Class Inequalities among Men and Women in Britain

Introduction

The debate on the extent and nature of inequalities in health has been largely restricted to men of working age and has concentrated on inequalities in mortality rather than morbidity (Fox, 1989; Wilkinson, 1986; Townsend, Davidson and Whitehead, 1988). This chapter examines class inequalities in chronic illness for both women and men over the life course. How chronic illness varies throughout life is particularly relevant to health policy and service provision.

Less attention has been given to class inequalities in women's than men's health, partly because of controversies over how to measure women's social class (Arber, 1989, 1991). Debates centre on the merits of using an 'individualistic' approach rather than using a 'conventional' approach (Arber, 1990; Goldthorpe, 1983, 1984; Siltanen, 1984). The latter approach classifies married women by their husband's occupation and other women by their own occupation. This chapter contrasts the 'conventional' approach with an 'individualistic' approach, which measures class based on the woman's own current (or last) occupation (Arber, 1990).

In most studies of ill-health, age is treated as a confounding variable to be controlled out of the analysis. However, it is important to analyse how class inequalities vary over the life course, and whether life course patterning varies for women and men. Existing analyses of inequalities in health within age groups have been restricted to broad age bands, such as 16-44, 45-64 and 65 and over, as in Aiach and Curtis (1990) and the General Household Survey annual reports (e.g. OPCS, 1988). Like gender, age should be treated as a sociological, not a biological, variable (Riley, 1987). There is a need to examine the sociological correlates of ill-health within narrow age groups, separately for men and women.

It is ironic that research on inequalities in health largely neglects those age groups with the greatest ill-health and highest use of health resources, namely elderly people. Health is of central importance to the lives of elderly people (Aronson, 1990; Palmore and Kivett, 1979), because it largely determines their ability to remain independent and autonomous. Since health is of such pivotal importance to elderly people, it is remarkable that the structural factors associated with good health in later life have been so little studied. The lack of research on inequalities in health in later life reflects an ageist image of elderly people as a homogenous group (Thane, 1988, 1989). Such ageist images blind us to both gender and structural differences, many of which derive from the elderly person's earlier biography, in particular their productive and reproductive roles in society.

A life course perspective allows us to begin to assess the relative importance of age, time and cohort. Elderly women spent their adult years in a very different world from that of younger women today. The majority were full-time homemakers and childrearers and few were in paid employment after marriage. Therefore elderly women's health may be affected more by their domestic and reproductive roles and less by their own labour market position. The majority of women in Britain still leave the labour market at the time of the birth of their first child, and subsequently return to part-time work when children reach school age (Arber and Gilbert, 1991). Many women suffer from occupational downgrading on reentry into the labour market following a break to have children (Martin and Roberts, 1984), and women's continuing family commitments reduce their likelihood of achieving promotion and equal occupational attainment (Arber and Gilbert, 1991). To the extent that a woman's long-term health status is influenced by the material conditions of the woman's home, it would be expected that the 'conventional' approach of measuring women's class using husband's occupation would be a more powerful determinant than a woman's own class.

The aims of this chapter are first, to analyse class differences in chronic illness over the life course, by examining the association between social class and limiting long-standing illness within ten year age groups for men and women under 65 and in five year age groups above age 65. Does the same pattern of inequalities exist throughout the life course or do inequalities diminish at certain ages, for example, among the elderly population? Second, to assess the most appropriate measure of class for women by comparing the 'conventional' approach, based on husband's occupation for married women and their own class for other women, with an 'individualistic' measure of class, based on the woman's own occupation, and to examine whether the pattern of the relationship with each measure varies at different ages in the life course.

Methodology

The General Household Survey (GHS) provides an annual nationally representative sample of about 10,000 British households (OPCS, 1988). Each adult aged 16 and over living in sample households is interviewed, with an overall response rate of 82% in 1985 (OPCS, 1988). However, non-response is likely to be higher among elderly people who are sick, including those temporarily in hospital. The sample omits elderly people living in residential establishments which represents a fifth of women over 85 and 13 percent of men (Arber and Ginn, 1991). Most of the analyses in this chapter use combined data from the 1985, 1986 and 1987 GHS, which represents nearly 30,000 men and women aged 16-64 and 11,000 elderly people (aged 65 and over).

Chronic illness in the GHS is a self-reported measure of whether individuals report any limiting long-standing illness. The respondent was asked 'Have you any long-standing illness, disability or infirmity?' (By long-standing I mean anything that has troubled you over a period of time or that is likely to affect you over a period of time). If the answer was 'Yes', the respondent was asked 'Does this illness limit your activities in any way?'. Those who answer 'Yes' to both questions are coded as having a 'limiting long-standing illness'. This measure is related to function

(Blaxter, 1985) and represents a self-assessment of the effect of any chronic ill health on daily life.

For people over age 65, an additional measure is used. A scale of functional disability was derived from the 1985 GHS based on the elderly person's ability to perform six activities of daily living (ADLs), namely climbing stairs, cutting toenails, walking down the road, washing all over/bathing, getting round the house and getting into and out of bed. It is comparable to the hierarchical scale developed by Kempen and Suurmeijer (1990), and like their scale used three possible answer categories per item. Each activity was coded 0 if the activity could be done easily, 1 if it could only be done with difficulty, and 2 if it could not be done unaided. These items were summed and formed a Guttman scale, which is hierarchical and cumulative, with the values 0 to 12, see Appendix A. A quarter of elderly people have 'moderate' or greater disability, defined as a score of three or more, and 11% have 'severe' disability, a score of 6 or more. The latter will generally be unable to walk down the road unaided, or bath or go up and down stairs without difficulty. Elderly people with 'severe' disability are high users of health and welfare services (Arber et al, 1988) and are most likely to require informal care (Arber and Ginn, 1991, 1992). The questions on activities of daily living were only asked in the 1985 GHS, so the analyses of functional disability are restricted to a single year of data.

Class is measured using current occupation, except for those not currently in paid employment who are asked about their last main occupation. In order to assess whether occupational characteristics have a comparable association with long-term illness for women and men, a ten-fold classification of occupations is used for adults aged 16-64, see Appendix B. In Britain, women and men work in quite different occupations, with men concentrated at the higher ends of both the non-manual and the manual labour markets (Table 1). Seven percent of men are in the higher professions compared with only one percent of women. Thirty percent of men are in skilled manual occupations compared with only five percent of women. Over a third of women are in junior non-manual occupations, mainly secretaries and clerical workers, compared with under eight percent of men. Women are also over represented in personal services, such as restaurant and bar work, 13 percent of women compared with only one percent of men. Classifying women using the 'conventional' approach (based on husband's occupation for married women) produces a similar occupational distribution for women and men under 65, but there is an over representation of women in junior non-manual work and in personal services.

Table 1 Socio-economic group of women by their own class, and 'conventional class', and of men, 16-64, Great Britain

	Men	Women Own Class	Women Conventional Class
Higher professionals	6.8	1.0	5.7
Employers & Managers	18.8	7.0	18.1
Lower professionals	6.8	12.7	8.4
Supervisory non-manual	2.4	4.7	3.2
Junior non-manual	7.5	33.6	14.0
Self employed (own account - manual)	8.0	2.9	6.5
Skilled manual	30.0	5.4	23.5
Semi-skilled manual	13.8	13.0	12.6
Personal service	1.2	13.1	4.3
Unskilled manual	4.6	6.6	3.7
	100%	100%	100%
N=	14732	15178	15202

Source: General Household Survey, 1985-87 (original analysis)

This ten-fold classification allows an assessment of the most appropriate way to regroup occupations for women into a smaller number of class categories, as well as providing sufficient detail to allow some insight into which occupations are associated with particularly good or poor health for women and men, and whether the same linear class ordering of ill health occurs for women as for men.

One reason why few researchers have examined class inequalities in the health of elderly people is because of difficulties in measuring the class of people who are no longer in the labour market.

For elderly men, class measured using last occupation may be considered too imprecise and error prone to be of value. For elderly women there are added concerns. Only a third of elderly women are married, and half are widowed. Therefore in the conventional method, husband's occupation cannot be used for two-thirds of elderly women. The alternative 'individualistic' approach may be considered invalid because many elderly women have not worked for several decades, often not since marriage. In addition, about a sixth of elderly women in Britain have never worked. Because of these problems, it might be expected that elderly women's own last occupation would have little association with their current life chances and health status. The chapter examines this assumption and assesses whether the 'conventional' method of class assignment has a clear advantage over the 'individualistic' method for elderly women. A five category class measure (see Appendix B), because of the small number of elderly people in some of the ten-fold class groups. An additional category of 'never worked' has been added.

Research on health inequalities among elderly people also needs to consider health selection since selective survival is related to class. If working class people aged 65 to 69 have poorer health and a higher mortality rate than middle class people of the same age, we would expect class differences in morbidity and mortality to narrow with advancing age. Such selective effects are exemplified by the 'racial cross-over' found in the United States (Jackson and Perry, 1989). Blacks over age 75 have a lower mortality than whites because of the higher mortality rate of blacks in adulthood and among the young elderly. Very elderly blacks are more healthy than whites of the same age. The problem of selective survival of the most healthy does not invalidate studies of class inequalities in health among elderly people, but means that any inequalities which are found, especially among the 'old elderly' would be considerably greater if it were not for the operation of selective survival.

The association between class and chronic illness is analysed in ten year age groups for men and women under 65 and five year age groups above 65. Logistic regression analysis, using the statistical package GLIM (Payne, 1985; Healy, 1988) is used to summarise the relationship between class and chronic illness, while preserving detailed age controls, and to assess the relative merits of the 'conventional' and the 'individualistic' approach when examining class inequalities in the ill health of women.

Using logit analysis, the dependent variable is the log of the odds of having the specified attribute. The odds ratios in Tables 2 and 3 are the ratio of the probability of someone with specified characteristics having a limiting long-standing illness compared to the probability that a person with the same characteristics does not. The odds ratios for each variable relate to a particular reference category: in Table 2 the reference categories are the 16-24 age group, and 'higher professionals'.

Chronic illness among adults under 65

There is a smooth gradient between class and chronic illness for men and for women (using the conventional class measure). The highest levels of chronic illness are among the unskilled and the lowest among higher professionals (Figure 1). This linear gradient is evident in each ten year age group from 25 to 64. The disadvantaged position of unskilled men aged 25-54 is particularly striking, for example three times more unskilled men aged 45-54 report limiting long-standing illness than higher professional men of the same age. The class differences are almost as great for women using the 'conventional' approach as for men.

Below age 25, the class differences are much more modest and are not entirely linear, although in each case young people in higher professional occupations have the best health and unskilled workers the poorest health. Among young adults the class basis of long-term ill health is beginning to form but is not as well-established as at older ages.

Figure 1 - % with chronic illness by social class and 10 year age groups

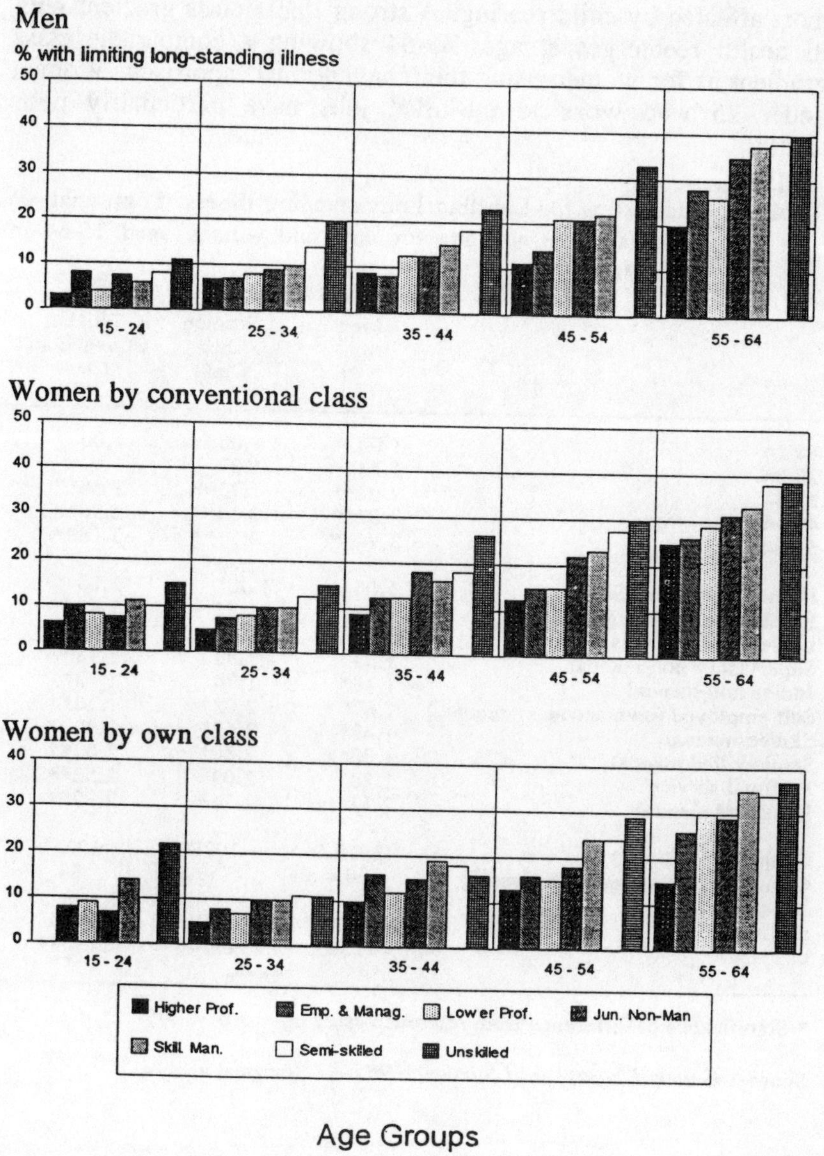

For women the 'individualistic' measure of class (based on their own current or last occupation) shows a non-linear class pattern, particularly at ages 35-44, which is the stage of the life course most affected by child rearing. A strong linear class gradient with ill health reemerges at ages 45-64 showing a comparable class gradient as for women using the 'conventional' approach. Women under 25 who work in unskilled jobs have particularly poor health.

Table 2 Odds ratios for Limiting Long-standing illness. Logit analysis of social class and age for men and women aged 16-64 in Great Britain.

	Men	Women Own Class	Women Conventional Class
16-24	1.00	1.00	1.00
25-34	1.53**	1.07	1.12
35-44	2.02**	1.73**	1.86**
45-54	2.82**	2.19**	2.36**
55-64	3.94**	3.53**	3.78**
Higher professionals	1.00	1.001	1.00
Employers & Managers	1.05	1.72	1.43*
Lower professionals	1.33	1.46	1.48*
Supervisory non-manual	1.33	1.83	1.73*
Junior non-manual	1.48*	1.74	1.72*
Self employed (own account - manual)	1.67**	2.08*	1.70*
Skilled manual	1.49*	2.62*	1.99**
Semi-skilled manual	1.80**	2.40*	2.07**
Personal service	1.28	2.09*	2.52**
Unskilled manual	2.32**	2.71*	2.99**
G squared	8918.0	10270	10251
Change in G squared with class	60.4	59	88
p <	.001	.001	.001
df	12303	13049	13049

* Significance of difference from reference category - * p < .05, ** p < .01

Source: *General Household Survey, 1985-87* (original analysis)

These analyses show that women's own occupational class has a marked association with long-term ill health below age 25 and above 45, but for women aged 25-44, the conventional approach, based on husband's occupation for married women and their own occupation for other women, shows a stronger class gradient.

Using logistic regression, the odds of reporting a chronic illness increase with age, as expected (Table 2). But for women, there is no significant difference between the likelihood of chronic illness at ages 16-24 and at 25-34.

The odds ratios clearly show a linear class gradient for men. The odds of ill health are comparable for higher professionals and 'employers and managers'. Lower professionals and supervisory non-manual workers also have similar levels of chronic ilness. Junior non- manual men have significantly poorer health than higher professionals and are comparable to skilled manual workers. The groups with the highest odds of ill health are unskilled workers, the semi-skilled and self employed own account workers, mainly skilled artisans. The small number of men who are personal service workers report relatively good health.

Using the 'conventional' approach for women, there is a linear gradient of chronic illness with all classes having significantly poorer health than higher professionals. Personal service workers occupy an intermediate position between unskilled and semi-skilled workers.

Using the woman's own occupation (an individualistic measure of class), none of the non-manual classes report significantly poorer health than higher professionals. Although, women 'employers and managers' are more likely to report chronic illness than professional women, confirming earlier work (Arber, 1989). For women, there is little difference between the odds of ill health for each of the three manual classes. This suggests that traditional skill distinctions are not reflected in differences in level of health for women, unlike for men. Women who are personal service workers have a lower chance of chronic illness than manual workers and a similar level to self-employed own account workers, the majority of whom are hairdressers.

A comparison of the improvement in fit of the model when class is added is provided near the base of Table 2. When 'conventional' class is added to the model in addition to age, there is a greater improvement in the fit (change in G squared of 88) compared with when the 'individualistic' measure of class is added (change in G squared of 59). Thus, for women under 65 the conventional measure of class has greater power in explaining differences in chronic illness than a woman's own class. However, this difference is mainly because of the poorer relationship between individualistic class and ill health for women aged 25-44 in Britain who because of childrearing are likely to occupy jobs which do not reflect their actual labour market potential.

Chronic illness among elderly people

There is less research on inequalities in health among elderly people than for other age groups, for example, the Black Report (DHSS, 1980) did not explicitly discuss inequalities in mortality or morbidity above age 65. Since then research has examined class differences in mortality of elderly men, but not women. Working class men aged 65-74 and over 75 have higher mortality than middle class men (Goldblatt, 1990; Fox et al, 1983).

There is some British research on class inequalities in health among elderly people, notably Taylor and Ford (1983; Taylor, 1988) and Victor (1989, 1991; Victor and Evandrou 1987) who showed working class elderly women and men have poorer health than their middle class counterparts. Blaxter's (1990) work on the Health and Lifestyle Survey has shown strong class differences for people aged over 70 in the more subjective dimensions of health - illness and psycho-social malaise, but little class difference on fitness and the presence of disease/disability. However, given the marked deterioration in health with advancing age, many of these studies are restricted by only using age controls of the 'young' elderly, aged 65-74, and the 'old' elderly, aged over 75.

The pattern of relationship between reporting limiting longstanding illness and class is much weaker in the five-year age groups above 65 (Figure 2) than for age groups below retirement age. For men in their late sixties and above 85 there is a curved relationship, but in the age groups 70-84 a linear pattern is largely maintained. Among these age groups differences between the higher middle class and unskilled workers are less pronounced than at younger ages. Except for women in their late sixties there is little evidence of a linear association between chronic illness and an elderly woman's own class.

Table 3 Limiting Long-standing illness of elderly women and men
Odds ratios for logit analysis of social class and age

	Men	Women Own Class	Women Conventional Class
Constant	.055**	.091**	.095**
65-69	1.00	1.00	1.00
70-74	1.41*	1.21	1.20
75-79	1.51*	1.49*	1.49*
80-84	1.86**	1.55*	1.55*
85+	1.37	2.29**	2.28**
High middle	1.00	1.00	1.00
Lower middle	0.75	0.99	1.00
Skilled manual	1.47*	0.97	0.93
Semi-skilled	1.40*	.122	1.15
Unskilled	1.70*	1.08	1.10
Never worked	1.19	1.02	
G squared	2489.5	4602.2	4604.4
Change in G squared with class	18.2	5.9	3.9
p <	.01	ns	ns
dF	4398	6486	6486

* Significance of difference from reference category - * p < .05, ** p < .01

Source: *General Household Survey, 1985-87* (original analysis)

Figure 2 - % with chronic illness by social class and 5 year age groups

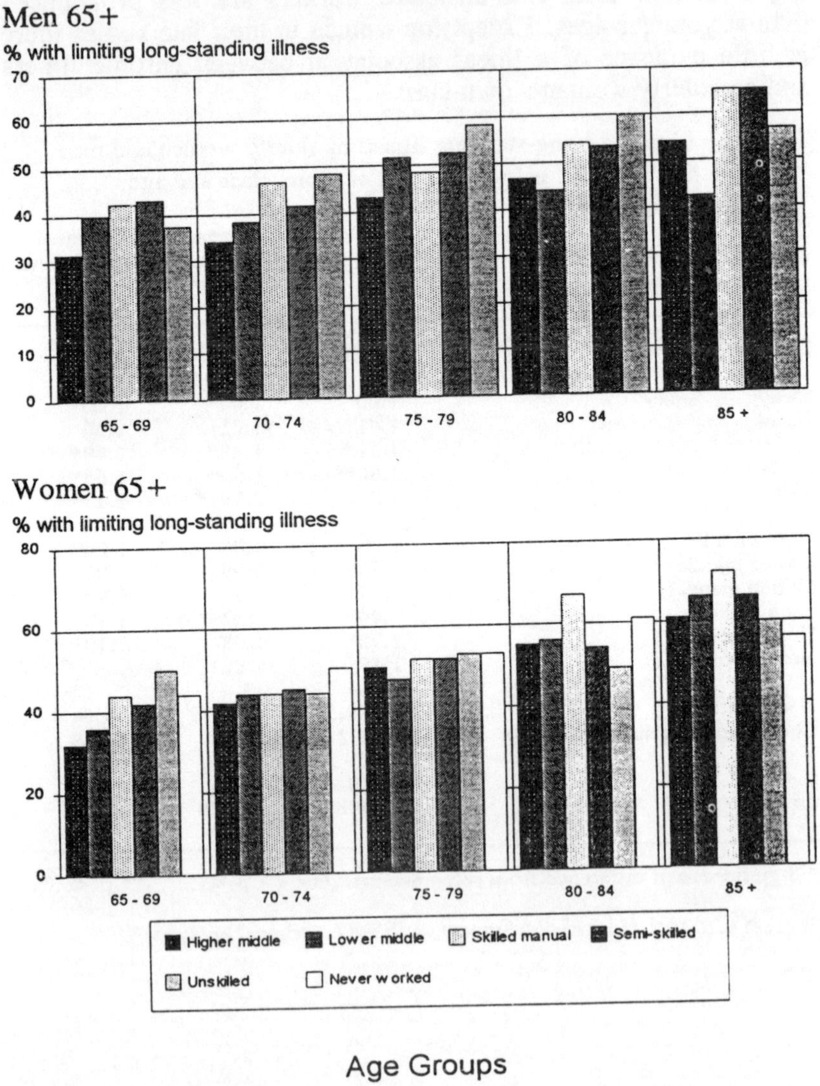

General Household Survey, 1985-87

To precisely measure the association between class and long-term illness for elderly men and women, Table 3 presents a logistic regression analysis, which analyses five-year age groups and class measured according to the conventional and the individualistic approach for elderly women. The odds of reporting chronic illness increase with age except among men over 85 who do not report a significantly higher odds than men in their sixties. For elderly men there is a statistically significant association between class and reporting chronic illness, after taking into account age. The relationship with class is broadly linear, although lower middle class men are less likely to report chronic illness than higher middle class men.

The logistic regressions show no significant association between class and reporting limiting long-standing illness for elderly women using either an individualistic or conventional measure of class. The change in G squared with the addition of class is not statistically significant in either cases, after controlling for age.

In order to assess whether these analyses reflect a lack of class inequality in ill-health in later life or the inadequacy of our measure of chronic illness at this stage of the life course, the next section examines class inequalities using a more objective measure of functional disability based on the elderly person's ability to perform six activities of daily living (see Appendix A).

Functional disability among elderly people

Unlike chronic illness, the class gradient with functional disability is strong for elderly women and men. Figure 3 shows what percentage of each five year age group above 65 have a disability score of three or more. Elderly women's own last occupation has a remarkably strong class gradient with disability for each age group under eighty. In their late sixties, only seven percent of higher middle class women compared to a fifth of unskilled women are functionally disabled, with a roughly two-fold differential between these groups of women maintained until age 80. Above eighty class is less clearly associated with functional disability. Selective survival has its greatest effect on these older age groups, but there is no evidence of a cross-over in class-associ-

Figure 3 - % with disability by social class for elderly men and women

Men

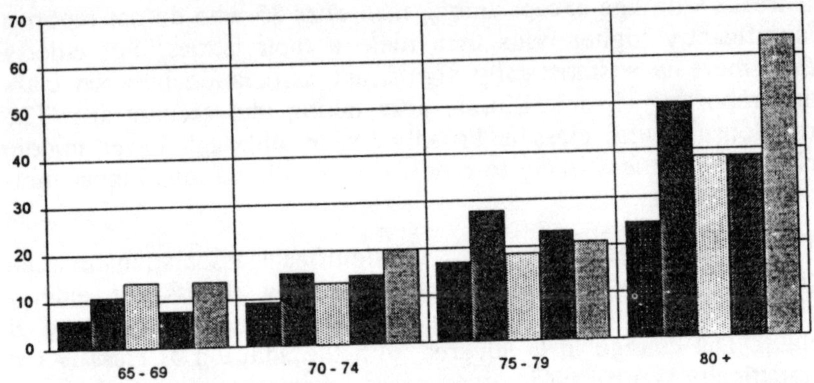

Women

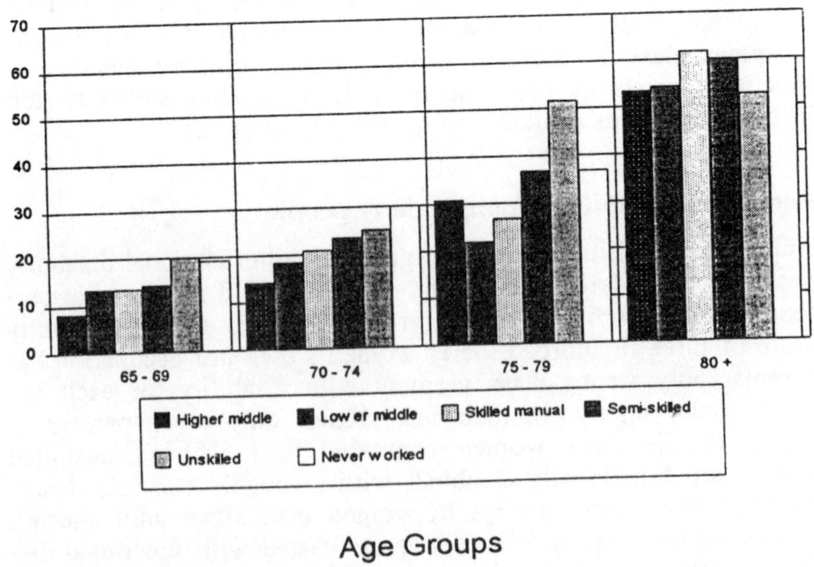

General Household Survey, 1985

Medical Sociology: Research on Chronic Illness

Table 4 Disability of elderly women and men
Odds ratios for logit analysis of social class and age

	Moderate (3+)			*Severe (6+)*		
	Men	Women Own Class	Women Conven Class	Men	Women Own Class	Women Conven Class
Constant	.078**	.119**	.125**	.032**	.35**	.40**
65-69	1.00	1.00	1.00	1.00	1.00	1.00
70-74	1.22	1.66*	1.69*	0.834	1.47*	1.46*
75-79	2.07**	3.06**	3.06**	2.30*	3.22**	3.25**
80-84	3.86**	5.99**	6.11**	2.40*	5.58**	5.70**
85+	8.50**	13.7**	13.7**	5.31**	12.7**	12.7**
High middle	1.00	1.00	1.00	1.00	1.00	1.00
Lower middle	1.92*	1.07	1.01	2.24*	1.46	1.20
Skilled man	1.71*	1.23	1.33	1.77*	2.01*	1.76*
Semi-skilled	1.66*	1.56*	1.42*	1.60	1.76*	1.36
Unskilled	5.00*	1.98	2.19*	2.89*	1.55*	1.75*
Never worked		1.68*	1.44		2.00*	1.73*
G squared	1220.8	2257.8	2256.5	699.5	1495.5	1495.
Change in G squared with class	19.5	19.8	21.1	9.1	10.6	10.6
p <	.01	.01	.01	.05	.05	.05
dF	1427	2083	2083	1427	2083	2083

* Significance of difference from reference category - * $p < .05$, ** $p < .01$

Source: *General Household Survey, 1985* (original analysis)

ated disability comparable to the US experience of a racial cross-over.

Within each age group of elderly men, occupational class is associated with disability. Higher middle class men are least likely to be disabled, and unskilled men have the highest levels of disability. Unskilled men are twice as likely as 'higher middle class' men to be disabled in most age groups. For example, over sixty percent of previously unskilled men in their eighties have this level of disability compared to a quarter of higher middle class men. At ages over 75, men who were previously in lower middle class occupations also have high levels of disability.

Logistic regression analyses show that the odds of being functionally disabled increase sharply with age, especially for women. They are thirteen times higher for women in their late eighties than in their late sixties. For elderly men between their late sixties and late eighties, the odds increase eight-fold for moderate or greater disability and five-fold for severe disability. There is no significant increase in the likelihood of being functionally disabled between the late sixties and early seventies, but then a sharp increase with each subsequent five years of age.

Class is significantly associated with disability for both elderly women and men after including age in the logistic regression models. Unskilled men have a five times higher odds of moderate disability than higher middle class occupations. The second highest odds ratio is for men who previously worked in lower middle class occupations. It is clear that elderly men who were previously in higher middle class are much less likely to be disabled than other elderly men. The class pattern for women shows little difference in disability between higher and lower middle class women, with the major divide between women previously employed in non-manual occupations, who are less likely to be disabled, and the higher level of disability of those previously in manual occupations or who never worked.

Overall, the association of class and disability is comparable for elderly women and men, although the class differentials are somewhat greater for men than for women. We conclude that class based on attachment to the labour market during working life is significantly associated with the disability of elderly men and women even among the oldest groups. This impact has hitherto largely been ignored by researchers and policy makers.

Turning to whether conventional class or an elderly woman's own class should be used in analyses of inequalities in health, it makes very little difference whether an elderly woman's own class or the more 'conventional' class measure is used. The change in G squared with the addition of class to the model containing age is virtually identical in each of the comparisons in Tables 3 and 4. These findings suggest there is no clear advantage in using the 'conventional approach' when analysing elderly women's health, probably because the difference in classification is only for married women, who represent only a minority of elderly women.

Discussion and conclusions

Long-term ill health is strongly associated with class measured by the individual's current (or last main) occupation in each ten year age group below 65, but is weakest among young adults (under 25). Other studies confirm the lack of association between chronic illness and class among young adults. Research on 15 year olds by Macintyre and West (1991) shows that in adolescence class gradients are not consistently apparent on most indicators of health including chronic illness. Power et al (1991) found that although the relationship between class and chronic illness was weak among 23 year olds, there was a very strong relationship between class and psycho-social health, such as malaise.

For women, the 'conventional' method of measuring class, whereby husband's class is used for married women and for all other women their own class, shows a significantly stronger and more linear association with chronic illness than the woman's own class.

Using the ten category class scale, the gradient is curved for women using class based on their own labour market position. Comparing gender differences in the association between own class and chronic illness suggests that the meaning of the same occupations differ between women and men, and that we should not assume that class gradients will be the same for women and men. For example, skill distinctions in manual work are associated with differences in health for men but not women, and women who are employers and managers report poorer health than professionals, but this is not the case for men.

Individualistic class is least clearly associated with ill health for women aged 25-44. This is interpreted as the effect of childrearing on women's labour market participation, which results in British women often taking part-time jobs which do not reflect their abilities and labour market potential (Martin and Roberts, 1984). As an increasing proportion of women remain full-time in the labour market throughout their working lives, we may see in future that an individualistic approach to measuring class becomes a more powerful tool than using the 'conventional' approach. In European countries where women traditionally maintain full- time attachment to the labour market, rather than taking part-time jobs, individualistic class may be a better predictor of chronic illness at all ages, unlike in Britain. Current work comparing Finland and Britain suggests that this is the case in Finland (Arber and Lahelma, 1992).

Few research studies have examined class inequalities in the health of elderly women and men. Chronic illness, measured by limiting long-standing illness, shows only a modest association with class for men and no significant association for elderly women. This could be interpreted as evidence of decreasing inequalities in health among elderly people. However, before accepting this conclusion, we analysed another measure of health status, namely functional disability.

Class based on the elderly person's previous labour market position, has a strong association with functional disability. In spite of elderly people having left the labour market a number of years earlier, higher occupational class continues to be associated with low functional disability. We conclude that limiting long-standing illness is a less valid measure of chronic ill health among the elderly than among younger age groups. It is a problematic indicator because elderly people may consider impairments associated with the ageing process as 'normal' for people of their age and not self-report a 'long-standing illness, disability or infirmity' as limiting their activities. If this is the case, we would expect a weaker association with class not because class inequalities in ill health are absent among elderly people but because a health measure which is valid for younger age groups is not sufficiently discriminating at older ages.

Functional measures of disability are most appropriate for capturing the differences in long-term health status among elderly people, particularly in the oldest age groups. Functional disability discriminated very well among the elderly population, with a thirteenfold increase in the odds of disability for women between the late sixties and above 85. This rapid increase in disability with five year age groups, also suggests that when analysing the health of elderly people it is essential to use detailed age controls, not simply split the elderly population into the 'young' elderly (65-74) and the 'old' elderly (75+).

The two alternative ways of assigning class to elderly women - the 'individualistic' approach based on the woman's own last occupation, and the 'conventional' approach - made little difference to the strength of association between disability and class. For elderly women as a whole either method of class assignment may equally well be used. This lack of difference contrasts with the stronger association of conventional class with chronic illness for women under 65. The major reason is because the two measures differ only for the one third of women over 65 who are still married.

Acknowledgements

For access to the General Household Survey data for 1985-87 I am indebted to the ESRC Data Archive, University of Essex, to the University of London Computer Centre, and to the Office of Population Censuses and Surveys for permission to use the GHS data. I am very grateful to Jay Ginn for collaboration on some of the research reported in this chapter, which was part of a research project funded by the Economic and Social Research Council (Grant No. R000231458).

Appendix A. *Construction of Disability Index from the 1985 General Household Survey*

Coded from answers to six questions: 'Do you usually manage to ..?'

Get up and down stairs and steps
Get around the house
Get in and out of bed
Cut your toenails yourself
Bath, shower or wash all over
Go out and walk down the road

The answers are scored:

0 On your own without difficulty
1 On your own, but with difficulty
2 Only with help from someone else, or not at all

These six items were summated to form a Guttman Scale, using the SPSS Guttman scale subprogram (version 1). The index has a coefficient of reproducibility of =.94 and a coefficient of scalability of 0.63.

Degree of Disability	*Scale* Value	Scale items as in Guttman Scale
None (49%)	0	None
Slight (26%)	1	Has difficulty cutting toenails
	2	Needs help/ cannot manage to cut toenails
	3	Has difficulty in going up and down stairs
Moderate (13%)	4	Has difficulty managing to go out and walk down the road
	5	Has difficulty having a bath/ shower or wash all over
	6	Needs help/ cannot manage to go out and walk down the road
Severe (11%)	7	Needs help/ cannot manage to go up and down stairs
	8	Needs help/ cannot manage to have a bath/ shower or wash all over
	9	Has difficulty in getting around the house
	10	Has difficulty in getting in and out of bed
	11	Needs help/ cannot manage to get in and out of bed
	12	Needs help/ cannot manage to get aound the house
100% (3691)		

Appendix B. *Social class classification*

The individual's current or last main occupation was classified into the Registrar General's socio-economic groups by the GHS and then grouped into social classes in the following ways. For women 'conventional' class was measured using the husband's last occupation for married women and the woman's own last occupation for all other women.

Measures of class for ages 16-64

Tables 1 and 2 (10 categories)	Figure 1 (7 categories)
Higher professionals	Higher professionals
Employers and managers	Employers and managers
Lower professionals	Lower professionals
Supervisory non-manual	& Supervisory non-manual
Intermediate and Junior non-manual	Intermediate and Junior non-manual
Self-employed (own account-manual)	Skilled manual
Skilled manual and foremen	
Semi-skilled manual and agricultural workers	Semi-skilled
Personal service workers	
Unskilled manual	Unskilled

Measure of class for age 65+ (6 categories)

Higher middle class:	Higher professionals
	Employers and Managers
	Lower professionals
Lower middle class:	Intermediate and Junior non-manual
Skilled manual:	Self employed own account workers
	Foremen
	Skilled manual workers
Semi-skilled:	Personal service workers
	Semi-skilled manual workers
	Agricultural workers
Unskilled:	Unskilled manual workers
Never worked:	For women who said they had never had a paid job

Literature

Aiach, P. and S. Curtis
1990 "Social Inequalities in Self-Reported Morbidity: Interpretation and Comparison of Data from Britain and France." *Social Science and Medicine*, 31(3): 267-274

Arber, S.
1989 "Gender and class inequalities in health: understanding the differentials." Pp 250-279 in A.J. Fox (ed) *Health Inequalities in European Countries*, Aldershot: Gower

1990 "Opening the 'Black' Box: Understanding inequalities in women's health." Pp 37-56 in P. Abbott and G. Payne *New Directions in the Sociology of Health*, Brighton: Falmer Press

1991 "Class, paid employment and family roles: making sense of structural disadvantage, gender and health status." *Social Science and Medicine*, 32(4): 425-436

Arber, S. and G.N. Gilbert
1991 *Women's Working Lives: Divisions and Change*, London: Macmillan

Arber S., G.N. Gilbert and M. Evandrou
1988 "Gender, household composition and receipt of domiciliary services by elderly disabled people." *Journal of Social Policy*, 17(2): 153-175

Arber S. and J. Ginn
1991 *Gender and Later Life: A Sociological Analysis of Resources and Constraints*, London: Sage

1992 "'In sickness and in health': care-giving, gender and the independence of elderly people." Pp 86-105 in C. Marsh and S. Arber (eds.) *Families and Households: Divisions and Change*. London: Macmillan

Arber, S. and E. Lahelma
1992 "Women, paid employment and ill-health in Britain and Finland." Paper presented to the British Sociological Association Annual Conference, University of Kent, April

Medical Sociology: Research on Chronic Illness

Aronson, J.
1990 "Women's perspectives on informal care of the elderly: Public ideology and personal experience of giving and receiving care." *Ageing and Society*, 10(1): 61-84

Blaxter M.
1985 "Self definition of health status and consultation rates in primary care," *Quarterly Journal of Social Affairs*, 1(2): 131-171

1990 *Health and Lifestyles*, London: Routledge/Tavistock

Department of Health and Social Security
1980 *Inequalities in Health*, The Black Report. London: DHSS

Fox, A.J.
1989 *Health Inequalities in European Countries*, Aldershot: Gower

Fox A.J. and P. Goldblatt
1982 *Socio-demographic mortality differentials from the OPCS Longitudinal Study 1971-75*, Series LS, no. 1, London: HMSO

Fox A.J., P. Goldblatt, and D.R. Jones
1983 "Social class mortality differentials: artefact, selection or life circumstances?" *Journal of Epidemiology and Community Health*, 39(1): 1-18

Goldblatt P.
1990 *Mortality and social organisation in England and Wales, 1971-1981*, Series LS, no 6, London: HMSO

Goldthorpe J.H.
1983 "Women and class analysis: In defence of the conventional view." *Sociology*, 17(4): 465-487

1984 "Women and class analysis: A reply to the replies." *Sociology*, 18(4): 497-499

Healy M.J.R.
1988 *GLIM: An Introduction*, Oxford: Oxford University Press

Jackson J.J. and C. Perry
1989 "Physical health conditions of middle-aged and aged blacks." Pp 111-176 in K.S. Markides (ed.) *Aging and Health: Perspectives on Gender, Race, Ethnicity, and Class*. Newbury Park, California: Sage

Kempen, G.I.J.M., and T.P.B.M. Suurmeijer
1990 "The Development of a Hierarchical Polychotomous ADL-IADL Scale for Noninstitutionalized Elders." *The Gerontologist*, 30(4): 497-502

Macintyre, S. and P. West
1991 "Lack of class variation in health in adolescence: an artefact of an occupational measure of social class?" *Social Science and Medicine*, 32(4): 395-402

Martin, J. and C. Roberts
1984 *Women and Employment: A Lifetime Perspective*, London, Department of Employment/OPCS

Office of Population Censuses and Surveys (OPCS)
1988 *General Household Survey*, 1985, London: HMSO

Palmore, E.B. and V. Kivett
1977 "Change in Life Satisfactions: A Longitudinal study of persons Aged 46-70." *Journal of Gerontology*, 32(3):311-316

Payne C.D.
1985 *The GLIM System release 3.77 Manual*, Oxford: Numerical Algorithms Group

Riley, M.W.
1987 "On the significance of age in sociology." *American Sociological Review*, 52(1): 1-14

Stanworth, M.
1984 "Women and class analysis: A reply to Goldthorpe." *Sociology*, 18(2): 159-170

Taylor R.
1988 "The elderly as members of society: an examination of social differences in an elderly population.". Pp 105-129 in N. Wells and C. Freer (eds.) *The Ageing Population: Burden or Challenge?*, London: Macmillan

Taylor R. and G. Ford
1983 "Inequalities in old age: an examination of age, sex and class differences in a sample of community elderly." *Ageing and Society*, 3(2): 183-208

Thane, P.

1988 "The growing burden of an ageing population?" *Journal of Public policy*, 7(4): 373-387

1989 "Old age: burden or benefit?" Pp 56-71 in H. Joshi (ed.) *The Changing Population of Britain* Oxford: Blackwell

Townsend, P., N. Davidson, and C. Whitehead

1988 *Inequalities in Health and the Health Divide*, Harmondsworth: Penguin

Victor, C.

1991a *Health and Health Care in Later Life*, Milton Keynes: Open University Press

1991b "Continuity or Change: Inequalities in Health in Later Life." *Ageing and Society*, 11(2): 252-269

Victor C. and M. Evandrou

1987 "Does social class matter in later life?" in S. di Gregorio (ed.) *Social Gerontology: New Directions*. London: Croom Helm

Wilkinson R. G. (ed)

1986 *Class and Health*, London: Tavistock

[13]

The Effects of Women's Employment: Personal Control and Sex Differences in Mental Health*

SARAH ROSENFIELD

Journal of Health and Social Behavior 1989, Vol. 30 (March):77–91

Married women have been found consistently to have higher rates of anxious and depressive symptoms than married men. Power explanations for this difference predict that employment for women, which is associated with greater power in the family, would reduce women's symptoms to approximate men's more closely. Results on the effects of women's employment, however, are inconsistent. One explanation for this inconsistency concerns role overload, or the greater demands experienced by women with employment. This paper proposes that overload creates greater symptoms for the same reason as low power; that is, through lowering individuals' sense of personal control. Thus employment for women is not consistently positive because it often trades one source of low control for another. We test a personal control explanation for the effects of women's employment, using community surveys of mental health. Results indicate that issues of personal control underlie the effects of both high demands and low power on sex differences in anxious and depressive symptoms.

One of the most consistent findings in the sociology of mental health is that women have higher rates of psychological distress and depression than men (Dohrenwend and Dohrenwend 1974, 1976; Dohrenwend, Dohrenwend, Gould, Link, Neugebaur, and Wunsch-Hitzig 1980; Weissman and Klerman 1977). These differences are found across cultures, over time, in different age groups, in rural as well as urban areas, and in treated as well as untreated populations. Researchers estimate that women have as much as twice the rate of distress and depression as men. Most recently the Epidemiological Catchment Area studies, which investigated the rates of mental disorders in the U.S. population, confirmed that women have higher rates of diagnoses of anxiety and depressive disorders (Myers, Weissman, Tischler, Holzer, Leaf, Orvaschel, Anthony, Boyd, Burke, Kramer, and Stoltzman 1984; Robins, Helzer, Weissman, Orvaschel, Gruenberg, Burke, and Regier 1984).

Power Explanations: The State of the Evidence

The differences between men and women in psychological distress, which includes both anxiety and depression, are greatest among married people. Thus social explanations of sex differences focus on gender roles within the family. A major explanation concentrates on the power differences between husbands and wives. One argument stresses women's relative lack of decision-making power within the family (Radloff 1975; Rosenfield 1980). Another argument is that the conventional feminine role of housewife is characterized by lower resources and prestige—two elements of power—than is the conventional masculine role of breadwinner (Gove and Tudor 1973; Horwitz 1982).

The mechanisms by which low power affects psychiatric symptoms are not clear, however. I suggest that low power implies less actual control over the environment and thus lower perceptions of personal control.

* Direct correspondence to Institute for Health, Health Care Policy, and Aging Research, Rutgers University, 30 College Avenue, New Brunswick, NJ 08903. This research was supported in part by a grant from the National Institute of Mental Health MH39105-01. I am grateful to Naomi Gerstel, Allan Horwitz, Mary Clare Lennon, Bruce Link, and three anonymous reviewers for their helpful comments.

With diminished assessments of their ability to act on and affect their social world, individuals experience greater psychological distress. Thus in general I propose that women have higher rates of anxious and depressive symptoms because their positions of lower power produce lower actual control and thus lower perceived control than those of men.

Such differences, however, vary across marriages. On the basis of a power explanation, one would hypothesize that the greater the power differences between husbands and wives, the greater the sex differences in symptoms of distress. Equal power would be associated with equal levels of symptoms. In testing this hypothesis, a major indicator of power relations in the family is employment among wives. Wives' employment is associated with greater decision-making power in the family (Blood and Wolfe 1960; Ferree 1976) and with a reduction in the amount of housework performed by women (Pleck 1984). Thus if low power is the reason why married women have higher rates of symptoms, employment among women should produce lower symptoms for women, reducing the sex differences.

Some research on married individuals does find reduced sex differences between husbands and wives when wives are employed (Kessler and McRae 1982; Rosenfield 1980). Research over time also shows that a decrease in sex differences from the 1950s to the 1970s is explained in part by the rise in women's employment (Kessler and McRae 1981; McLanahan and Glass 1985). Yet not all studies find lower sex differences with women's employment (Fendrich 1984; Roberts and O'Keefe 1981). Moreover, some that do reveal lower differences show that the reductions are due more to a rise in men's scores than to a decline in women's (Rosenfield 1980; Ross, Mirowsky, and Huber 1983b). In fact, men's scores are particularly high and exceed women's symptom levels when wives are employed in general (Rosenfield 1980) and when wives are employed but their husbands prefer them not to be employed (Ross et al. 1983b). Furthermore, studies comparing groups of women obtain inconsistent results. Some find positive effects for women when they are employed (Gore and Mangione 1983; Gove and Geerken 1977; Horwitz 1982; Kessler and McRae 1982; Radloff 1975), but others find no significant differences in anxiety and depression between employed women and housewives (Barnett and Baruch 1985; Cleary and Mechanic 1983; Pearlin 1975).

Taken together, these findings are difficult to interpret with a straightforward power explanation. Women's greater power, as indicated by employment, has an effect but it appears to change men's symptom levels for the worse rather than women's for the better; when employed women are compared to housewives, the results are equivocal. These inconsistent findings throw into question not only a power explanation in particular but also, insofar as women's employment represents a major change toward less traditional gender roles, social causation explanations for sex differences in general. Yet does this uncertainty suggest that we should abandon a power explanation with respect to the effects of employment? Instead we may find something about women's employment that places a heavier burden on women, although it involves greater power. Employment also involves increased demands; I suggest that just as the greater power associated with employment may increase women's sense of personal control, the demands associated with employment may diminish their sense of control. For this reason employment may fail to reduce women's psychological distress consistently. As a basis for this argument I explore a body of literature on role overload that would predict negative effects for employment.

Demands: The Role Overload Perspective

A role overload perspective is an alternative social causation explanation for sex differences in psychological distress (Aneshensel, Frerichs, and Clark 1981; Barnett and Baruch 1985; Cleary and Mechanic 1983; Gove and Geerkin 1977). Proponents of this perspective argue that women, either in caring for children per se or in combining children with employment, suffer from a greater level of demands than men. Although employed women do somewhat less housework than housewives, as noted above, men on average do not increase the amount of household tasks when their wives are employed (Pleck 1984). Thus women who are employed have the primary responsibility for housework and children in addition to their job demands. Combining the work of jobs and families, employed women average 15 hours more work per week and one-half hour less sleep per night than housewives (Pleck and Rustad 1980). Thus the increase in power with employment is often offset by a high level of demands. The frustrations and conflicts arising from these demands may contribute to women's higher rate of symptoms (Aneshensel et al. 1981; Cleary and Mechanic 1983; Gove and Geerken 1977; Ross and Mirowsky 1988).

There is some evidence for this perspective. Studies show that employed women with children in the home have higher symptoms levels than those without children (Kessler and McRae 1982; Radloff 1975). Other research also finds that women have significantly higher levels of anxiety than men when both are married, are employed, and have children in the home (Thoits 1986).

The more salient issue for role overload, however, is not the presence of children in the home per se but the level of demands and responsibility among employed women versus those among housewives and among men. To this point Kessler and McRae (1982), Ross et al. (1983b), and Krause and Markides (1985) find that the level of symptoms among employed women with the major responsibility for child care and/or housework equals the high levels of symptoms among housewives and exceeds those of employed women with fewer demands. Similarly, Ross and Mirowsky (1988) find that employed women who have difficulty arranging child care and who are totally responsible for child care have high depression levels. Further, Ross et al. (1983b) show that sex differences in depression are greatest in married couples in which wives are employed and are responsible for child care and housework. Women's scores equal men's when they have no difficulty arranging child care and husbands share in child care responsibilities (Ross and Mirowsky, 1988).

Integrating Power and Demands Explanations: The Importance of Personal Control

I argue that role overload and power may produce anxiety and depression by the same process and for the same reason: They affect individuals' psychological well-being by lowering their sense of personal control. Perceptions of personal control are emphasized increasingly as determinants of mental disorders. For example, the learned helplessness model of depression holds that a critical cause of depressive symptoms is the belief that the outcomes of one's actions are uncontrollable (Abramson and Sackheim 1977; Alloy, Peterson, Abramson, and Seligman 1984; Miller and Seligman 1973, 1975; Radloff 1975; Seligman 1975; Seligman, Abramson, Semmel, and von Baeyer 1979). Similarly, locus of control formulations hold that beliefs in external control—beliefs that events depend on forces outside oneself, such as luck or fate rather than one's own behavior—are related to anxious and depressive symptomatology (Abramowitz 1969; Burger 1984; Calhoun, Cheney, and Dawes 1974; Costello 1982; Evans 1981; Johnson and Sarason 1978; Leggett and Archer 1979; Mirowsky and Ross 1984; Molinari and Khanna 1981; Prociuk, Breen, and Lussier 1976; Rotter 1966). Arguments on fatalism connect the perception that one is "at the mercy of forces and people beyond one's control" to anxiety and depression (Kohn, 1972, p. 300; see also Wheaton 1980, 1983). Finally, mastery, which refers to perceptions of control over forces affecting individuals, is described as a fundamental goal to protect and enhance the self which is related to depressive symptomatology (Pearlin, Lieberman, Menaghan, and Mullen 1981).

Specific connections between personal control and anxiety and depression can be traced as follows. Feelings of lack of self-determination result in the perceptions of helplessness and hopelessness which are critical to anxious and depressive symptomatology. The perceived inability to affect one's environment also results in attributions of personal failure and thus in the attacks on self-worth which are central to anxiety and depression. In addition, attributing cause to environmental forces limits one's flexibility in responding to stressful circumstances (Thoits 1987). The feeling of having little control leads to a fearful view of social reality, which restricts using all options of action (Kohn 1972). Further, the sense that there is little connection between one's actions and the consequences limits the ability to learn from past experiences and thus to extinguish behavior with negative results (Mirowsky and Ross 1984; Phares 1962). Finally, when the point of coping efforts is unclear, there is less reason for coping behavior and thus fewer attempts and less persistence (Wheaton 1980, 1983).

These concepts and findings help to explain sex differences in anxiety and depression, insofar as women perceive themselves to have lower levels of personal control than men. As Radloff says about the origins of such differences, "Women are both more susceptible (i.e., have experienced more training in learned helplessness) and are more exposed to current situations of helplessness (i.e., where they have little control over what happens to them)" (Radloff 1975, p. 26). Thus women's perceptions of low control result in part from processes of childhood socialization and gender role training (Chodorow 1974, 1978). More important for this analysis, these perceptions largely come from and are reinforced by adult social conditions, which provide women with lower levels of actual control. Both low power and overload represent such conditions.

Power has an obvious effect on personal control, as positions of greater power imply greater effect or influence on one's environment. Weber (1954) defines power as "the possibility of imposing one's will upon the behavior of other people." Power within the family, with which we are concerned here, is defined as the real or potential ability of family members to change the behavior of other family members (Olson and Cromwell 1975). In connecting positions of actual power to perceptions of control, Kohn (1972) states that those lower in the social hierarchy have fewer options to act and thus little reason to feel in control. Because women are in positions lower in the social hierarchy in general and lower in marital power in particular, they perceive themselves to have less personal control over their social environment than men.

An excessive level of demands, or role overload, also produces feelings of lack of control which parallel the effects of structural positions of lower power. Role overload results from a level of demands which exhausts individuals' supply of time and energy (Coser 1974; Goode 1960) and produces "so many demands related to one's role(s) that satisfactory performance is improbable" (Barnett and Baruch 1985, p. 136). Resulting in the ability to meet any one demand fully, overload produces the feeling that one's life is out of control.[1] Thus the level of demands often experienced by women in combining employment and family roles compromises their sense of personal control. Like the effects of low power, overwhelming demands lead to feelings of helplessness as well as to perceptions of failure at the inability to accomplish objectives to the extent expected or desired.

In an alternative perspective to a role overload approach, however, others have argued recently that a greater number of social roles per se, regardless of the attendant level of demands, is associated with enhanced psychological well-being (Thoits 1986). By providing access to resources and alternative sources of gratification as well as by promoting social integration in general, a greater number of social roles is positive for mental health (Gove and Tudor 1973; Thoits 1986). I would also argue that the relationship between symptoms and multiple roles is mediated by issues of personal control. Multiple roles have been discussed as a major basis of power or control (Safilios-Rothschild 1970). Specifically, the existence of options increases control directly in terms of real or potential resources. The availability of alternatives also increases one's sense of personal control indirectly by decreasing dependency on any one object, activity, or individual.

According to a multiple roles perspective, women have a higher level of symptoms because they have fewer social roles than men. By equalizing the number of social roles, employment should lower women's symptoms to approximate men's more closely. Yet because women's employment has inconsistent effects on symptoms, it appears that neither a greater number of social roles nor greater power is sufficient to reduce women's symptomatology to equal men's. Rather it appears that when the demands associated with multiple roles are high, a greater number of roles does not necessarily lower symptoms. In fact, Thoits (1986) suggests that the relationship between multiple roles and symptoms may be curvilinear and that in situations of particularly high demands, multiple roles may be associated with greater symptomatology. Such conditions appear to exist among many married women who both are employed and have children in the home. Thoits's findings, as noted earlier, support this idea, as married employed women with children are significantly higher in symptoms than married employed men with children, in spite of the equal number of social roles. Therefore, this idea suggests that the high level of demands often experienced by women in combining familial and employment responsibilities compromises the greater personal control derived from employment in terms of both power and alternative roles.

In sum I propose that conditions both of low power and of role overload lower perceptions of personal control and heighten symptomatology as a result. Married women are higher in symptoms because they are more often either in positions of low power as housewives or in positions of high demands as employees. Work outside the home does not consistently reduce women's symptoms because gains in personal control in terms of power, or in terms of alternative roles, often are offset by the loss in control due to the overload in responsibilities from both jobs and family life.[2]

FIGURE 1. Outline of Predictions

Demands, Personal Control, and Sex Differences in Symptoms

Model:
Sex → Demands → Personal Control → Symptoms

Predictions:
1) Groups of women higher in demands (e.g., full-time employed women with children) have a higher level of symptoms than men.
2) A high level of demands (e.g., responsibility for child care) accounts for this difference.
3) Personal control accounts for the effects of demands on symptoms and thus for the sex differences.

Power, Personal Control, and Sex Differences in Symptoms

Model:
Sex → Power → Personal Control → Symptoms

Predictions:
1) Groups of women lower in power (e.g., housewives) have a higher level of symptoms than men.
2) Low power (e.g., lower resources in terms of relative income) accounts for sex differences.
3) Personal control accounts for the effects of low power on symptoms and thus for the sex differences.

Empirical Test of Predictions

To test this explanation for the effects of women's employment on sex differences, we can examine several predictions. Figure 1 summarizes these hypotheses.[3] The first model suggests that the higher the demands, the greater the symptom levels among women. Thus the groups under conditions of highest demands—women employed full time with children in the home—should be highest in symptoms. In addition, direct measures of high familial demands should account for the symptoms among these groups of women compared to men. The hypotheses predict further that issues of personal control account for the negative effects of demands on employed women. That is, issues of personal control are predicted to account for the higher rates of symptoms among high-demand groups and thus for sex differences between employed women in general and men. Further, issues of personal control should explain directly the effects of measures of demands on symptoms.

In explaining sex differences in general, the second model predicts that women in positions of low power, i.e. housewives, as well as women in positions of high demands are higher in symptoms than men. Direct measures of low power reduce these differences in symptoms. Personal control also mediates the effects of power on symptoms.

In addition, although these predictions focus on sex differences, we can derive from them comparisons between employed women and housewives. Employment fails to improve women's well-being because of the greater level of demands. This statement implies that employed women under high demands from job and family—the combination of which distinguishes them from housewives—are significantly higher in symptoms than housewives. It also implies that employed women under relatively low job and family demands are significantly lower in symptoms than housewives.

METHODS

Three data sets are used to test these predictions. These data sets allow the replication of certain tests of hypotheses as well as providing unique information on the relationships among power, demands, control, and symptoms. The first is the Fifty Communities Study, conducted in northern California in 1977 by Claude Fischer (Fischer 1982). The communities were selected randomly and represent the full spectrum from central city to small town. Within the communities, adults aged 18 years and older were selected randomly for inclusion in the study. Sampling procedures are described in detail elsewhere (Fisher 1982). The total N is 1050; the total N of married individuals used for this analysis is 554.

The second data set is the Americans View Their Mental Health Restudy, conducted by Joseph Veroff, Elizabeth Douvan, and Richard Kulka in 1976. A national sample of 2,264 adults aged 21 years and over was surveyed with a multistage probability area design (Veroff, Douvan, and Kulka 1981). The total number of married individuals in the sample for analysis is 1356.

The third data set is a survey of mental health made in 1985 as part of an ongoing study of Southern California residents by the author and Mark Baldassare. Five hundred adults aged 18 years and older in Orange County were interviewed by telephone. Random-digit dialing procedures were used in order to include both listed and unlisted numbers. Interviews averaged 25 minutes in length and focused on mental health, work, and family characteristics. The response rate for the survey was 65 percent. Comparisons with census data show that the sample is representative of the Orange County population in sex, age, and socioeconomic status. The total number of married individuals in the Orange County Study is 229.

Information on employment status will be used as one measure of power.[4] Each data set includes information on employment. Full-time employment consists of work outside the home occupying more than 30 hours a week. Part-time employment occupies 30 hours or less a week.[5]

As a direct measure of family power, we use the relative resources of husbands and wives in terms of income level. Relative income is computed as the percentage that the respondent's personal income from all sources contributes to the total family income. The Fifty Communities Study and the Orange County Study have information on individuals' total personal income from all sources as well as on total family income. This information provides a measure of relative resources which is applicable both to housewives and to employed women.

Overload is operationalized, first, by the presence of children in the household. In addition, the Fifty Communities Study and the Americans View Their Mental Health Restudy contain direct measures of perceived familial demands. The Fifty Communities Study includes an item on how often household members make demands: a lot of the time, some of the time, once in a while, or never. The Americans View Their Mental Health Restudy contains an item on child care demands which is asked of respondents who have any children under 12 years of age. Respondents are asked whether they do more of the child care, whether their spouse does more, or whether they share child care equally. For comparisons between employed women and housewives, the Fifty Communities data set also includes an item asking how frequently the job is demanding: much of the time, pretty often, occasionally, or almost never.

Personal control is measured by items in two of the data sets. The Americans View Their Mental Health Restudy contains the item, "Some people feel they can run their lives much the way they want to; others feel the problems in life are sometimes too big for them. Which one are you most like?" In the Orange County Study, this item was separated into two questions. Respondents were asked how often they feel the problems in life are too big for them and how often they feel they can run their life the way they want. These items are combined into a scale for analyses of personal control; the reliability of the scale using Cronbach's alpha is .56.

In measuring symptoms, the Fifty Communities Study includes a scale that covers a range of anxious and depressive symptoms. Depressive symptoms include how often the respondent feels depressed, avowed happiness, and how often the respondent feels pleased with what he or she is doing. Anxious symptomatology includes how often the respondent feels nervous or upset and how often the respondent feels tense. The study also includes items on how frequently the respondent feels frustrated. The reliability of this scale is .81.

The Americans View Their Mental Health Restudy and the Orange County Study use the Gurin Index, a 20-item symptom scale that includes the frequency of the following symptoms: trouble falling or staying asleep, being bothered by nervousness, being bothered by headaches, loss of appetite, being bothered by having an upset stomach, difficulty getting up in the morning, problems with ill health affecting work, shortness of breath when not exercising or working hard, heart beating hard, and drinking more than one should. Other symptoms include the frequency of spells of dizziness, being bothered by nightmares, losing weight when bothered by something, hands trembling enough to bother one, being troubled by hands sweating, inability to take care of things because one could not get going, being bothered by all sorts of pains and ailments, and feeling healthy enough to do what one would like. Two final items inquired whether respondents felt that they were going to have a nervous breakdown and whether they had any particular health trouble (Veroff et al. 1981). On the basis of Cronbach's alpha, the reliability of the Gurin Index is .83 in the Americans View Their Mental Health Restudy and .81 in the Orange County Study.

RESULTS

Analysis of covariance and regression techniques are used for testing the hypothesis. Symptom scales are transformed by means of square root in all analyses.[6] Age as well as social class variables of total family income and education are controlled for in the analysis.[7] Occupational status was related significantly to symptoms only in the Americans View Their Mental Health Restudy and thus is controlled for in analyses with this data set.[8] As in previous research (Cleary and Mechanic 1983; Kessler and McRae 1982; Radloff 1975), all comparisons between sexes are made between married women and full-time employed married men.

This section first shows results consistent with past research; thus overall sex differences and the analyses of employment are presented. Next we examine the effects of demands on symptoms with personal control as a mediating variable. Finally we investigate the effects of power on symptoms with personal control as a mediator.

Table 1 presents mean symptom scores of married women and full-time employed married men in the three studies.[9] In all three data sets, women have significantly higher symptoms than full-time employed men. These mean scores for men and for women provide information with which to compare results by employment status, controlling for demands, power, and personal control.

TABLE 1. Sex Differences in Symptomatology between Married Women and Men Employed Full Time

	Fifty Communities Study	Americans View Their Mental Health Restudy	Orange County Study
Full-time employed men	3.72	5.64	5.51
(N)	(183)	(520)	(94)
Women	3.82	5.88	5.73
(N)	(275)	(688)	(120)
F	6.200	42.427	6.372
p	.013	.000	.012

The Effects of Women's Employment

To test the effects of women's employment status on symptoms, we made comparisons between employed women and men and between housewives and men (see Table 2). As in previous research, housewives have a higher level of symptoms than men in all three data sets, although in the Orange County data the difference does not reach statistical significance. The effects of employment show that employed women have symptom scores somewhat lower than those of housewives in the Fifty Communities

TABLE 2. Sex Differences in Symptomatology among Employed Women, and Housewives, and Men Employed Full Time

	Fifty Communities Study	Americans View Their Mental Health Restudy	Orange County Study
Men employed full time	3.70	5.62*	5.49
(N)	(183)	(510)	(94)
Employed women	3.75	5.77	5.73
(N)	(121)	(248)	(67)
F	1.451	10.689	6.634
p	.229	.001	.011
Men employed full time	3.72	5.64	5.52
(N)	(183)	(520)	(94)
Housewives	3.86	5.94	5.69
(N)	(154)	(440)	(53)
F	7.470	50.610	2.188
p	.007	.000	.141

* The N for men is lower than the overall analysis of sex differences because data on occupational status are missing for 10 full-time employed men.

Study. Only in this study do employed women's scores equal the scores of men. Only in the Americans View Their Mental Health Restudy do employed women have a significantly lower level of symptoms (p=.009) than housewives; however, they are still significantly higher in symptoms than men. In the Orange County Study, employed women are slightly higher in symptoms than housewives; thus the sex differences are greater between employed women and men than between housewives and men.

Overall these results on women's employment mimic the inconsistency found in previous research. Thus, as in past research, a simple power explanation does not predict fully the effects of women's employment. Let us turn then to analyses of demands and personal control.

Demands, Personal Control, and Symptoms

I hypothesized that women's employment is associated with a high level of symptoms because of the high level of demands. Thus the groups highest in demands—women who work full time with children in the home—should be highest in symptoms in relation to men. In particular, sex differences should be greater between this group and men than between men and part-time employed women with children who have similar familial but fewer work demands, or women employed full time with no children who have similar work but fewer familial demands. As Table 3 shows, full-time employed women with children are the only employment group significantly higher in symptoms than men. When full-time employed women have no children or when women with children work part time, women are not significantly higher than men. In addition, there are no sex differences when all part-time employed women, both those with and those without children, are considered (findings not shown). It should be noted—and will be discussed further below—that part-time employed women with children have the lowest scores among these employment groups. In fact, in the Fifty Communities Study, part-time employed women with children are significantly lower in symptoms than men.

These analyses support a demands explanation, as the group highest in demands is highest in symptoms. Variations in samples in regard to demands could explain the inconsistencies in this and in previous research on women's employment. The greater the proportion of women in conditions of high demands—i.e., of full-time employed women with children in the home—the more negative the effects of women's employment.

Yet we still have not explained fully why employed women with children have a higher level of symptoms than men. Greater familial

TABLE 3. Sex Differences in Symptomatology among Women Employed Full Time with Children, Women Employed Part Time with Children, Women Employed Full Time with No Children, and Men Employed Full Time

	Fifty Communities Study	Americans View Their Mental Health Restudy	Orange County Study
Men employed full time with children	3.75	5.58	5.57
(N)	(118)	(344)	(51)
Women employed full time with children	3.96	5.80	6.03
(N)	(37)	(101)	(22)
F	7.463	7.861	8.528
p	.007	.005	.005
Men employed full time with children	3.75	5.60	5.59
(N)	(118)	(344)	(51)
Women employed part-time with children	3.57	5.67	5.56
(N)	(28)	(42)	(12)
F	5.038	.368	.031
p	.026	.544	.861
Men employed full time with no children	3.61	5.67	5.40
(N)	(65)	(166)	(43)
Women employed full time with no children	3.70	5.70	5.59
(N)	(45)	(90)	(26)
F	1.033	.599	2.744
p	.312	.758	.102

demands are expected to explain these differences; thus the differences between full-time employed women and men with children should be reduced to nonsignificance when demands are equalized. Table 4 shows results of analyses of covariance with items on familial demands in the Fifty Communities Study and in the Americans View Their Mental Health Restudy. The table shows differences in mean symptom scores of full-time employed women and full-time employed men with children, with perceived level of demands held constant. Both data sets support the hypothesis. In the Fifty Communities Study, when perceived demands are held constant, sex differences between full-time employed women with children and men disappear. In the Americans View Their Mental Health Restudy, when demands are equalized in terms of the division of child care between spouses, sex differences also are reduced to nonsignificance.[10] These reductions in sex differences are due more to the decrease in women's scores than to the increase in men's. Thus these analyses provide direct support for the hypothesis that greater demands account for the higher rates of symptoms among full-time employed women.[11]

Additional support comes from analyses of employed women versus housewives. These analyses use items on job and familial demands in the Fifty Communities Study. Although we cannot test for differences between employed women and housewives, controlling for demands, because there is no overall measure of demands with a common metric for these groups, we can compare employed women under different levels of

TABLE 4. Sex Differences in Symptomatology for Women Employed Full Time with Children and Men Employed Full Time, Controlling for Familial Demands

	Fifty Communities Study	Americans View Their Mental Health Restudy
Men employed full time with children	3.80	5.61
(N)	(118)	(257)
Women employed full time with children	3.80	5.70
(N)	(37)	(79)
F	.006	.524
p	.939	.470

TABLE 5. Sex Differences in Symptomatology between Women Employed Full Time with Children and Men Employed Full Time with Children, Adjusting for Demands and Personal Control: Americans View Their Mental Health Restudy

	F	p
Overall (N = 336)		
Sex	9.542	.002
Adjusting for Demands		
Sex	.524	.470
Demands	2.632	.073
Adjusting for Control		
Sex	.058	.810
Demands	1.567	.210
Control	54.338	.000

demands with housewives.[12] Employed women under both high work and high family demands are significantly higher in symptoms than housewives (p = .046). Employed women with both low work and low family demands, however, are significantly lower in symptoms than housewives (p = .001). Finally, when employed women are low in either source of demands—job or family—they are significantly lower in symptoms than housewives (p = .025 for job and p = .001 for family demands). Thus analyses within sex also indicate that employment may not be positive for women because of the high level of demands. When demands are relatively low, however, employment has beneficial effects on women's mental health.

In testing a personal control explanation for sex differences, we expect personal control to explain the effects of demands on symptoms. Here we can only compare employed women to men because the Fifty Communities Study—the only data set with information on housewives and on employed women's job and family demands—does not have information on personal control. To demonstrate control as a mediating factor, we expect demands to be related significantly to symptoms. Adjusting for demands should reduce sex differences found between full-time employed women and men with children to nonsignificance. When we enter personal control into the equation, sex differences should diminish further. In addition, adjusting for personal control should reduce the relationship between demands and symptoms to nonsignificance in order to explain the effects of demands.

Table 5 shows results of these analyses for

the measure of demands in the Americans View Their Mental Health Restudy. The hypothesis is generally supported. First, when we control for background variables of education, age, occupation, and total family income, and enter sex into the equation, we find significant sex differences in symptoms, as discussed earlier. Second, we enter perceived demands into the equation. The division of responsibility for child care is related to symptoms at the .07 level. In addition, when child care demands are controlled for, as shown above, the sex differences are reduced to nonsignificance. Third, we enter personal control into the equation. When personal control is adjusted for, sex differences are reduced further. In these analyses, holding personal control constant reduces to nonsignificance the relationship not only between sex and symptoms but also between demands and symptoms.

Overall, these results show that the impact of demands on sex differences in symptoms is mediated by personal control. Specifically, the analyses suggest that full-time employed women with children are higher in symptoms because the high demands they experience lead to perceptions of low personal control, which results in symptoms of anxiety and depression.

Power, Personal Control, and Symptoms

Finally, to investigate personal control as a general explanation for sex differences, we test hypotheses that issues of personal control underlie the effects of power as well as demands on symptoms. As Table 2 shows, housewives (that is, women in positions of low power) have higher levels of symptoms than men in all three data sets. To test more directly that personal control explains the effects of low power on symptoms, Table 6 presents analyses of relative income and personal control in the Orange County Study.[13] For this analysis, the total sample of women and men is used to provide greater variation in relative income. To support the hypothesis, relative income is expected to be related significantly to symptoms. When relative income is held constant, sex differences should be reduced. Entering personal control should reduce sex differences further. In order to explain the effects of relative income, adjusting for personal control also

TABLE 6. Sex Differences in Symptomatology between Married Individuals, Adjusting for Relative Income and Personal Control: Orange County Study

	F	p
Overall (N=214)		
Sex	7.721	.006
Adjusting for Relative Income		
Sex	4.002	.047
Relative income	5.112	.025
Adjusting for Control		
Sex	2.920	.089
Relative income	3.411	.066
Control	65.542	.000

should reduce the relationship between relative income and symptoms to nonsignificance. Results show, first, that overall sex differences are significant. In the second step, relative income is found to be related significantly to symptoms. In addition, controlling for relative income reduces sex differences, although these differences remain significant. When personal control is entered into the equation, sex differences are reduced to nonsignificance. Finally, in accounting for the effects of relative income, adjusting for personal control reduces the relationship between relative income and symptoms to nonsignificance. Thus personal control accounts for the higher symptoms among women in positions of low power as well as in positions of high demands.

DISCUSSION

Analyses both within sex and across sex show that differential levels of demands explain the inconsistent effects of women's employment. When familial demands are equal, employed women equal men in symptoms. When either job or family demands are low, employed women are significantly lower in symptoms than housewives. Under such conditions, women seem to benefit from the greater power and resources associated with employment. This point is illustrated further in analyses of power in terms of relative income. Women benefit in general from greater relative income and are more similar to men in symptoms when the relative contribution of income is equal. Because employment produces greater income for women, the power associated with employment is underscored further as beneficial for women's mental health.

These analyses also indicate that issues of personal control underlie the effects of both demands and power on symptomatology. Personal control is related strongly to symptoms in two independent data sets, giving evidence of the reliability of this relationship. Conditions of high demands and low power appear to raise women's rates of anxiety and depression by affording them lower actual control and thus a lower sense of control. On this basis, social positions of low control appear to explain women's higher rates of distress or demoralization. Because women are more often in positions of low power as housewives and in positions of high demands when employed, they continue to suffer higher rates of anxiety and depression than men.

As for the limitations in this analysis, the measures of overload, power, and personal control are restricted. The demonstrated importance of these variables in this analysis suggests that further research use more extensive measures of personal control and of overload. Future research also should include measures of familial power that focus on decision-making power of husbands and wives.

A second issue concerns the causal direction of the processes discussed here. Rather than demands and control resulting in symptoms, symptoms may cause changes in perceptions of control as well as in perceptions of demands. Because the data sets used for these analyses are cross-sectional, this possibility cannot be tested directly. Analyses with the more objective indicators, however, point to a causal direction *from* demands *to* symptoms. Specifically, it is unlikely that a higher level of symptoms results in married women entering the labor force, but a reverse causal direction in regard to symptoms and personal control remains a possibility. The results also would be interesting if only those forms of distress resulting in perceptions of low control were associated with power and demands.[14] To address these issues directly, however, with perceptions of control as well as demands, longitudinal analyses are necessary and are recommended for further research.[15]

In discussing these limitations, such longitudinal work would not be in order if these analyses had not suggested a mechanism for clarifying inconsistencies in past research. These inconsistencies in the effects of women's employment posed a threat to social causation explanations for sex differences in psychiatric disorders. The results reported here, replicated in several data sets, suggest that a personal control explanation integrates previous findings on employment which varied from sample to sample. Specifically, employment for women fails to have consistently positive effects because the greater personal control in terms of power is gained at the expense of the loss in control in terms of demands. Women who are employed have high symptoms for the same reasons as housewives: because of positions of low control, although from a different source. Thus the underlying cause of women's rates remains unchanged. That this situation is a result of actual control associated with social positions among women as housewives or workers is consistent with social causation explanations for sex differences in symptomatology. In this sense, although alternative explanations can be generated, this analysis offers a cogent set of findings that underscore the importance of social factors in explaining sex differences in psychopathology.

In addition, the positive effects of part-time work among women with children represent an empirical exception that supports the general rule. Part-time work for women with children represents more control in that it combines greater power with relatively lower demands. That is, part-time employment when children are in the home brings the benefits of greater familial power without the overload of work responsibilities, and thus may represent one ideal for maximizing control and minimizing distress for women, or for men. This employment status, however, alters the division of labor outside the household rather than inside. Lower symptom rates among women also can be achieved by changing the division of tasks within as well as outside the home, such as by sharing housework and child care and by making other arrangements that increase personal control in terms of both resources and demands for women and for men.

In conclusion, it appears that perceptions of personal control act to mediate certain chronic conditions of stress which characterize women's and men's social positions. Issues of personal control have been discussed as mediators of stressful life events as well as of chronic strains, both in general and in relation to sex differences (Kessler and Essex 1982; Thoits 1987; Turner and Noh 1983); but as Pearlin et al. (1981) argue, long-term chronic strains may be more damaging to the individual's sense of mastery than the more acute, more short-lived life events. Thus, in explaining sex differences, this analysis proposes the means or process by which the differential social positions of men and of women result in differential rates of symptomatology—that is, through the chronic strains associated with those positions which affect perceptions linked to mental health.

Power and the division of labor, the major dimensions by which gender roles are differentiated, have been dominant explanations for sex differences in anxiety and depression. A personal control explanation offers a parsimonious approach by integrating these diverse perspectives and by proposing the specific mechanisms through which they affect psychological well-being. In this sense, this perceptive can be generalized to explain differences in mental health among diverse populations. Specifically, a personal control perspective can be used to explain symptoms in population groups that differ in power or in demands. For example, there is evidence that differences by social class in symptomatology, the explanation for which has been a major source of controversy, may be explained in terms of personal control (Wheaton 1980). Similarly, racial differences in distress and depression can be explained from a control perspective. Therefore this approach offers a potentially general explanation for the effects of certain social positions on mental health, building on a conceptual framework which has received increasing theoretical attention and empirical support.

NOTES

1. As Epstein (1971) points out, women do not have the same means available as men to regulate the negative effects of high levels of demands, such as compartmentalization or socially defined hierarchies and priorities of demands. In keeping with this point, as Goode (1960) suggests, those with greater power have more mechanisms at their disposal to reduce role overload.
2. Greater power and alternative roles may not be the only positive aspects of employment for women. Employment also may be positive because it adds sources of social support and this increases coping resources. Past research, however, has not shown that employed women have more social support in regard to emotional support (Cleary and Mechanic 1983). Moreover, the Fifty Communities Study includes items on social support, including emotional and instrumental support. It shows no difference between employed women and housewives in the number of people to talk with about personal matters or to rely on for their judgment. The only difference in social support is that employed women have more people who help with household tasks. This difference may be a function of greater need and greater resources to pay for outside help rather than of greater support from coworkers.
3. The models presented in Figure 1 and the analyses offered here focus on the results of differential positions of actual control among men and among women for perceptions of personal control and therefore for symptoms. Thus sex affects perceptions of personal control through role overload and power. As discussed above, however, sex also could have a direct effect on perceptions of personal control through socialization processes and gender-role training.
4. It is recognized that employment is an indirect measure of power. As noted in the conclusion, I would recommend that future research include more direct measures in analyses of power and sex differences.
5. Items in the Americans View Their Mental Health Restudy also ask for personal and total family income. The item on personal income, however, asks how much the respondent earned in the last year. Thus for women who were not employed, any personal income from other sources is not obtained and analysis of relative income cannot be conducted with housewives.
6. Symptom scales are transformed because the distributions on the scales are skewed. The square root transformation of scale scores causes the distribution to be normal, satisfying the assumption of a normal distribution of the residuals for the statistical tests.
7. Analyses controlling for family income and education constitute a test of a power hypothesis. As Table 1 shows and in accordance with later findings, greater power among women in terms of family income and education lowers sex differences but the differences remain significant. Greater power appears to be a necessary but not a sufficient factor in reducing women's symptoms to equal those of men. These background variables of education and family income, as well as age, are controlled for because they have been shown both in previous research and in these

data to be related significantly to symptomatology. In regard to the analysis with relative income, controlling for total family income allows us to examine the effects of the percentage of total income contributed by a spouse regardless of the absolute amount of the total income.

8. Social desirability is not controlled for in this analysis. Although differences in expressiveness and in willingness to admit negative feelings have been proposed as an explanation for sex differences, Clancy and Gove (1974) and Gove and Geerken (1977) found that sex differences in symptoms remained after response biases of yea saying, nay saying, trait desirability, and need for approval were controlled.
9. Women are significantly higher than married men in general as well as full-time employed married men.
10. As mentioned above, the analyses on demands in the Americans View Their Mental Health Restudy are conducted on respondents with any children under age 12. Full-time employed women with children under 12 constitute 78 percent of full-time employed women with children in the home. Men with any children under 12 constitute 75 percent of full-time employed men with children. As for the overall symptom scores among these women and men, men with children under 12 and men with no children under 12 have the same mean scores (5.58). Women with younger children score somewhat higher (5.84) than women with no younger children (5.80). The sex differences for full-time employed women and for men with any younger children are significant at the .002 level.
11. Further tests of power in terms of relative income also were conducted in explaining the higher rates of full-time employed women with children. For both the Americans View Their Mental Health Restudy and the Orange County Study, differences between full-time employed women with children and men remain significant when relative income is controlled. For the Fifty Communities Study, sex differences are reduced but not as much as when demands are controlled. Therefore this finding gives further evidence that power alone is not sufficient to explain higher symptoms among employed women.
12. Employed women who report that the job is too demanding much of the time or pretty often and that household members make demands a lot or some of the time are categorized as under high demands. Employed women who report that work is too demanding occasionally or almost never and that household members make demands once in a while or never are categorized as under low demands.
13. Demands also were tested as a possible explanation for higher rates among housewives as compared to men. In the Americans View Their Mental Health Restudy, sex differences between housewives with children and men remain significant when items on responsibility for child care are held constant. In the Fifty Communities Study, sex differences are reduced when familial demands are held constant but less than when relative income is controlled. This finding gives further evidence that just as demands seem to explain higher rates of symptoms among employed women, lower power seems to explain the higher rates among housewives.
14. This point was suggested by an anonymous reviewer.
15. A related issue is the possible confounding of personal control with symptoms as to whether perceptions of personal control are part of anxious and depressive symptomatology. In addressing this issue, Pearlin et al. (1981) state that one way to show that control in terms of mastery is independent from depression is to demonstrate that they do not always covary. In their analysis they find that depressive symptoms are increased without a decrease in perceptions of mastery after stressful events which are out of an individual's control, such as severe illness or death of a child. Thus greater symptoms are not linked to lower perceptions of mastery in at least some situations, giving evidence that symptoms and perceptions of personal control are independent of one another.

REFERENCES

Abramowitz, Stephen I. 1969. "Locus of Control and Self-Reported Depression Among College Students." *Psychological Reports* 25:149–50.

Abramson, Lyn Y., and Harold A. Sackheim. 1977. "A Paradox in Depression: Uncontrollability and Self-Blame." *Psychological Bulletin* 84:838–51.

Alloy, Lauren B., Christopher Peterson, Lyn Y. Abramson, and Martin E. P. Seligman. 1984. "Attributional Style and the Generality of Learned Helplessness." *Journal of Personality and Social Psychology* 46:681–87.

Aneshensel, Carol S., Ralph R. Frerichs, and Virginia A. Clark. 1981. "Family Roles and Sex Differences in Depression." *Journal of Health and Social Behavior* 22:379–93.

Barnett, Rosalind C., and Grace K. Baruch. 1985. "Women's Involvement in Multiple Roles and Psychological Distress." *Journal of Personality and Social Psychology* 49:135–45.

Blood, Robert O., and Donald M. Wolfe. 1960. *Husbands and Wives*. New York: Free Press.

Burger, Jerry M. 1984. "Desire for Control, Locus of Control, and Proneness to Depression." *Journal of Personality* 52:71–89.

Calhoun, Laurence G., Thomas Cheney, and A. Stephen Dawes. 1974. "Locus of Control, Self-Reported Depression, and Perceived Causes of Depression." *Journal of Consulting and Clinical Psychology* 42:736–45.

Chodorow, Nancy. 1974. "Family Structure and Feminine Personality." Pp. 43–66 in *Women, Culture and Society*, edited by Michele Z. Rosaldo and Louise Lamphere. Palo Alto, CA: Stanford University Press.

———. 1978. *The Reproduction of Mothering*. Berkeley: University of California Press.

Clancy, Kevin and Walter Gove. 1974. "Sex Differences in Respondents' Reports of Psychiatric Symptoms: An Analysis of Response Bias." *American Journal of Sociology* 80:205–16.

Cleary, Paul, and David Mechanic. 1983. "Sex Differences in Psychological Distress Among Married People." *Journal of Health and Social Behavior* 24:111–21.

Coser, Lewis. 1974. *Greedy Institutions*. New York: Free Press.

Costello, Elizabeth J. 1982. "Locus of Control and Depression in Students and Psychiatric Outpatients." *Journal of Clinical Psychology* 36:661–67.

Dohrenwend, Bruce P., and Barbara S. Dohrenwend. 1974. "Social and Cultural Influences on Psychopathology." *Annual Review of Psychology* 25:417–52.

———. 1976. "Sex Differences in Psychiatric Disorders." *American Journal of Sociology* 81:1447–54.

Dohrenwend, Bruce P., Barbara S. Dohrenwend, Madeline S. Gould, Bruce Link, Richard Neugebaur, and Robin Wunsch-Hitzig. 1980. *Mental Illness in the United States*. New York: Praeger.

Epstein, Cynthia Fuch. 1971. Woman's Place. Berkeley, CA: University of California Press.

Evans, Ronald. 1981. "The Relationship of Two Measures of Perceived Control to Depression." *Journal of Personality Assessment* 45:66–70.

Fendrich, Michael. 1984. "Wives' Employment and Husbands' Distress: A Meta-Analyses and a Replication." *Journal of Marriage and the Family* 46:871–79.

Ferree, Myra Marx. 1976. "Working Class Jobs: Housework and Paid Work as Sources of Satisfaction." *Social Problems* 23:431–41.

Fischer, Claude. 1982. *To Dwell among Friends*. Chicago: University of Chicago Press.

Goode, William J. 1960. "A Theory of Strain." *American Sociological Review* 25:483–96.

Gore, Susan, and Thomas Mangione. 1983. "Social Roles, Sex Roles and Psychological Distress: Additive and Interactive Models of Sex Differences." *Journal of Health and Social Behavior* 24:300–12.

Gove, Walter R., and Michael Geerken. 1977. "The Effect of Children and Employment on the Mental Health of Married Men and Women." *Social Forces* 56:66–76.

Gove, Walter R., and Jeanette Tudor. 1973. "Adult Sex Roles and Mental Illness." *American Journal of Sociology* 78:812–35.

Horwitz, Allan. 1982. "Sex Role Expectations, Power, and Psychological Distress." *Sex Roles* 8:607–23.

Johnson, James H., and Irwin G. Sarason. 1978. "Life Stress, Depression, and Anxiety: Internal-External Control as a Moderator Variable." *Journal of Psychosomatic Research* 22:205–8.

Kessler, Ronald C., and Marilyn Essex. 1982. "Marital Status and Depression: The Importance of Coping Resources." *Social Forces* 61:484–507.

Kessler, Ronald C., and James McRae, Jr. 1981. "Trends in the Relationship Between Sex and Psychological Distress: 1957–1976." *American Sociological Review* 46:443–52.

———. 1982. "The Effect of Wives' Employment on the Mental Health of Married Men and Women." *American Sociological Review* 47:216–27.

Kohn, Melvin L. 1972. "Class, Family, and Schizophrenia: A Reformulation." *Social Forces* 50:295–304.

Krause, Neal, and Kyriakos S. Markides. 1985. "Employment and Psychological Well-Being in Mexican American Women." *Journal of Health and Social Behavior* 26:15–26.

Leggett, Jack, and Robert P. Archer. 1979. "Locus of Control and Depression among Psychiatric Inpatients." *Psychological Reports* 45:835–38.

McLanahan, Sara S., and Jennifer L. Glass. 1985. "A Note on the Trend in Sex Differences in Psychological Distress." *Journal of Health and Social Behavior* 26:328–36.

Miller, William R., and Martin E. P. Seligman. 1973. "Depression and the Perception of Reinforcement." *Journal of Abnormal Psychology* 82:62–73.

———. 1975. "Learned Helplessness, Depression and the Perception of Reinforcement." *Behavior Research and Therapy* 14:7–17.

Mirowsky, John, and Catherine E. Ross, 1984. "Mexican Culture and Its Emotional Contradictions." *Journal of Health and Social Behavior* 25:2–13.

Molinari, Victor, and Prabha Khanna. 1981. "Locus of Control and Its Relationship to Anxiety and Depression." *Journal of Personality Assessment* 45:314–19.

Myers, Jerome K., Myrna M. Weissman, Gary L. Tischler, Charles C. Holzer III, Philip J. Leaf,

Helen Orvaschel, James Anthony, Jeffrey H. Boyd, Jack D. Burke, Jr., Morton Kramer, and Roger Stoltzman. 1984. "Six Months Prevalence of Psychiatric Disorders in Three Communities." *Archives of General Psychiatry* 41:959–67.

Olson, David E., and Ronald E. Cromwell. 1975. *Power in Families*. New York: Wiley.

Pearlin, Leonard I. 1975. "Sex Roles and Depression." Pp. 191–207 in *Life-Span Developmental Psychology*, edited by Nancy Datan and Leon H. Ginsberg. New York: Academic Press.

Pearlin, Leonard I., Morton A. Lieberman, Elizabeth G. Menaghan, and Joseph T. Mullan. 1981. "The Stress Process." *Journal of Health and Social Behavior* 22:337–56.

Phares, E. Jerry. 1962. "Perceptual Threshold Decrements as a Function of Skill and Chance Experiences." *Journal of Psychology* 53:339–407.

Pleck, Joseph H. 1984. "The Work-Family Role System." In *Work and Family*, edited by P. Voydanoff. Palo Alto, CA: Mayfield.

Pleck, Joseph H., and Michael Rustad. 1980. "Husbands' and Wives' Time in Family Work and Pay Work: A 1975–76 Study of Time Use." Unpublished paper, Wellesley College Research Center for Women.

Prociuk, Terry, Lawrence Breen, and Richard Lussier. 1976. "Hopelessness, Internal-External Locus of Control and Depression." *Journal of Clinical Psychology* 32:299–300.

Radloff, Lenore. 1975. "Sex Differences in Depression: The Effects of Occupation and Marital Status." *Sex Roles* 1:249–65.

Roberts, Robert, and Steven O'Keefe. 1981. "Sex Differences in Depression Reexamined." *Journal of Health and Social Behavior* 22:394–400.

Robins, Lee N., John E. Helzer, Myrna M. Weissman, Helen Orvaschel, Ernest Gruenberg, Jack D. Burke, Jr., and Darrel A. Regier. 1984. "Lifetime Prevalence of Specific Psychiatric Disorders in Three Cities." *Archives of General Psychiatry* 41:949–58.

Rosenfield, Sarah. 1980. "Sex Differences in Depression: Do Women Always Have Higher Rates?" *Journal of Health and Social Behavior* 21:33–42.

Ross, Catherine E. and John Mirowsky. 1988. "Child Care and Emotional Adjustment to Wives' Employment." *Journal of Health and Social Behavior* 29:127–38.

Ross, Catherine E., John Mirowsky, and Patricia Ulbrich. 1983. "Distress and the Traditional Female Role: A Comparison of Mexicans and Anglos." *American Journal of Sociology* 89:670–82.

Ross, Catherine E., John Mirowsky, and Joan Huber. 1983. "Dividing Work, Sharing Work, and In-Between: Marriage Patterns and Depression." *American Sociological Review* 48:809–23.

Rotter, Julian B. 1966. "Generalized Expectancies for Internal versus External Control of Reinforcement." *Psychological Monographs* 80:1–28.

Safilios-Rothschild, Constantine. 1970. "The Study of Family Power Structure: A Review 1960–1969." *Journal of Marriage and the Family* 32:539–52.

Seligman, Martin E. P. 1975. *Helplessness*. San Francisco: Freeman.

Seligman, Martin E. P., Lyn Y. Abramson, Amy Semmel, and Carol von Baeyer. 1979. "Depressive Attributional Style." *Journal of Abnormal Psychology* 88:242–47.

Thoits, Peggy A. 1986. "Multiple Identities: Examining Gender and Marital Status Differences in Distress." *American Sociological Review* 51:259–72.

———. 1987. "Gender and Marital Status Differences in Control and Distress: Common Stress versus Unique Stress Explanations." *Journal of Health and Social Behavior* 28:7–22.

Turner, R. Jay, and Samuel Noh. 1983. "Class and Psychological Vulnerability among Women: The Significance of Social Support and Personal Control." *Journal of Health and Social Behavior* 24:2–15.

Veroff, Joseph, Elizabeth Douvan, and Richard A. Kulka. 1981. *The Inner American*. New York: Basic Books.

Weber, Max. 1954. *Max Weber on Law in Economy and Society*. Cambridge, MA: Harvard University Press.

Weissman, Myrna, and Gerald Klerman. 1977. "Sex Differences in the Epidemiology of Depression." *Archives of General Psychiatry* 34:98–111.

Wheaton, Blair. 1980. "The Sociogenesis of Psychological Disorder: An Attributional Theory." *Journal of Health and Social Behavior* 21:100–24.

———. 1983. "Stress, Personal Coping Resources, and Psychiatric Symptoms: An Investigation of Interactive Models." *Journal of Health and Social Behavior* 24:208–29.

SARAH ROSENFIELD is Assistant Professor of Sociology at Rutgers University. She is also a core member of the Institute for Health, Health Care Policy, and Aging Research. Her current research examines the effects of women's employment on the mental health of husbands and wives.

Part IV
Social Stress

[14]

The Sociological Study of Stress*

LEONARD I. PEARLIN

University of California, San Francisco

Journal of Health and Social Behavior 1989, Vol. 30 (September):241–256

This paper presents a critical overview of current concepts and analytic practices in stress research and considers how they can be changed to make the research more consistent with core sociological interests. An overarching concern of the paper is the analytic use of basic information about people's social and institutional affiliations and statuses. It is important that such information be treated not simply as data that need to be controlled statistically; we must examine the bearing of these data on each domain of the stress process: the exposure to and meaning of stressors, access to stress mediators, and the psychological, physical, and behavioral manifestations of stress. The conceptualization and measurement of stressors should move away from their focus on particular events or chronic strains and should seek instead to observe and assess over time constellations of stressors made up of both events and strains. Moreover, the effects of the mediators—coping and social support—are evaluated most fruitfully in terms of their effects in limiting the number, severity, and diffusion of stressors in these constellations. Finally, sociological stress researchers should not be bound to outcomes that better serve the intellectual interests of those who work with biomedical and epidemiological models of stress, nor should the research be committed exclusively to a single outcome.

Sociologists have an intellectual stake in the study of stress. It presents an excellent opportunity to observe how deeply well-being is affected by the structured arrangements of people's lives and by the repeated experiences that stem from these arrangements. Social research into stress is entirely consistent with a present-day social psychology that seeks to establish the unities between social structure and the inner functioning of individuals (House 1981a). Yet stress is not generally seen as part of a sociological mainstream, partly, I believe, because those of us who are engaged in stress research are not consistently attentive to the sociological character of the field. In this paper I attempt to identify what I regard as some of the conceptual and analytic issues that should be considered in bringing the study of stress closer to sociology.

Much of the paper is organized around what have come to be recognized as the domains of the stress process: stressors, stress mediators, and stress outcomes. There is considerable accumulated evidence that this process and its components largely arise from and are influenced by various structural arrangements in which individuals are embedded. To a large extent these arrangements determine the stressors to which people are exposed, the mediators they are able to mobilize, and the manner in which they experience stress. In view of its importance, the structural background of the stress process deserves a closer examination than it usually receives.

THE STRUCTURAL CONTEXTS OF THE STRESS PROCESS

Most research into stress starts with an experience—an exigency that people confront

* Direct all correspondence to Leonard I. Pearlin, Center for Social and Behavioral Sciences, 237; University of California; 1350 Seventh Avenue; San Francisco, CA 94143–0848. Support for this paper was provided by the National Institute of Mental Health, Grant MH AG42127; the Consortium for Research into Stress Processes, funded by the W.T. Grant Foundation; and the Network for Health Promotion and Disease Prevention, funded by the MacArthur Foundation.

and their perceptions of that exigency as threatening or burdensome. Many stressful experiences, it should be recognized, don't spring out of a vacuum but typically can be traced back to surrounding social structures and people's locations within them. The most encompassing of these structures are the various systems of stratification that cut across societies, such as those based on social and economic class, race and ethnicity, gender, and age. To the extent that these systems embody the unequal distribution of resources, opportunities, and self-regard, a low status within them may itself be a source of stressful life conditions. Thus it is quite understandable that the community studies conducted in the 1950s and 1960s consistently revealed powerful associations between people's statuses in stratified systems and indicators of their well-being (e.g., Gurin, Veroff, and Feld 1960; Hollingshead and Redlich 1958; Srole, Langner, Opler, and Rennie 1960). Interest in these statuses continues today, particularly as evidenced by the explosion of literature examining gender and stress (e.g., Gore and Mangione 1983; Kessler and McRae 1981; Thoits 1986).

Another important structural context is found in social institutions and their arrangements of statuses and roles. Incumbency in a major institutionalized role necessarily entails persistent encounters with a host of conditions and expectations that exert a structuring force on experience. Because the roles themselves persist in time, experiences within them tend to become a repeated feature of their incumbents' lives. When these experiences are threatening and problematic, they may result in stress. There are abundant indications that such experience is common among incumbents of occupational (e.g., Kahn 1973) and of family roles (see e.g., Pearlin 1983). Moreover, one does not act alone as an incumbent of a role. Instead, one role is part of a larger role set or of a constellation of complementary roles around which important interpersonal relations are structured. Thus one cannot be a husband without a wife, a parent without a child, a colleague without a fellow worker. Relationships formed by role sets are relatively enduring and stable, and typically are of considerable importance to the parties involved. Consequently, when such relationships are problematic and filled with conflict, they can produce considerable stress.

The importance of roles and role sets as sources of stress are elaborated in a later discussion of chronic strains. Here I wish to emphasize that interrelated levels of social structure—social stratification, social institutions, interpersonal relationships—mold and structure the experiences of individuals; these experiences, in turn, may result in stress. Therefore the structural contexts of people's lives are not extraneous to the stress process but are fundamental to that process. They are the sources of hardship and privilege, threat and security, conflict and harmony. In searching for the origins of stress, we may begin fruitfully by scrutinizing the social arrangements of society and the structuring of experience within these arrangements. This search, I believe, will reveal how ordinary people can be caught up in the disjunctures and discontinuities of societies, how they can be motivated to adopt socially valued dreams and yet can find their dreams thwarted by socially erected barriers, and how as engaged members of society they come into conflict with others and with themselves.

Certainly not all stress researchers are interested in the structural contexts of the stress process. As I noted above, most begin their work by looking directly at potential stressors that reside in individuals' experience without regard to the possible structural origins of the stressors. Sociological inquiry, however, does not have the option of ignoring these origins. The distinguishing mark of sociological inquiry is its effort to uncover patterns and regularities shared by people whose social characteristics and circumstances are similar. The essential element of the sociological study of stress is the presence of similar types and levels of stress among people who are exposed to similar social and economic conditions, who are incumbents in similar roles, and who come from similar situational contexts. There can be little, if any, sociological interest in randomly distributed problems or randomly distributed responses to the problems. Such random or idiosyncratic stress is of legitimate interest to clinicians or biologists, but not to sociologists. Therefore a salient feature of sociological stress research is its concern with the socially patterned distribution of components of the stress process: stressors, mediators, and outcomes. Such patterns provide a cue that individuals' potentially stressful experiences and the ways in which they are affected by these experiences may originate in the social orders of which they are a part.

Much of this discussion might appear to belabor the self-evident, particularly because virtually all social inquiry into stress collects information about people's backgrounds and situational circumstances that enables these social patterns to be detected analytically. Certainly current research cannot be faulted for its failure to assemble basic sociological data, but it can be faulted for failing to subject the data to sociological scrutiny. All too often, people's background and circumstantial attributes are either overlooked in analyses or receive only scant attention. Thus data that should be at the heart of sociological inquiry are frequently treated only as analytic noise that needs to be controlled statistically. Of course there is nothing wrong with the logic of controlling for the effects of social background characteristics; such controls can reveal whether a statistical relationship between other factors is spurious or independent of the possible effects of the social characteristics (Rosenberg 1968). Yet when social structural and contextual data are collected *only* so that they may be controlled, that treatment precludes the examination of their potentially important roles in the study of stress.

Information about structural contexts and people's links to those contexts should be analyzed at virtually every step of the stress process. Gender can be taken as an illustration because, as I noted earlier, this is a status on which a large and burgeoning research literature exists (see e.g., Pearlin and Aneshensel 1986). First, gender is a characteristic that influences the stressors to which people are exposed: women and men often experience different stressful circumstances (Pearlin and Lieberman 1978). In addition, even where exposure to stressors is similar for women and for men, the effects of these stressors on the outcomes may be conditioned by gender. Perhaps, for example, equivalent occupational hardships have different impacts on men and on women because of differences in the conditions that men and women face in other roles (Pearlin 1975a). Third, the personal and social mediating resources that can be mobilized to deal with hardships also may vary with gender (Pearlin and Schooler 1978). Finally, gender is a characteristic that can affect the ways in which stress outcomes are manifested. Thus, as I shall describe later, depressive symptomatology may be a more typical expression of stress among women, whereas drinking and other behaviors may be more typical among men (Aneshensel 1988).

The general point to be drawn from these examples is that the structural contexts of people's lives can affect each major phase of the stress process. When analytically we slight people's social and economic backgrounds, we necessarily neglect the sociological exploration of links that join broader dimensions of social organization to personal stress.

SOCIAL STRESSORS

Historically, stress research has been guided by two modal concerns: one having a primary interest in naturalistic stressors and the other in the mediation and outcomes of stress. As the preceding discussion suggests, sociologists have been and should be interested in the former. For other scientists, who are more concerned with stress outcomes and their psychological and biological dimensions, the nature and origins of the stressors are less important. To those researchers it makes little difference whether stress is controlled experimentally in the laboratory, is unique to individuals, or is anchored in highly unusual circumstances. From their viewpoint, the response of the organism to stress is legitimately of greater interest than the cause of the stress (Pearlin 1982). Sociological attention, by contrast, is more fixed on the stressors and their naturalistic sources.

Stressors, of course, refer to the experiential circumstances that give rise to stress. Although virtually all *social* scientists engaged in stress research are interested in stressors, they differ considerably as to how they conceptualize stressors and as to the importance they attach to different types of stressors. In recent years, attention generally has been divided between *life events*, on the one hand, and more enduring or recurrent life problems, sometimes referred to as *chronic strains*, on the other.

Life Events as Stressors

Life events have occupied by far the most research attention in the past 20 years. Indeed, in some circles life events inappropriately have become a metaphor for stress research. There are at least three reasons for the impressive surge of life events research in the past two decades. First, the pioneering work of Hans Selye (1982) provided an important theoretical foundation for events research. Second, in response to Selye's theoretical inspiration, a method was developed to assess in seemingly simple and objective fashion the magnitude of eventful change experienced by individuals. Third, interest in research into life events was spurred by its early success in showing relationships between the scope of eventful change and various indicators of health. All in all, stress researchers who attempted to identify and measure stressors found a theory to stimulate their work, a method by which to carry it out, and empirical results to reward their efforts.

Since the launching of life events research, however, its theory, its methods, and its findings have been called into question. It is not my purpose here to provide a review of life events research; others (e.g., Dohrenwend and Pearlin 1982; Thoits 1983) have done so. Instead I shall focus on a few of the more salient problems of this research.

With regard to underlying theory, it is now clear that a key assumption about life events as stressors is untenable. Following from the implications of Selye's observations of laboratory animals' responses to environmental changes, the theory held that *all* change is potentially harmful because all change requires readjustment. Sociologists should find this notion difficult to accept because change is a normal and inexorable feature of every level of social life and of aging. At any rate, the weight of current evidence shows that not change per se but the quality of change is potentially damaging to people. Specifically, changes that are undesired, unscheduled, nonnormative, and uncontrolled are most harmful (Fairbank and Hough 1979; Gersten, Langner, Eisenberg, and Simcha-Hogan 1977; Thoits 1981; Vinokur and Seltzer 1975). I believe that researchers no longer accept unquestioningly the assumption that change is categorically bad for people or that the magnitude of change is harmful independent of its quality.

Next, the instruments used to identify life events are misleading in crucial respects. Many events that typically appear on inventories such as the Holmes and Rahe Social Readjustment Rating Scale (1967) are simply markers or surrogate indicators of ongoing conditions; they do not represent free-standing or discrete life change. The loss of a home through foreclosure or a jail sentence, for example, is not an event that erupts unexpectedly. More likely, the event is merely an episodic segment of continuing problems. Because the event inventory allows us to see only the segment and not its history, we ignore the more extended life circumstances of which the event may be a part. Thus questions that presumably are asked about events may in fact elicit information about nonevents. Therefore the tools used to assess eventful change tend to confuse events with more enduring stressors.

This confusion, in turn, brings into question the meaning of past research findings showing relationships between events and health, relationships that have provided much of the empirical support for the interest in life events as stressors. To the extent that events are surrogate indicators of noneventful, ongoing circumstances, empirical relationships between events and health may be explained more accurately by the continuing circumstances in which the event is embedded. Thus in interpreting events-health relationships we are susceptible to exaggerating the importance of eventful change and to minimizing—or overlooking altogether—the problematic continuities of people's lives. The confusion between an event and a more chronic life strain, I submit, impedes a clear understanding of the social etiology of ill health and emotional distress.

In general, the theoretical assumptions, the methods, and the findings that gave life events research its early impetus have each come under critical scrutiny. It is encouraging that current sociological stress research is moving away from some of the early assumptions and confusions regarding events and their stressful impact. It is now common practice to distinguish events by their qualities, such as their desirability or their normative character. Even more promising and innovative is the work of Avison and Turner (1988), which seeks to separate events from the more enduring stressful circumstances in which the event may be embedded.

Earlier I emphasized that as sociologists we are interested in stress as it reveals patterned differences among groups and collectivities differentiated by their social and economic circumstances. Life events research generally has lacked this sociological character, although the reasons seem to lie more in the analytic treatment of events than in the inherent nature of the events. Past research tended to treat events as though they occurred willy-nilly, with no consideration of the social and economic situations of the people who experienced the event. Some events, of course, create havoc in a contextual vacuum, such as when one's house is destroyed by lightning (although even this random event may have nonrandom social and economic consequences). From a sociological perspective, events that are experienced idiosyncratically can be ignored. Often, however, events that in fact are rooted in people's social and economic circumstances are treated as though they are unrelated to these circumstances. To avoid treating these kinds of events as though they are capricious happenings, we must reveal their links to people's relevant social and economic characteristics. Some events under some conditions are powerful stressors that affect people's lives directly and indirectly; research into these stressors should not be abandoned, only rethought. The research needs to establish that events in fact are events and not proxy indicators of chronic hardships. Research also needs to be more selective in the events it studies, focusing particularly on those that illuminate the connections between social forces and individual well-being. This approach requires a sensitivity to events whose occurrence varies with people's key social and economic statuses, such as age and life stage, gender, race and ethnicity, occupational status, and economic class. The presence of relationships between these kinds of master statuses and potentially stressful events would bespeak the social character of eventful stressors.

Chronic Strains as Stressors

The second major type of stressor involves the relatively enduring problems, conflicts, and threats that many people face in their daily lives. The very number and diversity of this type of stressor and the formidable measurement problems that they entail are among the reasons why life event inventories, by comparison, are so inviting a research tool. One way in which sociologists can gain some conceptual control over the extensive array of potential chronic stressors is to focus their attention on problems that arise within the boundaries of major social roles and role sets. As I argued above, problems rooted in institutionalized social roles are often enduring, for the activities and the interpersonal relationships they entail are enduring. Moreover, when problems—or strains, as I refer to them—occur within roles, they are likely to affect their incumbents, because typically we attach considerable importance to our major roles. Difficulties in job, marriage, or parenthood have important effects because the roles themselves are important. Furthermore, the focus on role strains can reinforce the links between the contexts that largely structure people's activities, relationships, and experiences, and their well-being.

Several types of role strain were assessed in our earlier work (Pearlin 1983; Pearlin and Schooler 1978); only a brief review of those types is presented here. One type is *role overload,* a condition that exists when demands on energy and stamina exceed the individual's capacities. Role overload is found most commonly in occupational and homemaker roles as well as in specialized roles, such as among informal caregivers to seriously impaired relatives. *Interpersonal conflicts within role sets* are the type of chronic strain reported most often. This type of strain assumes many forms, but they all entail problems and difficulties that arise among those who interact with each other in sets of complementary roles, such as wife-husband, parent-child, or worker-supervisor. Still another type of strain, *inter-role conflict,* is found at the juncture of different roles. It entails the incompatible demands of multiple roles, especially demands of work and family. Commonly individuals cannot satisfy the demands and expectations of one of these roles without forsaking those of the other. A different strain involves *role captivity*, which exists when one is an unwilling incumbent of a role. People experiencing this type of strain include housewives or retirees who would prefer outside employment or employed workers who would prefer to be at home with young children. The roles that these people occupy might not be onerous or filled with conflict; the people simply prefer to be and to do things outside the confines of the unwanted role.

Finally, *role restructuring* is an important but overlooked type of strain that certainly deserves more attention. It is virtually inevitable that relationships in role sets undergo change. Although the actors and the role sets remain the same, either the aging process or extraneous exigencies force alterations in long-established patterns of expectation and interaction. This phenomenon can be observed in a variety of situations, such as the rebellious adolescent who complains that he is treated as a baby, the apprentice who grows restless with his mentor as he masters his craft, or adult children who must assume increasing responsibility for the care of aged parents. Often the restructuring of entrenched relationships is not easy; it can result in a sense of betrayal, status loss, and the violation of expectations. These kinds of strains may develop insidiously and may persist until people readjust to the new expectations and norms governing the relationships.

Not all severe strains are found within major roles. Living in or close to poverty, residing in neighborhoods where there is reason to fear crime or violence, and having a serious chronic illness are among the *ambient strains* that cut across roles and envelop people. Still other strains may arise in more informal and elective roles, such as in voluntary activities and associations or in dealing with friends and acquaintances. Thus the strains that people experience in their institutionalized roles by no means represent all chronic stressors.

Two methodological problems underlie the identification of chronic strains. One problem is that the chronicity of these strains is often inferred rather than established empirically. In my own work I have treated certain problems as chronic simply because they exist within a continuing relationship and are not of a sort that is likely to vary appreciably within a relatively short time. The absence of marital reciprocity is a case in point (e.g., Pearlin, 1975b). This problem is reflected in situations where one member of the marital pair feels that the other is not contributing equally to the relationship. Ideally, the chronicity of this kind of strain should be evaluated on the basis of information about the length of time for which the problem has been experienced. Yet because problems of this type can have insidious onsets, it may be difficult, if not impossible, to determine duration with reasonable confidence.

The second methodological difficulty concerns the possibility that measures of role strains are confounded with outcomes. That is, answers to questions about role strains and answers to questions about outcomes, such as depression, may be guided by the same underlying state of disaffection. Thus we must confront the nagging possibility that the robust correlations between measures of strain and measures of psychological distress reflect a lack of independence between the indicators of these constructs. There is no quick fix to this difficulty; obviously one must exercise care in wording the questions about strain so that they contain no language of distress, but to a large extent the independence of the measures must be established analytically. This can be done first by identifying people who are equivalent with regard to strain but who differ in the level of distress they express, and then by determining whether these differences can be explained systematically. For example, we might find that differences in the amount of distress experienced among people who report the same strains may be explained by variations in coping and social support. When uniform levels of strain joined to varying levels of distress can be explained in a theoretically meaningful way, the explanation bolsters our confidence in the independence of our measures of strain and of distress and in the significance of the relationships between them.

The Convergence of Events and Chronic Strains

Even if it were possible to overcome the difficulties in measuring and assessing both life events and chronic strains, our research still would be encumbered by conceptual blinders. A serious limitation of inquiry into stressors is the tendency toward "either-or" thinking. In searching for stressors, we usually focus either on life events or on chronic strains. As a result of this unwitting tendency we have missed opportunities to observe the ways in which events and strains converge in people's lives. There are at least three ways in which events and strains come together in stressful experience: 1) events lead to chronic strains; 2) chronic strains lead to events; and 3) strains and events provide meaning contexts for each other.

Consider first the capability of events to cause strains. Studies of events typically examine the events as direct causes of stress in individuals. Yet events also cause stress in an indirect manner by altering adversely the more enveloping and enduring life conditions. These conditions, in turn, become potent sources of stress in their own right—perhaps more potent than the precipitating event. This process, in which events adversely restructure social and economic conditions of life, has been demonstrated empirically for at least three events: involuntary job loss (Pearlin, Lieberman, Menagham, and Mullan 1981), divorce (Pearlin and Johnson 1977), and death of spouse (Pearlin and Lieberman 1978). These events commonly result in such circumstances as increased economic hardship, heightened interpersonal conflict, or greater social isolation. These kinds of circumstances, in turn, may be stronger antecedents of stress than the events that helped to create the circumstances.

Just as stressful chronic problems may be created by events, stressful events can be triggered by persisting problems. As I argued earlier, research into events usually does not separate the events from the strains that might have preceded them. Consequently there has been little study examining how enduring strains give rise to events. Some scattered evidence, however, suggests that this situation occurs. We know, for example, that continued marital conflict can result in separation and divorce (Menaghan 1982). Indeed, it is reasonable to speculate that in general, prolonged interpersonal conflict can precipitate events which mark the disruption of or withdrawal from the troubled relationships.

In the third way in which events and strains converge in stressful experience, each provides the meaning context for the other. Thus the nature of relevant conditions preceding the event may influence whether or not an event is experienced as stressful. It would be a mistake, for example, to assume that divorce is uniformly stressful without considering whether the couple's prior marital life was characterized solely by strife and frustration or whether it also contained fulfillment and satisfaction. Indeed, Wheaton (1988) shows that the intensity of the strains experienced in roles tends to govern the levels of stress that follow transitions out of the roles. Depending on prior circumstances, the same transitional events might be experienced either as liberating or as depriving. Moreover, just as *preceding* conditions color the meaning and the impact of the event, *consequent* conditions also may regulate the impact of the event. Retirement, for example, might have a negative effect on well-being if the retirement results in a loss of status or the atrophying of prized skills; it might have a positive effect if one finds in retirement the opportunity to pursue self-fulfilling passions that previously had been held in abeyance.

Events, then, typically do not stand as stressors separate from the durable stains that people experience, nor do the strains necessarily persist apart from the events they may precipitate. Events and strains often flow together in people's experiences, although researchers might see them as separate and unrelated. Events can create stressful strains; strains can precipitate stressful events; and events and strains each constitute the contexts that shape the meanings and the stressful effects of the other. Merely correlating events or strains with health outcomes fails to capture an accurate picture of an antecedent process that often involves a dynamic connection between events and relatively durable strains.

Primary and Secondary Stressors

Underlying the above discussion is the assumption that significant stressors rarely, if ever, occur singly. If people are exposed to one serious stressor, it is very likely that they will be exposed to others as well. One event leads to another event or triggers chronic strains; strains, for their part, beget other strains or events. Thus clusters of stressors may develop, each cluster made up of a variety of events and strains. Furthermore, the clustered stressors may be formed by problems that originated in different institutionalized roles (Wheaton in press): job loss may engender economic strains, occupational strains may create marital strains, and so on. It is reasonable that stressors should proliferate and diffuse within and across institutional lines, because the multiple sectors of people's lives are interrelated such that disruptions in one sector are likely to cause disruptions in others. Moreover, the stressors experienced by one individual often become problems for others who share the same role sets. Thus a married person who is in a difficult work situation probably has a spouse who is under stress as a consequence (Pearlin and McCall in press).

For the sociological stress researcher, the multiplication and the contagion of stressors means that studies must cast a wide net to capture the full array of stressors that are present in an individual's life. If we fail to discern all the appreciable stressors that are contemporaneous, we also will fail to interpret correctly the outcomes that we observe. Suppose, for example, we wished to study the relationship between serious physical injury and depression. Our inquiry would be incomplete, if not misleading, if we assumed that the injury was the only stressor present; in such a case we would ignore possible concomitant economic, occupational, family, and social problems. Variations in depression thus reflect not only the seriousness of the injury itself but also variations in the clustering of stressors. It is not an event or a strain that merits the sociologist's attention, but how the *organization of people's lives* may be disrupted in the stress process.

One step toward bringing this organization into view is to distinguish *primary* and *secondary* stressors. Primary stressors are those which are likely to occur first in people's experience. The stressor may be an event, especially one that is undesired and eruptive, such as the untimely death of a loved one, involuntary job loss, or injury; or it could be a more enduring or repeated stressor, such as those experienced in marriage or occupation. Whereas primary stressors can be conceptualized as occurring first in experience, secondary stressors come about as a consequence of the primary stressors. I do not refer to them as secondary because they are less potent than the primary stressors. On the contrary, once established, secondary stressors independently may become capable of producing even more intense stress than those we consider to be primary. They are secondary only on the basis of their presumed order in the stress process, not on the basis of their importance to the process.

Examples of secondary stressors resulting from more primary stressors may be drawn from our current studies of specialized caregiving roles, those involving the care of impaired relatives or friends (Pearlin, Semple, and Turner 1988; Pearlin, Turner, and Semple 1989). Informal caregiving to impaired people is an extreme instance of role restructuring: usually it occurs within established relationships, and when impairment is severe, prolonged, and progressive, the caregiving comes to dominate the interactions between actors whose previous relationships were organized in a very different way. A number of primary stressors, those involved directly in providing care to the impaired person, can be observed. They include the vigilance that may be required to monitor and control the patient, the psychological losses that accumulate with the patient's continued deterioration, and exhaustion and overload. Several secondary stressors stem from these primary problems. For example, increased conflict with others is quite common, as when the caregiver feels abandoned by family members. Caregivers holding outside jobs may find themselves unable to devote themselves fully to one activity without neglecting the requirements of the other. Economic strain arising from diminished income or increased expenditure is another frequently observed secondary stressor, as are the losses of desired social relationships and activities outside the caregiving situation. Once set in motion, these secondary stressors produce their own stressful outcomes.

These examples are intended to illuminate pivotal point: important life problems, whether in the form of events or of durable strains, do not exist in isolation from other problems. The very integration of individuals' activities and relationships means that disruptions in one area of their lives serve to create other disruptions. Therefore sociological stress researchers cannot confine their attention to a single event or to groups of events, nor can they examine only one role strain on the assumption that it is the only problem or the most important problem faced by the individual. Instead, the presence and the organization of constellations of stressors need to be discerned and measured independently. The discernment of this organization, in turn, may be enhanced by distinguishing primary and secondary stressors. This distinction will help to discriminate between people who may be similar with regard to their exposure to one stressor but who differ appreciably with regard to the array of stressors to which they are exposed. Such discrimination can go far in explaining why people who seem to be alike with regard to the problems that they face differ sharply with regard to the intensity and range of the stress outcomes that they manifest. People who are treated analytically as similar may, in fact, be different.

I would like to raise a final issue with regard to the identification and specification of stressors; this issue concerns values. As I have emphasized, a central task of research into stress is to explain why individuals exposed to stressor conditions that appear to be similar do not necessarily suffer the same outcomes. Part of this explanation lies in social values. By values I refer to what is defined socially as good, desirable, and prized or as something to be eschewed (Williams 1960, pp. 397–470). Although the importance of values to stress research has been recognized (Lazarus and Folkman 1984, pp. 77–81), their part in the stress process has not yet been examined systematically. Values, I believe, regulate the effects of experience by regulating the meaning and the importance of the experience (Pearlin 1988).

To understand the role of values in regulating the impact of stressors, one must understand that conditions are stressful when they are threatening. I use "threat" in the broadest sense to include reactions to such disparate constructs as loss, unfulfilled needs, violation of self-image, and blocked aspirations. Some conditions may be intrinsically threatening, as when one's life is at stake. More often, however, the threat that people experience from the circumstances they face depends to some degree on the values they hold—that is, on what they define as important, desirable, or to be cherished. An example can be provided from a study that showed that marital partners from unequal status backgrounds also tended to have higher levels of marital stress (Pearlin 1975b). Further analytic probing revealed that these inequalities were related to stress primarily among people who held certain status values. Specifically, hypogamous people—those who "married down"—were particularly vulnerable to marital stress, but only when they valued status enhancement and upward mobility. Others who also had married down but who were not status strivers were unaffected by their hypogamous marriage. Thus the cause of stress was neither a structural arrangement alone nor a value alone but a particular combination of the two.

Although other illustrations also could be mobilized, at this time we possess only scant evidence that certain values, when combined with certain social conditions, are especially productive of stress. We do not yet know, however, how to look systematically for these combinations. We can only assume that the kinds of values which will produce stressful effects must have relevance to the social conditions under study. At this stage of our work, however, sociological researchers must rely on their intuition to identify the stressful mix of circumstances and values, for there is no established theoretical guide to identification. At least this much is known: the relationships of social stressors to individual stress may be seen most clearly when we take into account social values that help to shape the meaning of the stressors. This line of inquiry is worth following by sociologists.

The careful study of stressors, then, should provide the researcher with an opportunity to learn something about social life as it bears on individual functioning. The sociological study of stressors can reveal the connections between social organization and the organization of lives. To find these connections, however, we cannot treat stress as stemming from unconnected happenings. Instead the antecedents of stress need to be understood in terms of process, whereby broad structured and institutional forces, constellations of primary and secondary stressors, and widely shared values converge over time to affect people's well-being. Most certainly, the sociological study of social stress does not rely on predictive models. We must guide our effort not simply by identifying and adding together all factors that might contribute to the variance of an outcome but also by asking how and why these contributions come about. Prediction alone does not make us wiser sociologists; for that purpose we need also to be good explainers and interpreters.

THE MEDIATORS AND THEIR INTERVENTIONS

I have already suggested two explanations for the fact that the same stressors do not necessarily lead to the same stressful outcomes: different configurations of unobserved stressors may surround the observed stressor, or different values may endow the same stressor with different meanings. Yet by far the largest responsibility for explaining outcome differences has been placed on constructs that I refer to collectively as mediators. They are mediators in the sense that they have been shown to govern (or mediate) the effects of stressors on stress outcomes. Coping and social support have received the most attention in the research literature; for this reason I shall confine my attention to these mediators. Other constructs, however, also have been cast analytically as mediators; in particular these include the self-concepts of self-esteem and mastery (Pearlin and Schooler 1978). These aspects of self represent personal resources and appear to serve as appreciable barriers to the stressful effects of difficult life conditions. In addition, personality constructs such as Type A, hardiness, and invulnerability are treated implicitly as mediators. Although such constructs possibly are useful in explaining differences among individuals in the effects of stressors, their utility in explaining differences among socially and economically demarcated groups has not yet been demonstrated. For this reason they have not attracted the attention of sociologists to the same extent as other types of mediators.

Although coping and social support certainly intersect, they are quite distinct; each has its own conceptual problems. Briefly and selectively I shall point out some of these problems. Then I shall consider strategies for evaluating mediating effects within the stress process.

Coping

Coping refers to the actions that people take in their own behalf as they attempt to avoid or lessen the impact of life problems (Pearlin and Schooler 1978). Although coping refers to individuals' actions and perceptions, it is of sociological interest because important elements of coping may be learned from one's membership and reference groups in the same ways as other behaviors are learned and internalized. Because interest in coping was rooted initially in clinical concerns, researchers tend to think of a person's coping repertoire as representing a clinical profile unique to the individual and to ignore the shared, normative basis of individual coping. Although aspects of one's coping indeed may be unique, it is likely that people who interact with each other and who share important life circumstances will also share coping behaviors. Consequently part of the sociologists' research agenda should be aimed at identifying the associations between people's social and economic circumstances and their coping repertoires.

Is coping a set of general dispositions activated when one is faced with threatening problems, or does it consist of more specific responses invoked selectively in dealing with specific kinds of problems? From a personality perspective, coping may be seen as a tendency to react in characteristic ways to threat, regardless of the nature of the threat or the context in which it arises. It is distinctly possible that there are general coping dispositions which cut across different situations. Perhaps, for example, people who engage in denial in one situation will do the same in a very different situation. Yet the sociologist finds it difficult to accept the notion that people cope with retirement from the job, for example, in the same way as with being fired from the job, or with conflict with one's boss in the same way as with conflict with one's child. There is simply no reason to assume that coping will be the same regardless of the nature of the impinging stressors, the institutional contexts in which they occur, or the relationships they might involve. Individuals have personalities that retain their integrity from one situation to another. Yet the coping responses that mediate the stressful impact of one situation may be entirely inappropriate to another. Therefore the researcher who is sensitive to the social and contextual origins of stressors also must be sensitive to the situation-specific character of coping.

Even so, the *functions* of coping are essentially the same in all situations, although the *forms* of coping might vary from one situation to another. As we described in detail elsewhere (Pearlin and Schooler 1978), all coping—regardless of the nature of the stressors—serves either to *change the situation* from which the stressors arise, to *manage the meaning* of the situation in a manner that reduces its threat, or to *keep the symptoms of stress within manageable bounds*. Therefore we possess a conceptual framework for the study of coping that has general application, even though the behavioral elements of coping are more specific to the particular stressor that is being experienced and vary with that stressor (Pearlin and Aneshensel 1986).

Social Support

It would appear that among the major

mediating constructs, social support should have the clearest and best established theoretical links to social theory. Somewhat surprisingly, however, this is not the case. Perhaps one reason is that sociologists who are interested in social networks tend not to be the same as those working in stress and social support. Networks refer more directly than supports to the structure of people's social attachments. These attachments, of course, differ in extensiveness and composition for different groups in the society. As Lin and his colleagues describe (Lin, Dean, and Ensel 1986, pp. 17–30, 53–70), most people's attachments include some mix of formal and informal, primary and secondary, and strong and weak ties; some attachments exist with friends and others with relatives; some involve frequent face-to-face interaction and others do not. The organization of one's social network mirrors the organization of one's engagement with the larger society.

Whereas the social network can be regarded as the totality of the social resources on which one potentially may draw, social support represents the resources that one actually uses in dealing with life problems (Pearlin 1985). In most instances, of course, one's sources of support in dealing with any given stressor will be much more restricted than one's total network. Consequently stress researchers tend to ignore network and its structure and to deal only with support as it is perceived by the individual. Certainly there is nothing wrong with data that bear on perceived support; studies indicate that perceived support indeed has a mediating function in the stress process (Turner 1983). Yet, when the study of perceived support is separated from the study of networks, we are unable to see how individuals' support is associated with their integration into various social institutions and contexts. The identification of the connections between individuals' social life and their inner well-being could be enhanced, I submit, by joining the study of social support more closely to the study of social networks.

Aside from its separation from network, the study of support lacks sociological substance for still another reason: typically it considers only the recipient of support and ignores the donors of support and their interactions with the recipient (Pearlin 1985; Pearlin and McCall in press). A construct that is inherently interactional is treated instead as an individual attribute. When the social and interactional nature of social support is ignored, we are left with an incomplete, if not distorted, picture of how it functions. The forms of support, its reciprocity, the connections between seeking and receiving support, its stability, and even whether or not it is welcomed depend not on the recipient alone but on the donor-recipient relationship.

Supporting relationships are found in virtually all institutional and social contexts: religion, occupation, family, neighborhood, voluntary associations, the medical care system, and elsewhere. Just as the forms and functions of support may vary with the nature of the relationship from which support is drawn, there is some evidence (House 1981b, 59–85) that the effect of support is constrained or enhanced by the context in which the relationships exist. Thus we need to learn more both about the interactional aspects of support and about the effects of social contexts on its forms, functions, and efficacy. Sociologists should be foremost among the contributors to this research.

How Do Mediators Mediate?

The very words "coping" and "social support" contain implicit consequences. Once a behavior is labeled as coping, we assume that it succeeds in relieving stress; if someone is labeled as the recipient of support, he is perforce supported. These assumed beneficial consequences, inherent in the very language we use to refer to stress mediators, inadvertently may have diverted us from asking whether in fact the mediators do mediate, and, if so, how. At any rate, insufficient effort has been devoted to evaluating the efficacy of the mediators, especially in the case of coping.

In raising this issue here, I am concerned less with the methodology of determining how much difference the mediators make than with where to look for these differences. In this regard it is useful to recall that stressful situations may contain constellations of primary and secondary stressors. Moreover, each type of stressor may contain multiple subtypes of stressors. This conceptualization of the stress process suggests ways to search for the effects of coping and social support that currently are not recognized. Specifically, we should expand our assessments of efficacy to include the ability of the mediators to inhibit the scope and severity both of the primary stressors and of the secondary stressors that follow. To whatever extent the mediators succeed in constraining the intensity, number, and diffusion of stressors, they also must succeed eventually in constraining the extent and intensity of stress outcomes. These *indirect* effects of the mediators may be every bit as instrumental in minimizing stress outcomes as the *direct* effects to which attention usually is limited.

The evaluation of indirect effects of mediators should help further to illuminate the question that now has been raised at several points of this paper: What accounts for variations in the outcomes of stressful life conditions? Our understanding of the variability of stress outcomes will be enhanced by observing how coping and social support affect each step of the process that precedes the outcomes. If we confine our assessment of the mediators solely to their direct effects on outcomes, we will not be able to detect their important indirect effects, those which are exercised through their regulation of antecedent conditions.

OUTCOMES

Outcomes refer to the manifestations of organismic stress. Many manifestations exist, and they are found at multiple levels of organismic functioning. Indeed, the multiplicity of stress indicators has led some researchers to question whether the very notion of stress is useful (Elliott and Eisdorfer 1982). A construct that subsumes such diverse (although presumably related) phenomena as the immunological and endocrine systems, the digestive and cardiovascular systems, anxiety, depression, and mental health—to name just a few—is bound to create confusion. The confusion is compounded understandably by the fact that several disciplines have developed their own distinctive approaches to the study of stress and its indicators. Yet despite its ambiguity, the notion of stress provides a framework sufficiently flexible to encompass the broad and diverse range of constructs found in sociological studies of stress and health. Thus for sociologists, an attractive feature of the stress concept is its ability to absorb the far-reaching notion of inseparability between the circumstances of social life and individual functioning.

In looking for indicators of individual stress that are sensitive to social circumstances, one is drawn inevitably to phenomena that traditionally have been the domain of biology and medicine. Thus sociologists must attain some usable knowledge of the research concerns that lie outside their own discipline. Although this knowledge is both necessary and desirable, preoccupation with the medical and biological markers of outcomes can come at the expense of attention to the social antecedents of the outcomes. Indeed, there are institutional pressures toward such preoccupation. Because these pressures arise out of prevailing economic and institutional conditions, I discuss them largely from a perspective of the sociology of knowledge.

In selecting the outcomes they will study, sociologists and others may be influenced subtly by the sources of funding for stress research. Most agencies that fund research in this area are organized around diseases—heart, cancer, mental, and so on—and the experts enlisted by these agencies to judge the merits of proposed research are typically oriented to biomedical models. Understandably these models place less importance on the social origins of stress than on the organismic manifestations. Thus in evaluating the merits of proposed research, the agencies may give more weight to the theoretical and methodological command of the biomedical outcomes than to that of the antecedent processes. In attempting to satisfy evaluative criteria, the sociologist may be drawn unwittingly into clinical, diagnostic, and epidemiological issues beyond the depth necessary to identify the social circumstances that affect well-being. I do not argue that limits should be placed on sociologists' expertise with regard to stress outcomes, but I do believe that this expertise should serve primarily to illuminate the organization of social life, the structure of experience, and the effects of these phenomena on individual health and functioning. Sociologists properly may be health researchers, but they also must be social researchers.

As Mirowsky and Ross (1989) have cogently discussed, sociological stress researchers who are interested primarily in mental health outcomes are currently encountering a special set of institutional constraints on the selection of outcome criteria. In psychiatry, attention is focused increasingly on pathologies likely to have a powerful genetic etiology, such as schizophrenia and bipolar depression. The study of these disorders fits comfortably within the medical model, its orientations to disease, and the identification of cases needing treatment. By contrast, the social scientist is more likely to be interested in dysfunctions that have a powerful social and experiential etiology, such as anxiety and subclinical depressive disorders. Moreover, these different orientations to outcomes require different tools. The medical researchers and the psychiatric epidemiologist need elaborate diagnostic instruments that can yield an accurate count of the prevalence and incidence of various disorders and that can identify cases in need of treatment. The social scientist, by contrast, needs symptom scales to rank people according to the intensity of their distress. Whereas the medical researcher and the epidemiologist are concerned with diagnostic tools that will help reliably in case identification, the sociologist is concerned with measures of distress that are reliably sensitive to antecedent processes.

These differences are reasonable and legitimate, and they should be maintained. Sociologists should avoid immersion in the medical and epidemiological models that emphasize diagnosis and case finding. Such immersion not only fails to serve the goals of social research; it may even hinder the achievement of those goals by diverting time and resources to issues that are extraneous to social inquiry.

What outcomes should be considered in sociological research into stress? Understandably, the answer to this query is based on the kinds of data to which sociologists have ready access as well as on their theoretical perspectives. For example, sociologists typically do not look at endocrine secretions or at the immunological system because they possess neither the skills nor the facilities to do so without the costly collaboration of others. Instead we usually examine outcomes that can be assessed through direct observation, medical records, or self-evaluations and reports. Examples of stress indicators found in sociological studies include health histories, symptoms of physical health, symptom scales measuring a variety of dimensions of mental health, the abuse of alcohol or of mind-altering drugs, inability to fulfill role obligations, and the disruption of social relationships. None of these outcomes has a compelling theoretical priority over the others, but there may be a theoretically compelling reason to avoid reliance on a single outcome in assessing the stressfulness of social conditions.

The observation of multiple outcomes is highly desirable because people having different social and economic characteristics also may have different modes of manifesting stress. As a result, we run the risk of seriously misjudging the effects of difficult life circumstances if we judge effect only on the basis of a single outcome. Gender differences again provide a telling illustration. It has been shown repeatedly that women more than men are host to depressive symptoms and emotional distress. In turn, this finding has led to speculation that women may be more vulnerable than men to certain stressful circumstances, such as network losses (e.g., Kessler and McLeod 1984). Yet before we can accept the assumption of vulnerability, we must be sure that we have considered a full range of relevant outcomes. Perhaps men and women do not differ in their overall vulnerability to stressors, but differ instead with regard to the particular outcomes to which they are vulnerable. This warning emerges from the work of Aneshensel (1988), who showed that apparent gender differences in vulnerability to the impact of events disappear when excessive drinking and other outcomes are considered along with depression. That is, the stressful events are no less harmful for men than for women, a fact that was obscured when only depression was examined. We must keep in mind that structurally demarcated groups may manifest stress in different ways. Unless multiple outcomes are considered, we can mistakenly exaggerate the vulnerability of some groups while underestimating at the same time the general impact of the stressors under examination.

SUMMARY AND DISCUSSION

In this paper I have not sought to lay out steps to be followed; rather, I have attempted to raise issues to be considered in the sociological study of stress. The overarching strategy of social research into stress is the identification of the many links that join forms of social organization to individual stress. I have suggested a number of conceptual and analytic perspectives that I believe will enable us to advance this agenda. One crucial element is the examination of statuses and other background circumstances at each step of the stress process. We need to know how these social factors bear on the kinds of stressors to which people are exposed, the personal and social resources to which people have access, and the emotional, behavioral, and physical disorders through which stress is manifested. This proposal contains nothing new; it deserves emphasis only because researchers tend either to limit the analyses of social background factors or to relegate them to serving as controls through which the independent effects of other conditions are established. Yet the sociological stake in stress research requires the careful and comprehensive analysis of information about the structural contexts of people's lives.

Many important life experiences, some of them stressful, are rooted in these contexts. Stressful experiences may take on different forms and configurations and it is unlikely that they can be fully captured by examining either life events or life strains separately and apart from each other. Over time, stressors typically surface as groups or constellations of stressors, some primary and others secondary, that blend events with more durable strains. This is a useful way to look at the antecedent process, and is consistent with available empirical evidence. It seeks stressors in the organization of lives and in the structure of experience rather than among unrelated "risk factors."

One of the analytic tasks of the stress researcher is to explain variations in stress outcomes. First, some of the variation in outcomes is to be found in the constellations of stressors. When we observe events and strains singly while ignoring broader clusters of primary and secondary stressors, we may incorrectly assume more similarity in exposure to stressful experience than actually exists. In other words, part of the unexplained variations in outcomes may be due to relevant stressors that are not being observed and whose effects therefore cannot be assessed.

Second, even though we have probably relied too heavily on the explanatory power of coping and support, nevertheless we may systematically have underestimated their mediating effects. We cannot appreciate the full capacity of these mediators until we examine their effects in limiting the number and severity of primary and secondary stressors. These are the indirect effects which soften stress outcomes but which are not in view when we concern ourselves only with the direct effects of the mediators on outcomes.

Finally, some of the difficulty encountered in analytically explaining variations in outcomes lies with the range of outcomes selected for study. Focusing exclusively on a single outcome, such as depression, may lead to the mistaken conclusion that some groups of people are affected adversely by stressors that leave others unaffected. These putative variations in vulnerability, however, may be an artifact of the ways in which different social and economic groups channel and manifest stress. Consequently the inclusion of a reasonable range of outcomes should prevent us from making inappropriate assumptions of differential vulnerability to common stressors.

However one thinks of the stress process, it obviously consists of multiple conceptual components; each component potentially has multiple aspects or dimensions. The richness and the complexity of the process invite us to phrase research questions in very different ways. One study, for example, may be concerned mainly with the epidemiological distribution of depression; another may have as its central question the buffering effects of social support on depression; a third might seek to evaluate the effects of a particular event or role strain on depression. Each question places a somewhat different set of issues at the center of its interests. Although the questions may generate overlapping data, the data essentially serve different research goals.

When studies start with questions about the parts played across the stress process by the social and economic arrangements in which people's lives are embedded, they produce knowledge that has a distinctive emphasis. Although studies of this type share with other approaches an interest in individuals' well-being, they also help to illuminate those aspects of social organization which pertain particularly to the differential exposure to and meaning of stressors, to differences in the various kinds of resources that people can mobilize in responding to stressful circumstances, and, finally, to differences in the manifestation of stress. The sociological study of stress, I believe, can contribute uniquely both to an understanding of social life and to an understanding of how the fates of individuals come to be bound to it.

In emphasizing some of the conceptual ingredients and analytic strategies of a sociology of stress, I do not wish to wave a banner of disciplinary parochialism. Yet it is of considerable importance to study social structures and their effects on individual well-being. If sociologists don't do this and do it well, who will?

REFERENCES

Aneshensel, Carol S. 1988. "Disjunctures between Public Health and Medical Models." Paper presented at the meetings of the American Public Health Association, Boston.

Avison, William R. and R. Jay Turner. 1988. "Stressful Life Events and Depressive Symptoms: Disaggregating the Effects of Acute Stressors and Chronic Strains." *Journal of Health and Social Behavior* 29:253–64.

Dohrenwend, Bruce and Leonard I. Pearlin. 1982. "Report on Stress and Life Events." *Stress and Human Health*, edited by G. Elliott and C. Eisdorfer. New York: Springer.

Elliott, Glenn R. and Carl Eisdorfer. 1982. "Conceptual Issues in Stress Research." Pp. 11–45 in *Stress and Human Health*, edited by G.R. Elliott and C. Eisdorfer. New York: Springer.

Fairbank, Dianne T. and Richard L. Hough. 1979. "Life Events Classification and the Event-Illness Relationship." *Journal of Health and Social Behavior* 19:41–47.

Gersten, Joanne C., Thomas S. Langner, Jeanne G. Eisenberg, and Ora Simcha-Hogan. 1977. "An Evaluation of the Etiologic Role of Stressful Life-Change Events in Psychological Disorders." *Journal of Health and Social Behavior* 18:228–44.

Gore, Susan L. and Thomas W. Mangione. 1983. "Social Roles, Sex Roles, and Psychological Distress: Additive and Interactive Models of Sex Differences." *Journal of Health and Social Behavior* 24:300–12.

Gurin, Gerald, Joseph Veroff, and Sheila Feld. 1960. *Americans View Their Mental Health*. New York: Basic Books.

Hollingshead, August B. and Fredrick C. Redlich. 1958. *Social Class and Mental Illness: A Community Study*. New York: Wiley.

Holmes, Thomas H. and Richard H. Rahe. 1967. "The Social Readjustment Rating Scale." *Journal of Psychosomatic Research* 11:213–18.

House, James S. 1981a. "Social Structure and Personality." Pp. 525–61 in *Social Psychology*, edited by M. Rosenberg and R.H. Turner. New York: Basic Books.

———. 1981b. *Work Stress and Social Support*. Reading, MA: Addision-Wesley.

Kahn, Robert L. 1973. "Conflict, Ambiguity, and Overload: Three Elements in Job Stress." *Occupational Mental Health* 3:2–9.

Kessler, Ronald C. and Jane D. McLeod. 1984. "Sex Differences in Vulnerability to Undesirable Life Events." *American Sociological Review* 49:620–31.

Kessler, Ronald C. and James A. McRae. 1981. "Trends in Sex and Psychological Distress." *American Sociological Review* 46:443–52.

Lazarus, Richard S. and Susan Folkman. 1984. *Stress, Appraisal and Coping*. New York: Springer.

Lin, Nan, Alfred Dean, and Walter Ensel. 1986. *Social Support, Life Events, and Depression*. Orlando, FL: Orlando Academic Press.

Menaghan, Elizabeth G. 1982. "Assessing the Impact of Family Transition on Marital Experience." Pp. 90–108 in *Family Stress, Coping and Social Support*, edited by H.I. McCubbin, A.E. Cauble, and J.M. Patterson. Springfield, IL: Thomas.

Mirowsky, John and Catherine E. Ross, 1989. "Psychiatric Diagnosis as Reified Measurement." *Journal of Health and Social Behavior* 30:11–25.

Pearlin, Leonard I. 1975a. "Sex Roles and Depression." Pp. 191–207 in *Life-Span Developmental Psychology: Normative Life Crises*, edited by N. Dalton and L. Ginsberg. New York: Academic Press.

———. 1975b. "Status Inequality and Stress in Marriage." *American Sociological Review* 40: 344–57.

———. 1982. "The Social Contexts of Stress." Pp. 367–79 in *Handbook of Stress*, edited by L. Goldberger and S. Breznitz. New York: Free Press.

———. 1983. "Role Strains and Personal Stress." Pp. 3–32 in *Psychosocial Stress: Trends in Theory and Research*, edited by Howard B. Kaplan. New York: Academic Press.

———. 1985. "Social Process and Social Supports." Pp. 43–60 in *Social Support and Health*, edited by Sheldon Cohen and Leonard Syme. New York: Academic Press.

———. 1988. "Social Structure and Social Values; The Regulation of Structural Effects." Pp. 252–64 in *Surveying Social Life*, edited by Hubert O'Gorman. Middletown, CT: Wesleyan University Press.

Pearlin, Leonard I. and Carol Aneshensel. 1986. "Coping and Social Supports: Their Functions and Applications." Pp. 53–74, *Applications of Social Science to Clinical Medicine and Health*, edited by L.H. Aiken and D. Mechanic. New Brunswick, NJ: Rutgers University Press.

Pearlin, Leonard I. and Joyce S. Johnson. 1977.

"Marital Status, Life Strains and Depression." *American Sociological Review* 42:704–15.

Pearlin, Leonard I. and Morton A. Lieberman. 1978. "Social Sources of Emotional Distress." Pp. 217–48 in *Research in Community and Mental Health*. Vol. 1, edited by R. Simmons. Greenwich, CT: JAI.

Pearlin, Leonard I. and Mary McCall. In press. "Occupational Problems and Marital Support." In *The Transmission of Stress Between Work and Family*, edited by J. Eckenrode and S. Gore. New York: Plenum.

Pearlin, Leonard I. and Carmi Schooler. 1978. "The Structure of Coping." *Journal of Health and Social Behavior* 19:2–21.

Pearlin, Leonard I., Shirley Semple, and Heather Turner. 1988. "Stress of Aids Caregiving." *Death Studies* 12:501–17.

Pearlin, Leonard I., Heather Turner, and Shirley Semple. 1989. "Coping and the Mediation of Caregiver Stress." In *Alzheimer's Disease Treatment and Family Stress: Directions for Research*, edited by E. Light and B. Liebowitz. Washington, DC: National Institute of Mental Health.

Pearlin, Leonard I., Morton Lieberman, Elizabeth Menaghan, and Joseph Mullan. 1981. "The Stress Process." *Journal of Health and Social Behavior* 22:337–56.

Rosenberg, Morris. 1968. *The Logic of Survey Analysis*. New York: Basic Books.

Selye, Hans. 1982. "History and Present Status of the Stress Concept." Pp. 7–17 in *Handbook of Stress*, edited by L. Goldberger and S. Breznitz. New York: Free Press.

Srole, Leo, Thomas S. Langner, Morris K. Opler, and T.A.C. Rennie. 1960. *Mental Health in the Metropolis: The Midtown Study*. New York: McGraw-Hill.

Thoits, Peggy A. 1981. "Undesirable Life Events and Psychophysiological Distress: A Problem of Operational Confounding." *American Sociological Review* 46:97–109.

______. 1983. "Dimensions of Life Events That Influence Psychological Distress: An Evaluation and Synthesis of the Literature." Pp. 33–103 in *Psychosocial Stress*, edited by H.B. Kaplan. New York: Academic Press.

______. 1986. "Multiple Identities: Examining Sexual and Marital Status Differences in Distress." *American Sociological Review* 51: 259–72.

Turner, R. Jay. 1983. "Direct, Indirect and Moderating Effects of Social Support on Psychological Distress and Associated Conditions." Pp. 105–55 in *Psychosocial Stress*, edited by H.B. Kaplan. New York: Academic Press.

Vinokur, Amiram and Melvin L. Seltzer. 1975. "Desirable versus Undesirable Life Events: Their Relationship to Stress and Mental Distress." *Journal of Personality and Social Psychology* 32:329–37.

Wheaton, Blair. 1988. "Life Transitions, Prior Role Problems and Mental Health: Where More Stress Is Stress Relief." Paper presented at meetings of the American Sociological Association, Atlanta.

______. In press. "Where Work and Family Meet: Stress across Social Roles." In *The Transmission of Stress between Work and Family*, edited by J. Eckenrode and S. Gore. Plenum.

Williams, Robin. 1960. *American Society*. New York: Knopf.

***LEONARD I. PEARLIN** is Professor of Medical Sociology, Department of Psychiatry, at the University of California at San Francisco. He has a long-standing interest in social structure and individual functioning.*

[15]

Soc. Sci. Med. Vol. 31, No. 10, pp. 1127–1134, 1990
Printed in Great Britain.
0277-9536/90 $3.00 + 0.00

LOW STATUS CONTROL, HIGH EFFORT AT WORK AND ISCHEMIC HEART DISEASE: PROSPECTIVE EVIDENCE FROM BLUE-COLLAR MEN

JOHANNES SIEGRIST,[1] RICHARD PETER,[1] ASTRID JUNGE,[1] PETER CREMER[2] and DIETER SEIDEL[2]
[1]Department of Medical Sociology, Medical School, University of Marburg, D-3550 Marburg, F.R.G. and [2]Department of Clinical Chemistry, Klinikum Grosshadern, University of Munich, 8000 Munich 22, F.R.G.

Abstract—An inverse relation between socio-economic class and occurrence of ischemic heart disease (IHD) in advanced societies is an often replicated finding from empirical studies. Yet, the processes which produce these effects remain an open question. One promising explanation concerns the prevalence of stressful working life, especially of distinct 'job strain' occupations. Based on these considerations, we develop a refined concept of work-related socio-emotional distress which considers a mismatch between high workload and low control over occupational status (e.g. job insecurity, poor promotion prospects, status inconsistency) as crucial distress-provoking conditions. Moreover, we assume that the effect of this condition on IHD risk is substantially increased by the presence of a distinct individual pattern of coping with work demand ('need for control').

Based on data from a 6.5 years prospective study on IHD incidence ($n = 21$) in a cohort of 416 middle-aged blue-collar men this concept is tested using logistic regression analysis. Results indicate that status inconsistency [multivariate odds ratio (o.r.): 4.4], job insecurity (o.r. 3.4), work pressure (o.r. 3,4) and 'need for control' (o.r. 4,5) independently predict IHD occurrence after adjusting for major confounding somatic and behavioral coronary risk factors. In conclusion, a refined model of work-related socio-emotional distress substantially contributes to the explanation of high IHD incidence among blue-collar men.

Key words—social epidemiology, ischemic heart disease, job insecurity, status inconsistency, work pressure, blue-collar workers

INTRODUCTION

Today we find a declining rate of mortality from ischemic heart disease (IHD) in a number of industrialized societies. However, IHD occurrence continues to be inversely related to social class. This was shown most convincingly for men in middle adulthood in several Western countries [1–5]. Only part of the excess mortality observed in lower social strata is explained by well-established behavioral risk factors such as unhealthy diet, overweight, cigarette smoking, heavy alcohol consumption or lack of physical exercise [2–4]. The contribution of other factors such as genetic predisposition or different medical treatment and compliance in explaining the social gradient of IHD needs to be studied further. Yet, in recent years, an alternative explanation was put forward and was substantiated by a growing body of evidence. This explanation concerns the role of distinct working and living conditions which produce chronic episodes of socio-emotional distress, and which are found to be more prevalent among lower social classes (for review see [6]). Chronic socio-emotional distress was shown to increase blood pressure [7, 8], atherogenic blood lipids [9, 10] and thrombogenic risk [11] which all contribute to the development of IHD [12].

This paper provides new evidence on the role of chronic socio-emotional distress in occupational life in explaining IHD morbidity and mortality among lower class men. Starting from a conceptual approach towards stress-producing working conditions it presents and discusses findings from a prospective study on IHD incidence in a sample of middle-aged blue-collar men.

A new conceptual approach

In pioneering research during the sixties and seventies a series of studies were conducted to conceptualize psychosocial stress at work and to demonstrate its adverse effects on cardiovascular health (for reviews see [6, 13–18]. In general, it was found that role conflicts at the worksite, high workload, job dissatisfaction and low social support at work were associated with a moderate increase in IHD risk factors, IHD morbidity or mortality. However, these approaches were limited in scope due to a lack of consensus concerning the relevant conceptual and empirical scales of assessing job stress. This situation changed when Robert A. Karasek and Töres Theorell introduced a two-dimensional model of job strain [19] which was based on a large body of evidence derived from psychophysiologic and psychoneuroendocrine studies [20, 21] as well as from occupational sociology [22]. This model "conceptualized job control (in the form of the factors "decision latitude" and "skill discretion") and job demand as interactive predictors of strain; jobs which combine low decision latitude with 'hectic work' and time pressure are seen as producing an imbalance which is manifest as psychological strain, and increased risk of mental and physical ill health" [23, p. 26] and especially of IHD. The same holds true for the combination "low skill discretion and high job demand" [24]. This approach which is now empirically well substantiated [19] can be considered a very significant contribution to the topic under study, and it has already shown a considerable impact on occupational policy.

Yet, two basic questions are not well answered by the job strain model. The first question relates to the long-term impact of low decision latitude and low skill discretion as indicators of low personal control. It is in line with general stress theory that experience of socio-emotional distress involves some element of threat [25]. Yet, the everyday job experience of low decision latitude or low skill discretion is likely to become routinized as part of a 'typical situation' to which workers in the long run may adapt both cognitively and emotionally [26]. It is evident that low status jobs in which low control over task is highly prevalent provide an increased risk of occupational threats, but it is unclear, both conceptually and empirically, to what extent adverse health effects are produced by the task control component of such occupational settings. For instance, one recent study found an association between high demand, low decision latitude and IHD among blue-collar workers, but not among white-collar workers [27]. The health-adverse effects of job strain to some extent may be confounded by undocumented, but relevant threats which are part of blue-collar working life (see below).

A second question relates to the issue of objective versus subjective control. Clearly, the job strain model considers control as an objective characteristic of the work situation. However, cognitive and affective responses of the workers to these characteristics vary considerably according to their individual patterns of appraisal and of coping [25]. For instance, generalized control believes were found to moderate the effects of objective job conditions on well-being [28]. Moreover, individual coping characteristics such as type A behavior [29], hostility [30, 31], or lack of hardiness [32] were associated with increased IHD risk. Such findings call for a conceptual clarification of the relationship between control-limiting job conditions and those personal characteristics which influence the perception of and the search for control.

Based on these considerations we have developed a model of work-related socio-emotional distress which defines threatening job conditions in terms of a mismatch between high workload (high demand) and low control over long-term rewards (low status control). Our emphasis on personal control in terms of long-term reward is explained by the fact that distressing experiences often result from basic threats to the continuity of a crucial social role. In adult life, this usually implies the occupational role. Most clearly, this is the case with job termination or job instability. However, related conditions of low reward and low security may also be identified, such as forced occupational change, downward mobility, lack of promotion prospects, jobs held with inconsistent educational background (status inconsistency). In many of these instances, personal control over objective job conditions is restricted, and adjustment to the potential threats caused by these conditions is difficult. We maintain that the mismatch between high workload and low status control, i.e. the interaction between demand and status control is critical in promoting stress-related cardiovascular pathology [33,34].

Moreover, according to our argument, the role of individual coping characteristics needs to be considered. In that respect we developed the concept 'need for control' as a distinct individual pattern of coping with work demands. This concept evolved from a critical analysis of the rather global pattern of type A behavior [35]. 'Need for control' specifies those cognitive, emotional and motivational components within the global concept of type A which are suspected of triggering enhanced arousal in demanding situations. The measurement of these components in the framework of a psychometric scale is discussed in the Method's section. However, it is important to note that 'need for control' defines a personal characteristic which is rather stable over time [36]. Thus, its measures do not merely reflect transient subjective states related to the situational conditions under study.

In summary, we suggest to analyze increased IHD vulnerability among members of low status occupations in terms of job conditions which define a mismatch between high workload (high demand) and low long-term reward (low status control). Secondly, we propose to combine these occupational conditions with individual coping characteristics (in terms of high need for control) to account for the risk of stress-related IHD morbidity and mortality in a substantial way. Accordingly, our hypothesis states that blue-collars exposed to high workload and low status control who also exhibit a high level of need for control are at elevated cardiovascular risk. Furthermore, we assume that associations of these psychosocial factors persist after adjusting for the effects of well-established behavioral and somatic coronary risk factors.

METHODS

The study sample

A prospective study on a cohort of 416 middle-aged male (25–55 years, mean: 40.8 ± 9.7) blue-collar workers followed over 6.5 years was performed to test our hypothesis. The study population was recruited from three industrial steel and metal plants in West Germany. The three plants were comparable in terms of size, type of production and composition of labor force. Sample criteria were age, occupational status (skilled, semi- or unskilled manual workers, foremen), daytime work and native speakers. Workers with documented coronary events as established by ECG were excluded after baseline screening. The sample was representative of the total labor force of the three plants meeting sample criteria with the exception of a slight underrepresentation of unskilled workers.

Four screenings took place over a 6.5 year period of observation. Medical data included blood pressure readings at all occasions, height, weight and resting ECG at the beginning and at the end, and blood samples during second and third screening. During the observation period a sample loss of 15% occurred. Compared to the initial group, the remaining sample was slightly biased with respect to only 2 out of 34 relevant characteristics examined: workers with high blood pressure and workers with high job instability were more likely to withdraw from follow-up.

Measurement of the components of the theoretical model

A structured interview including a psychometric test was applied to all participants at all four screenings to measure the components of the theoretical model specified below. In addition, socio-demographic and health-related information was collected through the interviews as well as information on social support at work and outside the working life and on recent life events [36]. Independent information on some of the core components of our model was obtained from companies' administrations. In the following description, this latter type of information is labeled 'contextual' (CI) whereas information obtained from the workers is labeled 'descriptive' (DI) or 'evaluative' (EI). Combining and comparing contextual and individual (descriptive, evaluative) information has the advantage of strengthening the validity of reported findings [37].

The following section briefly describes the measurement of the core variables of the model.

1. Components of status control and long-term reward

Occupational instability (CI). Membership in a plant with a high percentage (> 15%) of cut-down of personnel during observation period (yes/no).

Job insecurity (EI). Self evaluation of one's own job security (high, low).

Status inconsistency (CI-DI). A composed measure combining occupational grade with level of education. Status inconsistency defines people holding occupational grades with either too high or too poor educational background as compared to the majority of the workforce [38] (yes/no).

Promotion prospects (EI). Self evaluation of one's promotion prospects within or outside the company (fair, poor).

Level of wage (CI). Information on the system of wages based on qualification and job requirements is measured in three categories: high (essentially foremen), medium (essentially skilled workers), low (essentially un- and semiskilled workers).

Relative job deprivation (EI). Self evaluation of personal disadvantages at work relative to one's reference group (deprivation present, absent).

2. Components of workload

Piecework (CI). Workplace defined by individual or group piecework (yes/no).

Shiftwork (CI). Workplace defined by early or late day shift (night shift workers were excluded from this study) (yes/no).

Noise (CI). Workplace defined by high level of noise [< 85 dB (A)].

Work pressure (EI). Evaluation of frequency and intensity of self-perceived time pressure at one's work site [high work pressure defines workers who score 4 or 5 on a respective five point-Likert scaled item (yes/no)].

Increase of workload (EI). Evaluation of increase of workload over past year [due to cut-down in personnel, speeding up of production etc. (yes/no)].

3. *Assessment of individual coping characteristics*

The coping pattern 'need for control'. We measured this individual style of coping with demands at work by applying a psychometric scale. This scale contains 45 dichotomous items which represent the following 6 dimensions: 1—need for approval, coping with success and failure; 2—competitiveness, independence during challenge and latent hostility; 3—work commitment, hard driving; 4—perfectionism, need for making plans; 5—impatience and disproportionate irritability; 6—inability to withdraw from work obligations. Unidimensionality of each subscale was tested by the dichotomous probabilistic test model developed by Rasch [39]. By means of a confirmatory factor analysis, two latent factors were repeatedly found which are moderately correlated: the subscales 3 and 4 load on a factor labeled 'VIGOR', the other subscales on a second latent factor labeled 'IMMERSION'. According to our theoretical assumption, 'vigor' describes a state of active efforts with a high probability of positive feedback, whereas 'immersion' indicates a state of exhaustive coping reflecting frustrated, but continued efforts and associated negative feelings. We expect this latter factor to indicate an individual's increased vulnerability to experiences of high demand and low status control. The total score of 'immersion' is defined by 29 items. Scores in the upper tertile (ranging from 19 to 29 points) indicate a critically high level (for further details see [35]).

Whereas the pattern 'need for control' represents rather stable person characteristics additional information on individual coping was obtained which refers to transitional states. We are interested in the following indicators of critical states of coping:

Sustained anger. Self evaluation of feelings of anger and irritation over past 12 months (5 point Likert scaled item; workers scoring 4 or 5 are considered to exhibit sustained anger).

Sustained helplessness. Evaluation of feelings of helplessness and hopelessness over past 12 months (measured by a 5-point Likert scaled item; workers scoring 4 or 5 are considered to exhibit sustained helplessness).

In addition to these indicators of emotional well-being we were interested in complaints about sleep disturbances and short sleeping time. As explained elsewhere in detail distinct types of sleep disturbances can be interpreted as indicators of critical states of socio-emotional distress [40].

Poor sleep. Evaluation of frequency of problems with maintaining sleep and with waking up too early in the morning, in combination with total sleeping time per night (6 hr or less) (poor sleep present, absent).

4. Measurement of coronary risk factors

Blood pressure readings were performed by sphygmanometry according to WHO criteria at standardized diurnal time.

Total serum cholesterol and triglycerides were determined enzymatically [41]. Lipoproteins were

Table 1. Coronary risk factors [means and standard deviation (SD)] (left side) and frequency (right side) at entry ($n = 416$, blue-collar men)

Variable	Mean ± SD		%
Age (yr)	40.8 ± 9.7	Regular cigarette smoking	34.8
BMI (kg/m²)	27.3 ± 3.4	Lack of physical exercise	78.8
Systolic blood pressure (mmHg)	139.1 ± 16.2	Hypertension**	31.6
Diastolic blood pressure (mmHg)	89.6 ± 9.6	Hyperlipidemia***	24.8
Total cholesterol* (mg/dl)	235.9 ± 38.5	Co-manifestation of hypertension and hyperlipidemia	10.8
LDL-cholesterol* (mg/dl)	155.9 ± 32.9		

*Serum lipids were assessed at second screening (one year later; $n = 356$).
**SBP > 160 mmHg and/or DBP > 95 mmHg.
***LDL-cholesterol > 180 mg/dl and/or ratio between LDL- and HDL-cholesterol > 4.0.

measured by quantitative lipoprotein electrophoresis (for details see [10]) and by available precipitation techniques for quantification of low density lipoprotein and of high density lipoprotein -cholesterol [42, 43]. In addition to lipoprotein quantification, the main protein components of HDL and LDL, Apo A1 and Apo B were assessed. All analyses were performed blind by the department of clinical chemistry. Further information on risk factors was obtained from interviews. It included cigarette smoking (number of cigarettes smoked per day, years of smoking), physical exercise in leisure time (frequency, duration, intensity), family history of IHD (parents or siblings, age of onset, diagnosis), treatment of diabetes or of hyperuricemia and age.

5. Measurement of outcome variables (IHD)

Expert judgments on primary endpoints [definite or probable letal or non-letal acute myocardial infarction (AMI) or sudden cardiac death (SCD) (ICD 410–414)] are based on the criteria defined below* [44]. Information on primary endpoints was obtained from 85% of the initial sample.

Statistical analysis

The contribution of the described variables in terms of identifying workers who experience IHD during follow-up as opposed to workers who remain free from IHD is analyzed using univariate and multivariate (logistic regression) analysis [45–47]. The model fit of the most parsimonious model is tested by the likelihood ratio difference test in a bottom-up procedure. Regression coefficients, standard errors, multivariate odds ratios and the 95% confidence intervals are indicated in respective tables. All calculations were performed on personal computers using SPSS-PC [48] and GLIM [49] programs for data analysis.

*Criteria for definition of IHD (primary endpoints): judgments of primary endpoints [definite or probable letal or non-letal acute myocardial infarction (AMI) or sudden cardiac death (SCD) (ICD 410–414)] are based on the following criteria: 1. ECG [Minnesota Code evaluated independently by two physicians (cardiologists)]; in case of discordance (about 5%), a third physician was asked to give his judgment. 2. History taking according to WHO MONICA protocol [44] (overt cases resulting almost always in hospital admission where positive enzyme signs were an additional criterion to establish the diagnosis AMI). 3. Official cause of death. Definite AMI was coded if clear ECG signs and unequivocal additional information (criteria 2 or 3) were present. Probable AMI-SCD was coded if clear ECG-signs, but no definitively reliable additional information was present (in some of those cases silent AMI may have occurred). Letal and non-letal cerebrovascular events and noncardiovascular causes of death were recorded as well, but this information is not analyzed in the present report.

RESULTS

The blue-collar cohort under study is exposed to unfavorable working conditions. As far as workload is concerned, 31% are confined to piecework, and the workplaces of every fourth blue-collar exhibit noise levels beyond 85 dB(A). High work pressure is present in 18% of the sample, and 22% indicate that they suffer from an increase of workload during past year. With respect to long-term rewards, 14% work under conditions of low occupational stability and only 30% indicate fair or good promotion prospects. Status inconsistency prevails in 16% of the sample and relative job deprivation in 42%. Thus, the sample under study shows considerable mismatch between high workload and low status control.

Before exploring the relationship between these two distinct components of occupational stress and future IHD, coronary risk factors at baseline are examined. As can be seen from Table 1, the present blue-collar sample is at increased coronary risk. For instance, 31.6% are manifest hypertensives as compared to 18% in a comparable age group of West German men recruited from all social strata [50]. Part of this high prevalence is attributable to the frequent occurrence of obesity and of physical inactivity. Furthermore, there is a powerful interaction between elevated lipid levels and high blood pressure: 32% of all hypertensives exhibit levels of LDL-cholesterol which require medical treatment. Every fourth worker is at risk of hyperlipidemia. This is reflected in a very high mean level of LDL-cholesterol. Mean levels of HDL-cholesterol, APO A1 and APO B, not presented in Table 1, indicate a comparable atherogenic risk. The only major coronary risk factor whose prevalence was well comparable to the one observed in the general population of the respective age groups was cigarette smoking.

Next, we analyze the risk profile of workers who experience IHD during the 6.5 years follow-up in comparison with the remaining group*. Twenty-one workers (5.9%) suffered from a definitive or probable acute myocardial infarction, two of them died suddenly.

Table 2 presents information on means (or frequencies) of coronary risk factors in the group of cases as compared to non-cases. The group of non-

Table 2. Coronary risk factors [mean and standard deviation (SD) of frequencies (%)] in future victims of IHD and in men who remain free from IHD

Variable	Cases ($n = 21$)	Non-cases[a] ($n = 293$)	t-Test or chi²
Age	46.6 ± 7.3	40.7 ± 9.9	2.65**
BMI (kg/m²)	26.9 ± 2.5	27.4 ± 3.3	0.57
Systolic blood pressure (mmHg)	151.1 ± 19.8	140.9 ± 16.6	2.84**
Diastolic blood pressure (mmHg)	95.3 ± 12.3	89.3 ± 12.1	2.26*
Total cholesterol (mg/dl)	254.7 ± 25.0	233.0 ± 36.8	2.65**
LDL-cholesterol (mg/dl)	178.8 ± 24.2	155.7 ± 33.9	3.01**
Regular cigarette smoking	28.5%	33.7%	0.60
Lack of physical exercise	90.0%	77.7%	1.03
Status inconsistency	33.3%	14.4%	5.40*
Low promotion prospects	90.5%	69.8%	3.21
Job insecurity	19.0%	8.9%	2.33
High work pressure	33.3%	13.4%	4.72*
Immersion (% upper tertile)	28.6%	8.3%	6.89**
Poor sleep	61.9%	35.5%	4.81**

**$P < 0.01$; *$P < 0.05$.

[a]Participants with cerebrovascular events ($n = 6$), with non-ischemic heart disease ($n = 7$), with advanced coronary artery disease not meeting criteria of primary endpoint ($n = 21$), and with non-cardiovascular cause of death ($n = 5$) were excluded from analysis.

cases has been restricted to men who were definitely free from advanced coronary artery disease, from cerebrovascular events and from non-ischemic heart disease. Moreover, non-cardiovascular causes of death were excluded. Due to missing data, the total number of persons whose data are included into multivariate analysis is somewhat smaller than the 314 men (21 cases; 293 non-cases) defined according to these criteria. Table 2 indicates that blue-collar men who suffer from IHD are significantly older. They exhibit significantly higher levels of blood pressure (both systolic and diastolic) and significantly higher levels of total cholesterol and LDL-cholesterol. Lack of regular physical exercise is more prevalent, but the difference is not significant. Two additional findings are in contrast to our expectation, although they both do not reach statistical significance: future IHD victims have a somewhat lower body weight and there are slightly less smokers in this group as compared to the remaining group. This latter finding is explained by the fact that nearly half of the non-smokers within the group of future cases were ex-smokers at baseline screening after a history of obviously excessive smoking.

Turning to psychosocial indicators we find that 5 variables are clearly more prevalent among the group of IHD cases as compared to the remaining group. Two of these indicators relate to conditions of low status control (status inconsistency, low promotion prospects), one to workload (work pressure), and two to personal coping characteristics [the latent factor 'immersion' of the concept need for control and an indicator of a critical state of coping (poor sleep)].

Twice as many future victims of IHD suffer from personal job insecurity as compared to the remaining group. However, this finding is not statistically significant in univariate analysis.

In a next step, multivariate analysis is performed using logistic regression analysis in search of the most parsimonious prediction model. In a 'bottom-up' procedure with the likelihood ratio difference test as a selection criterion a model is found which is composed by four biobehavioral and four psychosocial variables listed in Table 3. Table 3 displays the unstandardized regression coefficients of these variables, their standard error, the multivariate odds ratios adjusted for each factor in the model and the 95% confidence intervals. The model is highly significant. In view of the small number of cases, large confidence intervals are inevitable, but multivariate odds ratios nevertheless indicate that these variables can be interpreted as risk factors contributing to the prediction of IHD occurrence in the sample. Whereas all other variables are associated with IHD risk in a positive direction, body weight is negatively associated with IHD risk.

It is in line with established knowledge in cardiovascular epidemiology that blood lipids and systolic blood pressure result as the most powerful somatic risk factors. However, four important indicators of a psychosocial coronary risk constellation contribute to the model in a substantial way: status inconsistency, low job security, high workload (work pressure) and high scoring on a critical component of the individual coping pattern 'need for control' (immersion).

Analysis so far is restricted to models that include only main effects of single predictors. Yet, the theoretical model outlined in the introduction implies that a cumulative effect of indicators of high effort (work

Table 3. Logistic regression analysis of factors associated with IHD incidence among blue-collar workers ($n = 263$)[a]

Variable	Regression coefficient[b]	Multivariate odds-ratio	95% CI
Age	1.09 (0.57)	2.98	0.97–9.16
BMI	−1.13 (0.55)	0.32	0.11–0.95
Systolic blood pressure	2.11 (0.83)	8.22	1.63–41.5
LDL-cholesterol	2.45 (1.14)	11.60	1.24–108.8
Status inconsistency	1.48 (0.60)	4.40	1.36–14.2
Job insecurity	1.23 (0.74)	3.41	0.81–14.5
Work pressure	1.24 (0.65)	3.45	0.97–12.3
Immersion	1.51 (0.70)	4.53	1.15–17.8
Constant	−6.23 (1.58)***		
Deviance $df = 254$	105.01		

***$P < 0.001$.

[a]The reduced number of subjects is due to selective missing data.

[b]All variables in model. Each factor adjusted for each other factor in the model. Standard error of parameter given in parentheses.

pressure, immersion), and of low status control (status inconsistency, job insecurity) is required in order to substantially improve prediction of IHD. Thus, a logistic regression model is calculated with the biobehavioral variables defined in Table 3 and with the combined psychosocial variable 'low reward/high effort' defined as follows (see Table 4): 1—no psychosocial risks at all; 2–indicator(s) of either low reward *or* high effort; 3—indicator(s) of low reward *and* of high effort. In 38% of the future IHD cases a co-manifestation of the two critical indicators is observed, but only in 7.4% of the remaining group (chi square = 20.31; $P < 0.0001$). Table 4 indicates that this model again is highly significant. Beta coefficients are all significant.

Expected probability of IHD incidence is calculated for each combination of the variables under study (see respective equation in Table 4). Results are displayed in Fig. 1. As can be seen, the expected probability of IHD is substantially increased if conditions of low status control *and* of high effort are present. However, this finding holds true only under conditions of cumulated biobehavioral risk factors. Thus, our findings support the notion of a synergism of biobehavioral and psychosocial factors in producing IHD onset.

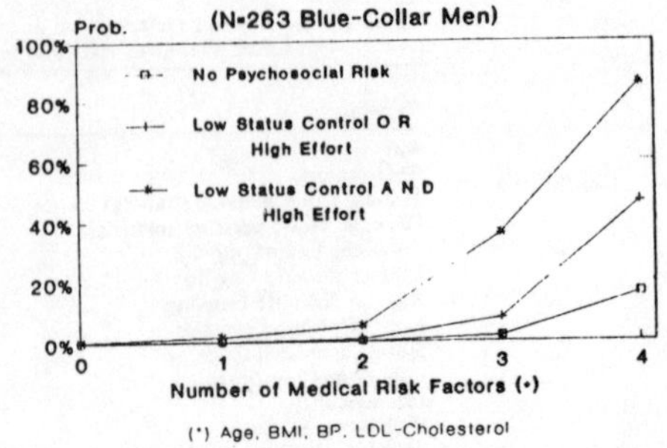

Fig. 1. Expected probability of IHD incidence (6.5 yr) in a logistic regression model using medical and psychosocial variables.

DISCUSSION

The results reported in this paper indicate that occurrence of IHD in a cohort of middle-aged blue-collar men followed over a 6.5 years period is successfully explained by a model which combines information on biobehavioral and work-related psychosocial risk factors. Results underscore the significant role of stressful working conditions in explaining increased IHD morbidity and mortality among middle-aged blue-collar men. More specificially, they point to the critical role of a mismatch between high workload and low status control, and they indicate that individual patterns of coping with work demands, namely high need for control, need to be considered to better explain an elevated IHD risk.

In terms of more differentiated models of stress the present findings suggest that stress-related research in social epidemiology and medical sociology should further specify formerly used global explanatory concepts. In particular, social class [51], social status [1–4] or work stress should be operationalized in form of two- or three-dimensional models. These models enable us to identify otherwise undetected subgroups at risk within the larger socio-economic strata. One such two-dimensional model, the job strain model, was briefly discussed in the Introduction. In our own approach, we too have used a two-dimensional sociological model, but our focus was on status control rather than on task characteristics such as decision latitude and skill discretion. Furthermore, we have analyzed the interaction between objective and subjective control by introducing the concept 'need for control'. We maintain that effort spent at work is analyzed more accurately if demand characteristics (e.g. workload) and characteristics of individual coping with these demands (need for control) are combined.

Recently, a three-dimensional model of job strain was suggested, integrating the dimension of social support at work [27]. In our study, we could not find any effect on IHD incidence produced by social support, regardless of whether support at work or support outside the workplace was considered. At present, it is unclear whether this is due to the specific measurement of social support in our study or whether the possible protecting effect of social support is simply overridden by the potent effects exerted by occupational stressors and individual coping characteristics.

In recent past, several studies found type A behavior to be more prevalent among middle-class populations than among lower socio-economic groups [29, 52]. Yet, this finding is difficult to reconciliate with the established inverse social grade of IHD [1–5]. In contrast, several studies showed 'need for control' measures rather unaffected by social class [36]. Thus, patterns of coping can be identified which are not in contrast with the established inverse social grade of IHD.

The concept 'need for control', and especially its latent factor 'immersion' is not only related to some of the components of the global type A behavior, but also to the concept of vital exhaustion. This latter approach was elaborated most impressively by the Maastricht group, and it was shown to be predictive of increased IHD risk in several studies [53]. We are currently exploring the relation between the two concepts in cross-cultural studies.

Table 4. Logistic regression analysis with a combined psychosocial variable ('low reward/high effort, see text)

Variable	Regression coefficient[a]
Age	1.13 (0.56)*
BMI	1.17 (0.56)*
Systolic blood pressure	2.32 (0.87)**
LDL-cholesterol	2.34 (1.10)*
'Low reward/high effort' (2)	1.51 (0.60)*
'Low reward/high effort' (3)	3.42 (0.83)***
Constant	−7.46 (1.53)***
Deviance	103.92
df	256

*$P < 0.05$; **$P < 0.01$; ***$P < 0.001$.

[a] All variables in model. Each factor adjusted for each other factor in the model. In parenthesis: standard error of parameter.

Expected probability of IHD incidence is calculated according to the equation: $p = \exp(\mu)/1 \pm \exp(\mu)$, $\mu = \beta_0 + \beta_{1 \times 1} + \beta_{2 \times 2} \cdots \beta_{i \times i}$.

Some comment is in order with respect to the relative importance of our psychosocial predictors. In quantitative terms, LDL-cholesterol and hypertension remain the most important factors analyzed. Although we have shown elsewhere that high levels of atherogenic lipoproteins in this cohort to some extent are explained by indicators of severe socio-emotional stress at work [10], lifestyle characteristics such as unhealthy diet, poor weight control, lack of physical exercise, alcohol consumption and smoking are probably more effective in producing hyperlipidemia [54]. Non-compliance is a further possible reason for the high prevalence of hyperlipidemia and especially hypertension. Even after informing participants of our screening results including leaflets on health education, only 46% of all manifest hypertensives in our study adhered to antihypertensive treatment [55].

Other factors not analyzed in our study, e.g. thrombogenic factors, may have contributed to the observed high rate of IHD incidence [11]. Cardiotoxic effects of chemical substancies related to steel and metal production were reported in the literature although their dose may be negligeable in the group under study [56].

In view of the relatively few cases of IHD and the respective large confidence intervals more information on the validity of reported findings is needed. There are two ways of dealing with this issue: first, additional analysis of subclinical IHD in the sample, and, secondly, independent replication of findings. Both strategies are briefly discussed. First, in the present analysis of differences between cases and non-cases we excluded a group of 21 men whose ECG showed signs of advanced coronary artery disease and/or of left ventricular hypertrophy without meeting criteria of primary endpoints [44—see footnote to Table 2]. Although a usual procedure in epidemiologic analysis, this approach fails to analyze the role of psychosocial variables in explaining subclinical IHD. A replication of findings reported from the group of cases by data from the subclinical IHD group would strengthen the validity of our results. In fact, two of the four psychosocial predictors of clinical IHD were significantly associated with subclinical IHD. Furthermore, multivariate analysis revealed a strong, highly significant independent effect of the core predictor 'low reward/high effort' on combined subclinical and clinical IHD status. Thus, results indicate that the psychosocial variables analyzed in this study explain both subclinical and clinical IHD. Furthermore they demonstrate that the explanatory power of psychosocial factors is closely linked to the presence of biobehavioral coronary risk factors such as hypertension and hyperlipidemia.

Turning to the second argument, we now have first results from an independent replication of findings from a second, much larger prospective study based on 4820 men aged 40–60 years. These men so far were followed prospectively over 2.5 years. A questionnaire containing an abbreviated version of some psychosocial measurements reported in this study was applied. Preliminary statistical analysis indicates that the group of future IHD cases exhibits a significantly higher mean score of immersion, a significantly higher percentage of high workload and of sleep disturbances. These findings provide some first independent support of the role of coping characteristics in explaining IHD.

In conclusion our results indicate that simultaneous occurrence of high effort at work and low control over occupational status defines an independent risk configuration in the prediction of IHD in middle-aged blue-collar men. The findings provide further evidence on the observed relationship between stressful working life, low socio-economic position and high IHD occurrence. Moreover, they illustrate the contribution of more differentiated theoretical concepts derived from sociology and social psychology to social epidemiology. Finally, the present findings may also have important implications for health policy. Reducing the burden of high workload at specific blue-collar production sites and increasing reward and security associated with status control in the long run could result in a sizeable reduction of IHD risk. In addition, individual prevention may be directed at reducing inappropriate ways of coping with work demands and at strengthening the regenerative potential available within and among individual workers. The inverse relation between social grade and one of the major chronic degenerative diseases in advanced societies is not a fate but a societal challenge.

Acknowledgements—The authors gratefully acknowledge help of a number of experts and collaborators in this study, most importantly of the former members of the research team: Herbert Matschinger, Ph.D., Karin Siegrist, Ph.D., Ingbert Weber, Ph.D., and Daniela Klein, Ph.D. Furthermore, we thank the physicians, nurses and members of the administrative staff of the companies under study for their assistance. Thomas Abel, Ph.D., provided substantial comments on an earlier version of this paper. The technical help of Adjuta Bertsch and Annemarie Harms in producing the present manuscript is also acknowledged.

Supported by the German Research Foundation (Si 236-5).

REFERENCES

1. Antonovsky A. Social class and the major cardiovascular diseases. *J. chron. Dis.* **21**, 65, 1968.
2. Marmot M. G., Shipley M. and Rose G. Inequalities in death—specific explanation of a general pattern? *The Lancet* **1**, 1003, 1984.
3. Holme I. *et al.* Socio-economic status as a coronary risk factor: The Oslo Study. *Acta med. scand.* Suppl. **660**, 147, 1982.
4. Buring J. E. *et al.* Occupation and risk of death from coronary heart disease. *J. Am. med. Ass.* **258**, 791, 1987.
5. Ruberman W. *et al.* Psychosocial influences on mortality after myocardial infarction. *New Engl. J. Med.* **311**, 552, 1984.
6. Marmot M. and Theorell T. Social class and cardiovascular disease: the contribution of work. *Int. J. Hlth Serv.* **18**, 659, 1988.
7. Weiner H. *The Psychobiology of Essential Hypertension.* Elsevier, New York, 1979.
8. Cottington E. *et al.* Occupational stress and diastolic blood pressure in a blue-collar population: the Pittsburgh Noise-Hypertension Project. *Am. J. Epidem.* **118**, 442, 1983.
9. Dimsdale J. E. and Herd A. Variability of plasma lipids in response to emotional arousal. *Psychosom. Med.* **44**, 413, 1982.
10. Siegrist J. *et al.* Atherogenic risk in men suffering from occupational stress. *Atherosclerosis* **68**, 211, 1988.

11. Markowe H. L. *et al.* Fibrinogen: a possible link between social class and coronary heart disease. *Br. med. J.* **291**, 1312, 1985.
12. Beamish R. E., Singall P. K. and Dhalla N. S. (Eds) *Stress and Heart Disease*. Nijhoff, Boston, MA, 1985.
13. House J. S. *Work Stress and Social Support*. Addison-Wesley, Reading, MA, 1981.
14. Caplan R. D. *et al. Job Demands and Worker Health.* U.S. Government Printing Office, Washington, DC, 1975.
15. Cooper C. L. and Payne R. (Eds) *Stress at Work*. Wiley, New York, 1978.
16. Gentry W. D., Benson H. and De Wolff C. J. (Eds) *Behavioral Medicine: Work, Stress and Health*. Nijhoff, Dordrecht, 1985.
17. Steptoe A. and Appels A. (Eds) *Stress, Personal Control and Health*. Wiley, Chichester, 1989.
18. Sauter S. L., Harrell J. J. and Cooper C. L. (Eds) *Job Control and Worker Health*. Wiley, New York, 1989.
19. Karasek R. A. and Theorell T. *Healthy Work*. Basic Books, New York, 1990.
20. Henry J. P. and Stephens P. M. *Stress, Health and the Social Environment*. Springer, Berlin, 1977.
21. Frankenhaeuser M. Psychoneuroendocrine approach to the study of emotions related to stress and coping. In *Nebraska Symposium on Motivation* (Edited by Howe D.). University of Nebraska Press, Lincoln, NE, 1979.
22. Kohn M. L. and Schooler C. *Work and Personality*. Ablex, Norwood, NY, 1983.
23. Parkes K. E. Personal control in an occupational context. In *Stress, Personal Control and Health* (Edited by Steptoe A. and Appels A.), p. 21. Wiley, Chichester, 1989.
24. Theorell T. Personal control at work and health: a review of epidemiological studies in Sweden. In *Stress, Personal Control and Health* (Edited by Steptoe A. and Appels A.), p. 48. Wiley, Chichester, 1989.
25. Lazarus R. S. and Folkman S. *Stress, Appraisal and Coping*. Springer, New York, 1984.
26. Schutz A. *Collected Papers*, Vols I–III. Nijhoff, The Hague, 1962–1966.
27. Johnson J. V. and Hall E. M. Job strain, work place, social support and cardiovascular disease. *Am. J. publ. Hlth* **78**, 1336, 1988.
28. Spector P. E. Interaction effects of perceived control and job stressors on affective reactions and health outcomes for clerical workers. *Work & Stress* **1**, 155, 1987.
29. Rosenman R. H. Current and past history of type A behavior pattern. In *Biological and Psychological Factors in Cardiovascular Disease* (Edited by Schmidt T. H., Dembroski T. M. and Blümchen G.), p. 15. Springer, Berlin, 1986.
30. Williams R. B. *et al.* Type A behavior and angiographically documented coronary atherosclerosis in a sample of 2289 patients. *Psychosom. Med.* **50**, 139, 1988.
31. Koskenvuo M. *et al.* Hostility as a risk factor for mortality and ischemic heart disease in men. *Psychosom. Med.* **50**, 230, 1988.
32. Kobasa S. C., Maddi S. and Zola M. A. Type A and hardiness. *J. behav. Med.* **6**, 41, 1983.
33. Siegrist J., Siegrist K. and Weber I. Sociological concepts in the etiology of chronic disease: the case of ischemic heart disease. *Soc. Sci. Med.* **22**, 247, 1986.
34. Siegrist J. and Matschinger H. Restricted status control and cardiovascular risk. In *Stress, Personal Control and Health* (Edited by Steptoe A. and Appels A.), p. 65. Wiley, Chichester, 1989.
35. Matschinger H. *et al.* Type A as a coping career: towards a conceptual and methodological redefinition. In *Biological and Psychological Factors in Cardiovascular Disease* (Edited by Schmidt T. H. *et al.*), p. 104. Springer, Berlin, 1986.
36. Siegrist J. *et al.* Der Einfluß sozialer Belastungen und ihrer Verarbeitung auf die Entwicklung kardiovaskulärer Risiken. Unpublished Research Report, Marburg, 1987.
37. Mechanic D. Medical sociology: some tensions among theory, method, and substance. *J. Hlth soc. Behav.* **30**, 147, 1989.
38. Vernon S. W. and Buffler P. A. The status of status inconsistency. *Epidem. Rev.* **10**, 65, 1988.
39. Rasch G. *Probabilistic Models for Some Intelligence and Attainment Tests*. Nielsen & Lydiche, Copenhagen, 1960.
40. Siegrist J. Sleep disturbances in pre-infarction patients. In *Predisposing Conditions for Acute Ischemic Syndromes* (Edited by v. Arnim T. H. and Maseri A.), p. 42. Steinkopff, Springer, Darmstadt, 1989.
41. Cremer P., Seidel D. and Wieland H. Quantitative Lipoproteinelektrophorese. *Lab. Med.* **9**, 39, 1985.
42. Wieland H. and Seidel D. Quantitative lipoprotein electrophoresis. In *Handbook of Electrophoresis II* (Edited by Lewis L. A.), p. 83. CRC Press, Boca Raton, FL, 1983.
43. Wieland H. and Seidel D. A simple and specific technique for precipitation of low-density lipoproteins. *J. Lip. Res.* **24**, 904, 1983.
44. World Health Organization. *Monica Manual*. Unpubl. Report, Geneva, 1986.
45. Efron B. The efficiency of logistic regression compared to normal discriminant analysis. *J. Am. Statist. Ass.* **70**, 892, 1975.
46. Press S. I. and Central W. Choosing between logistic regression and discriminant analysis. *J. Am. Statist. Ass.* **73**, 699, 1978.
47. Nelder J. A. and Wedderburn R. W. M. Generalized linear models. *J. Natn. Statist. Soc. Am.* **135**, 370, 1972.
48. Norusis M. J. *SPSS-X Advanced Statistics Guide*. McGraw–Hill, New York, 1985.
49. Andress H. J. *GLIM—Verallgemeinerte Lineare Modelle*. Vieweg, Braunschweig, Wiesbaden, 1986.
50. Stieber J., Döring A. and Keil U. Häufigkeit, Bekanntheits- und Behandlungsgrad der Hypertonie in einer Großstadtbevölkerung. Ergebnisse der Münchner Blutdruckstudie I. *Münch. Med. Wochenschr.* **35**, 747, 1982.
51. Liberatos P., Link B. G. and Kelsey J. L. The measurement of social class in epidemiology. *Epidem. Rev.* **10**, 87, 1988.
52. Härtel U. and Chambless L. Occupational position and Type A behavior: results from the first MONICA Survey, Augsburg, FRG. *Soc. Sci. Med.* **29**, 1367, 1989.
53. Appels A. and Mulder P. Excess fatigue as a precursor of myocardial infarction. *Eur. Heart J.* **9**, 758, 1988.
54. Kannel W. B. *et al.* Optimal resources for primary prevention of atherosclerotic diseases. *Circulation* **29**, 157A, 1984.
55. Siegrist J., Matschinger H. and Motz W. Untreated hypertensives and their quality of life. *J. Hypertens.* Suppl. 1 **5**, 15, 1987.
56. Kristensen T. S. Cardiovascular diseases and the work environment: a critical review of the epidemiological literature on non-chemical factors. *Scand. J. Work Environ. Hlth* **15**, 165, 1989.

Part V
Health Behaviour

A. d'Houtaud and Mark G. Field

The image of health: variations in perception by social class in a French population

Abstract In order to determine how a population defines the meaning of health, a study was made using a sample of 4,000 respondents from Lorraine, in the north-eastern part of France. The respondents, all of whom were undergoing a health examination, were asked to respond to an open-ended question on what health meant to them. A total of 6,172 replies were obtained whose contents were classified into 41 main themes themselves regrouped under 10 heading (or groups of themes).

The responses were clearly linked to the socio-economic class position of the respondents, which was the most discriminating variable, and the one discussed here. There was a gradient from the higher, non-manual classes to the lower manual classes, the former conceiving health more in personalized, positive and expressive terms, and the latter more in negative, socialized and instrumental terms, thus reflecting the complementary positions of social classes as mediated through the occupational structure.

Introduction[1]

Critical, in any examination of a health-care system, and indeed in any evaluation or planning for such a system, is the attitude of the population to be served concerning health, and the position that health occupies in that population's scheme of priorities. Inasmuch as such an attitude is likely to determine health-care seeking behaviour, i.e. the utilization or non-utilization of medical and allied services, it is an important bit of datum. Furthermore, as populations in industrial societies are rarely homogeneous but tend to be stratified primarily along socio-economic dimensions, it is necessary to identify these dimensions or classes and to determine the differences (if any) in the attitudes of their members toward health. Such an identification theoretically allows us to understand better the various sub-cultures that may exist within a population, and pragmatically it should permit us to shape a health-care system that is more differentiated and thus more sensitive to the health-care seeking activities of such a population.

Sociology of Health and Illness Vol 6 No. 1 1984

This kind of approach is relatively infrequent [1 to 7] when compared to the more common subjects of sociological investigation which have tended to address two major topics: the relationship of health to its opposite, illness, and the services meant to restore health, either partly or totally. And yet, in addition to the opinions, attitudes and behaviours[2] that one observes in populations on the subject of health, there is an even more fundamental question: it is that of representations,[3] in the sense used by Durkheim, or basic consciousness or general world-view that underlie these opinions, attitudes and behaviours.

Access to that world of representations is, however, narrowly limited to the modes and capacities of written or oral expression and to that relatively narrow semantic field that health occupies in the large territory of language. This is indicative of difficulties and the complexities in apprehending the image of health. In this paper we shall limit ourselves, in an exploratory manner, to the cultural universe of the French language in two recent investigations in two different geographical areas of France.

The oldest such study in France is that which Claudine Herzlich [12] published on social representations of both health *and* illness, which she carried out simultaneously in the Parisian region and in a village of Normandy. To this end, she undertook a series of 80 interviews only with members of the middle and intellectual classes because, as she wrote, '. . . of the dynamic role that one may attribute to these classes . . . in the origins, in the transformation, in the renewal of the ideologies in our society'. In particular, after having reviewed the respective merits of anthropological and psychosociological approaches, and after having referred to the analyses of Freud and Parsons, Herzlich examined the problem of the social representation of health and illness. According to her, the experiences of each person on the one hand, the values and information available in society at large on the other, are integrated in that representation. The relationship of the individual to his health or illness *and* to his society are crystallized in that same representation. In that dual relationship, the individual defends himself simultaneously against illness and against society: from his viewpoint, illness is caused by the life style imposed by society.

In a more recent investigation, carried out at a health centre in Vandoeuvre-les-Nancy (France) with a sample of 4,000 persons that included manual workers (997 industrial and 125 rural workers), 797 employees, as well as 680 members of the middle, and 534 members of the higher socio-economic classes, and 867 persons not gainfully employed in the labour force (primarily students, housewives and retired persons), we preferred considering health itself[4] (without associating it with illness) as perceived by our population such at least as it appears in the written responses of our respondents to an open-ended question.[5]

Because of its objective of looking only at health, and because its methodology in administering a written questionnaire to a larger sample comprising members of different social classes, our approach is complementary to that of Herzlich. It also helps to explain why the conclusions of these two investigations include both similarities and differences. We shall return to these when we discuss our results. We have already reported the results of this work in the first part of a doctoral dissertation [8] and in [13, 14]. In this paper, intended for an English-speaking audience, we will present these results, concentrating on the essential aspects of this work, and referring the reader for methodological discussions and for greater details to the three previously mentioned publications [8, 13, 14] and to [15] from which we shall borrow the six tables presented here.

It may be noted, before we proceed further, that a follow-up to the research presented here is in the process of being carried out. In that second stage of our work, utilizing an even larger sample of the population from the Health Centre, the instrument we use is a structured question. With that instrument we examine the most synthetic elements of the responses obtained with the open-ended question administered in the first stage and reported here. We shall limit ourselves here to the already complex results obtained in that stage. We shall, later on, report on a comparison of the results of the two stages and of the two methods used (open-ended and structured question) and we shall more generally discuss all the questions of methodology and of conceptualization raised by our total approach to representations of health.[6]

This is also why we deal here only with a conceptual and methodological comparison of the research of Herzlich and the first stage of ours. Indeed, that limited comparison is indicated because of a certain similarity between the interview method used by Herzlich and the open-ended question we used in our work.

In the first part of this paper, we shall then succinctly define our methodology. In the second and longer part, we shall report the major results obtained with our open-ended question.[7] In the third part, we shall critically discuss these results as well as the implications of our methodological choices, a discussion which, as we have already indicated, will acquire all its significance when we will broaden it in the light of the more recent results derived from structured questions.

Methodological presentation of the research

The sample

The psychosociological investigations we undertook using the above defined population (a sample of 4,000 male and female adults, selected from the 72,515 who underwent a health examination between 21 January 1971 and 15 May 1974) represent, in a way, experimental conditions analogous to those of a laboratory: they consist of the population of a relatively new centre in Vandoeuvre-les-Nancy, which we rigorously defined in our earlier work [8].

Briefly, the members of the sample were selected randomly from among those registered in the catchment area of the social security of Nancy, as well as in accordance with legislative regulations, from volunteers of that same region. Since those who were selected and invited (to undergo a health examination) were equally free to refuse or to accept, we obviously obtained a population concerned with health and a health examination: however, a compensatory element to this bias was produced by the fact that the majority of those who were invited and who neglected to signal their acceptance in time, came on their own a few months later. Consequently, our sample can be understood as being representative, in the strict sense of the term, only of the population undergoing a health examination from which it is drawn, but in fact remains very close to that of the region of those who were invited. We have attempted to measure the nature of that bias in a pilot study drawn from a larger area than surveyed here [13]: the greatest difference resulting from comparing these two studies concerns primarily the group of themes relative to the value of health and prevention (see below).

At any rate, we intend to retain here, in order to respect the rigour of our method, only the parameter which, in that comparison, appeared in the two samples as the most discriminating at the level of perceptions of health: that of socio-economic category (S.E.C.).[8] However, we reserve the right to mention briefly, toward the end of this paper, the parameter of age in a brief comparison of diachronic and synchronic comparisons: the impact of age on the S.E.C. was examined in Chapter 10 in [8].

To summarize we shall relate our dependent variable, representations of health, only to one independent variable, socio-economic category, the other variables not being controlled.

The open-ended question as an instrument

In order to reconnoitre the terrain, in our first stage of research, we explored the question of the image of health with an open-ended question whose advantages and disadvantages compared to a close-ended question have already been discussed in detail [8]. Let us add that our open-ended question came toward the end of the health examination after three open-ended questions concerning the individual's motivation for coming to the examination, his impressions and his suggestions. It was formulated as follows: 'What is, according to you, the best definition of health?' At first, such a formulation has the inconvenience of appearing rather abstract. One could have, for example, preferred to ask: 'What is health?' However, that second formulation, certainly more concrete, might have in our opinion, the risk of orienting informants toward less varied, more stereotyped, even tautological responses of the type: 'To feel well'. By contrast, the formulation we retained concretely elicited numerous and well-differentiated responses that we shall examine using content analysis.

Content analysis

We have preferred to place, in note 9 the definition and description of our methods for content analysis. Let us only note here that our informants had all the latitude to give more than one element of response. This explains why we collected 6,172 such elements, an average of 1.5 per informant. In fact, problems of quantification were fairly easy to resolve, given that most responses were formulated in a few terms or rather standardized expressions, some (less frequently) being surrounded by structured expresssions of a more sophisticated discourse.

The elements of responses were, little by little, classified into more synthetic themes which, in accord with the title of the question, we shall also call definitions. The regrouping of the elements of responses by theme was effected around the keywords of the constellations of terms spontaneously used by the respondents.

When we speak of spontaneity, we intend only to emphasize the introspective manner by which informants perceive their action in their response to an open-ended question. By contrast their initiative appears *to them* less obvious and their contribution more directed in a close-ended or structured question. In fact, what the informants (knowingly) believe they say spontaneously is an unequally reliable reflection of the multiple and complex social influences that affected them in the course of their education, notably the influences of their different milieux (family, school, occupation, cultural groups) and the increasingly more pervasive influences of the mass media.

In our tabulated results, we only kept the frequency of each theme by S.E.C. expressed in a percentage. We preferred to calculate these percentages on the basis of the totals at the bottom of the columns.

As to the average frequencies for the 4,000 informants, they are, in the right-hand column, calculated on the basis of the 6,172 mentions. It is precisely in relation of this average frequency by theme that the predominance in one or more S.E.C. has been defined: that (or those) showing a percentage equal or superior to 0.2 per cent above the average of all informants. In that total are included those respondents who are not gainfully employed or are otherwise inactive, although they are not always specifically mentioned as such (for example, in Tables I and II) given their heterogeneity and the diversity of their membership in other categories. Furthermore, we preferred to retain from the listing of S.E.C. of the Institut National de la Statistique et des Etudes Economiques (I.N.S.E.E.) only a simplified series, allowing us to contrast manual with non-manual categories: superior cadres (higher class), middle classes, employees, workers, agricultural workers.

The only independent variable taken into consideration in this paper (S.E.C.) having thus been defined, it is now our task to present our results according to the only dependent variable considered here, the perception of health. We shall intentionally abbreviate the presentation of the quantitative aspects of our results, in order to give more importance to the qualitative aspects of the interpretation.

Major results

Because health is also (and indeed first of all) the concern of everyone in any society, whatever its form or political structure, the question 'What is health?' must be asked of each person, whether well or sick, and irrespective of age, sex, occupation, income and educational level.

In other words, parallel to the conceptions of politicians and economists, there is a specific place for a sociopsychological investigation whose purpose is to delineate the images, the analogies, the symbols with which the population defines, for itself, what is meant by 'health'.

This then is the purpose of the open-question we submitted to our sample of 4,000 adults mentioned earlier.

Within the 6,172 responses we obtained, we find a considerable dispersion of themes. This is why, after listing them in a decreasing order of frequencies, then classified according to socio-economic class, we felt the need to group them into ten dominating groups (see Table III).

36 d'Houtaud and Field

A classification according to the frequency of themes mentioned

	Frequency	%	Frequency	%
• More than 400 mentions (Two definitions)				
No. 1 : Not to be sick	472	7.6		
No. 2 : To be at the top of one's form	401	6.5		
Sub-total			873	14.1
• Between 300 and 400 mentions (Three definitions)				
No. 3 : Good physical equilibrium (1)	360	5.8		
No. 4 : Good mental equilibrium	356	5.8		
No. 5 : Joy of living	324	5.2		
Sub-total			1,040	16.8
• Between 200 and 300 mentions (Seven definitions)				
No. 6 : To have a regular preventive examination	263	4.3		
No. 7 : To watch oneself	257	4.2		
No. 8 : To be regularly under medical supervision	251	4.1		
No. 9 : To know oneself well	248	4.0		
No. 10 : The essential	231	3.7		
No. 11 : The greatest wealth	214	3.5		
No. 12 : Life without constaint	208	3.4		
Sub-total			1,672	27.1
• Between 100 and 200 mentions (Twelve definitions)				
No. 13 : Good equilibrium	181	2.9		
No. 14 : Happiness	174	2.8		
No. 15 : Not to feel one's body	169	2.7		
No. 16 : To have a good morale	162	2.6		
No. 17 : To feel well in one's skin	156	2.5		
No. 18 : To have a regular life	155	2.5		
No. 19 : To be able to work	150	2.4		
No. 20 : To lead a healthy life	141	2.2		
No. 21 : To benefit from life	122	2.0		
No. 22 : 'It is better to prevent than to cure'	114	1.8		
No. 23 : Avoid excesses	102	1.8		
No. 24 : To have a balanced diet	100	1.6		
Sub-total			1,726	28.0

Variations in perceptions by social class in a French population 37

		Frequency	%	Frequency	%
	• Between 50 and 100 mentions				
%	(Eight definitions)				
	No. 25 : To be able to face all problems	92	1.5		
	No. 26 : Not to think of illness	78	1.3		
	No. 27 : To be in a good mood	73	1.2		
14.1	No. 28 : A healthy mind in a healthy body	72	1.2		
	No. 29 : Engage in sports	62	1.0		
	No. 30 : Equilibrium in the family	53	0.9		
	No. 31 : Optimism	52	0.8		
	No. 32 : To have a good appetite	52	0.8		
	Sub-total			534	8.7
16.8	• Less than 50 mentions				
	(Nine definitions)				
	No. 33 : To live as much as possible in the open air	49	0.8		
	No. 34 : To see the physician as little as possible	41	0.7		
	No. 35 : Not to fear the future	41	0.7		
	No. 36 : To sleep well	40	0.6		
	No. 37 : Personal unfolding	37	0.6		
	No. 38 : Sobriety	35	0.5		
	No. 39 : Dynamism	32	0.5		
	No. 40 : To rest	27	0.4		
	No. 41 : To live as long as possible	25	0.4		
27.1	Sub-total			327	5.3
	N =			6,172	100.0

Note: The frequent mention of the term 'equilibrium' has permitted us to differentiate sub-themes according to the modifiers used by the respondents. It is precisely this procedure that will allow us to observe variations according to age and S.E.C.

On first sight, the negative definition of health (No. 1) i.e. not to be sick, predominates (472 mentions); if to this we add another definition (No. 26), *sickness* or *illness* is mentioned 550 times. References to *life* are more numerous: No. 5 *Joy of living* (329 mentions); No. 12 *Life without constraint* (208 mentions); No. 21 *To benefit from life* (122 mentions). This gives a total number of mentions of 654, to which one could add No. 33 *To live as much as possible in the open air* (49 mentions), No. 41 *To live as long as possible* (25 mentions), as well

28.0

as the meanings of No. 18 *To have a regular life* (155 mentions), No. 20 *To lead a healthy life* (141 mentions) we come to a total of 1,014 mentions referring to life or one-sixth of all the responses (6,172), almost twice as many as references to sickness or illness. By the same token, the totality of the explicit references to *equilibrium* (Nos 3, 14, 13, 30) yield 950 mentions. The *body* and the *skin* (Nos 15, 17, 28) are mentioned 397 times, and the *physician* (Nos 8, 34) 292 times.

It does not seem to be most productive to regroup these themes *according to their terminological affinities*. For example, the 292 mentions of the physician are not homogeneous: *to be regularly under medical supervision* (251 mentions) and *To see the physician as little as possible* (41 mentions) have an opposite meaning.

This then leads us to a second attempt at an empirical classification of these themes along a socio-economic dimension.

An empiricial classification of themes of health by S.E.C.

Arraying across Table I the simplified series of S.E.C. defined above, we distributed on the vertical axis the 41 synthetic definitions (or themes) so that those that predominate among the higher, then the middle S.E.C. appear at first and those that predominate among manual workers (urban, then rural) are located at the bottom of the list. To facilitate access to the results, we shall first consider only those S.E.C. where each theme is dominant. Thus constituted, Table I reveals three major areas:

– that of the higher and middle S.E.C. alone (A)
– that of the manuals alone (C)
– that of those S.E.C. where the distribution of themes is more complex (B).

At this stage of our presentation, the reader of Table I has every opportunity to familiarize himself, in this entirely empiricial classification, with the 41 themes that were retained; then, before being influenced by our interpretations, to imagine for himself diverse possible systems for a logical organization of the 41 definitions of health.

A logical and scalar classification of health definitions by S.E.C.

We propose in Table II a logical classification of the 41 main definitions of health, such that one could at the same time relate them in more synthetic regroupings and to put in evidence the underlying scalar structure of Table I.

This structure, thus regrouped under 10 headings, gives us Table III. The three first headings predominate among the higher and middle S.E.C. alone and the three last ones among the manuals alone; the

Table I The 41 themes of health and the socio-economic classes zones of their predominance

Socio-economic class (S.E.C.):

	Socio-economic status → / The 41 themes of health ↓	higher-class	middle class	employees	urban workers	rural workers
	1 To see the physician as little as possible	⊕				
	2 Life without constraints	⊕	+			
	3 Not to think of illness	⊕	⊕			
	4 Good physical equilibrium	⊕	+			
	5 Good mental equilibrium	⊕	+			
A	6 Not to feel one's body	+	+			
	7 A healthy mind in a healthy body	⊕	+			
	8 Personal unfolding	⊕	⊕			
	9 Dynamism	⊕	⊕			
	10 To benefit from life		⊕			
	11 Not to fear the future		⊕			
	12 Good equilibrium	+	⊕	+		
	13 To feel well in 'one's skin'	⊕	+	+		
	14 To be able to face all problems		⊕	+		
	15 Optimism		⊕	+		
	16 Equilibrium in the family	+	+			⊕
	17 The greatest wealth			⊕		+
B	18 The essential			+	+	⊕
	19 To watch oneself			+	+	⊕
	20 To have a regular life			+	+	⊕
	21 To be at the top of one's form			+	+	⊕

40 d'Houtaud and Field

Table I (cont.):

Socio-economic class (S.E.C.):

	Socio-economic status→ / The 41 themes of health ↓	higher-class	middle class	employees	urban workers	rural workers
	22 To be in a good mood			⊕	+	
	23 To live as much as possible in the open air			+	⊕	
B	24 To sleep well			⊕	⊕	
	25 To live as long as possible			⊕	+	
	26 Joy of living			⊕		
	27 Happiness			⊕		
	28 To have a balanced diet			⊕		
	29 To have a good morale				⊕	
	30 To lead a healthy life				⊕	
	31 Engage in sports				⊕	
	32 To have a good appetite				⊕	
	33 To rest				⊕	
	34 'It is better to prevent than to cure'				⊕	
	35 Not to be sick				⊕	
C	36 Avoid excesses				+	⊕
	37 Sobriety				+	⊕
	38 To have a regular preventative health examination				+	⊕
	39 To know oneself well				+	⊕
	40 To be regularly under medical supervision				⊕	+
	41 To be able to work				+	⊕

A cross + indicates socio-economic classes where the definition has a percentage superior to the general average. ⊕ indicates the category whose percentage is the highest.

Table II Logical classification of themes of health according to socio-economic class (6, 172 themes from 4,000 individuals who visited the Centre de Médecine Préventive from January 1, 1971 to May 15, 1974)

S.E.C. →	higher class	middle class	employees	urban workers	rural workers	not gainfully employed	TOTAL
Life without constraints	5.0	4.6	2.6	2.4	2.0	2.9	3.4
To benefit from life	1.9	3.0	1.6	1.4		2.2	2.0
Not to think of illness	1.6	2.3	0.9	0.6	0.6	1.2	1.3
See the physician as little as possible	0.9	0.5	0.6	0.8	0.6	0.6	0.7
HEDONISTIC USE OF LIFE	9.4	10.4	5.7	5.2	3.2	6.9	7.4
Good physical equilibrium	9.9	7.5	5.5	2.8	3.2	5.1	5.8
Good mental equilibrium	9.0	7.7	5.8	2.6	3.2	5.2	5.8
Good equilibrium	3.4	3.6	3.3	1.6	0.6	3.3	2.9
Equilibrium in the family	1.3	1.1	0.7	0.6	2.7	0.5	0.9
EQUILIBRIUM	23.6	19.9	15.3	7.6	9.7	14.1	15.4
Not to feel one's body	3.5	3.3	1.8	1.5	1.3	4.0	2.7
To feel well 'in one's skin'	4.4	2.9	2.7	0.8	1.9	2.4	2.5
'A healthy mind in a healthy body'	1.9	1.6	0.9	0.7		1.1	1.2
REFERENCE TO THE BODY	9.8	7.8	5.4	3.0	3.2	7.5	6.4
To be able to face all problems	1.6	2.0	1.8	0.9	0.6	1.3	1.5
Optimism	0.7	1.2	1.1	0.5	0.6	0.7	0.8
Not to fear the future	0.6	1.2	0.8	0.5	0.6	0.3	0.7
Personal unfolding	0.9	0.9	0.5	0.2	0.6	0.5	0.6
Dynamism	0.7	0.7	0.2	0.5		0.5	0.5
VITALITY	4.5	6.0	4.4	2.6	2.4	3.3	4.1

Table II (cont.):

S.E.C. →	higher class	middle class	employees	urban workers	rural workers	not gainfully employed	TOTAL
Joy of living	3.9	4.8	6.1	5.3	5.3	5.8	5.2
Happiness	2.4	2.7	3.3	2.9	2.6	2.7	2.8
To have a good morale	1.5	1.9	2.7	3.5	1.9	3.4	2.6
To be in a good mood	0.7	1.0	1.6	1.4	0.6	1.0	1.2
PSYCHOLOGICAL WELL-BEING	8.5	10.4	13.7	13.1	10.4	12.9	11.8
To have a regular life	1.7	2.3	2.7	2.4	2.6	3.4	2.5
To lead a healthy life	2.1	1.7	2.4	2.8	1.3	2.4	2.4
Avoid excesses	1.6	1.5	1.6	2.3	2.7	1.1	1.8
To have a balanced diet	1.4	1.3	2.0	1.7	0.6	1.7	1.6
Engage in sport	0.8	0.8	1.1	1.2		1.2	1.0
To have a good appetite	0.3	0.8	0.9	1.4		0.8	0.8
To live as much as possible in the open air	0.4	0.3	1.0	1.1	0.6	1.0	0.8
To sleep well	0.2	0.7	0.9	0.9		0.7	0.6
Sobriety	0.4	0.4	0.5	1.0	1.3	0.3	0.5
To rest	0.5	0.3	0.2	0.9		0.3	0.4
HYGIENE	9.4	10.1	13.3	15.7	9.1	12.9	12.4
The essential	2.2	3.5	5.0	4.2	5.9	3.0	3.7
The greatest wealth	3.5	3.6	4.7	2.0	4.5	3.6	3.5
VALUE OF HEALTH	5.7	7.1	9.7	6.2	10.4	6.6	7.2

Continued overleaf

Table II (cont.):

To have a regular preventive health examination	2.8	2.9	3.4	7.0	9.7	4.0	4.3
To watch oneself	3.4	2.9	5.0	5.2	5.2	3.9	4.2
To know oneself well	4.5	4.0	2.7	4.9	5.8	4.0	4.0
'It is better to prevent than to cure'	1.9	1.5	1.9	2.3	1.3	1.7	1.8
To live as long as possible	0.2	0.1	0.9	0.7		0.1	0.4
PREVENTION	12.8	11.4	13.9	20.1	22.0	13.7	14.7
To be at the top of one's form	6.6	5.7	6.7	7.0	9.7	5.9	6.5
To be able to work	2.3	2.1	2.0	2.9	7.1	2.3	2.4
PHYSICAL APTITUDES	8.9	7.8	8.7	9.9	16.8	8.2	8.9
Not to be sick	5.9	6.7	6.6	10.1	6.5	8.4	7.6
To be regularly under medical supervision	1.5	2.4	3.4	6.5	5.8	5.5	4.1
ABSENCE OF SICKNESS	7.4	9.1	10.0	16.6	12.3	13.9	11.7
	100.0	100.0	100.0	100.0	100.0	100.0	100.0
Number of mentions	953	1189	1279	1317	154	1280	6172
Number of respondents	534	680	797	997	125	867	4000

Shaded areas are those where the themes predominate.

other four constitute an intermediate zone of transition analogous to that of (B) in Table I.

Table III The 10 headings of the themes of health and the socio-economic zones of their predominance

S.E.C. / Headings (thematic groupings)	higher class	middle class	employees	urban workers	rural workers
1 Hedonistic use of life	+	⊕			
2 Equilibrium	⊕	+			
3 Reference to the body	⊕	+			
4 Vitality	+	⊕	+		
5 Psychological well-being			⊕	+	
6 Hygiene			+	⊕	
7 Value of health			+		⊕
8 Prevention				+	⊕
9 Physical aptitudes				+	⊕
10 Absence of sickness				⊕	+

A cross + indicates the S.E.C. where the group has a percentage higher than the average.
• indicates the S.E.C. where the percentage is the highest.

Let us remark, incidentally, that the way of labelling the 10 headings comes from the interpretation of the investigator, whereas those of the 41 fundamental definitions reflect the language of the respondents. Thus, there manifests itself, in the course of the analytical process, a methodologically interesting tension between the empirical data where the diversity is uneasily rejoined by the procedures of perception of the observer desirous to remain neutral, and the rational redistribution of the data, where the more abstract schemes of conceptualization of the interpreter impose *a priori* structures, however creative of meaning. In other words, the process of interpretation, while seemingly constricting the original richness of the empirical data, brings a final wealth of meaning: in giving meaning, the interpretation intervenes as a bridge between the demands of reality in its fundamental diversity, and that of the rational in its indispensable simplification.

Critical discussion

Now that the reader has progressively discovered and analysed the major mentions that were gathered and the three different ways to classify them, it is important to come back to our central question: what is the meaning of health in the eyes of the population we surveyed?

To do this, we shall sketch, basing ourselves on the two other tables (IV and V), more synthetic views of the total data gathered. On the one hand, a somewhat bipolar interpretation seems satisfactory to interpret most of the data. On the other, some of the data that seem to resist a bipolar interpretation, suggest a more differentiated approach using a tripartite classification. We shall thus examine, one after the other, these two complementary approaches, before asking ourselves, thirdly, what are the limits of the present investigation and what avenues of further research they suggest.

The 10 synthetic regroupings of the definition of health: an attempt at a bipolar interpretation

The three preceding tables reveal a similar structure which appears most clearly in Table II: the first categories of themes are clearly much more predominant among higher and middle S.E.C. The last categories predominate among manual workers, urban or rural.

Table IV Two parallel classifications on the ten groupings of themes of health

	Series A	Series B
	Predominance of the 'I', of internalization, of personal norms	Predominance of the 'one',* of externalization, of social norms
1 Objective criteria	Hedonistic use of life	Value of health
2 Subjective criteria	Reference to the body	Psychological well-being
3 Means	Equilibrium	Hygiene Prevention
4 Objectives	Vitality	Absence of sickness Physical aptitudes

*in French *on* equivalent to the German *man*

Two series of groupings

Such a disparity among the themes and groupings of themes by S.E.C. serve as a basis for their distribution into two series (Series A and

46 d'Houtaud and Field

Series B), i.e. precisely the ones that Table IV brings out into clear relief.

Series A characterizes mainly the higher and middle S.E.C., whose objective criteria of health are centered on the *hedonistic use of life*, whereas those of the others, in Series B, are based on the *value of health*. The subjective criteria of the higher and middle classes are related to the body, whereas those of the others are to psychological well-being. As means, the higher and middle classes prefer *equilibrium*, the others *hygiene* and *prevention*. Finally, against *vitality* as an objective of the higher and middle classes, *absence of sickness* and *physical aptitudes* are the objectives of the others.

The associations that Table IV proposes have the advantage of referring to the totality of the 10 headings of themes. But one can, in these more partial associations, emphasize, for example, the *reference to the body* among the higher and middle classes and *physical aptitudes* among the others.

At the level of the 41 themes (Table II), one can bring together the absence of sickness among the employees and manuals (*'not to be sick'*, *'to be regularly under medical supervision'*) with two of the four definitions of the *hedonistic use of life* among the higher and middle classes (*'not to think of sickness'*, *'to see the physician as little as possible'*). In the first case, the average frequency of the two themes is close to 12 per cent, in the second case it is only 2 per cent. On one side a positive formulation, on the other a negative one. These differences explain why we have preferred not to combine the four themes into a single whole, but to associate the two euphemisms of the higher and middle classes with the grouping of the *hedonistic use of life*, whose global orientation they correctly reflect, and to emphasize the negativity of the two perceptions of health which predominate among the manuals: health defined by the negation of sickness and by the control of the physician. In this respect, the grouping of the *hedonistic use of life* among the higher and middle classes which we made to correspond in Table IV so that of the *value of health* among the manuals could equally have been contrasted to that of non-sickness, as two complementary ways of characterizing health.

The bipolar interpretation

Whatever the various possibilities to correlate groupings or definitions, the bipolar interpretation that we just proposed in Table IV has the advantage of associating, in the A series, themes where the 'I', the internalization, the personal norms predominate, whereas, in the B series, the 'one' (*on* in French), the externalization, the social norms predominate. In other words, against the more personalized conception of the higher and middle classes which emphasizes the realization of the self for the self, there corresponds among the manuals a more socialized conception, where it is rather a question of the integration of the self into society and into the tasks which society demands of individuals. It is not difficult to discern in such complementary representations of health the *reflection of the corresponding roles of mastery on the one hand and of the execution of social tasks on the other*.

Let us also use the opposition which the Romans used to differentiate their activities by the two terms of *uti* and *frui*. The first one characterizes activities oriented toward the utilitarian, i.e. what is concerned with, what is aimed at something else; the second one is typical of activities which are an end in themselves, which suggest a certain form of detachment and bring to the author real enjoyment. In the first perspective, health becomes utilitarian behaviour: it is the means to reach other ends. In the second perspective, health is envisaged as a value (the Latin term *valere* means primarily 'to be in good health'), i.e. it makes the individual a value in himself: man is then interested in health for itself and seeks it for himself.

In sum, we have two polar conceptions of health, between which individuals and social groups oscillate, and between which the different socio-economic classes array themselves according to the benefits which they derive from society or which they contribute to it. It is perfectly understandable that those who manage social tasks tend also to appropriate their health and to cultivate it for their own purposes, whereas those who perform these tasks tend to alienate themselves from their health, and to place it mainly at the disposal of society, which usually requires their labour.

The preceding paragraph has presented what, in Table IV, leads to the establishment of a bipolar interpretation of the 41 themes culled, let's remember, from the 6,172 elements of answers provided by our 4,000 respondents. But it also has attempted to impose restrictions to this interpretation, by revealing limits. However, several of these go in the direction of a tripartite structure in function of which Table V proposes another possible reorganization of ten regroupings of definitions according to four perspectives at three levels.

The extreme level opposes the manuals (urban and rural workers) to the higher and middle classes, whereas the intermediate level is characterized by the employees to which are added, for certain themes, the urban workers: This corresponds to urban informants who are not of the higher and middle classes.

Two perspectives with a tripartite structure

The first perspective implicitly responds to the question: *How does one recognize being in good health*? One would thus move from an objective negative criterion, *non-illness*, to two subjective positive criteria, *psychological well-being*, then to the *hedonistic use of life*. The urban manuals (see Table II) clearly dominate for *non-illness* when compared to rural workers, and place themselves in a second position for *psychological well-being* behind the employees; as to the *hedonistic use of life*, middle classes precede higher class, employees being on this point much closer to the manuals. Level 1 verifies the usual embarrassment in perceiving and positively defining what health is:[10] one resorts openly to notions of the vocabulary of illness, either the contrary of health (illness itself) or what permits one to verify the state of non-illness (the control or check-up of the physician). Level 2[11] resorts to responses that are already more personalized, but only the psychic being escapes social dispossession. Health is then evoked with sentiments which appear in the happy moments of life. We are dealing here with city-dwellers of a rather modest social standing altogether. At Level 3, we arrive to the superior hierarchical elements of society and to ego-centric attitudes of a more radical appropriation of health. Illness appearing as a radical constraint, health receives here the image of freedom and becomes an integral part of the individual personality, of the *ego*.

Table V Perceptions of health according to four perspectives, by three social levels

S.E.C. 4 perspectives	(Level 1) Rural workers	(Level 2) Employees	(Level 3) Higher and middle class
	↑ Urban workers →	↑	
1st perspective . . .	non-illness	psychological well-being	hedonistic use of life
2nd perspective. . .	prevention	hygiene	equilibrium
3rd perspective . . .	physical aptitudes		reference to the body
4th perspective . . .	↑ value of health →	↑↑ vitality →	↑

The underlying question in the second perspective is this one: *How does one have access to health*? According to the order of the three levels, one would pass from *prevention* to *hygiene*, then to *equilibrium*. Rural workers and, in second position, urban workers highly dominate over the others at Level 1 (cf. Table II). Urban workers precede employees at Level 2. *Equilibrium* is clearly a prerogative of the higher and middle classes at Level 3, particularly the higher classes:

their frequency is triple that of urban workers, that of the middle classes, which comes after it, being double that of rural workers. As a preference of the most-favoured social strata of modern societies, *equilibrium* refers either to an interior harmony of the individual (for example between the physical and the mental), or to an exterior harmony (for example with the surrounding milieu: cosmos or society). As to *hygiene*, it is the response required by urbanization where infectious diseases have, for a long time, spread more easily; it presumes individuals who are convinced of its merits. In any case, it is less felt as a requirement by the rural workers, whose attraction to preventive health examinations and to a good knowledge or supervision of health explains its dominance in the area of prevention. *Hygiene* and *prevention* intervene as precautions, whereas *equilibrium* is a latent reference to social organization of which the higher and middle classes are the privileged beneficiaries.

Certainly one should not exclude the fact that, in part, these different terms may be interpreted as referring to the same meaning and that, by the same token, the three different meanings fulfil here, at the various cultural levels of society, equivalent functions. Nevertheless, even with this hypothesis, it is significant that health is perceived and represented as equilibrium in proportion to the degree of integration of individuals in the economic and cultural life of a country.

Two perspectives with a bipolar structure

The last two perspectives represent what is irreducible in the bipolar interpretation: in one case, the employees remain rather behind manuals and the higher and middle classes (3rd perspective); in the other, on the contrary, they are associated with both (4th perspective).

In the 3rd perspective, it is the role of the body in health that is explicit: *To what end is the body a privileged point of application of health*? One finds again, at the bottom of the social scale, what was in the course of previous millennia the absolute priority: to survive through physical force, today chiefly from working, earlier from hunting and from warring, in particular. Therefore we find among manuals the reference to health as *physical aptitudes* (whether it is *to be at the top of one's form* or *to be able to work*) where the body is only an instrument for the individual working simultaneously for himself and for society. By contrast, the improvement and the emancipation of the higher and middle classes in social life also involve the cultivation of their own bodies as of their own health. Since then, attention has focused on what to do with that body thus rendered available, if not to place it at the centre of personal life and specially at the centre of leisure. All at once, the body is less destined to exercise an instrumental role than to localize the *I* in the living body: in this case health appears as a quality permitting the body to be able to improve each individual *ego* toward greater self-realization and better well-being, toward expressive use. There remains the 4th perspective: *What is the value of health*? The only time when employees and rural workers dominate together is at the level of the two definitions presenting health as a value: one observes a stronger insistence of the workers for the definition that views health as *the essential* and, correspondingly, a stronger insistence on the part of the higher and middle classes for the other view which considers health as the *greatest wealth*. One is then justified to ask, does health not appear more to those who are privileged as *wealth* and to those who are more disadvantaged in social life as *the essential*. In the measure to which those who insist most on *the greatest wealth* are employees and the most insistent on the *essential* are rural workers one should differentiate more: the most inclined to compare health to wealth would be those who expect more improvement in their income.

Anyway, whether it appears *the essential* or the *greatest wealth*, health well verifies the etymology, already mentioned above, of the Latin verb *valere* (to be in good health): it is the fundamental value whereby other goods acquire more value, and without which they lose all their value. This is why, in that last perspective, higher and middle classes prefer to place more emphasis on the definitions which we have regrouped under the theme of *vitality* and according to which health is not only *personal unfolding* and *dynamism*, but particularly among the middle classes which are trailed here by the employees, *optimism, to be able to face all problems*, and *not to be afraid of the future*. One could not more clearly place health in relation to its role of purveyor of survival, i.e. with a function of salvation.[12] This grouping of vitality manifests precisely an affinity and a continuity with that of the *hedonistic use of life*, in the measure to which it expresses the individual *will-to-live* whereas, dominating among rural workers and employees, health takes up again the two formulas of folk wisdom which rejoin that of a French manuscript of the fifteenth century: 'Who has health, has everything; who does not have health, has nothing.'

Why three levels?

Thus, following Table IV, Table V permits a complementary interpretation of Table II. One assuredly can ask oneself *What do the three levels represent*?

Is this only a logical ordering in the classification of 10 headings of definitions? Is one justified to recognize there, in addition, an order of chronological succession in the evolution of individuals and groups?

In other words, are we dealing with an average evolution in the course of transition from the countryside to the city or in the course of social mobility, beginning with the manuals and going to the higher and middle classes? Our sample, drawn only from Lorraine, permits us to pose the question, but not to answer it in a completely satisfactory manner. We have attempted elsewhere [8] to give it a partial answer, in confronting the synchronic perspective of the classes, presented here, with the diachronic perspective of age groups. It seems that a correspondence exists for certain themes (themes common to manuals and the aged, others to higher and middle classes and the young), but not for all themes. It is sufficient here to suggest that the problem, which poses again an important aspect of the interpretation of the tripartite structure, is complex and should be the object of further research.

Limits and expectations of the present research

The problem of the correspondences between the synchronic and diachronic perspective does not constitute the only limitation, which suggests a continuation of the research undertaken. We would like to consider below three other points, equally objects of discussion: the quantification utilized, the difficult semantic problem of the terms used in different classes, and the contribution of our research to the notion of representation.

Quantification of responses

The statistical approach that we utilized to distinguish the classes (as, incidentally, the groups by sex, by age, by successive group of 500 informants), has certainly led to highly significant differences, but at the level of the 10 groupings of themes or headings i.e., when definitions by similar socio-economic predominance accumulate small differences: it is here, as we have noted, that the interpretation is a process external to the data, bringing to the latter a significance that is the rational work of the researcher. On the other hand, at the individual level of the terms and of themes coming from the respondents, the differences among categories (and groups) do not impose themselves so manifestly. The meaning brought by the interpretation is obvious only at the level of the elaborated structures to which finally one adapts reality at the expense of its diversity.

On this point, our contribution has, at least, allowed us better to pose that problem of quantification; for, starting from its results, one is in a better position to propose research hypotheses in function of which one will then be able more rigorously to organize the collection of the data, then their handling. For example, it would be better not to take up the entire population without prior selection, because too many individual situations do not lend themselves easily to the S.E.C. classification of the I.N.S.E.E., but to select, at the major levels of the social scale, some categories whose internal homogeneity is not questionable, on which to confirm or disconfirm whether there is a predominance of the definitions taken in isolation, before proceeding, secondly, to the regrouping of the only definitions that present the same individual socio-occupational predominances and logical affinities.

The significance of the terms according to different categories

Even if, with a more satisfactory quantification of the definitions, one were able to extract the most specific terms of each category, the problem of the contents of the expressions and of the significance would remain whole. Clearly, do some terms receive in different milieux the same acceptance? Is the same term employed in different milieux with different meanings? These are two questions that singularly complicate the study of the representations of health. Up to now we have hardly tackled the problem. Here, in the discussion, it is important to formulate it as clearly as possible.

Let us say, briefly, that the research that we have undertaken has certainly led to some results such that they have permitted us positively to locate the elements of the problem, but that it was not conceived to resolve it. In other words, the materials we have collected pose that question at the level of their handling: they do not lend themselves to a completely satisfactory elucidation. For even a partial elucidation we can, within the framework of this article, only refer the reader once more to our doctoral dissertation [8]. For an even better elucidation, it would be necessary to envisage the mounting of a supplementary investigation. For example, as a follow-up to an inquiry of the type that the preceding paragraph proposes, it would be important, through a multi-disciplinary team of linguists, psychologists, sociologists, to subject a small sub-sample of respondents to interviews meant to explore the semantic contents of several supposedly interchangeable terms and to bring out the terms that have presumably different contents in different milieux.

The notion of representation applied in the health sector

The more the access to the S.E.C. is difficult, and the more the access to the meaning of terms poses questions, the more uncertain becomes the notion of representation, at least in its possible applications in the domain that health occupies in the immense territory of the language.

Every social representation contains cognitive elements and a reference to behaviours, and confronts the experience of the individual with the norms and the information that are current in the cultural universe where he lives.

The representation of health verifies the remark of S. Moscovici in his preface to the work of Herzlich [12]: 'The map of social interactions is legible through images, information and symbols.' Indeed, even if we have not pinpointed the process of the most pertinent quantification nor elucidated all the questions that the semantic analysis poses to our terminological material, at least let us dare to hope a justification of our exploration of the area in the fact that it has led us to rejoin the complementary social roles of the manuals and of the higher and middle classes through their unequal emphasis on themes relating to health.

On her part, Herzlich has observed that 'the representation of a particular object is part of that, ampler (representation), of the society in its entirety.' Yet, we have noted that two extreme conceptions in the bipolar structure of representations of health make it (health), either a means to better align oneself with the very purposes of society even at the expense of the individual personality, or the additional instrument of recovery of society for the purposes of the individual: the appropriation and the alienation of health go together with work and its fruits. Is this not a verification that the representation of health is as much a model of behaviour meant to be applied to social reality as a cognitive reflection of the values and of the knowledge current in society? Is this not as much the concrete reaction of the individual who integrates himself more with his social environment, or of the one who chooses to dominate it for his advantage, as it is communication among the members of a community? Is it not a faithful witness of the conflicts that oppose social partners and their manner of perceiving their reciprocal interests?

More specifically, it is here that we find again what distinguishes the approach of Herzlich from our own. Everything derives from the fact that hers is interested at the same time in illness *and* health, whereas ours takes into consideration health alone, and that she has on the other hand carried out her investigation among members of the privileged classes, whereas we have listened both to manuals as well as to non-manuals. Precisely on that last point, their relationship to society has appeared to us basically different. In a privileged class, health is indeed appropriated by the individual and illness attributed to life styles imposed by society. Whereas in the disadvantaged categories, health is utilized for the benefit of the purposes of society; it is alienated from the individual.

A second divergence has to do with the body, whose role in the

Table VI Socio-economic classes (S.E.C.) as used in this study

Categories used in the tables (French categories)	Includes the following:	Categories in French – Numbers correspond to those used in the Liste des Groupes et des Catégories Socio-Professionnelles, published by the Institut National de la Statistique et des Etudes Economiques, Code des Catégories socio-professionnelles, 1977, 6th edition, pp. 15-60
higher class (cadres supérieurs)	owners and higher managers of industry, trade; owners of smaller enterprises (includes artisans) professionals; professors	33 Ingénieurs 30 Professions libérales 32 Professeurs 34 Cadres administratifs supérieurs 21 Industries 22 Artisans 27 Petits 26 et gros commerçants
middle class (cadres moyens)	teachers and technicians; middle managers; medical and social workers	43 Techniciens 42 Services médicaux et sociaux 41 Instituteurs 44 Cadres administratifs moyens
employees (employés)	office employees, in private business and public services; clerical workers; white-collar employees; librarians, etc.	53 Employés de commerce 51 Employés de bureau

Continued overleaf

Table VI (cont.):

urban workers (ouvriers)	foremen; workers of all types; mechanics; service personnel; apprentices; waiters; domestics; etc.	60 Contremaîtres 61 Ouvriers qualifiés 63 Ouvriers spécialisés 67 Apprentis ouvriers 68 Manoeuvres, etc . . .
rural workers (agriculteurs)	farm owners; gardeners; salaried agricultural workers; cattle breeders; forest workers	00 Agriculteurs exploitants 10 Salariés agricoles
not gainfully employed (non actifs)	students; housewives; retired persons (all categories)	91 Etudiants 98 Femmes au foyer 93 Retraités, etc . . .

sample of the 80 persons interviewed by Herzlich, [12] is limited to that of a localization of illness. What has, by contrast, struck us in the responses of our 4,000 respondents, is the importance of the body, whether for some it is placed at the service of society during work, thanks to non-illness, under medical control, or whether among others it serves as a support to health in a perspective for the development of the individual personality and for the enjoyment of life.

Finally, is the analysis of Herzlich not altered by the absence of manuals? And is not the representation of health that she obtains narrowly subordinate to that of illness – not to say obliterated by it – which is only the other side of the same coin, if not the exception that confirms the rule, in the sense that L.S. Kubie wrote that health is a rare state which is, however, not pathological? In the same way that we have preferred the instrument of the open-ended question, because it gives access to a large number of individuals coming from all social categories, to the interview, which certainly deepens the data provided, but with only a very restricted number of subjects: by the same token we have chosen to investigate what is health by itself and for itself alone, rather than what it becomes in the shadow of its opposite (illness), so overwhelming in societies where it lends itself to exploitation. Would this not be the reason for which, in our 41 themes, we have come across so many terms connected with life, with well-being, with a healthy use of our environment, and so few terms which evoke the obsessive image of illness or of the physician who treats it?

It is possible from now on for the reader to reflect ahead to all the implications of our choices as to the notion itself of representation. This representation also appears, in particular, to be a point either of revelation or of concealment of the insidious interference of the investigator or of the interpreter of the oral or written responses.

Summary

According to the bipolar interpretation, it is possible to organize our 10 headings of health definitions into two socio-economic areas, which distinguish themselves through numerous traits: that of the manuals along the line of utility, of the *one*, and of the social; that of the higher and middle S.E.C. along the line of the enjoyment, of the *I*, of the personal. Following the tripartite structure, these 10 groupings or headings of themes of health array themselves in three levels along four perspectives. Globally, one would go from the manuals (level 1) to the higher and middle classes (level 3) through the intermediary of the town dwellers (level 2) who are employees, who are joined by workers for certain themes where they distinguish themselves from the rural workers. Thus one would go from *absence of sickness* to *psychological well-being*, then to the *hedonistic use of life*, when it is a question of characterizing health. Similarly, one would go from *prevention* to *hygiene*, then to *equilibrium* when it is a question of access to health or to improving it.

The limits of our sample (it is from Lorraine and is tied to preventive health examinations) have only allowed us to pose here the problem of the perception of health by analysing certain methodological aspects of the psycho-social approach utilized in such research.

Institut National de la Santé et de la Recherche Medicale
Nancy, France
and
Department of Sociology
Boston University

Notes

1. This paper is the result of the collaboration of the two authors in the following sense: the research, the analysis and the results are those of the senior author. The English translation and version were done by the junior author, in consultation, and indeed negotiation with the senior one. The translation posed certain thorny problems, raised by cultural differences, in the meaning of the terms and expressions that did not have their precise English equivalents. The process of translation served, at the same time, to refine, re-define and sharpen certain of the concepts, findings and conclusions.
2. For a definition of the terms *représentation, attitude, opinion, conduite* (behaviour) we refer the reader to [8].
3. The concept of 'representations' was developed particularly in French sociology by Emile Durkheim ('social life consists essentially of representation') he wrote in his sociological study of suicide [9, p. 352], by Mauss [10], by Moscovici [11], and by Herzlich [12].
4. The English translation of the image or representation of health caused considerable difficulties, a reflection of the fact that such representations are deeply embedded in the total culture and do not benefit from a standardized definition such as is found in the International Classification of Diseases. For example, we translated 8 – *Epanouissement* as 'personal unfolding'. Actually the term means blooming, expanding; perhaps expansiveness or development would have done. 9 – *Dynamisme* was translated as 'dynamism', again, not a completely accurate rendering of the connotation of the term. Perhaps drive or energy would have done better. 13 – *Se sentir bien dans sa peau* we translated literally to 'feel well in one's skin', though the meaning is one of ease and physical well-being, perhaps being comfortable with oneself. 21 – *Pleine*

forme was translated as 'To be at the top of one's form', might have been translated into the more American vernacular as 'firing on all cylinders'.

5. We have already discussed the respective advantages and the disadvantages of the open-ended versus the structured question in our state dissertation [8].
6. Whereas Herzlich speaks of a social representation in the *singular* according to a perspective that Moscovici had already made familiar, we intentionally use the *plural* (representaions or images of health) to locate our analysis at a methodological level quite distinct here.
7. For the two parts of this paper, we follow quite closely the outline of our publication [14] to which we refer the reader, specially for a more complete development of the critical discussion. It is understood that we did not hesitate to introduce here certain modifications suggested by a new reflection on the subject and particularly by the beneficial demands of translation into English.
8. For an explanation of the socio-economic classes (S.E.C.) used in this study, and for French–English equivalents, see Table VI.
9. Generally speaking, classical research methods (historical, literary, juridical, psychological, etc.) are primarily qualitative, relying chiefly on the intuitive and global perceptions of observers: they present all the pitfalls of non-systematic research. The more recently developed procedure of contents analysis seeks to substitute for the personal impressions of the observer a more standardized procedure for gathering data susceptible to scientific treatment.

   In quantitative analysis, the number of times is the criterion; in qualitative analysis what is important may be sought in the novelty of the themes, the interest they present, even if their frequency is low. Both types of analysis may focus on what is latent in the manifest language, for example in symbols. At the initial stage a qualitative analysis may furnish the necessary categories for a rigorous quantitative analysis at a further stage (see Grawitz [18], 628–72).

   Without denying the practical utility of this analytical procedure, which must satisfy, just like the other techniques of the social sciences, criteria of objectivity, reliability, validity, generalizability, one must recognize at the same time the reality and the limits of its scientific value.

   In the specific case of our research, it is a matter of a psycho-social investigation of an exploratory character, having as its goal the creation of written communication materials by means of an open-ended question on health. The unit of analysis chosen has been the response to each open-ended question.

   The constitution of the categories was realized, step by step, starting from the first thousand responses: from the first hundreds, the researcher gathered the great variety of terms and expressions through which the respondents gave their opinions; little by little, a process of regrouping of the terms took place around those most apt to express the themes that emerged; in a few instances, we had, on the contrary, to subdivide numerically very important themes (for example, that of equilibrium) into sub-themes comprising quite distinctive variations (for example, good equilibrium, physical equilibrium, mental equilibrium, equilibrium in the family) or into formulations indicative of a well-differentiated manner of perceiving reality (for instance, not to be sick, not to think of illness). In this manner, an empirical list of 41 themes (or definitions) of health was obtained, which was the subject of several trials according to the affinities of meanings.

   It is in proceeding to the constitution of the grid of Table II that we very quickly noted the scatter of the definitions between the two poles corresponding to the higher and middle classes and manual (urban and agricultural) workers. In associating, along the scale thus obtained, the distribution of the definitions by their socio-economic variables we hypothesized that some among them could constitute an intermediary grouping between those that clearly characterize higher and middle classes and those that clearly characterize manual workers. This led to the idea of tripartite structure explicit in Table V that goes beyond the bipolar distribution expressed in Table IV.

By associating the 41 definitions of health at the level of the 10 groupings that were finally adopted, we have obtained the highly significant differences below (cited in our Dissertation [7] Vol. II, page 58).

10. See, for example, the popular proverb, 'He who is in good health is rich without knowing it.'
11. Cf. the adjective *bon* (good) in *bonheur* (happiness), *bon moral* (good morale), and *bonne humeur* (good spirits).
12. In Latin the same word *salus* designates religious salvation as it does health, as well as salutation; one finds this again in the Germanic languages with *heil*, *heilen*, *heilig* [16, 17].

References

1. Estes, C.L. and Gerard, L.E., 'Social Research in Health and Medicine: A Selected Bibliography,' in Freeman, H.E., Levine, S. and Reeder, L.G., *Handbook of Medical Sociology* (3rd ed.), Englewood Cliffs, N.J., Prentice Hall, 1979, part II, 479–88.
2. Koos, E., *The Health of Regionville: What the People Thought and Did About It*, Hafner, New York, 1954 and 1967.
3. Kirscht, J.P. et al., 'A national study of health beliefs', *Journal of Health and Human Behaviour*, 7, 248–54, Winter, 1966.
4. Nall, F.C. II and Speilberg, J., 'Social and cultural factors in the responses of Mexican-Americans to medical treatment', *Journal of Health and Human Behaviour*, 8, 200–308, December 1967.
5. Stacey, M. and Homans, H., 'The sociology of health and illness: its present state, future prospects and potential for health research', *Sociology*, 12, 281–307, 1978.
6. Stacey, M., 'Main theoretical and methodological orientations in contemporary sociology: the case of the sociology of health and illness in Britain', Presented at the International Sociological Association, Research Council Meeting, Jablonna, Poland 1980 (mimeo).
7. Straus, R., 'Sociological determinants of health beliefs and behavior', *American Journal of Public Health*, 20, 105–10, January, 1970.
8. d'Houtaud, A., *Recherches en Lorraine sur les facteurs psycho-sociaux de la santé*, Thèse de doctorat ès Lettres et Sciences humaines, Dijon, Librairie H. Champion, Paris, 3 vols, 1977.
9. Durkheim, E., *Le Suicide, étude de sociologie*, Alcan, Paris, 1972; Routledge & Kegan Paul, London.
10. Mauss, M., 'Divisions et proportions des divisions de la sociologie', *Année Sociologique*, 2, 98–176, 1925.

11. Moscovici, Sa., *La Psychanalyse, son image et son public. Étude sur la représentation sociale de la psychanalyse*, PUF, Paris, 1976.
12. Herzlich. C., *Santé et maladie: analyse d'une représentation sociale* (Preface de S. Moscovici), Mouton, Paris-LeHaye, 1969. An English translation is also available.
13. d'Houtaud, A., 'Les représentations de la santé – recherches dans un centre de bilans de santé en Lorraine', *Rev. Int. Education pour la santé*, 19, 99–118 and 173–88, 1976.
14. d'Houtaud, A., 'L'image de la santé dans une population Lorraine: approche psycho-sociale des représentations de la santé', *Rev. Epidem et Santé Publ.*, 26, 299–320, 1978.
15. d'Houtaud, A., Poulizac, H., Senault, A., 'A la recherche d'une pédagogie de la santé: enquête d'opinions et d'attitudes à propos d'un bilan familial de la santé', *Rev. Int. Education pour la santé*, 16, encart de 48 pages, 1973.
16. d'Houtaud, A., 'Santé et salutation: pour une approche historique et sémantique du terme santé', *Rev. Int. Education pour la santé*, 1978, 21 (4), 277–83.
17. d'Houtaud, A., 'Santé et salut', *Rev. Int. Education pour la santé*, 22 (1), 49–56, 1979.
18. Gravitz, M., *Méthodes des sciences sociales*, Paris, Diffusion française, 1976 (3rd edition).
19. Michelat, G., 'Sur l'utilisation de l'entretien non-directif en sociologie', *Rev. fr. Sociologie*, 16, 229–47, 1975.

[17]

Social Stratification and Health Lifestyles in Two Systems of Health Care Delivery: A Comparison of the United States and West Germany*

WILLIAM C. COCKERHAM
University of Illinois at Urbana-Champaign

GERHARD KUNZ
University of Cologne (West Germany)

GUENTHER LUESCHEN
Technical University of Aachen (West Germany) and University of Illinois at Urbana-Champaign

Journal of Health and Social Behavior 1988, Vol. 29 (June):113–126

This study compares health lifestyles among a sample of Americans in Illinois and West Germans in Northrhine-Westphalia. There was a general lack of difference between Americans and West Germans, as well as between social strata in the two countries, with respect to participation in health lifestyles that take place outside the health care delivery system. A more paternalistic system of health benefits (West Germany) does not appear to undermine personal incentives to stay physically fit in comparison to persons living in a more individualistic system (United States).

The purpose of this paper is to examine whether significant differences exist between Western populations with comprehensive health care benefits provided through their government (West Germans) and those generally lacking such guarantees (Americans) in regard to participating in health lifestyles. We wish to determine whether persons who do not have the security of a state-sponsored health insurance program work harder to stay healthy than those who have access to this resource. Research investigating this situation has important implications for health policy in that it assesses whether or not a welfare system with a tradition of providing comprehensive health coverage undermines individual incentives to participate in lifestyles that promote health.

We will pursue this line of inquiry with data collected in the United States and in the Federal Republic of Germany. Both countries are Western democracies with high standards of living, healthy populations, and advanced systems of health care delivery, but each is distinctive with respect to culture and the provision of health services. As Burns (1986, p. 39) explains, most Germans believe in an extensive welfare state and support relatively close governmental regulation of the economy, whereas Americans are less highly committed to government welfare programs and support greater involvement by private

* Direct all correspondence to William C. Cockerham, Department of Sociology, University of Illinois, 702 South Wright Street, Urbana, IL 61801.

Support for this study was provided by the Volkswagen Foundation, Hannover, West Germany, the Graduate College Research Board, Department of Sociology, and College of Medicine, University of Illinois at Urbana-Champaign; the Institute for Sports Science, Technical University of Aachen; and the Seminar for Social Science, University of Cologne. Data were collected in the United States by the University of Illinois Survey Research Laboratory and in West Germany by the Institute of Sports Science in Aachen and the Seminar for Social Science in Cologne. Thomas Abel and Jin-Ho Rha assisted in the preparation of data. The authors wish to acknowledge the particularly insightful comments of three anonymous reviewers for *JHSB*.

enterprise in dealing with economic and social problems.

Recent research by Pescosolido, Boyer, and Tsui (1985) on public evaluation of medical care in eight countries, including West Germany and the United States, illustrates this difference. West Germans rated government performance lower if they believed that the government was taking less responsibility for providing health care. Americans, conversely, were not as negative about this situation. These differing perspectives form the background for our comparison.

THEORETICAL PERSPECTIVE

Before analyzing the specific situation of West Germany and the United States, we will discuss some theoretical issues that need to be considered in the study of health lifestyles. Sociological research dealing with the emergence of modern industrial societies has focused on such processes as integration, social control, secularization, and emancipation—to name several of the most prominent themes. Such concepts, connected to the work of Durkheim, Marx, and Weber, implied notions of social change. The efforts of modern industrialized societies to promote their own integration and prosperity and the civil rights of their members generally have resulted in gains for their citizens' well-being. Equality before the law, unemployment insurance, child benefits, and the right to education are such developments, as is the provision of adequate health care for everyone. Social welfare as a charity in the modern welfare state has evolved into a public right (Marshall 1964).

With the exception of Great Britain, where social class distinctions remain strongly pronounced (Hollingsworth 1981; Reid 1981; Ryder and Silver 1985), explanations of health-related behavior in the northern and central welfare states of Western Europe, including West Germany, do not appear to be as strongly grounded in socioeconomic differences as in the United States (Cockerham, Kunz, Lueschen, and Spaeth 1986a; Heidenheimer and Elvander 1980; Sidel and Sidel, 1983). Therefore, in the face of greater equality in material conditions and equal access to medical resources, a person's state of health in relation to patterns of social stratification may be explained best theoretically by Weber's (1958) concept of status groups and the lifestyle dimension, along with system levels of culture (Cockerham et al. 1986b). The classical Marxian model, with its focus on material life chances and social class as a strict reflection of economic position, fails to account adequately for the full relationship between lifestyles and socioeconomic status.

Nevertheless, Marxist theory, as seen in the recent works of Waitzkin and Navarro, provides an important statement on health lifestyles. Waitzkin (1983) maintains that the capitalist system is exonerated by attempts to displace responsibility for health in capitalist medical systems from social institutions and physicians as a group to individuals through an emphasis on health lifestyles. Although not denying that individual lifestyles are important determinants of health, Waitzkin points out that individuals often lead unhealthy lives as a result of social inequality. When the burden of responsibility for staying healthy is shifted to the individual, the system itself is not at fault if individuals become sick or die early deaths because of adverse social conditions.

Navarro (1986, p. 57) agrees that the strategy of individual responsibility for health assumes that the fundamental cause of an individual's health problem is the individual, not the system. In this context the individual and his or her lifestyle, rather than society and its health sector, constitute the primary solution for coping with threats to health. Yet Navarro argues that this focus on individual lifestyles assumes an illusory degree of independence and freedom for the individual. A person's psychological orientation and lifestyle are shaped by his or her relationship to the means of production. Yet Navarro maintains that it is a condition of capitalism that workers have no control over their work or their lives, including their health. Consequently, lifestyles are not left to the individual's discretion but are shaped by the work environment which is controlled by the upper class and organized to protect their socioeconomic advantage.

The merit of the Marxist perspective on health lifestyles, as advanced by Waitzkin and Navarro, is its emphasis on the fact that many health problems (the most obvious are those problems that stem from poverty) have roots in the structure of society which cannot be addressed by individual lifestyles alone. This observation implies a reconsideration of social policy and societal-level responsibility for the health of the individual in the United States. But a problem with the Marxist interpretation of health lifestyles is its assumption that health behavior in particular and social behavior in general are determined not by the individual's choice and decision but by the socioeconomic structure of society and by the ideology that underlies it. Nevertheless people do have some choices, no matter how limited, in whether or not they want to live as healthy as possible given their circumstances. Decisions about smoking, alcohol use, and exercise fall ultimately on the individual. What is needed for our analysis is a theoretical approach that takes individual as well as societal factors into account with respect to health lifestyles.

In our view a Weberian perspective meets this requirement best because Weber emphasizes the role of choice, intention, goals, and social values in shaping individual behavior. In fact, Weber (1978) explains that even a socialist economic system needs to be understood in terms of what lies behind the actions of the individuals who are involved in it. Weber provides us with a framework for analysis through his concept of status groups and the function of lifestyles in such groups. Whereas Weber views class strictly as a reflection of the marketplace, signifying a person's level of income, property, or economic skill, he depicts status groups as communities of people with similar status, social class backgrounds, and political power. He sees status groups as originating through a sharing of similar lifestyles or as a means to preserve a particular style of life. People belonging to the same status group recognize each other as more or less equal; they have the same social standing, as reflected in their manner of living.

Therefore Weber (1978, p. 54) suggests that while classes are formed in accordance with relations of production and the acquisition of wealth, status groups are formed according to the principles governing their consumption of goods in the context of specific lifestyles. Lifestyles are based on what one consumes, rather than on what one produces. Inherent in Weber's view of lifestyles are aspects of participation determined at individual levels (motives and goals) and at group or societal levels (norms and values), as well as by social structural conditions (income and social class position).

In the case of health lifestyles, a person is attempting to produce good health on the basis of his or her degree of motivation and capability. The aim of this activity, however, is ultimately one of consumption. Thus people attempt to maintain or enhance their health in order to use it for some end, such as a longer life or enhanced enjoyment of their physical being. In the research of d'Houtaud and Field (1984) in France, for example, we see that health was viewed as something to be cultivated for increased vitality and enjoyment of life among members of the upper and middle classes, and for the ability to continue to work among lower-class respondents. Yet in both situations, health was something that was to be consumed, not simply produced.

Moreover, as Bendix (1960) observes, Weber held that lifestyles can spread beyond the groups in which they originate. A strong example is Weber's (1958) analysis of the manner in which the Protestant ethic became part of Western culture and influenced the rise of capitalism as a generally shared belief system. Consequently, certain lifestyles not only set people apart, but also can be incorporated into the mainstream culture of society. In the case of health lifestyles, Cockerham and his associates (1986b) suggest that health-advancing activities, promoted through the mass media and public health campaigns, have indeed spread throughout the United States. This observation is consistent with the findings of Harris and Guten (1979), who suggest that virtually everyone engages in some sort of health-protective behavior. Thus Weber's notion of status groups helps us to understand the central role of lifestyles in producing both differences and similarities between social strata, and guides our approach to this study.

Because the mass media and health professionals in both the United States and West Germany promote participation in health lifestyles, and because of the tendency, as Field (1987) notes, toward similar cultural and social lifestyles generally in Western society, there may in fact be little or no difference between American and West German health lifestyles. Featherstone (1987) observes that some lifestyles grounded in consumerism (namely, certain choices of clothes, leisure activities, consumer goods, and bodily dispositions) are not fixed to specific status groups. Featherstone disagrees, however, that the emergence of these lifestyles is evidence of a dramatic change in class structure. Instead he maintains, along with Bourdieu (1984), that this development is a new movement within the existing class hierarchy consisting of an expansion and legitimation of upper middle-class lifestyles. This evolution features the notion that everybody has choices and should seek self-improvement regardless of age and class origin. Both Featherstone and Bourdieu identify body maintenance as a major focus of this cultural trend.

This review of the literature suggests that neither the social structure of modern Western nations nor the organization of different systems of health care delivery may necessarily promote significant differences between social strata with respect to participation in health lifestyles. Weber's analysis of the spread of the Protestant ethic demonstrated how a class-specific lifestyle became part of the general culture of Western society. We suggest that this is also the case for health lifestyles.

APPLICATION TO WEST GERMANY AND THE UNITED STATES

The United States is the only industrialized nation in the world that does not provide financial coverage for the medical care of a majority of its citizens. The dominant values in American medicine at present are commercial, as Cassell (1986, p. 40) observes, with medical services viewed as a commodity and physicians as purveyors of that commodity. Thus medical care in the United States is and has been more of a privilege than a right of citizenship, with access to quality care determined largely by one's ability to pay.

In West Germany, conversely, medical care has been more of a right than a privilege. A distinctive psychological effect of this circumstance can be found in the concept of *Anspruchsdenken*. This term cannot be translated literally into English, but essentially it means a "mentality of entitlement." It signifies a readiness on the part of the individual to claim and use the welfare benefits to which he or she is entitled by law. As Scheuch (1987a) explains, the current welfare system in the Federal Republic of Germany makes it possible for citizens to demand the most in all welfare programs. Thus West Germans, on the average, appear to have a different mentality from Americans about health care. They can use this service whenever and as long as it is necessary; therefore, West Germans are able to approach health care providers with an exceptionally strong sense of personal entitlement. The fact that *Anspruchsdenken* has no equivalent in English underscores the lack of a corresponding mentality in American society.

The historical basis for this orientation dates from Bismarck's social reforms in 1883. These reforms, which were initiated to thwart the influence of socialist politicians, to secure the loyalty of an expanding working class, and to express Bismarck's view that the state has the duty to provide for the welfare of its subjects, included a compulsory system of national health insurance (Light 1986; Stone 1980). Politics, however, were never far from Bismarck's thinking; there can be little doubt that he was aware of the advantage that might be gained from a public insurance program in his struggle against socialism (Craig 1982, p. 151). Schmoller (Wehler 1985) described these measures as the quintessence of social politics. Bismarck was a Prussian, and Prussia had a tradition of state responsibility for the health and welfare of its citizens in return for their obedience and allegiance. Not only was a program of national health insurance for all of Germany consistent with this tradition, but it offered Bismarck an opportunity to promote the state at the expense of socialist politicians and workers' trade unions. Socialist members of the Reichstag were caught in a dilemma, and eventually supported Bismarck's plan in order to avoid being accused of overlooking the needs of the working class.

Yet as Light (1986, p. 429) reminds us, medical care and health services are acts of political philosophy; therefore, political and social values underlie the choices made, the institutions formed, and the levels of funding provided. Bismarck was forced to make concessions because of the strong opposition of employers and workers' mutual-aid societies established by centuries-old guilds, who objected to a government takeover of health care. Compromise was reached with employers and employees assuming the responsibility for managing and financing health-care benefits through sickness funds or insurance groups. "Thus," Light comments, "Bismarck succeeded in tying workers to employers and preventing unions from taking over health care, but he failed to get a system run and financed by the state" (Light and Schuller, 1986, p. 5). Funds to support the program are collected through employers and are provided to insurance groups to pay for services. Physicians typically are paid through financial service companies, who bill the insurance groups on behalf of the doctor. Fees are determined through a payment schedule negotiated by the insurance groups in cooperation with doctors and the organizations representing them. The government's role is one of regulation and rule making to resolve any conflicts between providers and consumers.

According to Stone (1980) and Light (1986), this form of health service organization is termed *corporatism* and represents a unique contribution by Germany to the provision of health care. Corporatism in the German context consists of compulsory membership in a national health plan and a set of institutions situated between the government and its citizens with the authority to manage health care under government auspices.

For individuals, the program that was established consisted of compulsory health insurance, free health services, and sick benefits such as payment for salary lost because of illness or injury. Employees, the self-employed, the unemployed, students, old-age pensioners, and certain categories of household workers who provide infant and child care, home help, and similar services are all required to be insured by one of several hundred health insurance funds. Depending on where one lives, 11 to 13 percent of a person's income goes to pay for public health insurance. Approximately seven percent of the West German population is excluded from coverage, but these are persons with the highest incomes; private health insurance is available for them.

In contrast to corporatism, the American system is described by Light (1986) as a professional model with an emphasis on fee for service and professional autonomy. Both the American and the West German systems have fee for service (with set fees for government-sponsored programs) and professional autonomy. Autonomy is greater in the United States because of less government regulation and the absence of a general requirement to negotiate with other parties. Individuals in both societies are free to choose their own physician and to decide when to use professional health services. An essential difference, however, is that in West Germany the state is ultimately responsible for the health of all but the most affluent, while in the United States the government is obligated directly only to the poor and the aged through Medicaid and Medicare public health insurance. Thus the majority of West Germans have greater personal security with respect to health benefits. In the United States the patient's ability to pay is the decisive factor in determining how care is obtained and in establishing the range of its quality.

With some 93 percent of the West German population participating in a government-sponsored system of payment for medical services, as compared to 19 percent of the American people, a sense of government paternalism for health seems more likely to exist in West Germany. We see this situation when we observe that except for the aged, participation in a government welfare system is not considered normative in the United States. Those Americans who receive welfare tend to be stigmatized and devalued socially (Mead 1985). In West Germany, in distinct contrast, providing welfare and social security for the general public, not only for the poor and the elderly, is a normal feature of the state's role. This contrast implies a fundamental difference between the value systems of the two countries: the Americans emphasize individualism and the Germans manifest a high regard for the state.

Bismarck's concept of mandatory public health insurance, for example, was based on the idea of the state organizing and providing security for its citizens; the notion of self-sufficiency for workers and other members of society was absent (Childs and Johnson 1981). In present-day West Germany the state provides comprehensive health insurance, featuring free medical and dental treatment, drugs, and hospitalization for an indefinite period of time. Sick or injured workers also receive full wages from their employers for six weeks; they receive their approximate take-home pay from public health insurance for 78 weeks thereafter. Other benefits are available for more protracted illnesses and for permanent disability. Extensive maternity and death benefits also are paid through public health insurance. In general, the West Germans have considerably more health benefits than the Americans.

This difference is consistent with the fact

that in regard to national culture, Americans are more oriented toward individual independence and free enterprise than are the West Germans (Gatzke 1980). Since the nineteenth-century reforms of von Stein and Bismarck, and as expressed in Hegel's philosophical perspective, the idealization of the state as a moral entity has been a major characteristic of German social thought (Freund 1979) despite its misuse during the Nazi period. Individualism and free enterprise receive less emphasis in this context because of the state's paternalistic role. Laqueur (1985) notes that Germans tend to be perfectionists; although few individual Germans are likely to apply the same standards of competence, altruism, and morality to themselves that they desire of their social and political institutions, the perfectibility of such institutions nonetheless is expected. Laqueur explains that Germans tend to feel the shortcomings of their society more acutely than others and to experience greater disappointment and disillusionment when the political system fails to meet their expectations.

Thus Marxist ideology and political/ecological pressure groups like the Greens seem to find more support in West Germany than in the United States as a means of criticism. The West German health care system does not lack problems, however; the high cost of care has produced a severe strain on the medical system as it competes for subsidies with other systems of the welfare state (Scheuch 1987a, Stone 1980). Yet the adequacy and the responsiveness of the West German system of health care delivery have not been a major target of social criticism. The intended paternalism of the system appears to be consistent with public expectations. This is not the case in the United States, where criticism of the medical profession and of its lack of responsiveness to public interest is common (Freidson 1975; Navarro 1986; Starr 1982; Stevens 1971; Waitzkin 1983). Therefore it is not surprising that West Germans evaluate their public insurance program for medical care more positively than do Americans (Pescosolido et al. 1985).

This discussion suggests that West Germans are more dependent on the state for meeting their health needs than are Americans. In the German system health benefits under a state-sponsored program are conceptualized as a right and as a normative feature of societal membership. This situation not only promotes the *Anspruchsdenken* mentality but also enhances the paternalistic image of the state. Even though business corporations in the United States may provide extensive health benefits to their employees, corporate paternalism is grounded in profits (employee recruiting and work motivation) and in maintenance of the labor force, not in a humanistic concern for general welfare (Brown 1979). Not only is a sense of paternalism likely to be weakened (or absent), but Americans have out-of-pocket costs for some services like cost-sharing deductibles, office visits to physicians, drugs, and other items. Moreover, the West German system has the advantage of linking government paternalism with national pride in the general quality of available medical care. In the United States, corporations and public institutions in the civilian sector ultimately do not have responsibility for the individual's health. In the final analysis, Americans tend to be more on their own in securing health care.

Yet what about those activities related to health maintenance that take place outside government programs? Do West Germans show a high degree of initiative in health-protective activities in everyday life, or do Americans, who generally do not participate in a paternalistic system of state-sponsored health benefits, work harder to keep themselves fit? The lessened health security of Americans, combined with a tradition of greater individuality in the United States indeed could influence Americans to work harder to stay healthy.

Our discussion in the previous section, however, took the position that health care lifestyles have spread throughout the general culture of Western society. This observation would suggest that there is no difference between Americans and West Germans in regard to participating in health lifestyles outside the health care delivery system. That is, the health lifestyles characteristic of modern Western culture, which the two countries share, would override differences in the provision of medical care and in the public mentality associated with it. Therefore we will test the following hypothesis:

> There is no significant difference in general between Americans and West Germans, or between social strata in the two countries, with respect to participation in health

lifestyles that take place outside the health care delivery system.

DATA AND METHODS

Data for this study consist of 1,606 telephone interviews conducted in the states of Illinois (N = 804) in the United States and in Northrhine-Westphalia (N = 802) in West Germany in 1985. Illinois, with a population of over 11 million in 1980, is a major business, agricultural, and manufacturing state which includes Chicago, the nation's third largest city, with seven million people in its metropolitan area. Northrhine-Westphalia in West Germany contains the Ruhr industrial region, the West German capital of Bonn, and Cologne, West Germany's fourth largest city, with a population in 1982 of 971,000. Over 17 million people lived in Northrhine-Westphalia in 1982.

With 97 percent of all households in Illinois having telephones, practically all households in the state had the same probability of being included in the sample. Because of the larger number of unlisted telephone numbers in the Chicago area, the survey employed random-digit dialing in that locale and used systematic sampling from telephone directories in the rest of the state. Systematic sampling from telephone directories was employed throughout Northrhine-Westphalia, where 90 percent of the households had telephones in 1985. For each household, respondents were selected on the criteria of being 18 years of age or older and of having the most recent birthday (the latter method was employed to select randomly the member of the household to be interviewed).

A limitation of collecting data by telephone, however, is that only households with telephones can be included in the sample. Usually homes with the lowest incomes are the most likely to be without the necessary equipment, but in West Germany, this assumption is only partially correct because of public subsidies for telephones for low-income and elderly persons and for students. This situation reduces considerably the detrimental effects of telephone interviewing. In Illinois the proportion of households without telephones is only 3 percent—not large enough to affect statistical analysis significantly.

The sample in Illinois was 43 percent male and 57 percent female. Racial composition was 77 percent Anglo or non-Hispanic whites, 12 percent Hispanic, 10 percent black, and one percent other. Ages ranged from 18 to 84 years, with a mean of 42. Mean family income for 1984 was $29,500; mean level of education was 13.2 years.

Some 98 percent of the sample in Northrhine-Westphalia represented German households; the remaining 2 percent were foreign workers. The sample was 44 percent male and 56 percent female. Ages ranged from 18 to 74 years, with a mean of 47. Family income for 1984, computed in dollars at the exchange rate for that period, shows a mean of $18,000. Mean level of education was 10.2 years.

Some comment is in order with respect to differences in family income and age. The Americans had higher incomes, but it also was more likely that both husbands and wives were wage earners in the same household. In addition, one must account for the fluctuating exchange rates, which (as of April 1987) placed the average German family income in this sample at $26,000. This latter figure does not differ especially from that for American households. As for the age difference, it is consistent with demographic trends. With the lowest birthrate in the world, the West German population is not only declining but is becoming older on the average.

We used nine independent variables in our analysis. Three of these variables reflect socioeconomic status: 1) education, indicated by years of formal schooling completed; 2) income, indicated by total household income before taxes in 1984; and 3) occupational status, as measured by the Treiman scale in both the United States and West Germany. The four sociodemographic variables employed in the analysis are 4) age in years; 5) gender, coded as female = 1, male = 0; 6) minority status, coded as black, Hispanic, or other in the United States = 1, non-Hispanic white = 0; non-German resident in West Germany = 1, German = 0; and 7) nationality, coded American = 0, German = 1. As indicators of the effect of the larger social system on health lifestyles, we included two additional variables: 8) PRIVINS (private insurance), which pertains to the type of health insurance each respondent has, coded as private insurance = 1, public insurance = 0; and 9) BESTCARE, in which the respondent was asked whether he or she "had access to first-rate hospitals and doctors." Responses were coded as strongly agree = 4, agree = 3, disagree = 2, and strongly disagree = 1.

We constructed six indices to serve as dependent variables and measures of health lifestyles. SPORTEX (sports and exercise) is the sum of the number of sports and exercise activities in which the respondent participated. Responses were coded from 0 (none) to 19 activities for basketball or volleyball, bicycle riding, gymnastics, calisthenics or aerobics, dancing, fishing or hunting, football, hiking or walking, jogging or running, racquetball, winter sports (e.g., skiing), softball or baseball, swimming, tennis, sailing or surfing, weight lifting, and any three other sports not on our list. SMOKE (smoking) measures use of cigarettes and is coded as current smoker = 3, former smoker = 2, and nonsmoker = 1. ALCOHOL (alcohol use) measures drinking habits; the total number of alcoholic drinks consumed in a typical week is summed to determine a respondent's score.

FOOD (food selection) is a four-point Guttman scale for investigating the respondent's approach in selecting food. Each respondent was asked how important it was to him or her that the food they eat "is not fattening," "has no artificial additives," "is low in cholesterol," and "fills you up." The last item ("fills you up") was reverse scored for Americans but not for Germans because it has a negative connotation among Americans and is positive for Germans. Among Americans, the item suggests overeating; among Germans, it suggests satisfaction and a personal feeling of security. Responses were coded as very important = 4, important = 3, not so important = 2, and not at all important = 1. Each respondent's score was determined by summing the total point value of each response.

APPEAR (appearance) is a four-point Guttman scale in which the respondent was asked how important it is to "have a good appearance," "look attractive to the opposite sex," "have a healthy complexion," "have good posture," and "fix yourself up so that you look like yourself." Responses were coded as very important = 4, important = 3, not so important = 2, and not at all important = 1. APPEAR is included as a measure of health lifestyle because looking healthy is an important characteristic of being healthy and feeling good about it.

The sixth index, RELAX (relaxation), consists of responses to two items asking the respondent how often he or she "takes a rest at noon or lies down at some other time during the day" and "uses the weekend for pure relaxation." Responses were coded as often = 4, sometimes = 3, seldom = 2, and never = 1.

In addition to the six lifestyle variables we included a seventh dependent variable, HEALTH (health status), as a measure of the respondent's subjective sense of physical health. This variable consists of the respondent's self-rating of his or her general level of health on a continuum of very good = 5, good = 4, satisfactory = 3, not so good = 2, and bad = 1.

Data were analyzed by multiple regression. Correlation coefficients, means, and standard deviations for the data are shown in Table 1.

FINDINGS

Table 2 presents regression results for the health lifestyles and self-assessments of health status for the American sample. This table, which considers together the three socioeconomic status variables (education, income, and occupational status), shows only modest effects for SES on health lifestyles. Education is the best predictor of health lifestyles; Table 2 shows that more highly educated Americans participate significantly more in sports and exercise (SPORTEX) and in the selection of healthy foods (FOOD). Less well educated Americans, in contrast, smoke more and are more interested in their appearance (APPEAR). Income is significant only with respect to relaxation (RELAX); the direction of the data shows that lower-income persons relax significantly more. Occupational status, however, does not have significant effects on any of the lifestyle variables or on self-rated health status (HEALTH). High education and income, on the other hand, promote higher self-assessments of health. Yet despite the tendency of better educated and more affluent persons to rate their health more positively, the results suggest that overall, SES does not produce extensive differences in participation in health lifestyles.

Table 2 also shows that age is significant in

TABLE 1. Correlation Coefficient, Means, and Standard Deviations (N = 1,606)

	1	2	3	4	5	6	7	8	9	10	11	12	13	14	15	16
1 SPORTEX	1.00															
2 SMOKE	−.10															
3 ALCOHOL	.06	.16														
4 FOOD	.14	−.17	−.15													
5 APPEAR	.13	.01	−.02	.14												
6 RELAX	−.06	−.03	−.06	.17	−.05											
7 HEALTH	.24	−.04	−.03	−.10	.14	−.17										
8 EDUCATION	.24	.04	−.02	−.06	.02	−.17	.29									
9 GERMAN	−.04	.02	.10	.12	−.25	.20	−.29	−.44								
10 INCOME	.15	.00	.09	−.06	.14	−.17	.29	.42	−.38							
11 OCCUPATION	.16	−.06	.02	−.01	−.05	−.03	.11	.53	−.09	.32						
12 AGE	−.27	−.13	−.12	.18	−.18	.26	−.32	−.26	.12	−.17	−.00					
13 GENDER	−.08	−.21	−.34	.20	.15	.05	−.08	−.10	−.01	−.17	−.10	.13				
14 MINORITY	.00	.04	−.05	.04	.17	−.01	.02	.09	−.29	−.00	−.04	.12	−.01			
15 PRIVINS	.09	−.03	.00	−.05	.13	−.16	.24	.40	−.52	.36	.18	−.11	−.01	.10		
16 BESTCARE	.06	−.04	−.03	.03	.07	.01	.09	.05	−.07	.17	.07	.07	.00	−.13	.09	1.00
MEAN	.12	.90	4.71	1.80	3.25	1.53	3.77	11.74	.50	23.81	44.15	44.50	.56	.11	.76	1.95
SD	.07	.87	7.64	.53	.53	.87	.99	3.33	.50	15.31	11.44	17.55	.50	.32	.93	.55

relation to five of the six health lifestyle variables and in the self-assessment of health. Younger Americans are more likely to participate in sports and exercise, to drink alcohol, to emphasize appearance, and to rate their health significantly higher. Older Americans, on the other hand, are more careful about their food selection and relax more. As for gender, Table 2 shows that males exercise more, smoke more, and drink alcohol more than females, but that females are more careful about their food and their appearance. Minority status shows that minorities are more selective about their food, emphasize their appearance more, and relax more, but that nonminorities rate their health higher. PRIVINS (private health insurance) makes no difference whatever for the Americans on any of the health lifestyle variables or on the self-rating of health status, while BESTCARE (belief that one has access to the best medical care) is significant only in that such persons

TABLE 2. Unstandardized (b) and Standardized (Beta) Regression Coefficients for American Data

	SPORTEX	SMOKE	ALCOHOL	FOOD	APPEAR	RELAX	HEALTH
Education	.44	−.52	−.21	.19	−.26	−.22	.33
	(.15)***	(−.16)***	(−.01)	(.09)**	(−.14)**	(−.07)	(.10)*
Income	.19	.83	.19	.44	.34	−.38	.94
	(.00)	(.01)	(.04)	(.01)	(.12)***	(−.08)*	(.18)***
Occupation	.95	−.17	−.30	−.21	−.21	.35	−.32
	(.01)	(−.02)	(−.05)	(−.04)	(−.05)	(.05)	(−.04)
Age	−.15	−.23	−.66	.54	−.50	.10	−.11
	(−.33)***	(−.05)	(−.15)***	(.17)***	(−.17)***	(.21)***	(−.21)***
Gender	−.41	−.30	−3.83	.19	.12	.57	−.83
	(−.02)	(−.17)***	(−.25)***	(.17)***	(.12)***	(.00)	(−.04)
Minority	−.47	.90	1.18	.19	.20	.18	−.23
	(−.02)	(.04)	(−.06)	(.14)***	(.17)***	(.09)*	(−.10)**
PRIVINS	.12	.16	−.17	.25	.43	−.32	.33
	(.01)	(.02)	(−.02)	(.04)	(.01)	(−.03)	(−.03)
BESTCARE	.11	.50	.42	.40	.71	.35	.75
	(.07)*	(.03)	(.03)	(.04)	(.07)*	(.02)	(.04)
Constant	.10	1.75	9.62	1.07	3.67	1.08	3.87
R^2	.18	.06	.10	.07	.09	.07	.15
N =	802	802	801	777	798	796	802

* p<.05, ** p<.01, *** p<.001, two-tailed tests.

participate more in sports and exercise and emphasize their appearance.

Table 3 shows the results for the West German sample. In the first column in Table 3, the results for SPORTEX display strong effects for the SES variables. West Germans with high education, income, and occupational status are significantly more likely than those at the lower end of the social scale to participate in sports and exercise. Age also is significant in that younger persons show greater participation. This finding suggests that participation in sports and exercise has not spread throughout West German society to the degree found in the United States. According to Scheuch (1987b), jogging and aerobic exercise have been a major interest among West Germans for only a limited time, but tennis, a sport more common among the more affluent, has been popular for a much longer time and attracts large numbers of participants. Thus our finding that sport participation is related to higher SES is not surprising.

Yet Scheuch (1987b) observes that the number of West Germans participating in sport and exercise is impressive and that a plateau has not been reached; even larger increases in participation are predicted. Kimmerle (1987) finds likewise that jogging as a means to enhance health is developing into a social movement in West Germany similar to the pattern that evolved in the United States. Therefore it appears that in West Germany participation in sports and exercise is likely to spread across the social strata to a much greater degree than is true today.

Even so, the finding that SES has a strong effect on sports and exercise participation does not mean that SES differences in relation to health lifestyles are more extensive overall in West Germany than in the United States. Quite the contrary; with the exception of sports and exercise, SES differences are negligible. Table 3 shows that smoking, food selection, relaxation, and self-rating of one's health are unaffected by socioeconomic status. Other than SPORTEX, education (low) affects only appearance, income (high) affects only alcohol use and appearance, and occupational status has no other effects. Therefore, the data shown in Table 3 indicate that SES does not have a strong overall effect on the health lifestyle variables.

As for the other independent variables in Table 3, age is significant in that younger respondents are more likely to participate in sports and exercise, to smoke, to emphasize appearance, and to rate their health the highest. Older respondents are more careful

TABLE 3. Unstandardized (b) and Standardized (Beta) Regression Coefficients for West German Participation in Health Lifestyles

	SPORTEX	SMOKE	ALCOHOL	FOOD	APPEAR	RELAX	HEALTH
Education	.27	.10	−.17	.75	−.32	.83	.13
	(.13)**	(.04)	(−.01)	(.05)	(−.19)***	(.03)	(.04)
Income	.61	−.14	.10	.34	.57	−.82	.11
	(.09)*	(−.01)	(.13)***	(.06)	(.10)**	(−.01)	(.00)
Occupation	.62	−.47	−.40	.42	.32	−.64	.58
	(.10)*	(−.06)	(−.06)	(.01)	(.07)	(−.01)	(.06)
Age	−.47	−.99	−.17	.54	−.69	.13	−.20
	(−.12)**	(−.20)***	(−.00)	(.18)***	(−.23)***	(.27)***	(−.34)***
Gender	−.26	−.41	−5.97	.23	.28	.38	.70
	(−.02)	(−.23)	(−.38)***	(.22)***	(.26)***	(.02)	(.00)
Minority	.19	.26	1.01	.15	.54	.30	.13
	(.00)	(.04)	(.02)	(.04)	(.01)	(.00)	(.02)
PRIVINS	−.15	−.73	1.36	.36	.81	−.55	.10
	(−.01)	(−.05)	(.11)**	(.04)	(.01)	(−.04)	(.06)
BESTCARE	.61	−.57	1.18	.32	.91	.67	.13
	(.05)	(−.04)	(.09)**	(.04)	(.10)**	(.05)	(.08)*
Constant	.65	1.86	10.77	1.27	3.19	.92	3.74
R^2	.09	.12	.20	.09	.12	.08	.14
N=	787	778	801	741	775	766	801

* $p<.05$, ** $p<.01$, *** $p<.001$, two-tailed tests.

about their food and relax more. Gender is significant in that males drink more (in fact, males produced 17% of the 20% variance in the r-square for ALCOHOL), while females are more careful about food and appearance. Minority status has no significant effects; PRIVINS (private health insurance) is significant only in that persons with such insurance consume more alcohol. The finding in Table 3 that private health insurance and high income are both related to greater alcohol use is consistent with the fact that private insurance is required in West Germany only for persons with the highest incomes. Finally, BESTCARE is significant for alcohol use, appearance, and self-rating of health.

With the exception of age, the independent variables have no marked effects on the health lifestyles in Table 3 for the West Germans. Nor can a strong case be made that the SES variables of education, income, and occupational status have significant overall effects. The only exception to this statement for West Germans is SPORTEX; the literature cited suggests that participation in sport and exercise is just beginning to spread throughout the country's social structure in the same manner as in the United States. Otherwise pronounced differences in health lifestyles do not appear currently to exist between social strata in West Germany.

Table 4 presents regression results for the combined West German and American data sets in order to determine differences between the two countries. The SES variables shown in Table 4 are not strong predictors of participation in health lifestyles, as would be expected from the separate analyses of the West German and American samples. Table 4 shows that more highly educated persons in the combined sample participate more in sports and exercise and in the selection of healthy food. Less well educated persons, in contrast, are more interested in their appearance. Higher-income persons drink significantly more alcohol and are also more concerned about their appearance; lower-income persons, on the other hand, are more likely to relax. Occupational status is significant only in that higher-status respondents participate more in sports and exercise. None of the SES variables shown in Table 4 were significant for smoking. Overall, the results show that SES does not produce extensive differences in participation in health lifestyles.

TABLE 4. Unstandardized (b) and Standardized (Beta) Regression Coefficients for Combined American and West German Participation in Health Lifestyles

	SPORTEX	SMOKE	ALCOHOL	FOOD	APPEAR	RELAX	HEALTH
Education	.34 (.16)***	−.15 (−.05)	.18 (.01)	.11 (.07)*	−.28 (−.17)	−.63 (−.02)	.26 (.09)**
Income	.16 (.03)	−.30 (−.00)	.34 (.07)*	.13 (.04)	.40 (.11)*	−.36 (−.06)*	.75 (.12)***
Occupation	.38 (.06)*	−.39 (−.05)	−.19 (−.03)	−.99 (−.02)	.12 (.00)	.19 (.02)	−.52 (−.01)
Age	−.98 (−.24)***	−.60 (−.12)***	−.35 (−.08)**	.52 (.17)***	−.58 (−.19)***	.11 (.23)***	−.15 (−.26)***
Gender	−.35 (−.02)	−.36 (−.20)***	−4.92 (−.32)***	.20 (.19)***	.19 (.18)***	.20 (.01)	−.51 (−.02)
Minority	−.17 (−.01)	.82 (.03)	−.78 (−.03)	.19 (.11)***	.19 (.11)***	.18 (.07)**	−.21 (−.07)**
PRIVINS	.11 (.01)	−.71 (−.01)	.39 (.05)	.67 (.01)	.61 (.01)	−.37 (.04)	.51 (.05)
BESTCARE	.86 (.07)***	−.23 (−.01)	−.48 (−.03)	.35 (.04)	.70 (.07)***	.47 (.03)	.10 (.06)*
German	.12 (.04)	.18 (.01)	2.16 (.14)***	.20 (.19)***	−.23 (−.22)***	.24 (.14)***	−.33 (−.17)***
Constant	.83	1.75	8.48	1.13	3.59	.88	3.96
R^2	.12	.07	.14	.09	.15	.11	.21
N=	1589	1580	1602	1518	1573	1562	1603

* p<.05, ** p<.01, *** p<.001, two-tailed tests.

For self-rated health status, however, Table 4 shows that high education and income promote a higher perceived state of health. Thus Germans and Americans with higher SES characteristics tend to *think* that they are especially healthy, but they do not appear to be particularly different in doing things to stay healthy.

Table 4 also shows that age affects each dependent variable significantly. Younger persons are more likely to participate in sports and exercise, to smoke, to drink alcohol, to emphasize appearance, and to rate their health the highest. Older persons are more careful about their food, and relax more often. As for gender, males are more likely to smoke and to drink alcohol, while females select better food and take a greater interest in appearance. In addition, Table 4 shows that minority persons emphasize food selection, appearance, and relaxation, but that nonminority persons are prone to rate their health significantly higher.

An independent variable of particular interest is PRIVINS; the results show that Germans and Americans with private health insurance are not significantly more likely to participate in any of the health lifestyles or to rate their health higher than persons with public health insurance. Respondents simply do not differ on the basis of type of insurance. This finding suggests that having public health insurance does not undermine participation in health lifestyles outside the health care delivery system, and that having private health insurance does not particularly promote such participation.

For BESTCARE we noted some differences. Persons who reported that they could obtain the best medical care are more likely to participate in sports and exercise and to emphasize appearance. They also rate their health higher.

Finally, with respect to differences between Germans and Americans, Table 4 shows that Germans are more likely to drink alcohol, to select healthy food, and to relax. Americans in turn, are more likely to emphasize appearance and to rate their health more positively. Of the six health lifestyles, Germans participate more in two (food selection and relaxation). German respondents also are significantly more likely to use alcohol, but in this case the response signifies greater rather than lesser use; it is not regarded as health-advancing because it indicates significantly higher consumption.

We found no significant differences between the two nationalities with respect to smoking and participation in sports and exercise. As for exercise, even though SES characteristics are significant within the German sample, the two variables producing the greatest variance for both Germans and Americans are education and age. Well-educated and younger persons are more likely in both societies to participate in sports and exercise than are less well-educated and older persons. Consequently, when the data are combined, we find no significant difference between Germans and Americans.

Overall, the differences between the two nationalities are not extreme. These data cannot be used to make a strong case that Americans and West Germans differ especially in health lifestyles. Therefore our hypothesis is supported: in general there is no significant difference between Americans and West Germans, or between social strata in the two countries, with respect to health lifestyles that take place outside the health care delivery system.

As an additional comment, it is not surprising that West Germans tend to drink more alcohol and to relax more. The greater use of alcohol appears to be a cultural matter; beer drinking historically has been identified as part of Germany's tradition, and recent data reported by Feuerlein (1984) show that the West Germans continue to rank first in the world in beer consumption. Feuerlein indicates that only six percent of the adult West German population abstains completely from drinking. Most alcohol is consumed at home, and beer is the most common drink; some 39 percent of the population reports that they drink beer daily. Moderate drinking without drunkenness appears to be socially acceptable. Abstainers, Feuerlein points out, tend to have a "bad image" in society. This pattern suggests that widespread alcohol use is not abnormal among Germans.

As for relaxation, West Germans are provided with greater opportunity in that they have more vacation days on the average than Americans (30 days compared to 12) and more legal holidays (13 to 16 holidays compared to nine). Almost all businesses are closed from early afternoon on Saturday until Monday morning. The number of working hours per year is lower in West Germany than elsewhere in Western Europe or in the United States and Japan (Burns 1986).

This does not mean that West Germany is a utopia. A recent decline in the economy has led to growing unemployment, increased discrimination against foreign workers, limited job opportunities for youth, and debate over whether the strength of the work ethic is declining (see Burns, 1986; Laqueur 1985; Noelle-Neumann and Strumpel 1984). Yet our data indicate that the West Germans may be catching up to Americans in smoking reduction and that, as noted, participation in sports and exercise may become more widespread in the future. In regard to smoking, Wetterer and von Troschke (1986) found a clear decline in the proportion of male smokers in West Germany and a continual but less substantial decrease in female smokers, similar to trends in the United States. The West Germans, according to our data, also are more careful about what they eat. The latter development is consistent with findings that detail a significant improvement in the West German diet since 1955 (Scheuch 1987b) and greater obesity among Americans than among West Germans (Lueschen, Cockerham, and Kunz 1987). Even though West Germans consume significantly more alcohol than Americans, the evidence suggests that the welfare system does not undermine the incentives of West Germans generally to pursue a healthy lifestyle outside the health care delivery system.

CONCLUSION

Weber's critique of Marx led him to identify the importance of lifestyles in distinguishing between status groups, but he also recognized that aspects of a group's lifestyle could spread into the mainstream culture. Our findings are consistent with Weber's perspective: these data show that health lifestyles practiced outside the health care delivery system have become common both between social strata and cross-culturally in the United States and West Germany. Adoption of healthy lifestyles has been encouraged through the mass media and by health professionals in both countries, and such behavior seems to have been accepted widely.

We base this conclusion on our finding that socioeconomic variables did not produce extensive differences among the social classes and nationalities in our study. This result carries an important policy implication: if the United States should adopt some form of national health insurance, it would not undermine or reduce incentives to continue practicing the health-advancing behavior that people follow on their own. That is, a more paternalistic system of health care does not seem to remove individual incentives for health. Whether one has private or public health insurance in either the United States or West Germany makes absolutely no difference with respect to health lifestyles. West Germans, with their more extensive state-sponsored health benefits, appear to work just as hard to stay fit as do Americans, who have more individual responsibility for obtaining and maintaining coverage for health services. A country's provision of national health insurance does not necessarily encourage careless health practices by that country's citizens.

REFERENCES

Bendix, Reinhard. 1960. *Max Weber: An Intellectual Portrait*. New York: Doubleday.

Bourdieu, Pierre. 1984. *Distinction*, translated by R. Nice. London: Routledge and Kegan Paul.

Brown, E. Richard. 1979. *Rockefeller Medicine Men: Medicine and Capitalism in America*. Berkeley: University of California Press.

Burns, Arthur F. 1986. *The United States and Germany: The Vital Partnership*. New York: Council on Foreign Relations.

Cassell, Eric J. 1986. "Ideas in Conflict: The Rise and Fall (and Rise and Fall) of New Views of Disease." *Daedalus* 155:19–41.

Childs, David, and Jeffrey Johnson. 1981. *West Germany: Politics and Society*. London: Croom, Helm.

Cockerham, William C., Gerhard Kunz, Guenther Lueschen, and Joe L. Spaeth. 1986a. "Symptoms, Social Stratification, and Self-Responsibility for Health in the United States and West Germany." *Social Science and Medicine* 12:1263–71.

______. 1986b. "Social Stratification and Self-Management of Health." *Journal of Health and Social Behavior* 27:1–14.

Craig, Gordon A. 1982. *Germany, 1848–1945*. New York: Oxford.

d'Houtaud, A., and Mark G. Field. 1984. "The Image of Health: Variations in Perception by Social Class in a French Population." *Sociology of Health and Illness* 6:30–59.

Featherstone, Mike. 1987. "Lifestyle and Consumer Culture." *Theory, Culture & Society* 4:55–70.

Feuerlein, Wilhelm. 1984. *Alkoholismus—Missbrauch und Abhängigkeit*. Stuttgart: Thieme.

Field, Mark G. 1987. "The Comparative Evolution of Health Systems: Convergence, Diversity, and Cross-cultural Issues." Paper presented to the International Symposium on Health Conduct and Health Care in the Modern Welfare State: United States and FRG. Bad Homberg, West Germany.

Freidson, Eliot. 1975. *Doctoring Together*. New York: Elsevier-North-Holland.

Freund, Julien. 1979. "German Sociology in the Time of Max Weber." Pp. 149–86 in *A History of Sociological Analysis*, edited by T. Bottomore and R. Nisbet. London: Heinemann.

Gatzke, Hans W. 1980. *Germany and the United States: A Special Relationship?* Cambridge: Harvard University Press.

Harris, Daniel M., and Sharon Guten. 1979. "Health-Protective Behavior: An Exploratory Study." *Journal of Health and Social Behavior* 20:17–29.

Heidenheimer, Arnold J., and Nils Elvander (eds.). 1980. *The Shaping of the Swedish Health System*. New York: St. Martins.

Hollingsworth, J. Rogers. 1981: "Inequality in Levels of Health in England and Wales, 1891–1971." *Journal of Health and Social Behavior* 22:268–83.

Kimmerle, Roland. 1987. "Jogging—zur Entstehung und Entwicklung einer kollektiven Bewegüng im Sport." *Sportwissenschaft* 17:121–50.

Laqueur, Walter. 1985. *Germany Today*. Boston: Little, Brown.

Light, Donald W. 1986. "Comparing Health Care Systems: Lessons from East and West Germany." Pp. 429–43 in *The Sociology of Health and Illness*, 2nd edition, edited by P. Conrad and R. Kern. New York: St. Martins.

Light, Donald W., and Alexander Schuller (eds.). 1986. *Political Values and Health Care: The German Experience*. Cambridge: MIT.

Lueschen, Guenther, William C. Cockerham, and Gerhard Kunz. 1987. "Deutsche und amerikanische Gesundheitskultur—oder What They Say When You Sneeze." *Medizin Mensch Gesellschaft* 12:56–69.

Marshall, Thomas H. 1964. *Class, Citizenship, and Social Development*. New York: Free Press.

Mead, Lawrence M. 1985. *The Social Obligations of Citizenship*. New York: Free Press.

Navarro, Vicente. 1986. *Crisis, Health, and Medicine*. New York: Tavistock.

Noelle-Neumann, Elisabeth, and Burkhard Strumpel. 1984. *Macht Arbeit Krank? Macht Arbeit Glucklich? Eine Aktuelle Kontroverse*. Munich: Piper.

Pescosolido, Bernice A., Carol A. Boyer, and Wai Ying Tsui. 1985. "Medical Care in the Welfare State: A Cross-National Study of Public Evaluations." *Journal of Health and Social Behavior* 26:276–97.

Reid, Ivan. 1981. *Social Class Differences in Britain*. 2nd edition. London: Grant McIntyre.

Ryder, Judith, and Harold Silver. 1985. *Modern English Society*. London: Methuen.

Scheuch, Erwin K. 1987a. "Entwicklung der Bevölkerungsstruktur and unser Gesundheitswesen." *Medizin Mensch Gesellschaft* 12:135–43.

———. 1987b. "Recent Social Changes and Their Consequences for the Health Care System." Paper presented to the International Symposium on Health Conduct and Health Care in the Modern Welfare State: United States and FRG. Bad Homberg, West Germany.

Sidel, Victor W., and Ruth Sidel. 1983. *A Healthy State: An International Perspective on the Crisis in United States Medical Care*. Revised edition. Boston: Beacon.

Starr, Paul E. 1982. *The Social Transformation of American Medicine*. New York: Basic Books.

Stevens, Rosemary. 1971. *American Medicine and the Public Interest*. New Haven: Yale University Press.

Stone, Deborah. 1980. *The Limits of Professional Power*. Chicago: University of Chicago Press.

Waitzkin, Howard. 1983. *The Second Sickness: Contradictions of Capitalist Health Care*. New York: Free Press.

Weber, Max. 1958. *From Max Weber: Essays in Sociology*. New York: Oxford University Press.

———. 1978. *Weber: Selections in Translation*, edited by W. Runciman and translated by E. Matthews. Cambridge: Cambridge University Press.

Wehler, Hans-Ulrich. 1985. "Das Deutsche Reich, 1871–1918." Pp. 203–404 in *Deutsche Geschichte*, Vol. 3, edited by R. Rürup, H. Wehler, and G. Schulz. Göttingen: Vaudenhoeck and Ruprecht.

Wetterer, Angelika, and Jürgen von Troschke. 1986. *Smoker Motivation*. Berlin: Springer.

[18]

Fitness and the Postmodern Self*

BARRY GLASSNER
University of Connecticut

Journal of Health and Social Behavior 1989, Vol. 30 (June):180–191

This essay suggests that contemporary fitness practices share aesthetic and ideological commitments with other activities that have been classified as postmodern. *The aesthetic similarities are evident in the use of pastiche and simulation by manufacturers of exercise machines and videotapes. In terms of ideology, the pursuit of fitness is promoted as an opportunity for individuals to avert several of the risks to selfhood thought to be present in modern social organization. Implications for G.H. Mead's theory of the self are discussed.*

Over the past couple of decades, national surveys (Caspersen, Christenson, and Pollard 1986; Gurin and Harris 1987) and the consumer marketplace have documented a widespread and growing interest among middle and upper class Americans in the pursuit of fitness. Health clubs grossed $5 billion in 1987, exercise equipment $738 million (up from $5 million ten years earlier), diet foods grossed $74 billion, and vitamin products $2.7 billion (Brand 1988). Frequently throughout the 1980s, exercise video cassettes have appeared on weekly *Billboard* lists of the ten top selling home video products (Morse 1987–88), and magazines such as *American Health*, *Prevention*, and *Self* each report circulations in excess of one million.

One readily can identify structural shifts which might account for this interest. The large and relatively prosperous "baby boom" cohort has entered middle age, and its members have begun to encounter signs of their own physical decline. The major illnesses they and their elders encounter are chronic and degenerative rather than infectious, and hence susceptible in some measure to prevention and treatment by means of exercise and diet.

Concurrently, as the consumer market for fitness goods and services has expanded, economic factors have come into play which serve further to legitimate fitness practices. In particular, corporate collaborations have become commonplace since the mid-1970s. Several hundred hospitals have invested in the construction of exercise facilities on site in an effort to derive additional revenues and in-patient referrals at a time when occupancy rates have reached historic lows (Cole 1986; *Business Week* 1986; letter from the American-Hospital Association). During this same recent period, approximately 50,000 U.S. corporations made available exercise, diet, and other "wellness" programs to their employees in hopes of reducing insurance, absentee, and inefficiency costs at a time when many were "downsizing" their workforces (Conrad 1988; Glassner 1988, p. 221–227).

Yet while these and related factors could help to explain why fitness has achieved a privileged position in American public discourse—and they deserve a close examination in their own right—the present paper addresses a correlative question. How do the practices, products, and ideological positionings of the fitness industry derive their appeal; what is their sociocultural aesthetic?[1] Structural explanations can spell out why a social trend takes root when it does, but cultural explanations are required to explain how the trend took the particular shape it did.

* Direct all correspondence to Barry Glassner, Department of Sociology, Box U-68, University of Connecticut, Storrs, CT 06268.

For helpful comments on earlier drafts I thank Howard S. Becker, Peter Conrad, Paul DiMaggio, Julia Loughlin, Steven Mailloux, Robert Perinbanayagam, Barry Schwartz, David Silverman, Manfred Stanley, David Sylvan, and anonymous reviewers for this journal.

A first step is to examine the concept itself, whereupon one discovers that "fitness" refers to the general state of a person's psycho-physical well-being—mind as well as body. Thus, the subtitle of *American Health* magazine is "Fitness of Body and Mind." A direct mail advertisement from Time-Life Books, for a series of volumes on exercise, diet, stress, and toning proclaims that "if you're ready to enter the new age of fitness . . . ," with their help, "[y]ou'll go beyond exercise to experience a dimension of health, vitality and confidence you've never known before."

A hybridization of potentially independent matters also can be found in many of the most successful commercial programs in the body improvement industry. A major selling point in Weight Watchers advertisements has been their Quick Start Plus Exercise Plan; and Nautilus, the manufacturer of exercise machines, markets to health clubs its Nautilus Diet, which "consists of three-times-per-week supervised Nautilus workouts combined with a descending-calorie diet."

Although some fitness enthusiasts distinguish between "fitness" and "health," the two have become generally synonymous in everyday usage. Each of the activities (diet, exercise, stress reduction, etc.) implies the others. The longer expression, "health and fitness," is used primarily when the speaker wants to draw attention specifically to non-exercise components. Packages of Nabisco Shredded Wheat, for example, recently featured a mail-in coupon for an exercise video by Jane Fonda. The advertising copy referred to Fonda as "one of America's favorite health and fitness advocates." In so doing, Nabisco made an association to their own product, which is positioned as a health(ful) food. ("It's the natural goodness of whole wheat and has no added sugar or salt.")

Therein lies one of several warrants for the central argument of this paper: that fitness is a *postmodern* pursuit. Both the material products of the fitness industry and their practical uses resemble in important regards other cultural activities that have been labeled postmodern.

Among the similarities is the use of pastiche, a borrowing from diverse imagery, styles, and traditions, including both high and low, commercial and artistic, and past, present, and future, wherever these seem usable. Such pastiche is a form of context-less quotation (see Jameson 1984; Clarke 1985; Venturi 1966; and Venturi, Brown, and Izenour 1972). The pastiche quality of fitness is evident even where the concept is used to refer primarily to exercise. More than mere movement is generally involved, after all, in exercise programs. The typical exercise video (like its live counterparts at health clubs) involves also dance, nostalgic or futuristic imagery, and commercial tie-ins. One video, selling briskly at the time this paper was being prepared, "Esquire's Dance Away—Get Fit With the Hits of the 50's," includes on the side cover, without explanation, the Tampax Tampons emblem. The tape itself features workouts performed to songs including "Rock Around the Clock" and "Blue Suede Shoes."

In the pages that follow, I will elaborate further upon the theme of fitness as pastiche and will suggest additional aesthetic features of fitness products and practices which prompt a consideration of them as *postmodern*. By using the term postmodern, I do not intend, however, to engage in what is coming to be called postmodern social theory (Denzin 1986; Ashley in press), which attempts to deconstruct modernist texts of the social sciences nor do I intend to engage in metatheory. Rather, my use of the term is a matter of convenience for crossing disciplinary boundaries. For better or worse, postmodern has become the currency in several scholarly literatures to refer to certain aesthetic practices and attendant ideological positions.

From a socio-historical perspective, postmodern is a somewhat unfortunate concept. As Hassan (1987, p. 87) noted, "it evokes what it wishes to surpass or suppress, modernism itself" and "it denotes temporal linearity and connotes belatedness, even decadence, to which no postmodernist would admit." With hindsight, one might suggest *dismodern* as a better choice, evoking as it does many English words describing the transfiguration of modernity attempted over the past couple of decades (disabuse, disarm, dissemble, dissolve, disjunct, etc.).

Whether or not postmodern movements in fact succeed at gaining independence from the modern—and authors have raised considerable doubts (e.g., Ghirardo 1984–5; Hab ermas 1981; Laffey 1987; Venturi and Brown 1984, pp. 104–116)—in contrast with Daniel Bell (1978, pp. 53–4), we can recognize more in postmodern social action than nihilism, narcissism, and "anything goes." The postmodern pursuit of fitness is a case in point. Fitness activities afford many Americans the opportunity to disenthrall their selves from the perceived shortcomings of everyday life in modern culture—in particular, from constraining dualities such as expert versus amateur, self versus body, male versus female, and work versus leisure.

SYMBOLIC INTERACTIONS WITH THE MODERN

Modernity resulted in the first place, according to a Weberian analysis, from the collapse of religious authority and the rise of a rationalized, bureaucratic social order. Within this order, separate groups of professionals, each with special technical abilities, are granted responsibility for separate spheres of activity. Scientists oversee nature, lawyers administer justice, critics orchestrate taste, physicians regulate health, and so forth. The hope, beginning with the philosophers of the Enlightenment, was that this specialization and rationalization "would promote not only the control of natural forces, but would also further understanding of the world and of the self, would promote moral progress, the justice of institutions, and even the happiness of human beings" (Habermas 1981, p. 9). Instead, by the late 1960s and 1970s many middle-class Americans had come to believe—whether correctly or not—that the activities of modernity resulted in a *loss* of control over nature (evidenced, for example, by the prevalence of heart disease, cancer, and environmental pollution), a loss or splintering of selfhood, entrenched immorality in public institutions, and ever-inflated false promises of consumer happiness.

Americans were losing faith in machine age science and technology. Toward medicine, in particular, considerable disillusionment was expressed during the late 1960s and the 1970s, as exemplified in popular books by Ivan Illich (1975), Thomas Szasz (1966), and others. The implicit message of these works was that one's best hope for mental and physical health was to be found outside modern medicine; and a group of physician-critics suggested what that alternative might be. George Sheehan, Kenneth Cooper, and several lesser known authors proposed aerobic fitness as the mode of salvation from both the disappointing health care institutions and the stressful, sedentary ways of life common in the modern age.

In her analysis of the social factors which elicited the early jogging craze of the late 1960s, Muriel Gillick (1984) underlines two. First was the recognition that medicine could not be relied upon to prevent death. A majority of heart attack victims died before receiving medical attention, and even the new and highly publicized coronary care units saved only a small percentage of lives. Second, there was a public discourse underway about collective immorality and social disintegration, centering on rights and Vietnam War issues. Jogging served as a response to these conditions. "The pursuit of physical fitness was seen by some as a means by which individuals could improve America. By ridding us of the stress and tension, the competitiveness and sleeplessness which are ruining our society, so the argument goes, running can help us pull ourselves up by our bootstraps."[2]

Even at this inaugural stage, the contemporary fitness movement departed, in its form of commentary on American society, from earlier health and fitness movements. At the end of the 19th century and beginning of the 20th, progressiveness served as a guiding motif for the fitness movement, as it did also in modernist artistic and political movements of the time (Brown and Clignet 1988, pp. 3–4). Those advocating exercise and healthful diets spoke of "regeneration" and preparing Americans for a bright new day. They also evoked notions—which had been deployed in health movements earlier in the 1800s—of a citizenry that had recently been strong and virtuous but was going flabby as the result of too much affluence (Green 1986; Schwartz 1986).

In contrast to those earlier movements, fitness talk of the late 1960s through '80s is not primarily about a happier recent past, progress, or the perils of wealth. Rather, what must be exorcised now are the deficiencies of the modern era. Fitness is portrayed as a way to protect oneself from characteristic ills of modern culture such as drug abuse, depression, and eating disorders. Biographical vignettes such as the following from *Weight Watchers Magazine* about 35-year-old Kathy Smith (whom *Time* called "The Beverly Hills

Fitness Guru") are standard fare in articles and books promoting exercise:

> When she was in college, her parents died within a year and a half of each other—her father of a heart attack, her mother in a plane crash. "My whole emotional foundation had been destroyed. It was the lowest point in my life," she recalls. Always outgoing and bubbly before, Smith withdrew into a shell of confusion, depression and fear. Unfortunately, there was no one to crack that shell—her only living relative, a sister, turned to drugs and alcohol for solace. At first, Smith turned to food to ease her despair: She'd binge on sweets one day, then, feeling guilty, fast the next day . . . . Running eventually helped her to climb out of her depression. "I found solace, real peace while running," she says . . . (Fain 1987, p. 47).[3]

The article goes on to describe how Smith has brought exercise to the aid of others who suffer with the problems she and her relatives experienced. "When she's not working out, Smith keeps her mind off the bathroom scale by joining in the fundraising efforts of such nonprofit organizations as the American Heart Association and Fitness Against Drug Abuse" (p. 47).

For another example, consider the premise of Chris Pepper Shipman's book, *I'll Meet You at the Finish!* (1987): that in these times of high divorce rates and marital unhappiness, couples who exercise together stay together. Shipman details how her own marriage improved substantially once she took up marathon running with her husband.

To paraphrase an observation Andreas Huyssen (1986, p. 180) made about postmodern artists, fitness enthusiasts hold an "ostentatious self-confidence" that there can be "a realm of purity" for the self, if that self will maintain a proper regimen. By means of vital, rationalized, and self-directed action, the practitioner of fitness strives to construct an integral biography during a time when roles and collective morality are inconsistent and rapidly changing (cf., Brown and Clignet 1988, p. 4).

FITNESS AND THE MEADIAN SELF

At the level of experience, what the practice of fitness promises to achieve is nullification of a fundamental polarity. That polarity was described succinctly by Mead in *Mind, Self and Society:*

> We can distinguish very definitely between the self and the body. The self has the characteristic that it is an object to itself, and that characteristic distinguishes it from other objects and from the body. It is perfectly true that the eye can see the foot, but it does not see the body as a whole. We cannot see our backs; we can feel certain portions of them, if we are agile, but we cannot get an experience of our whole body (1934, pp. 136).

Yet precisely that experience is what fitness is said to offer. The self "in touch with," "caring for," "in control of" the body,[4] no longer need experience the body as but another object out in the world (Mead 1934, p. 164).

Moreover the fit body holds a signal position in contemporary American culture—as locus for billions of dollars of commercial exchange and a site for moral action (Stein 1982; Crawford 1984). As a result the body which is fit or in the process of becoming so is no longer an "object to which there is no social response which calls out again a social response in the individual" (Mead 1938, p. 292; and see pp. 445–53). Fitness activities frequently are performed with others in group programs, so that the body becomes a focus of interaction and hence a key constituent of the "me"—that experience of self in which the vision of the community is vitally present (Mead 1934, sections 22 and 25). Even where fitness is pursued privately, in one's own home, the body is commonly experienced by way of conceptual looking glasses—by how it is interpreted in disciplines such as medicine (cf., Foucault 1970 and 1977) and in comparison to images of bodies in the media (cf., Brown and Adams 1979), and eventually, by how it is commented upon by significant others (cf., Freedman 1986).

If in modernity, "Through self-consciousness the individual organism enters in some sense into its own environmental field; its own body becomes a part of the set of environmental stimuli to which it responds or reacts" (Mead 1934, p. 172), in postmodernity this encounter has been radicalized. The person experiences his or her own body within the context of a media environment of repeating images (see Baudrillard 1987, pp.

70–72), from the time the infant is first mesmerized by the bodies in the exercise video its mother watches.

The exercise video is a quintessential postmodern object, not only in its pastiche quality as noted above, but in at least two other defining regards as well. First, it reverses the usual structure of representation. Rather than the image being a copy of the real, in the exercise video, the real strives to become a copy of the image. The viewer mimics the images on the tape and strives to alter her or his appearance to resemble them (Morse 1987/88).

In addition, an exercise video is constructed of simulacra—representations for which there are no originals. In an interview (cited in Morse 1987/88, p. 49), the director of a Jane Fonda exercise video described how it was made. From the point of view of the home viewer, the tape is simply a recording of Fonda leading a class in aerobics. According to the director, however, the video required three days to shoot in order to get all the angles right; it was shot without music, the soundtrack dubbed in later; and the "class" was recorded separately, without Fonda present.

Many of the exercise machines found in health clubs and for home use are simulacra as well. Like the bodies to which their users aspire, they are technologically induced copies of copies. Stationary bicycles resemble ordinary bikes and sometimes afford a similar feel when one "rides" them, but they do not achieve the traditional function of a bicycle, which is to transport a person from one location to another. Newer "ergometers," which involve the same motions, often look more like metal ducks than traditional bikes. As for rowing machines: "People who are serious about rowing don't own rowing machines," reports a designer of these contrivances (Jacobs 1987, p. 95), so far from the original experience is the simulation.

Some popular machines are nearly pure simulacra: they bear virtually no resemblance to their ancestors. The Bow-Flex, for instance, is a bench with "power rods" atop, each of which provides a different amount of tension. By modeling the postures displayed in the instruction manual, the Bow-Flex can be used like a bench press, rower, or skiing device, and for several dozen other types of movements as well. "In a sense, what the Bow-Flex does is simulate other simulators," reports an architectural design author (Jacobs 1987, p. 98).[5]

Ironically, the more nearly bodies become present to selves in primarily third-hand, reflective, machine-made ways, the more ostensibly intrinsic to selfhood they are. The analytic distinction Maines (1978, p. 242) made "between *bodies*—the physical fact of human existence, and *identities*—social categories through which people may be located and given meaning in some organizational context" has become less apposite to many people's everyday lives. A statement such as the following, made by Joe Daddona, mayor of Allentown, Pennsylvania, and quoted in *Prevention* magazine, no longer seems preposterous: "I began to wonder, how well can I possibly manage a city when I do such a lousy job managing my health."

If, as Stone (1962, p. 101) suggested, "in appearances . . . selves are established and mobilized," through fitness, selves are truly embodied. The physique has become a cardinal sign of the self in a way which add-ons such as fashion and cosmetics (the appearance-enhancer signs of modernity) no longer can. The information a person gives off by being fit is meant to be both economical and globally favorable for the self, in the manner upon which Goffman (1963, p. 35) remarked in a different context:

> Although an individual can stop talking, he cannot stop communicating through body idiom; he must say either the right thing or the wrong thing. He cannot say nothing. Paradoxically, the way in which he can give the least amount of information about himself—although this is still appreciable—is to fit in and act as persons of his kind are expected to act.

If the advertisements and publications of the fitness industry are to be believed, a great advantage of a fit body is that it can be entrusted to perform competently and reliably; it bespeaks a contemporary version of Goffman's "bureaucratization of the spirit." Not merely a well-oiled machine (as modernists understood it), the fit body-cum-self is cognized as an information-processing machine, a machine which can correct and guide itself by means of an internal expert system. When information from the medical and psychological sciences or from health crusaders is received via exercise and diet instructors or the media, the self-qua-information-processor is able to use that information to change its own behavior for the better. Thus, as part of their effort to recruit and retain members, many health clubs offer computerized analyses of "risk factors" for various diseases, along with quantified prescriptions for exercise and diet protocols intended to reduce individuals' levels of risk.

A commitment to fitness puts in perspective, too, the phenomenal information contents of the body itself. Aches, pains and wrinkles are, if not meaningful each in their own right, at least occasions for constructive further action. For women, especially, there is the promise of a more intentional selfhood. "Femininity is no longer proposed as nature, but is read as cultural, as work, a machinated body produced by a woman's consciousness" (Morse 1987/88, p. 24).

Taken to its logical limit, this version of selfhood virtually equates the self with fitness activities—as can be seen in autobiographical accounts by fitness-obsessed people (e.g., Sabol 1986; Elman 1986). In a less extreme way, this is also the vision of the self in the mass-market magazine, *Self*. Not only are many of the articles in *Self* about how to exercise and diet, but those articles which address other topics often resolve matters by means of fitness. In the November 1987 issue, for instance, the lead article on the page devoted to pop psychology is headlined, "How staying in shape yourself can help keep your relationship in shape, too." In the same issue, atop the page on parenting appears an article and photograph on how to strap an infant safely to one's chest in preparation for riding a stationary bicycle. And a fashion feature answers the question, "How to fit your fitness life into a decent-size bag that's *not* a dingy duffel?"

The advertisements, too, treat the tasks of everyday life in fitness frames. The advertisement for Lubriderm, a skin cream, lists as "the bare necessities" for arising in the morning—exercise, soap and Lubriderm. A new product from Kotex is said to stay in place in "your shortest shorts, latest leotards, and active afternoons." Even the cigarette advertisers, who are required by law to include a warning from the surgeon general about health risks of smoking, evoke fitness imagery. Their products are called "Lights" or "Ultra Lights," the copy is about low "tar" content, and the photographs feature models in sporting clothes or engaged in active endeavors.

Perhaps Faurschou (1987, p. 72) is not out of line when she identifies postmodernity as "no longer an age in which bodies produce commodities, but where commodities produce bodies: bodies for aerobics, bodies for sports cars, bodies for vacations, bodies for Pepsi, bodies for Coke . . ." Nonetheless, some fitness partisans bristle at the sight of cigarette advertising in magazines devoted to healthy living. But viewed from the perspective advanced in this essay, the inclusion of such advertisements is unexceptional. In a modernist context, one expects consistency and a clear distinction between good and bad, positive and negative, pure and dirty. In a postmodernist context, on the other hand, contradiction and complexity are the order of the day (Venturi 1966).

POSTDUALISTIC SELFHOOD

Quite apart from how closely the material products and byproducts of the fitness industry call upon aesthetic features common to the production of other objects which have been categorized as postmodern, it is this attempted blurring of polarities—self and body being perhaps primary among them—which earmarks contemporary fitness practices and their attendant ideologies as postmodern.

The impulse towards "the defusing of polarities, the short-circuiting of every differential system of meaning, the obliteration of distinctions and oppositions . . . ." (Baudrillard 1980, p. 142) is generally regarded as a defining characteristic of postmodern social action (Brown and Clignet 1988, p. 9; Collins 1987, p. 16; Hebdige 1986, p. 85–6; Huyssen 1986, pp. 216–7; Mainardi 1987, p. 35; Zukin 1988, p. 6).

In "Post-Modern Man," a 1970 paper in *Social Problems* (and apparently the earliest sociological account of postmodernity), Vytautas Kavolis wrote: "I would define the "post-modern" personality as one characterized by the sense that *both* polarities of a great many . . . dilemmas are contained, in an unresolved form, within one's own experience (at least as potentialities), in the organization of one's personality" (p. 445). His list of 'dilemmas' engendered by modernist social organization included the following: mastery versus impotence (resulting from technological growth); vividness versus numbness (engendered by the media environment); and the "participation of 'specialists' " versus the "alienation of 'innocents' " (deriving from the modern division of labor).[6]

From our vantage point nearly two decades after Kavolis offered his analysis, we can point to a great deal of activity that has been directed at the disavowal or deconstruction of these tensions. The most ready examples, not surprisingly, have been in the arts, in which postmodernist creations are "designed to reconcile contradictions" (Mainardi 1987, p. 35). This they do by de-structing (see Spanos 1987) rather than formalizing or abstracting, by quoting between genres and eras, and by intermixing male and female body parts, articles of clothing, and other gendered media (see Kent and Morreau 1985), among other ways.

In social theory, too, one finds that the transition from modernism to postmodernism involves an abandonment of structuralisms (both of the Saussure/Levi-Strauss and Parsonian varieties), with their formal analyses of bipolarities (Sylvan and Glassner 1985)—those listed in the previous paragraphs being the most fundamental or generative—in favor of deconstructionism and a return to pragmatism (Denzin 1986; Kellner 1988).[7]

The manner in which fitness ideologies and practices are positioned to dissolve polarities (or more precisely, their warrant to segment experience) is undeniably less explicit than in some arts movements. Indeed, in certain regards, there persists within the contemporary fitness movement a residual modernism. This is particularly evident in the valuation of traditionally masculine attributes such as strength, endurance, and rational self-control; and most fundamentally, in the vision of the body as existing in an either-or state (i.e., one is said to be either "in shape" or "out of shape," fat or thin).

Nonetheless, a resolution of many of Kavolis' 'dilemmas' is promised by those who promote fitness programs. They suggest that by exercising and eating correctly, one will achieve professional-quality mastery, not just of one's appearance and health, but of one's position in the labor and mate markets (Freedman 1986, pp. 146–191; Glassner 1988), and that one will feel alive, in charge, and a full participant in life (e.g., Cooper and Cooper 1972).

Beyond Kavolis' early considerations, several other principal dualities that have served to structure the experience of everyday life in modernity are likewise partly decomposed in the discourse on fitness. Let us consider, briefly, three:

Male and female. Jane Fonda and others have suggested that fitness activities are a route to empowerment for women. Even if such claims prove falsely optimistic (Chapkis 1986, pp. 8–14), the contemporary fitness movement does differ in a significant regard from body improvement movements of the nineteenth and earlier centuries, and even those of the 1920s. In those cases, prescriptions for men and women differed (Green 1986; Schwartz 1986), whereas typically the prescriptions for fitness in the 1970s and 80s are nearly the same for both men and women. Both should exercise in qualitatively the same ways (with the same movements, using the same equipment or games) and in the same quantities, they should eat the same healthful foods, and subscribe to the same values, such as naturalness, self-control, and longevity.

Even where male-female distinctions are made early on, soon enough they become blurred. For instance, calcium supplements were targeted to women at first, but cereal and vitamin packages and advertising soon stopped specifying gender. Cholesterol reduction, until lately regarded as a worry primarily for men, is now promoted for the entire population. When concerns about exercise "addiction" and "overuse" injuries surfaced, much attention was paid to women's symptoms (e.g., the disruption of menstrual cycles), but soon enough both genders were encouraged to exercise less intensively.

Moreover, for women, one result of the fitness movement has been a new ideal of the feminine physique which involves a pulling together of several cultural antitheses: strength with beauty, muscularity with thinness, and hardness with curvaceousness (Morse 1987/88, p. 25).

Inside and outside. Over the past hundred or so years, "Within consumer culture, the inner and the outer body became conjoined: the prime purpose of the maintenance of the inner body [became] the enhancement of the appearance of the outer body" (Featherstone 1982, p. 18). Within fitness practice the reverse applies: enhancement of the outer body is undertaken in the service of the inner body, as witness magazine articles on fitness which equate an "outer glow" with mental and physical health. We can observe, as Brown and Clignet (1988, p. 6) have done with regard to artists, "By literalizing the belief that spirit can shape matter, postmodernists reduce surface and depth to a relativized sameness."

In some forms of talk about fitness, one encounters an outright merger of outer and inner. An advertisement for a cosmetic surgery practice in California (reproduced in Dull and West 1987) features a photo of an attractive woman, and beneath it the caption: "It's important for me to look and feel the best I can. That's why I eat the right foods and exercise. And, that's why I had plastic surgery." Whether or not the average fitness devotee would readily endorse that conjunction, this advertisement illustrates how, within the semantics of fitness, acts which earlier predicated either 'vanity' or 'health' can be made interchangeable (and see Schwartz 1986 and Morse 1987/88).

Work and leisure. In modernity, "Work strengthens conscience; leisure facilitates impulse" (Wheelis 1958, quoted in Kavolis 1970). But at the postmodern health club—filled with glimmering machines which disaffirm their modernism by being labor-*making* devices (Jacobs 1987, p. 60)—leisure is work, impulses are harnessed into repetitions-per-minute, and the conscience, now of the body as much as it is of the soul, is only as strong as its owner's heart and as firm as her thighs.

In David Riesman's classic argument, consumerism and "workism" were juxtaposed. The distinction provided one of the marks of American cultural modernism, one which fitness and other postmodern constructions deconstruct. But just what is the consumer of fitness working towards? Not a singular, rational goal, but a mosaic of physical, emotional, economic, and aesthetic transformations, a potpourri of ends-and-means. The headline atop the cover of *Working Woman* (October 1986) reads: "*Aiming for the Top?* How To Stay Fit & Look Great At Every Age"—thus combining some of the most difficult choices many white middle class women have been told they must make during the last century or so: beauty versus brains, sexuality versus achievement, health versus fashion, and aging versus attractiveness.

For men also, a modernist distinction *par excellence* has partly collapsed under similar pressures: namely, that between work time and work values, on the one hand, and leisure, on the other. As already mentioned, many corporations encourage their employees to engage in fitness activities by making these available at little or no cost. The vast majority of these corporate fitness programs began during the 1970s and 80s, with some firms, such as Xerox, Pepsi, Kodak and Campbell Soup, building large, state-of-the-art health clubs (Castillo-Salgado 1984; Howe 1983; McCallum 1984). These programs send a couple of messages to employees: that to be out-of-shape is to be expensive to the corporation by way of health care costs, inefficiency, and damage to the collective company image (Crawford 1978); and as a corollary, that the space between work time and private time has narrowed (Conrad 1987). By means of new claims upon the employee's body, the corporation holds title to more of the employee's selfhood.

CONCLUSION

If recent movements in the arts which have been classified as postmodern attempts to "counter the modernist litany of the death of the subject by working toward new theories and practices of speaking, writing and acting subjects" (Huyssen 1986, p. 213), so, too, does the fitness industry retheorize selfhood. By becoming fit, persons are said to achieve a degree of independence from medical professionals and medical technology.[8] They also achieve protection against temptations to alienated or marginalizing forms of deviancy such as obesity, drug abuse, and psychological depression, and a set of frames within which information from and about the body can be effectively reduced and catalogued.

The fitness industry purveys concurrently the dissolution of several cardinal polarities of experience in modern society. The body-self distinction as described by Mead, for example, is attenuated in the process of constant comparisons with ideal images in the media. So, too, do the borders between male and female, inside and outside, and work and leisure, founder.

In short, the contemporary fitness mode incarnates, through practical beliefs and behavioral prescriptions, some elemental premises and aspirations of a postmodern cultural order. It is therefore unsurprising to find that those who market fitness make use also of production ploys found in other reputedly postmodern objects. Exercise videos and workout equipment, in particular, evidence the qualities of pastiche and take the form of simulacra.

While a sociological understanding of the discourse on fitness is not exhausted by identification of its postmodernist turn, this effort serves to situate what is otherwise viewed as merely fad or fancy, as a constituent part of the ongoing process of culture production.

NOTES

1. To pose the question in this manner is to sidestep a preemptive, "rational man" argument, which holds that the fitness industry has prospered because it carries the imprimatur of Science. Although fitness spokespersons do invoke scientific studies to support their claims, they also roundly criticize the medical science establishment. Moreover, there are sharp disagreements in the scientific literature about the health benefits of exercise, weight control, and changes in diet (Becker 1986; Goodman and Goodman 1986; Hughes 1984; LaPorte et al. 1985; Schwartz 1986; Solomon 1985).
2. These themes are evident in writings by running advocates such as George Sheehan and Kenneth Cooper, and in articles about running which appeared in popular magazines (e.g., Lynch 1978).
3. In quoting this and other material from popular magazines, my intent is to display some of the ways in which these magazines portray fitness acts and beliefs, not to imply that the chosen excerpts provide data indicating general behavioral tends. The choice of excerpts results from my ethnographic content analysis (Altheide 1987; Glassner and Corzine 1982) of approximately 300 books and articles on fitness published between 1978 and 1988. Theoretical sampling (Glaser and Stauss 1967) was employed, toward the specific goal of discovering modernist and postmodernist themes in the texts.
4. These are phrases heard time and again in open-ended interviews with fitness enthusiasts (Glassner, 1988).
5. Notwithstanding their thrice-removed quality, machines like Bow-Flex and Nautilus do serve to unify the body with the self by helping to mold the body into a closer copy of ideal bodies as displayed in the media, but they also fragment the body. Depending upon the health club, there can be a dozen or more machines, one for each group of muscles. Finer distinctions about muscular design are made in this context than in any other that people ordinarily encounter.
6. Kavolis failed to take note of the developing postmodernist art of the 1960's, which did address itself, at times, to the 'dilemmas' he mentions. Examples can be found in novels by John Barth, Donald Barthelme, and John Hawkes, plays by Sam Shepard and Tom Stoppard, music by Steve Reich and John Cage, dance by Twyla Tharp and Trisha Brown, as well as Robert Venturi's and Michael Graves' buildings (Trachtenberg, 1985:263–292).
7. Once again, there is no compelling evidence that any of these postmodernist movements, whether in the arts, social theory, or personal health, *succeed* in undermining dualities. The following pages should not be read to imply, for instance, that members of health clubs make less fine distinctions than others between male and female, or inner and outer body (though that possibility might make for an interesting empirical study).
8. Whether this assumption is accurate remains to be tested. Quite possibly, fitness enthusiasts actually utilize more medical services than others, given their heightened attention to their bodies and injury rates from athletic pursuits (see Solomon 1984).

REFERENCES

Altheide, David L. 1987. "Ethnographic Content Analysis." *Qualitative Sociology* 10:65–75.

Ashley, David. forthcoming. " 'Postmodernism' and the End of the Individual: From Repressive Self-Mastery to Ecstatic Communication." *Current Perspectives in Social Theory* 10.

Balsamo, Anne. 1987. "Un-wrapping the Postmodern: A Feminist Glance." *Journal of Communication Inquiry* 11:64–72.

Baudrillard, Jean. 1980. "The Implosion of Meaning in the Media and the Information of the Social in the Masses." Pp. 137–48 in *The Myth of Information: Technology and Post-Industrial Culture*. Madison: Coda Press.

______. 1983. *Simulations*. New York: Semiotext(e).

______1987. *Forget Foucault*. New York: Semiotext(e).

Becker, Marshall H. 1986. "The Tyranny of Health Promotion." *Public Health Reviews* 14:15–25.

Bell, Daniel. 1978. *The Cultural Contradictions of Capitalism*. New York: Basic.

Bowman, Stanley J. 1985. "Photography." Pp. 177–208 in *The Postmodern Moment*, edited by Stanley Trachtenberg. Westport, CT: Greenwood.

Brand, David. 1988. "A Nation of Health Worrywarts?" *Time*, July 25, p. 66.

FITNESS

Brody, Jane. 1987. "Research Lifts Blame From Many of the Obese." *The New York Times*, March 24, C1.

Brown, Beverly and Parveen Adams. 1979. "The Feminine Body and Feminist Politics." *m/f* 3:39–50.

Brown, Richard and Remi Clignet. 1988. "The Emergence of Post Modernism." Paper presented at the meetings of the Eastern Sociological Society, Philadelphia, March.

Bruno, Giuliana. 1987. "Ramble City: Postmodernism and 'Blade Runner.' " *October* 41:61–74.

Business Week (no author listed). 1986. "The Health Industry Finally Asks: What Do Women Want." August 25:81.

Caspersen, Carl J., Gregory Christenson, and Robert Pollard. 1986. "Status of the 1990 Physical Fitness and Exercise Objectives," *Public Health Reports* 101:587–92.

Castillo-Salgado, 1984. "Assessing Recent Developments and Opportunities in the Promotion of Health in the American Workplace." *Social Science and Medicine* 19:349–58.

Chambers, Iain. 1986. "Waiting for the End of the World?" *Journal of Communication Inquiry* 10:99–103.

Chapkis, Wendy. 1986. *Beauty Secrets*. Boston: South End Press.

Chen, Kuan-Hsing (ed.). 1986. "Special issue on MTV." *Journal of Communication Inquiry* 10.

Clarke, Garry E. 1985. "Music." Pp. 157–176 in *The Postmodern Moment*, edited by Stanley Trachtenberg. Westport, CT: Greenwood.

Cole, Galen. 1986. "A Systems Perspective for Hospital-Based Health Promotion," *Optimal Health*, November/December:24–28.

Collins, James. 1987. "Postmodernism and Cultural Practice: Redefining the Parameters." *Screen* 28:11–26.

Conrad, Peter. 1987. "Wellness in the Workplace: Potentials and Pitfalls of Worksite Health Promotion." *Milbank Quarterly* 65:255–75.

———. 1988. "Health and Wealth: Notes on the Rise of Worksite Wellness Programs." Draft.

Cooper, Mildred and Kenneth Cooper. 1972. *Aerobics for Women*. New York: Bantam.

Crawford, Robert. 1978. "You Are Dangerous to Your Health." *Social Policy* 8:11–20.

———. 1984. "A Cultural Account of 'Health.' " Pp. 198–214 in *Issues in the Political Economy of Health Care*. London: Tavistock.

Crimp, Douglas. 1980. "The Photographic Activity of Postmodernism." *October* 15:91–101.

Denzin, Norman K. 1986. "Postmodern Social Theory." *Sociological Theory* 4:194–204.

Doubiet, Susan. 1984. "I'd Rather Be Interesting." *Progressive Architecture* 2:65–69.

Dull, Diana and Candace West. 1987. " 'The Price of Perfection': A Study of the Relations Between Women and Plastic Surgery." Paper presented at the meetings of the American Sociological Association.

Elman, Judith B. 1986. "The loneliest of the long-distance runners." *Runner's World* 21 (July):34–39.

Ewen, Stuart and Elizabeth Ewen. 1982. *Channels of Desire: Mass Images and the Shaping of American Consciousness*. New York: McGraw-Hill.

Fain, Jean. 1987. "Kathy Smith: Making Fitness Fun for Every Body." *Weight Watchers Magazine*, December, 47–50.

Faurschou, Gail. 1987. "Fashion and the Cultural Logic of Postmodernity." *Canadian Journal of Political and Social Theory* 11:68–82.

Featherstone, Mike. 1982. "The Body in Consumer Culture." *Theory, Culture and Society* 8:18–33.

Folkins, Caryle H. and Wesley E. Sime. 1981. "Physical Fitness Training and Mental Health." *American Psychologist* 36:373–89.

Fonda, Jane. 1981. *Jane Fonda's Workout Book*. New York: Simon and Schuster.

Foucault, Michel. 1970. *The Order of Things: An Archaeology of the Human Sciences*. New York: Random House.

———. 1977. *Discipline and Punish*. New York: Pantheon.

Freedman, Rita. 1986. *Beauty Bound*. Lexington MA: Lexington Books.

Freund, Peter E.S. 1982. *The Civilized Body*. Philadelphia: Temple University Press.

Frampton, Kenneth. 1986. "Some Reflections on Postmodernism and Architecture." Pp. 26–29 in *Postmodernism*, edited by Lisa Appignanesi. London: ICA Documents.

Frisby, David. 1986. *Fragments of Modernity: Theories of Modernity in the Work of Simmel, Kracauer and Benjamin*. Cambridge, MA: MIT Press.

Ghirardo, Diane. 1984–85. "Past or Post Modern in Architectural Fashion." *Telos* 62:187–96.

Gillick, Muriel R. 1984. "Health Promotion, Jogging, and the Pursuit of the Moral Life." *Journal of Health Politics, Policy and Law* 9:369–87.

Giovannini, Joseph. 1988. "The Limit of Chaos Tempts A New School of Architects." *The New York Times*, February 4, pp. C1 and C12.

Glaser, Barney G., and Anselm L. Strauss. 1967. *The Discovery of Grounded Theory: Strategies for Qualitative Research*. New York: Aldine.

Glassner, Barry. 1982. "An Essay on Iterative Social Time." *Sociological Review* 30:668–81.

———. 1988. *Bodies*. New York: G.P. Putnam.

Glassner, Barry and Jay Corzine. 1982. "Library Research as Fieldwork: A Strategy for Qualitative Content Analysis." *Sociology and Social Research* 66:305–19.

Glassner, Barry and Jonathan Moreno. In press.

The Qualitative-Quantitative Distinction. The Hague: D. Reidel.

Goffman, Erving. 1963. *Behavior in Public Places: Notes on the Social Organization of Gatherings*. Illinois: Free Press.

———. 1974. *Frame Analysis*. New York: Harper and Row.

Goodman, Lenn E. and Madeleine J. Goodman. 1986. "Prevention: How Misuse of a Concept Undercuts Its Worth." *Hastings Center Review* 16:26–38.

Green, Harvey. 1986. *Fit for America: Health, Fitness, Sport, and American Society, 1830–1940*. New York: Pantheon.

Gurin, Joel and T. George Harris. 1987. "Taking Charge." *American Health*, March, pp. 53–57.

Habermas, Jurgen. 1981. "Modernity versus Postmodernity." *New German Critique* 22: 3–14.

Hassan, Ihab. 1987. *The Postmodern Turn: Essays in Postmodern Theory and Culture*. Columbus, OH: Ohio State University Press.

Hebdige, Dick. 1986. "Postmodernism and 'The Other Side.' " *Journal of Communication Inquiry* 10:78–98.

Herron, Jerry. 1987/88. "Postmodernism Ground Zero, or Going to the Movies at the Grand Circus Park." *Social Text* 18:pp. 61–77.

Holzner, Burkart and John H. Marx. 1979. *Knowledge Application: The Knowledge System in Society*. Boston: Allyn and Bacon.

Howe, Christine. 1983. "Establishing Employee Recreation Programs." *Journal of Physical Education, Recreation, and Dance* 54:52–53.

Hughes, John R. 1984. "Psychological Effects of Habitual Exercise." *Preventative Medicine* 13: 66–78.

Huyssen, Andreas. 1986. *After the Great Divide: Modernism, Mass Culture, Postmodernism*. Bloomington: Indiana University Press.

Illich, Ivan. 1975. *Medical Nemesis*. New York: Pantheon.

Jacobs, Karrie. 1987. "Making Work." *Metropolis*, November:58–63 and 95–98.

Jameson, Frederic. 1983. "Postmodernism and Consumer Society." Pp. 111–125 in *The Anti-Aesthetic*, edited by Hal Foster. Port Townsend: Bay Press.

———. 1984. "Postmodernism, or the Cultural Logic of Late Capitalism." *New Left Review* 146:53–92.

Kamm, Thomas. 1988. "Are They Copies or Are They Fakes? Art World Diverges." *The Wall Street Journal*, January 12, 1988:pp. 1 and 12.

Kavolis, Vytautas. 1970. "Post-Modern Man: Psychological Responses to Social Trends." *Social Problems* 17:435–48.

Kellner, Douglas. 1988. "Postmodernism as Social Theory: Some Challenges and Problems." *Theory, Culture and Society* 5:239–69.

Kent, Sarah and Jacqueline Morreau. 1985. *Women's Images of Men*. London: Writers and Readers.

Klotz, Heinrich. 1984. *Postmodern Visions: Drawings, Painting, and Models by Contemporary Architects*. New York: Abbeville.

Kroker, Arthur and David Cook. 1987. *The Postmodern Scene*. New York: St. Martin's.

Kuhn, Annette. 1985. *The Power of the Image*. London: Routledge and Kegan Paul.

Laffey, John. 1987. "The Politics at Modernism's Funeral." *Canadian Journal of Political and Social Theory* 11:89–98.

LaPorte, Ronald E., Stephen Dearwater, et al. 1985. "Cardiovascular Fitness: Is It Really Necessary?" *The Physician and Sports Medicine* 13:145–50.

Leymore, Varda. 1982. "Structure and Persuasion: The Case of Advertising." *Sociology* 10: 337–89.

Lynch, Maureen. 1978. "The Beauty of Running." *Ladies Home Journal* (April):114.

Lyotard, Jean-Francois. 1984. *The Postmodern Condition: A Report on Knowledge*. Minneapolis, MN: University of Minnesota Press.

———. 1986. "Defining the Postmodern." Pp. 6–7 in *Postmodernism*, edited by Lisa Appignanesi. London: ICA Documents.

Mainardi, Patricia. 1987. "Postmodern History at the Musee d'Orsay." *October* 41:31–52.

Maines, David. 1978. "Bodies and Selves: Notes on a Fundamental Dilemma in Demography." Pp. 241–266 in *Studies in Symbolic Interaction*, volume 1, edited by Norman K. Denzin. Greenwich, CT: JAI.

McCallum, Jack. 1984. "Everybody's Doin' It: Getting Into the Fitness Business, That Is." *Sports Illustrated*, December 3, 72–86.

McRobbie, Angela. 1986. "Postmodernism and 'The Other Side.' " *Journal of Communication Inquiry* 10:108–16.

Mead, George Herbert. 1938. *The Philosophy of the Act*. Chicago: University of Chicago Press.

———. 1934. *Mind, Self and Society*. Chicago: University of Chicago Press.

Melville, Stephen W. 1986. *Philosophy Beside Itself: On Deconstruction and Modernism*. Minneapolis: University of Minnesota Press.

Morse, Margaret. 1987/88. "Artemis Aging: Exercise and the Female Body on Video." *Discourse* 10:19–53.

O'Neill, John. 1985. *Five Bodies*. Ithaca, NY: Cornell University Press.

Paoletti, John T. 1985. "Art." Pp. 53–80 in *The Postmodern Moment*, edited by Stanley Trachtenberg. Westport, CT: Greenwood.

Ritenbaugh, Cheryl. 1982. "Obesity as a Culture-bound Syndrome." *Culture, Medicine and Psychiatry* 6:347–61.

Sabol, Blair. 1986. *The Body of America*. New York: Arbor House.

Sawchuk, Kim. 1987. "A Tale of Inscription/

Fashion Statements." *Canadian Journal of Political and Social Theory* 11:51–67.

Schwartz, Hillel. 1986. *Never Satisfied: A Cultural History of Diets, Fantasies and Fat*. New York: Free Press.

Shabe, John. 1987. "Taking Fitness in Stride." *Syracuse Post Standard*, June 26.

Shipman, Chris Pepper. 1987. *I'll Meet You at the Finish*. New York: Kinetics.

Silverman, David and Brian Torode. 1980. *The Material Word*. London: Routledge and Kegan Paul.

Solomon, Henry A. 1984. *The Exercise Myth*. New York: Harcourt, Brace, Jovanovich.

Spanos, William. 1987. *Repetitions: The Postmodern Occasion in Literature and Culture*. Baton Rouge: Louisiana State University Press.

Stein, Howard. 1982. "Neo-Darwinism and survival through fitness in Reagan's America." *The Journal of Psychohistory* 10:163–87.

Stimpson, Catherine R. 1985. "The Somagrams of Gertrude Stein." Pp. 30–43 in *The Female Body in Western Culture*, edited by Susan Rubin Suleiman. Cambridge MA: Harvard University Press.

Stone, Gregory P. 1962. "Appearance and the Self." Pp. 86–118 in *Human Behavior and Social Processes*, edited by Arnold M. Rose. Boston: Houghton-Mifflin.

Stutman, Fred A. 1986. *Walk Don't Die*.Philadelphia: Medical Manor Books.

Sylvan, David and Barry Glassner. 1985. *A Rationalist Methodology for the Social Sciences*. New York and London: Blackwell.

Szasz, Thomas. 1966. *The Myth of Mental Illness*. New York: Dell.

Topousis, Tom. "Walkers Outpace Joggers." *USA Today*, May 28, 1987.

Trachtenberg, Stanley (editor). 1985. *The Postmodern Moment: A Handbook of Contemporary Innovation in the Arts*. Westport, CT: Greenwood.

Turner, Bryan S. 1984. *The Body and Society*. London: Blackwell.

Venturi, Robert. 1966. *Complexity and Contradiction in Architecture*. New York: Museum of Modern Art.

Venturi, Robert and Denise Scott Brown. 1984. *A View From The Campidoglio*. New York: Harper and Row.

Venturi, Robert, Denise Scott Brown, and Steven Izenour. 1972. *Learning From Las Vegas*. Cambridge MA: MIT Press.

von Moos, Stanislaus. 1987. *Venturi, Rauch and Scott Brown: Buildings and Projects*. New York: Rizzoli.

Weschler, Lawrence. 1988. "Onward and Upward with the Arts (Boggs—Parts I and II)." *The New Yorker* January 18, pp. 33–56, and January 25, pp. 88–98.

Zukin, Sharon. 1988. "The Postmodern Debate Over Urban Form." Paper presented at the annual meetings of the American Sociological Association, August, Atlanta Georgia.

***BARRY GLASSNER** is Professor and Chair, Department of Sociology, University of Connecticut. His recent books include* Bodies *(Putnam, 1988),* Drugs in Adolescent Worlds *(with Julia Loughlin; St. Martins, 1987), and* A Rationalist Methodology for the Social Sciences *(with David Sylvan; Blackwell, 1985). His articles have appeared in* American Sociological Review, Social Problems, American Journal of Psychiatry, *and elsewhere.*

Part VI
Illness Behaviour

[19]

Soc. Sci. Med. Vol. 33, No. 9, pp. 1011–1022, 1991
Printed in Great Britain.

0277-9536/91 $3.00 + 0.00

SELF CARE: JAPAN AND THE U.S. COMPARED

MARIE R. HAUG,[1] HIROKO AKIYAMA,[2] GEORGEANNA TRYBAN,[3] KYOICHI SONODA[4] and MAY WYKLE[1]

[1]Center on Aging and Health, Case Western Reserve University, Cleveland, OH 44106, U.S.A., [2]University of Michigan, Ann Arbor, MI 48109, U.S.A., [3]Indiana State University, Terre Haute, IN 47809, U.S.A. and [4]University of Tokyo, Hongo, Bunkyo-ku, Tokyo, Japan

Abstract—Experience of common symptoms and subsequent self care behaviors among older adults are compared between Japan and the United States, two industrial countries with different cultural backgrounds and health insurance systems. Based on a modification of the Health Belief Model, perceived susceptibility to illness and belief in the efficacy of physician care were selected as major explanatory concepts for the decision to use self care for a complaint. Among 900 respondents in Japan and 728 in the United States, in three communities of varying size, self evaluations of good health, an indicator of low susceptibility, were very similar. Although Japanese respondents claimed fewer experiences of physician error, they still expressed lower preference for physician care than did those in the U.S. In addition, the Japanese reported far fewer symptoms than their U.S. counterparts during a three month period, and were more likely to use self care, even for symptoms they considered more serious. Disparate effects of such variables as good health behaviors, presence of a chronic condition and desire for autonomy are discussed in terms of cultural differences in the two countries.

Key words—elderly, self treatment, Japan, United States

INTRODUCTION

In all parts of the world, self care is the most common form of response to perceived symptoms of illness [1, 2]. In the past, 'medicine without doctors' was widely practiced and still continues to characterize the preponderance of sickness care. Although intensive research into self care behaviors has begun recently [3–6], it is still a largely untapped area of health behavior and little is known about its content, range and determinants.

The definition of self care varies. The one adopted in many prior studies encompasses a broad range of activities that a lay person undertakes to maintain and promote health, and to prevent, detect, and treat health problems [4, 7, 8]. Although this multifaceted definition is useful in many ways, it is obvious that the behaviors bundled together (e.g. health promotion and self-treatment of symptoms), will have quite different determinants and consequences. Diffuseness in self care research, mainly due to this broad definition of self care, has hindered researchers in comparing and discussing their findings. Our definition of self care is much more specific. We define it in terms of response behavior to a perceived symptom without the involvement of physicians. Responses include deciding to do nothing, resting, taking over-the-counter medicine and resorting to various forms of self-treatment and care provided by lay persons, such as family members, without concurrent medical advice. It should be noted that although care provided by lay persons, for example taking chicken soup prepared by a family member for a cold symptom, is sometimes categorized in the literature as 'informal care' separately from 'self care', our definition includes all response behaviors to a symptom that do not involve a physician.

The theory underlying the analysis in this paper is that of the Health Belief Model [9, 10]. This model, originally developed to explain preventive care, posits that perceived seriousness of an experienced symptom, perceived susceptibility to it, and belief in the efficacy of professional help will account for health behavior. Within the framework of the Health Belief Model, Haug and her associates developed a new model that was designed specifically to explain self care behavior, in the presence of signs of illness. For more information on the construction of the conceptual model, see the authors' earlier paper [5].

This model of self care postulates that self care action is explained by two major concepts. The first, preceived susceptibility, relates to the respondent's mental and physical health status and daily health practice. Individuals who perceive their health to be good and who are not plagued by psychological distress would have confidence in their own resilience and be ready to care for their ailments without resorting to professional help. Conversely, individuals with chronic conditions or who experience high numbers of symptoms could view themselves as basically in poor health and thus in need of a doctor's advice for any new ailment. In brief, positive health facilitates self care. Similarly individuals who are vigilant about their health, and who engage in good health practices with regard to diet and exercise, should be able also to distinguish between symptoms that require a physician's attention and those best treated by home remedies.

The second explanatory concept is the individual's attitude concerning the efficacy of physician care. This concept encompasses faith in doctors, claimed experience with medical error and self reliance in health care. The concept again borrows from the Health Belief Model, but in a reverse sense. Instead of belief in the benefits of normative action, namely consultation with a health professional, belief in the ineffectiveness of such action is substituted and triggers self treatment. In brief, negative views of physician care favor a choice of self care.

This model was developed in connection with an empirical study of self care among older adults that Wykle and Haug conducted in the United States [5]. The model was shown to account for self care decisions in response to symptoms perceived as mild as well as those viewed as serious, and to explain more variance than found in many studies using the Andersen's Health Behavior Model, once the effect of need was factored out. The study reported in the present paper was constructed to provide a replication in Japan of the Wykle and Haug study, but also to explore cultural differences in self care.

Cross-cultural studies of self care, particularly between a Western society and a non-Western society, are virtually non-existent. Caudill has noted that, "Culture and social structure are interrelated with the occurrence of disease and its treatment. This is true for both major and minor illnesses, and for the attitudes, beliefs and behaviors that make up the everyday care of the body" [11, p. 159]. The health behavior patterns and underlying principles identified in United States society may not be observed in other socio-cultural contexts. Comparative studies are essential to establish the generalizability of research findings and the validity of interpretations beyond a single culture. By conducting research in different cultures, we can often increase the range of variation in variables beyond that which is obtainable within a single setting, which enables a better understanding of the relationships among the variables. Consequently, it leads us to a much better sense of the robustness of research results [12].

The United States and Japan are leading Western and Eastern industrial societies, with very different historical backgrounds and belief systems. The two nations are similar in their basic economic structures, levels of industrialization, medical technologies, medical care organization and delivery systems, and epidemiological statistics. Like the United States, Japan is a capitalist, technologically advanced, urban, industrialized society. The population is stable, its general health standards are high, and the epidemiology of disease is similar to that in Western industrial societies [13]. In contrast with many European countries, but similar to the United States, the majority of medical care in Japan is delivered by health care providers in private practice. Furthermore, virtually all persons in Japan are covered by a national health insurance scheme, with medical care costs mostly reimbursed based on the fee-for-service system and people free to choose their health care providers. Japan's development, social structure and formal medical care system make Japan, except for the universal insurance feature, the most similar Asian society to compare with the United States.

In counterpoint to its developmental and structural similarities, Japan presents several contrasts that affect health behaviors. First, Japan has a unique medical history. Long ago Chinese medical practices were imported to Japan and flourished beside traditional folk practices [14]. In general, such Eastern health beliefs and practices attribute health problems primarily to the imbalance in body homeostasis and focus their therapeutic efforts on restoring the balance by holistic methods. Self-reliance is encouraged in Eastern medicine which requires more active involvement of patients and their families in therapy compared to the Western medical model. Since Western medicine became the officially recognized and approved system of health care in 1883, it has gradually gained influence. Currently, partly because insurance coverage for non-Western medicine is quite limited, Western medicine is the dominant power in professional health care in Japan, although recent publicity concerning iatrogenic diseases related to synthetic drugs have eroded faith in the Western medical model. However, Eastern health beliefs and practices are still deeply rooted in Japanese health care, particularly in self care. Ohnuki-Tierney [15] offers an excellent discussion on medical pluralism in contemporary Japanese society.

A second counterpoint is the differing role of American and Japanese families in making health care decisions. Approximately two-thirds of older Japanese live with their adult children and only ten percent live alone. In comparison, as many as 40% of older urban Americans live in single person households [16]. Such differences in living arrangements affect the behavior of older persons in two primary ways. Family care, which in most cases is care by lay persons, is more readily available to people who live with family members than to those who live alone. For example, middle aged daughters-in-law usually undertake the major responsibility of house-work in Japanese multi-generation families. Under such living arrangements, a sudden illness of an older person would not affect his/her daily life as much as it would affect the life of a person who lives alone. On the other hand, living with a family could facilitate physician use, through the advice of relatives and their assistance in physical and financial access. These issues require empirical test.

All of these cultural differences are expected to affect personal health care decisions in the two countries. This paper describes similarities and variations in self care practices among older persons in the United States and Japan. More specifically, it addresses four questions:

(1) What are the differences between American and Japanese older persons in the experience of physical symptoms?
(2) What are the differences between American and Japanese older persons in the use of self care for such symptoms?
(3) What are the differences between the two countries in the factors that could account for the use of self care to deal with these symptoms?
(4) What are the differences between the two countries in the joint effects of these factors on the use of self care?

A comparison of the choices made by these older populations with respect to self care will test the generalizability of the conceptual model of self care beyond a single society, and, at the same time, offer clues to the social and cultural factors implicated in personal health care decisions.

METHODOLOGY

Overall model

The conceptual scheme for the study is based on the Health Belief model. It diagrams the effect upon treatment action, namely self care practices, of perceived susceptibility to ill health and belief in physician efficacy, as modified by demographic controls (Fig. 1). The variables used to measure each concept are those for which congruent items were included in the data collection in Japan and the United States.

Socio-economic status is omitted from the model because it was considered impossible to rate occupations in a comparable fashion in the two countries. Fortunately education, useful as a surrogate for socio-economic status, could be measured identically in Japan and the U.S. Description of all measures is supplied below. Age, gender, education and social support were included as controls on the grounds that each has been shown to affect health behavior in the face of perceived illness. Consistent with the Health Belief model, the conceptual design includes perceived susceptibility to illness and belief in the utility of professional assistance as predictor variables, and differentiates resulting behavior on the basis of perceived seriousness of the complaint.

Samples

Answers to the research questions are derived from data collected in comparable surveys in these two countries. In the United States, 900 persons in three age groups (45–59, 60–74 and 75 and over), and in three communities of a Midwest state (major metropolis, midsized industrial city, and small rural town) were selected by random digit dialing. Following this computerized telephone process of identifying the random sample of subjects, face-to-face interviews were conducted, yielding an 81% response rate, with 728 cases for analysis. This study was completed in 1987. In Japan the data were collected in 1988 by contract with a major survey organization in Tokyo. A sample of 900 persons in the same age groups and community sizes were selected in the central part of the main island, by a process that involved random selection of a household from a stratified list of randomly selected neighborhoods in the comparative sized communities. Interviews were then secured from this household as a starting point until the quota from the neighborhood was attained. Thus absent persons and refusals were replaced on the basis of the randomly selected neighborhood and household. The procedure assured that a total of 900 interviews be completed, so that this number is available for comparative analysis. Major variables in the two studies were identical, with question wording congruent as assessed by back translation of the Japanese version.

MEASURES

Dependent variables

Self care rates. Each respondent was asked individually whether any of a list of 29 symptoms had been experienced in the past three months, and if so what action had been taken to deal with the symptom, including both self treatment and professional care. In the United States the first response was open-ended, followed by specific probes concerning the two types of care. In Japan, since the availability of open-ended response time was limited by the data collection agency, closed ended items based on these probes, were substituted. Thus a response that occurred in the United States, initially 'doing nothing' about a symptom, was not available in Japan. However it is reassuring that data from a subset of 124 respondents in Japan who kept daily health diaries for one month revealed that doing nothing as the sole response to a complaint was a very rare occurrence.

In both countries, respondents were also asked if they considered the symptom mild or serious. The symptom list contained complaints that fit potentially into either category. Among the less serious symptoms were running nose with fever, frequent sneezing, waking up stiff in the morning and upset stomach. Potentially serious symptoms included dizziness,

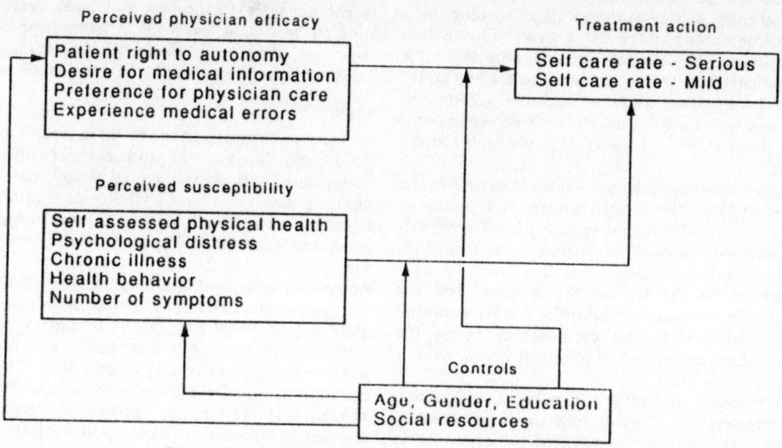

Fig. 1. Conceptual model for explaining self care practices.

chest pains, shortness of breath after light activity and swelling of extremities. It will be noted that symptoms rather than diagnoses were listed, for example frequent sneezing rather than allergy [see Appendix for full list of symptoms].

Finally each individual reporting a symptom in Japan was also asked if he or she consulted a physician, either Eastern or Western, about the symptom. Self care rate for each respondent was then calculated by dividing the number of symptoms for which no physician was consulted by the total number of symptoms experienced. The results were placed in three categories for each respondent: all symptoms were responded to by physician utilization; all symptoms were responded to by self treatment; some symptoms were responded to with physician care while others received self treatment. This procedure was repeated separately for symptoms considered mild and those considered more serious. Since persons with multiple complaints often considered some mild and some serious, there was overlap in the results, so that mild and serious self care rate totals exceeded the total number of persons with symptoms.

Independent variables

Perceived physician efficacy. Nineteen items concerning attitudes to physicians and their care were factor analyzed using the data from Japan. The items were those developed in prior work by Haug and Lavin [17], augmented by selections from Krantz, Baum and Wideman [18]. Three factors emerged with eigenvalues greater than 1. The first, entitled *Right to Autonomy*, with six items, encompassed statements concerning the right to make decisions about accepting treatment, to leave a hospital against advice, and the advisability of curing one's own illnesses. Reliability was 0.60. *Preference for Physician Care*, also including six items, involved confidence in physician care, the risks of eschewing medical advice, and the benefits of professional services. Alpha was 0.59. Finally, *Desire for Medical Information*, the third factor, contained seven items, three of which concerned the desire for full explanations of treatments and risks, as well as the utility of reading one's own medical records and securing views of more than one physician. The rationale for including this scale is that patients who secure information are in a better position to question their physician's recommendations and to act autonomously if those recommendations are considered ineffective. Cronbach's alpha was 0.65.

The same items were factor analyzed earlier in the self care study in the United States, and produced different factors. Given that cross-national comparisons would only be possible with identical measures, the factor analysis results from the Japanese data were applied to the United States data, and are reported here. Although reliabilities for the resulting United States scales were considerably below the Japanese, the requirement of identical scales made it necessary to use them.

An additional indicator of belief in physician efficacy was reports of prior *Experiences of Medical Error* as evaluated by the respondent. Three items made up the scale; belief that there had been mistakes in care, that the physician had caused harm, and that care had come late. Reliability was 0.80.

Perceived susceptibility. Five scales were used to measure this concept. *Self Assessed Health* was a summated scale, ranging from very poor to excellent (0–9). It combines assessment of own health in the last month, from poor to excellent, comparison of own health to that of age peers—worse, same or better—and extent to which health interfered with activities, from a great deal to not at all. Alpha reliability was 0.67. *Psychological Distress* combined yes/no answers to seven items from the Langner scale into four categories from low (1) to very high (4) distress. The seven items were selected from those used in the Cleveland GAO study as non-somatic based on factor analysis [19]. They included difficulty in 'getting going', being a 'worrier', not feeling 'worthwhile', and being 'isolated'. Internal consistency reliability was 0.66. *Chronic illness* was assessed as a dichotomy, with 0 measuring no chronic condition and 1 representing one or more conditions. The Health Behavior scale combined indicators of adequate sleep, eating breakfast daily and not snacking, low or no use of cigarettes and alcohol, and engaging in one or more physical activities, ranging from fishing to active sports. This scale was originally developed by Berkman and Breslow [20] in the Alemeda County study, and has a bio-medical theoretical base. The elements of sleep, eating practices, substance use and exercise were considered to be cross-nationally relevant, since they did not include specific dietary elements that vary widely between countries. Note that good health behaviors do not necessarily correlate with self assessed good health. For example, sedentary drinkers and smokers who are not currently ill could believe themselves to be quite healthy. The scale was grouped into five categores with 1 equaling very poor and 5 very good Health Behaviors. Cronbach's alpha assessed reliability as 0.39, suggesting the multi-dimensionability of the scale.

Total *Number of Symptoms* was also included as indicating perceived susceptibility, on the grounds that persons who had reported many conditions might consider themselves in fragile health, easily prey to becoming seriously ill from symptoms that the more robust could throw off. Accordingly resorting to self treatment might be considered risky.

Controls

Age was categorized in the three sampling groups: 45–59, 60–74, and 75 and over. *Gender* was a dichotomy, with female scored 0 and male 1 in the analysis. *Education* was trichotomized into less than 8 years of schooling, from 8 to 12 years or high school level, and more than 12 years of education or beyond high school. The Social Resources scale combined household composition, ranging from living alone, the least supportive, to living with spouse and children, the most supportive; frequency of contact with family and friends, availability of a confidante, loneliness, and availability of care if ill. This scale is an adaptation of the social resources section in the OARS [21]. The major revision involved type of contact with family or friends. Although frequency of telephone contact questions were the same, queries about frequency of visits to others' homes were expanded for Japan, to include meeting with and going out together with others outside the home, since this is a more common form of social interaction in that country. Each element was coded from 0 (not supportive) to 3 (most supportive) and the seven elements summed. Responses, which ranged from scores of 1–21, were grouped into six categories, from very low support (score of 1–5) to very high (score of 19–21).

Analysis. Comparisons between the U.S. and Japan on all variables were evaluated by chi-square. The joint effects of the susceptibility and efficacy indicators on self care rates, as modified by the controls, were assessed by multiple regression. The rationale for this procedure is discussed further below.

Findings

The samples in the United States and Japan were not entirely similar demographically. In age groupings the United States had somewhat fewer of the very old, those 75 and above. Moreover in Japan, the procedures used produced a 50/50 male/female split, whereas in the United States close to two thirds of the respondents were women, reflecting both their predominance among the elderly and perhaps their greater willingness to be interviewed. In level of education, on the other hand, the two samples were virtually identical, with a third in both countries having more than the equivalent of a high school education. With respect to social support, the findings showed that in both countries the modal level was the next to the highest. Thirty-eight percent in the United States and 32% in Japan reported strong social support.

In response to the first research question on differences between the two countries in symptom experience, the results revealed the most marked difference in the percentage of respondents who claimed they had experienced *none* of the 29 listed symptoms. It will be recalled that the list included common complaints like cold symptoms or stomach upsets, as well as potentially more serious problems such as dizziness and chest pains. Only 10% of the United States respondents reported experiencing none of the symptoms in a prior three month period, compared to 47% of the Japanese with no reported complaints (Table 1).

The fear that this disparity was due to language differences in the instruments was allayed by the fact that the Japanese data were similar to those found in

Table 1. Number of symptoms experienced in a three month period, based on a list of 29, comparing the United States and Japan

	U.S. ($N = 728$) %	Japan ($N = 900$) %
None	10	47
1 or 2	26	38
3 or 4	21	10
5 or 6	15	3
7 or 8	11	1
9 or more	18	1
Total	101	100
Total symptoms reported	3577	1274

χ^2, df 5 = 520.89, $P < 0.0000$, $V = 0.57$.

Table 2. Differences in reported symptom frequency for ten common complaints, comparing the United States and Japan

	Percentage with reported symptom of those with any symptom U.S. %	Japan %
A. Japan rate higher than U.S.		
Cold signs for two days	9	11
Frequent backaches	27	32
B. U.S. rate at least 25%, and higher than Japan		
Shortness of breath	25	9
Insomnia	26	19
Joint or muscle pain	29	11
Memory problems	29	7
Swelling of arms, legs, feet	30	5
Nervousness	37	4
Waking up exhausted	40	17
Waking up stiff	40	8

national government surveys of health in that country, and were consistent with results on studies of other complaints (e.g. Lock [22]). Moreover, those who claimed to have experienced a symptom were much more likely to have reported multiple ailments in the United States than in Japan. Forty-four percent of those in the United States reported five or more complaints compared to only 6% of those in Japan. In the United States 3577 symptoms were reported by 655 persons (an average of 5.5) compared to 1274 in Japan for 475 persons (an average of 2.7).

The pattern of symptom experience was diverse as well. Among the 29 complaints about which the subjects were interviewed only two showed a higher incidence over three months in Japan than in the United States. Cold symptoms lasting at least two days were reported by 9% in the United States and 11% in Japan, while frequent backaches occurred among 27% in the United States and 32% in Japan. In all other cases, the United States showed higher rates than Japan (Table 2). Among the eight complaints that 25% or more respondents reported in the United States, only insomnia showed a rate near that in Japan. The most marked disparity was in reported nervousness 37 vs 4% in the two countries, and in waking up stiff in the morning, 40 vs 8%.

Behaviors in response to symptoms were also markedly different. The answer to question two regarding self treatment showed that among those who had experienced symptoms, 50% of the Japanese used self care only, compared to only 27% of those in the United States who relied exclusively on non-professional treatment (Table 3). In Japan, use of both Eastern and Western practitioners was counted as physician care, since doctors of both persuasions are accredited as medical professionals.

Because a person's beliefs about the seriousness of a symptom could affect his or her treatment actions, rate of self care in connection with symptoms perceived as serious was compared with symptoms perceived as mild. The results for symptoms believed to be only mild again revealed a higher rate of self care in Japan than in the United States. Nearly two-thirds of persons in Japan relied entirely on self treatment if they considered their symptom mild, while in the United States only about a third with the same symptom evaluation did so (Table 4A).

Table 3. Rate of self care for 29 symptoms comparing the U.S. and Japan

Self care rate	U.S. ($N = 657$) %	Japan ($N = 475$) %
No self care (100% MD use)	11	26
Mixed self care and MD use	62	24
Self care only	27	50
Total	100	100

χ^2, df 2 = 163.63, $P < 0.0000$, $V = 0.38$.

Differences were somewhat less marked with respect to symptoms the respondents evaluated as more serious. In these circumstances 24% of the United States persons compared to 31% of the Japanese relied solely on self treatment (Table 4B).

The factors considered to account for self care, as posed in research question three involve both belief in physician efficacy and in one's own susceptibility to illness. Ideas about the right to autonomy in doctor–patient relationships, patients' desire for medical information, preference for physician care when ill, and experience of medical error are viewed as four indicators of perceived physician efficacy. It should be noted in presenting these and the variables assessing respondents' health, frequencies are provided only for those who claimed symptoms. However their characteristics did not differ significantly from those of the total number of respondents.

With respect to belief in patient autonomy, some older adults in Japan were a bit more likely than those in the U.S. to think they had little right to an autonomous relationship with a physician (15 vs 8%). The implication is that lay persons are less able than professionals to deal with illness, and should defer to their greater skill (Table 5A). However about half in each country were on the higher end of this distribution, demonstrating a desire to maintain patient rights. The fact that differences by country are statistically significant is due more to the size of the samples than the size of the differences.

Further in Japan a similar minority of older adults with symptoms were less likely to be interested in securing information on their condition than those in the United States, 20% in Japan in the lowest information seeking categories, compared to 2% in these

Table 4

A. Rate of self care for symptoms considered mild comparing the U.S. and Japan

Self care rate	U.S. ($N = 632$) %	Japan ($N = 393$) %
No self care (100% MD use)	11	19
Mixed self care and MD use	54	18
Self care only	34	64
Total	99	101

χ^2, df 2 = 135.02, $P < 0.000$, $V = 0.36$.

B. Rate of self care for symptoms considered more serious comparing the U.S. and Japan

Self care rate	U.S. ($N = 302$) %	Japan ($N = 173$) %
No self care (100% MD use)	43	56
Mixed self care and MD use	33	13
Self care only	24	31
Total	100	100

χ^2, df 2 = 28.86, $P < 0.0000$, $V = 0.25$.

Table 5

A. Belief in patients' right to autonomy: United States and Japanese elderly with symptoms

	U.S. ($N = 654$) %	Japan ($N = 451$) %
Low (0, 1)	8	15
Moderate (2, 3)	42	37
High (4, 5)	43	40
Very High (6)	7	8

χ^2, df 3 = 16.06, $P < 0.005$, $V = 0.12$.

B. Belief in medical information seeking: United States and Japanese elderly with symptoms

	U.S. ($N = 653$) %	Japan ($N = 475$) %
Low (0, 1, 2)	2	20
Moderate (3, 4)	50	32
High (5, 6)	46	38
Very High (7)	2	10

χ^2, df 3 = 154.94, $P < 0.0000$, $V = 0.37$.

categories in the United States (Table 5B). Again it is noteworthy that 48% in each country have a high or very high belief in the right to information. This attitude is consistent with adherence to autonomy *vis-à-vis* the physician, since knowledge of one's condition is an asset in dealing on an equal footing with a medical professional.

In the United States, symptomatic respondents were more likely to prefer a physician's services when ill: 23% strongly preferred this care compared to 14% in Japan (Table 6A). Again a sizable minority, from 24 to 32% were not so sure they wanted medical attention.

These preferences existed in the face of the fact that persons in the United States were much more apt to claim having experienced a physician making an error in their care, than were persons in Japan (46% compared to 26%) (Table 6B). Whether this finding reflects higher quality of care in Japan, or a tendency of Americans to complain about their medical outcomes cannot be determined from these self-reports.

The second set of factors that could account for turning to self care were entitled perceived susceptibility and included both mental and physical health, as well as commitment to good health practices,

Table 6

A. Preference for physician care when ill: United States and Japanese elderly with symptoms

	U.S. ($N = 648$) %	Japan ($N = 475$) %
Low (0, 1)	4	5
Moderate (2, 3)	20	27
High (4, 5)	53	55
Very high (6)	23	14

χ^2, df 3 = 19.24, $P < 0.000$, $V = 0.13$.

B. Perceived physicians' past errors: United States and Japanese elderly with symptoms

	U.S. ($N = 655$) %	Japan ($N = 460$) %
None	54	74
Some	46	26

χ^2, df 1 = 45.40, $P < 0.0000$, $V = 0.20$.

Table 7
A. Level of psychological distress: United States and Japanese elderly with symptoms

	U.S. ($N = 655$) %	Japan ($N = 473$) %
Low (1)	32	43
Moderate low (2)	44	39
High (3)	16	14
Very high (4)	9	4

χ^2, *df* 3 = 22.81, $P < 0.000$, $V = 0.14$.

B. Self assessed health: United States and Japanese elderly with symptoms

	U.S. ($N = 655$) %	Japan ($N = 474$) %
Very Poor (0, 1, 2)	10	9
Poor (3, 4)	10	12
Fair (5, 6)	27	25
Good (7, 8)	42	45
Excellent (9)	11	9

χ^2, *df* 4 = 3.70, ns, $V = 0.06$.

Table 8
A. Prevalence of chronic conditions

Chronic condition	U.S. ($N = 655$) %	Japan ($N = 475$) %
None	33	64
Some	67	36
Total	100	100

χ^2, *df* 1 = 108.12, $P < 0.0000$, $V = 0.31$.

B. Good health behaviors: United States and Japanese elderly with symptoms

Health behavior	U.S. ($N = 657$) %	Japan ($N = 475$) %
Very poor 1	4	3
2	11	14
3	21	31
4	33	35
Very good 5	32	17
Total	101	100

χ^2, *df* 4 = 36.39, $P < 0.0001$, $V = 0.18$.

presence of one or more chronic conditions, and frequency of symptom reporting. These could indicate a person's perceived low likelihood of getting worse and thus willingness to forego reliance on professional help. On the measure of psychological distress, 43% of these Japanese older adults reported little or no distress, compared to 32% of the United States respondents, and in the same vein 25% in the United States elders admitted to high or very high distress, compared to 18% of the Japanese (Table 7B). These results suggest more psychological well-being among the Japanese than the American respondents.

With respect to the scale combining three facets of self assessed physical health, evaluations were about equal. Fifty-four percent of those in Japan considered their health very good or excellent, compared to 53% of those in the United States with the same view (Table 7A). However, not consistent with these findings, respondents in the two countries were dissimilar with respect to the presence of chronic conditions. About a third reported one or more chronic ailments in Japan, but in the U.S. two-thirds claimed such conditions (Table 8A). The lower rate in Japan matches the lower incidence of experienced symptoms in that country as compared to the United States.

The index of Good Health Behavior, which combined indicators of adequate sleep, reasonable diet, low use of alcohol and cigarettes, and physical exercise, suggested an orientation to maintaining one's good health. On this measure, the United States outshone the Japanese respondents, with 32% reporting very good behavior, compared to only 17% in Japan (Table 8B).

Also used as an indicator of health status was the number of symptoms reported in the prior three months. The rationale is that persons with more symptoms are likely to consider their health fragile. As reported above, persons in Japan claimed fewer symptoms than those in the United States.

To determine the answer to question four, concerning Japanese and American differences in the joint effects of attitudes toward physician efficacy and beliefs in own mental and physical health on use of a self care, multiple regression was employed, controlling for age, gender, education and social resources. The trichotomous outcomes, rates of self care, are not normally distributed, it will be noted, but ordinary least squares are considered robust in the face of departures from normality. Also factors reaching statistical significance at the 0.10 level are reported, as being indicative of trends in the data. Since persons reporting multiple symptoms could have considered some mild and some serious, the variable of symptom seriousness could not be used in the regression, because it did not apply exclusively to some subjects. Accordingly separate regressions were run with self care for symptoms considered mild and for symptoms considered more serious, as two distinct outcomes, along with a regression for the total set of symptoms, which perforce omitted seriousness as a measure.

Table 9. Regression of self care rate for all symptoms on health and attitude variables, with demographics controls, comparing the U.S. and Japan

	U.S. β	U.S. P[a]	Japan β	Japan P[a]
Chronic condition	0.072	<0.09	−0.129	<0.01
Good health behavior	−0.076	<0.06	−0.102	<0.03
Self assessed health	0.094	<0.06	0.127	<0.02
Total number of symptoms	−0.086	<0.07	—	—
Desire for information	—	—	0.081	<0.08
Social resources	—	—	−0.078	<0.10
Education	−0.089	<0.03	—	—
Adjusted R^2	0.03		0.05	
	$F_{5,642} = 5.49$, $P < 0.001$		$F_{5,445} = 5.67$, $P < 0.0001$	

[a]Probabilities of <0.10 are reported to indicate trends in the data.

Table 10. Regression of self care rate for symptoms considered mild on health and attitude variables, with demographics controls, comparing the U.S. and Japan

	U.S. β	U.S. P^*	Japan β	Japan P^*
	($N = 624$)		($N = 373$)	
Total number of symptoms	−0.139	<0.01	—	—
Chronic condition	0.073	<0.09	−0.142	<0.01
Psychological distress	0.095	<0.05	—	—
Education	−0.068	<0.10	—	—
Right to autonomy	—	—	0.10	<0.07
Adjusted R^2	0.03		0.04	
	$F_{5,618} = 5.19$, $P < 0.001$		$F_{1,370} = 5.53$, $P < 0.01$	

*Probabilities of <0.10 are reported to indicate trends in the data. In the U.S. Health Status entered at the 0.14 level, while in Japan Right to Information entered at the 0.12 level.

Explanatory patterns showed both similarities and differences between the two countries. In both the United States and Japan, factors related to self care use for the total set of symptoms included better self assessed health, and fewer good health behaviors although technically these factors qualified only as trends in the United States. In Japan absence of a chronic condition encouraged self treatment while in the United States a trend toward presence of chronic ailments related to self care, as did a trend to fewer perceived symptoms. Only one attitude variable, desire for information, was relevant to self care, but it was limited to a trend in Japan. Also, in Japan, fewer social resources were related to self treatment. Lower education was the most significant predictor of self care in the United States sample, but had no effect in Japan (Table 9). Explained variance in self care rate was minimal; R^2 was 3% in the U.S. and 5% in Japan respectively. But it should be noted that these results did not include a variable of 'need', and in this respect explained variance was similar to that remaining in utilization studies after 'need' has been ruled out (e.g. Ref. [23]).

Regression results for symptoms believed to be mild exhibited less cross-national congruence. Chronic condition, the only common explanatory factor was again opposite in effect; absence of chronicity was significant in Japan, in contrast to a trend for presence of chronicity fostering self care in the United States. Fewer symptoms experienced and greater psychological distress along with lower education related to self care rate in the United States, but only belief in the right to autonomy had a similar effect in Japan. Again explained variance was small, 3 and 4% respectively (Table 10).

As for symptoms believed to be serious, only less good health behavior among the Japanese respondents, and lower preference for physician care among the United States respondents had any effect on their self care rates. Moreover the explained variance was trivial, 1% in the U.S. and 2% in Japan (Table 11).

DISCUSSION

In response to research questions one and two, concerning cross-cultural differences in symptom experience and self care behavior, the findings show that older adults in Japan, as compared to those in the United States, report fewer symptoms and are more likely to use self treatment for perceived symptoms, even if they are considered more serious. The most meaningful variations in attributes that might explain these differences, as posed in question three, are the Japanese lower rate of emotional ill-health, lower desire for health information, and less preference for physician care, despite fewer claimed experiences of physician error. On the other hand, older adults in the two countries were almost identical in evaluations of their own state of health, although in the Japanese society the respondents were less likely to engage in good health practices.

In answer to question four about the joint effect of these variables, results revealed that different sets of factors explain the use of self care in these two countries. In the United States fewer symptoms and lower education were related to more use of self care, while greater desire for information and fewer social resources applied only to Japan. This lends some support to the suggestion that family involvement facilitates physician utilization, in Japanese culture. The result is intriguing, and the role that social resources play in self care needs to be explored in future studies. Japan and the United States shared three explanatory factors. In both countries persons with higher self-assessed health more frequently relied on self care. In contrast, it was also those persons who practiced fewer good health behaviors who used more self care. Finally, although the presence of

Table 11. Regression of self care rate for symptoms considered more serious on health and attitude variables, with demographics controls, comparing the U.S. and Japan

	U.S. β	U.S. P^*	Japan β	Japan P^*
	($N = 297$)		($N = 166$)	
Good health behavior	—	—	−0.17	<0.03
Preference for MD care	−0.10	<0.10	—	—
Adjusted R^2	0.01		0.02	
	$F_{1,296} = 2.86$, $P < 0.10$		$F_{1,165} = 5.01$, $P < 0.03$	

*Probabilities of <0.10 are reported to indicate trends in the data.

chronic conditions had a significant impact on self care, the variable expressed itself in opposite directions in the two cultures. In the United States the presence of chronic conditions led to more self care, but in Japan the opposite was true.

For mild symptoms, in the United States less psychological distress was explanatory, while a desire for autonomy affected use of self care in Japan. For serious symptoms, only low preference for M.D. care was effective in the United States, while in Japan poor health behavior was explanatory. The low amount of explained variance for total, mild and serious symptoms reveals that many explanatory factors were missing in the research. Furthermore, there are apparent contradictions in the data. The presence of a chronic condition fosters self care in the United States, but its absence relates to self care in Japan. The Japanese report fewer symptoms but engage in less good health behavior, and they use both more physician care and more self care than found in the United States data.

The disparate effect of chronic illness may well be a result of cultural differences. In the United States the need to cut health costs, particularly among the elderly and the focus on patient responsiblity for the management of chronic illnesses, along with an increasing emphasis on consumerism [17] argues for self treatment. In Japan the presence of a chronic condition may be decisive in drawing the individual into the network of repeat visits and monitoring that is characteristic of the Japanese biomedical system [15]. On the other hand, being free of a chronic ailment, in terms of the Health Belief model, indicates confidence in ones low susceptibility to disease and thus assurance that self treatment will work.

The Japanese place a high priority on health and medical care and they report themselves as being in good health both objectively and subjectively [24]. The research reported here confirms this finding and shows that the Japanese, compared to a U.S. sample, report fewer symptoms in a three month retrospective, but in apparent contradiction claim less good health behavior. The contradiction can be resolved through the recognition that the effects of poor dietary habits, indulgence in cigarettes and alcohol and lack of exercise do not necessarily result in immediate ill health, even if they have a negative impact on cardiovascular disease and cancer in the long run. If anything, the report of poor health behavior appears incompatible with personal autonomy, the decision to take charge of ones own health and well-being, a disparity that is discussed further below. The greater use of both physician care and self care in Japan than in the United States depending on the seriousness of a condition, is not really an anomaly, but instead indicative of a focus on good health that is more central to the culture of Japan than it has been in the United States. The Japanese are very sensitive to the condition of the body, and the management of its care [11] and will selectively use professional and/or lay care as they consider appropriate for a specific bodily change.

One line of logic argues that good health results from speedy professional attention to any symptoms of ill health. This reasoning would lead us to expect our Japanese sample to report high rates of physician utilization for the symptoms they did experience. As already noted above, Japan has a national health care system that, since 1961, has covered its entire population at a relatively low cost to the consumer. In addition, its urban areas, in particular, are well supplied with physicians, making ambulatory care at local clinics easy to obtain [25]. Furthermore, Lock [26] argues convincingly that the medical institution and its medicalization of (especially women's) socially induced psychosomatic problems serves to satisfy important non-medical needs. Secondly, the cultural pattern of recommended or required revisits is present, due primarily to the financial rewards of over-scheduling patients [15]. Indeed the rate for those receiving medical care has been increasing, though this is due in part to the aging of the population.

On the other hand, the national health care system is unlikely to account for the much lower rate of reported symptoms in Japan. One speculation is that the Japanese are in fact healthier, as evidenced by their lower prevalence of chronic conditions, and their self assessed emotional well being, as well as government statistics on symptom prevalence [27]. A counter view is that older Japanese are more reticent about admitting to psychological distress or ill health, or may have a different conception of when a bodily change can be considered a symptom.

The Japanese, when compared to Americans, do show a higher rate of exclusive physician consultation. However, this is coupled with an even larger reliance on self care. This occurs in spite of the fact that Americans and Japanese report similar preferences for physician care and even fewer instances of physician error in Japan. In other words, Japanese, unlike Americans, seem to do one or the other.

One key to this pattern lies in the doctor–patient relationship in Japan, which, as is true of all countries, is embedded in culture, and thus embodies aspects not present in the American relationship. It is highly non-verbal [15, 26] and hierarchical [25, 28], and may be subject to manipulation, as for example the use of gift giving by patients to establish a reciprocal, not wholly dependent relationship with the physician [29, p. 41]. Patients do not expect to be equal participants, or involved in health care decision-making. Indeed this has led to growing patient dissatisfaction, but without the possibilities for change through confrontation that exist in the consumer movement in the U.S. [26]. This acceptance of the cultural definition of the role of the physician can be seen in the data on information seeking. This would seem to indicate a low desire for knowledge about one's medical condition or health. However, the Japanese are avid consumers of medical information [26]. A deconstruction of the scale coupled with cultural knowledge suggests a different conclusion: that the scale accurately reflects the Japanese acceptance of cultural norms prohibiting discussion as indicative of lack of faith and respect that could even put the continued relationship with the physician in jeopardy [25]. This leads to the conclusion that due to their recognition of the loss of autonomy once the hierarchical doctor–patient relationship is entered, the Japanese prefer to avoid use of physicians except in response to the more serious symptoms. This allows them the autonomy of self care through published materials and over the counter and kanpo medications that flourish in Japan [30]. Only if the symptom is deemed really serious, and the patients feel their lay knowledge is inadequate, are they willing to forego autonomy, and place themselves fully in the hands of the doctor [31].

Although there is a statistically significant difference favoring patients' rights in the U.S., as pointed out in the results section, this significance is primarily an artifact of the large sample size, since about half in each country support the value of patient autonomy in dealing with physicians. In fact the degree of similarity of Japanese and U.S. views on autonomy is arresting given the established physician belief that patients have no 'right' to know their diagnosis and prognosis in the case of terminal illness [32], and should be protected from such knowledge by their physician. Debate on the ethics of such denial of information was intensified by the emperor's death in 1990 from cancer, and the controversy about the non-disclosure of his diagnosis, and has continued with his cousin's insistence in 1991 on disclosure of his cancer diagnosis.

A close examination of the nuances of the items in the Right to Autonomy Scale shows that it contains references to the level of autonomy a person has in decision making once the physician–patient relationship is established as well as the person's right to terminate that relationship. Thus autonomy may express itself in two ways. One dimension is patients' belief or perception of the level of autonomy that will be afforded them, or that they can legitimately expect, ... an expectation that as Antonovsky [29] shows is at least in part culturally based. The cultural factors that produce this particular role definition will influence the patients' perception of the appropriate role behaviors and rewards from the autonomy within that role. In Japan, noted for its emphasis on hierarchical relationships in general and in the medical profession as a mirror of society [28], the physician–patient relationship is seen as one in which one's dependency must be expressed, making it simultaneously opportunity and obligation [25].

A second dimension of autonomy, that was not originally conceptually distinct but whose distinction is urged by the results, is personal autonomy as the rejection of passivity in regard to the body's health. This involves the individual's awareness of physical states and response to his/her symptoms, and it stands in contrast to the relational autonomy that one experiences within interpersonal relationships. While relational autonomy is low in the physician–patient context there is support in this study as well as others [14, 15, 26, 27] that personal autonomy in regard to health is high. This distinction may help to explain the autonomy and self care findings from these data.

An apparent contradiction to personal autonomy is the lower score on good health behaviors, particularly smoking and drinking alcohol, to which the Japanese would be expected to adhere. However, the negative effects of neglecting good health behaviors have only recently been publicized, and health education for prevention, beyond the areas of cancer and hypertension, is not yet well coordinated or widespread [25]. In practical terms the Japanese already practice an important good health behavior, walking, which no doubt contributes to the lower level of some of their particular symptoms, such as shortness of breath, stiffness, and edema of the legs. Activity in the form of walking is an integral part of Japanese daily life as well as the most popular sports activity for the elderly [33]. In contrast to American society, Japan's reliance on public transportation and daily food shopping at a local market necessitate a greater amount of routine daily walking, not for sport but as transportation to the bus stop and market. Furthermore, many Japanese elderly still prefer to sit on a tatami floor rather than a Western style sofa [33] and this, combined with the use of squat toilets and lower incidence of obesity, results in Japanese with greater physical flexibility. On the other hand, the different seasons in which interviewing was done (January–March in Japan and July–September in the United States) can account for the slightly higher incidence of colds in the Japanese population.

Another pathway that could be explored in future research on Japan concerns differences between those who report symptoms, and those who do not. Data not reported here show that those who do not claim to have experienced symptoms are no different from the symptomatic in attitudes toward autonomy, physician care and the desire for medical information. But they are less likely to have a chronic condition and to report psychological distress. Comparisons between the symptomatic and asymptomatic in the United States were not possible because, unlike the situation in Japan, nearly everyone reported having experienced a complaint. Differences in defining bodily changes as symptoms offer fruitful areas for cultural variations in health perceptions.

In conclusion, Japanese cultural patterns of activity and interpersonal relationships explain much of their desire to rely on self care. The Health Belief Model's explanatory variables of perceived efficacy of physician care, and perceived susceptibility to illness take different forms in the United States and Japan, although they are still related to self care actions. Cultural variations in levels of personal and relational autonomy in every day life styles and attitudes about the body are most critical in describing cross-national differences in health behavior. Although differences in the structure of health care delivery play a role, they take second place to the impact of the cultural milieux of the two industrial countries.

Acknowledgement—Support for this project was provided in part by National Institute on Aging, RO1-AGO5876.

REFERENCES

1. Levin L. S. and Idler E. L. *The Hidden Health Care System: Mediating Structures and Medicine*. Ballinger, Cambridge, 1981.
2. Williamson J. D. and Danaher K. *Self Care in Health*. Croom Helm, London, 1978.
3. Fleming G. V., Giachello A. L., Andersen R. M. and Andrade P. Self care: Substitute, supplement or stimulus for formal medical care services? *Med. Care* **22**, 950, 1984.
4. Dean K. J. (1986) Self care behavior: Implications for

aging. In *Self Care and Health in Old Age* (Edited by Dean K., Hickey T. and Holstein B. E.), pp. 58–93. Croom Helm, Dover, NH.

5. Haug M. R., Wykle M. L. and Namazi K. H. Self-care among older adults. *Soc. Sci. Med.* **29,** (2), 171–183, 1989.
6. Rakowski W., Hickey T. and Dengiz A. N. Consequence of health and treatment perceptions among older patients and providers of primary care. *Int. J. Aging Hum. Dev.* **25,** (1), 63–77, 1987.
7. Levin L. S., Katz A. H. and Holst E. *Self Care: Lay Initiatives in Health*. Prodist, New York, 1976.
8. Hickey T. *Health and Aging*. Brooks/Cole, Monterey, CA, 1980.
9. Becker M. H., Brachman R. H. and Kirscht J. P. A new approach to explaining sick role behavior in low-income populations. *Am. J. Publ. Hlth* **64,** 205, 1974.
10. Janz N. K. and Becker M. H. The Health Belief Model: A decade later. *Hlth Educ. Q.* **11,** 1, 1984.
11. Caudill W. The cultural and interpersonal context of everyday health and illness in Japan and America. In *Asian Medical Systems: A Comparative Study* (Edited by Leslie C.), pp. 159–177. University of California Press, Berkeley, 1976.
12. Triaudis H. G. and Breslin R. W. Cross-cultural psychology. *Am. Psychol.* **39,** (9), 1006–1016, 1984.
13. Japan Ministry of Health and Welfare. *Annual Report on Health and Welfare for 1989, October*. Ministry of Health and Welfare, Tokyo, Japan, 1989.
14. Lock M. M. *East Asian Medicine in Urban Japan*. University of California Press, Berkeley, 1980.
15. Ohnuki-Tierney E. *Illness and Cultural in Contemporary Japan*. Cambridge University Press, London, 1984.
16. Ford A. B., Haug M. R., Jones P. K., Roy A. W. and Folmar S. J. Race-related differences among elderly urban residents: A cohort study, 1975–1984. *J. Geront.* **45,** (4), S163–S171, 1990.
17. Haug M. R. and Lavin B. *Consumerism in Medicine*. Sage, Beverly Hills, CA, 1983.
18. Krantz D. S., Baum A. and Wideman M. V. Assessment of preferences for self treatment and information in health care. *J. Person. Soc. Psychol.* **39,** 977–990, 1980.
19. Haug M., Breslau N. and Folmar S. J. Coping resources and selective survival in mental health of the elderly. *J. Geront.* **2,** (4), 468–491, 1989.
20. Berkman L. and Breslow L. *Health and Ways of Living: The Alameda County Study*. Oxford University Press, New York, 1983.
21. Duke University Center for the Study of Aging and Human Development. *Multidimensional Functional Assessment: The OARS Methodology*, 2nd edn. The Center for the Study of Aging and Human Development, Durham, NC, 1978.
22. Lock M. Cultural construction of the menopausal syndrome: The Japanese case. *Maturitas* **10,** 317–332, 1988.
23. Coulton C. and Frost A. K. Use of social and health services by the elderly. *J. Hlth Soc. Behav.* **23,** 330–339, 1982.
24. Steslicke W. E. The Japanese state of health: A political-economic perspective. In *Health, Illness, and Medical Care in Japan* (Edited by Norbeck E. and Lock M.), pp. 24–65. University of Hawaii Press, Honolulu, 1987.
25. Powell M. and Anesaki M. *Health Care in Japan*. Routledge, London, 1990.
26. Lock M. M. Protests of a good wife and wise mother: The medicalization of distress in Japan. In *Health, Illness, and Medical Care in Japan* (Edited by Norbeck E. and Lock M.), pp. 1–23. University of Hawaii Press, Honolulu, 1987.
27. Japanese Ministry of Health and Welfare. *Annual Report on Health and Welfare for 1983, October*. Ministry of Health and Welfare, Tokyo, 1983.
28. Long S. O. Health care providers: Technology, policy, and professional dominance. In *Health, Illness, and Medical Care in Japan* (Edited by Norbeck E. and Lock M.), pp. 66–88. University of Hawaii Press, Honolulu, 1987.
29. Antonovsky A. A model to explain visits to the doctor: With specific reference to the case of Israel. *J. Hlth Soc. Behav.* **13,** 446–454, 1972.
30. Sonoda K. *Health and Illness in Changing Japanese Society*. University of Tokyo Press, Tokyo, 1988.
31. Long S. O. The ins and outs of doctor-patient relations in Japan. *Am. J. Chinese Med.* **VIII,** (1), 37–46, 1980.
32. Long S. O. and Long B. D. Curable cancers and fatal ulcers: Attitudes toward cancer in Japan. *Soc. Sci. Med.* **16,** 2101–2108, 1982.
33. Hakuhodo Institute of Life and Living. *Changing Lifestyles in Japan 4: Japanese Seniors, Pioneers in the Era of Aging Populations*. Tokyo, Japan, 1987.

Appendix (Symptom List) overleaf

APPENDIX

Symptom List

These symptoms are grouped by possible type of classification, but will be put in random order in the questionnaire. For each symptom, respondents will be asked if it was experienced in the past four months, and if so (1) what action was taken in response, and (2) if s/he considered it mild, fairly serious or very serious. Data from prior work of the investigators are included, as evidence of subjects' understanding of the symptoms as an illness.

	Number of persons reporting symptom	% using some form of self care as first response*	% considering symptom fairly or very serious
Digestive system:			
Diarrhea for more than one day	28	86	43
Abdominal pains, for at least a couple of days	77	94	36
Repeated indigestion or upset stomach	105	98	19
Trouble moving bowels regularly	118	100	16
Heart and circulation:			
Repeated pains in or near the heart	70	90	40
Shortness of breath, even after light work	162	80	26
Swelling of feet, legs or hands	198	82	20
Dizziness	124	84	14
Muscular-skeletal system:			
Pain or swelling in any joints or muscles during the day	191	82	29
Waking up with stiff or aching joints or muscles	260	90	23
Frequent backaches	179	95	32
Infections:			
Sore throat or running nose with a fever as high as 100°F for at least two days	61	94	43
A cough anytime during night or day which lasted for several weeks	103	82	34
Any infections, irritations or pain in the ears	62	79	29
Any infections, irritations or pain in the eyes	116	84	27
Sneezing for two weeks or more	46	52	6
General tiredness:			
Feeling tired for weeks at a time for no special reasons	84	82	33
Sudden feelings of weakness or fainting	144	100	25
Getting up some mornings tired and exhausted even with the usual amount of rest	261	78	14
Not otherwise classified:			
Frequent headaches	88	88	38
Unexpected bleeding from any part of the body	57	82	30
Skin rash or breaking out on any part of the body	119	84	19
A burning sensation when urinating	30	73	17
Itching, bleeding or pain of the rectal area	66	79	18

*The balance either used 'nothing', followed by self care, or immediately visited a physician.

[20]

Sociology of Health & Illness Vol. 15 No. 2 1993 ISSN 0141–9889

Reshaping of self: a pendular reconstruction of self and identity among adults with traumatic spinal cord injury

Karen K. Yoshida

(University of Toronto)

Abstract This paper describes the impact of chronic illness on self and identity among 35 adults with traumatic spinal cord injury (paraplegic), living in the community. The reconstruction of self and identity post spinal cord injury is conceptualised as a pendulum. The pendulum of self represents a dynamic model of identity reconstruction. The pendulum suggests that identity reconstruction is a process that swings back and forth like a pendulum between the nondisabled and disabled aspects of self. The pendulum depicts five predominant identity views (outcomes). These are: 1) the former self; 2) the supernormal identity; 3) the disabled identity as total self; 4) the disabled identity as an aspect of the total self; and 5) the middle self. These identity views are influenced by five experiences (processes). These are: 1) loss; 2) sustainment; 3) integration; 4) continuity and 5) development of the self. It is suggested that frameworks of identity reconstruction or reconstitution which include both process and outcome components may elucidate more clearly the impact of chronic illness on self and identity. In addition, this pendulum model of identity reconstruction is an alternative approach to traditional sociological conceptions of identity reconstruction.

Introduction

This paper examines the consequences of chronic illness and disability for self and identity. The importance of the life reconstruction process makes understanding the impact of chronic illness on self and identity a fundamental concern (Conrad 1987: 11–12). Both Mead (1934) and Blumer (1969) have identified the centrality of the self as the medium through which people interpret situations and take action.

A number of authors have examined and conceptualised the self generally and in relationship to chronic illness and disability. Both Goffman (1959; 1961) and Strauss (1969) have illustrated the active nature of individuals in controlling the definition of self and the social situation. Goffman has extended this analysis to individuals who are 'stigmatised' and has discussed the negotiation between individuals' social and personal identities (Goffman 1963: 42–102).

Recent work on the reconstruction of self in the illness experience literature can be organised into 'process' and 'outcome' frameworks and constructs. With respect to process, both Bury (1982) and Williams (1984) examined how individuals achieved or attempted to achieve a sense of order of their past biography resulting from the onset of rheumatoid arthritis. Bury describes this process as a 'biographical disruption' (Bury 1982: 169), while Williams uses the concept of 'narrative reconstruction' (Williams 1984: 177–80) to illustrate how respondents accounted for their arthritis. Corbin and Strauss (1987; 1988) have also examined the 'process' of identity reconstruction among individuals with a variety of chronic conditions. They believe that conceptions of self refer to the individual's personal identity concerning his/her life course or biography. The total self is formed by the integration of various aspects of 'self into a more inclusive whole' (Corbin and Strauss 1987: 264). This conception of self is formed through four types of biographical work; one form of work focussing on identity reconstitution. The specific process of identity reconstitution appears to focus on the continuity of the self prior to the chronic illness or disability and integration of 'new aspects of self' (Corbin and Strauss 1987: 272). While this 'process' literature on identity reconstruction describes in a variety of ways the means by which self and identity may be reconstructed, it lacks specificity regarding what emerges through identity reconstitution.

Other authors have attempted to delineate the 'outcomes' of identity reconstitution. Loss of self is a fundamental consequence of chronic illness (Charmaz 1983; Fontana and Smith 1989; Orona 1990: 1254). Fontana and Smith (1989: 43–5) describe further what aspects of selfhood remain after the deteriorating effects of Alzheimer's disease. They believe that socially constructed aspects of self remain, maintained by the actions of others. Charmaz (1987: 284) has illustrated a potential range of outcomes of reconstituted identities for individuals with chronic progressive deteriorating conditions. She argues that individuals aspire to construct preferred personal and social identities. Charmaz conceptualises this striving for self as an identity hierarchy consisting of identity levels. These identity levels are: 1) the supernormal social identity, an identity where extraordinary feats are commonplace in the conventional world; 2) the restored self, a reconstruction of previous identities prior to the illness; 3) a contingent self; which is a potential, but uncertain identity because of the possibility of future illness; and 4) the salvaged self, which is retaining a past identity based upon a valued activity or attribute while becoming physically dependent. Movement through the hierarchy with respect to progressive deteriorating illness often means, 'reducing identity goals and aiming for a lower level in the identity hierarchy' (Charmaz 1987: 285).

While there is a substantial literature in this area, there are a number of omissions and assumptions. First, there is an absence of conceptualisation of identity reconstitution that considers both 'process' and 'outcome' components. Frameworks which include both may elucidate more clearly the consequence of chronic illness for self and identity. Related to this concern is that while the sociological literature depicts identity reconstitution as linear and nonlinear processes of change, it is the continued explicit development of nonlinear models of identity reconstruction which will further our understanding of living with disability. This is important as living with chronic illness or disability is a continuous adaptive process (Strauss and Glaser 1975; Gallagher 1976; Anderson and Bury 1988). Current conceptualisations of identity reconstruction also focus either on the self prior to the chronic illness, ie the nondisabled self, or on the disability, the disabled self. There is little explicit work that reveals how the disability 'fits' into the total self. This latter point is not just an academic concern; individuals with disabilities are grappling with how encompassing the disability should be to their individual and collective identities (Hahn 1990; Groch 1990).

The purpose of this paper is to describe the emerging self among individuals who have sustained traumatic spinal cord injuries. This analysis takes into consideration the notions of a non-linear transformation of identity, 'process' and 'outcome' elements of identity reconstruction, and how the disability merges with the nondisabled self. This emerging selfhood among individuals post spinal cord injury has been conceptualised here as a pendular reconstruction of self.

Post-disability identity reconstruction

The concept of self is derived from a symbolic interactionist perspective (Blumer 1969). While the self is seen as a reflexive process and not a structure per se, it is an organisation that is sustained by the appraisals of the individual, other individuals and by the shared meanings that arise from social interaction. Similar to Charmaz (1987: 284), it is argued here that people may have more than one identity and that identities are formed through the above processes of self-definition and social interaction. Individuals hold personal and social identities which influence and shape an evolving self (Goffman 1963). The self, then, is 'an emergent structure or organisation as it may shift or change as the person reflexively interprets the identifications and images that self and others confer upon him or her (Charmaz 1987: 284).

Pendular shape and identity reconstruction

The form of this identity reconstruction among individuals with traumatic spinal cord injuries is best described as a pendular shape. The metaphor of a pendulum has been used to depict the dynamic process of identity reconstruction as revealed by the respondents in this study. The metaphor of a pendulum is used as respondents illustrated through their accounts how they moved back and forth between their nondisabled and disabled aspects of the total self, in speaking about how they reconstructed their lives post injury. The pendular shape of identity reconstruction among individuals with traumatic spinal cord injuries represents an oscillation between conceptually distinct, but empirically overlapping types of identities which encompass nondisabled and/or disabled aspects of self. Central to the pendular shape is the expression of identity reconstruction as a dual directional process. Using a pendular shape to denote this adaptation to living with a disability is in contrast to current sociological concepts of trajectory (Glaser and Strauss 1964) and career (Hughes 1958) which have been used to describe the process of living with chronic illness and disability.

The sociological concept of trajectory was first articulated by Glaser and Strauss (1964) in the context of research on dying in hospitals. The term dying trajectory reflected the perceived course of dying from the patient's perspective. A dying trajectory was a concept denoting a unidirectional passage through time and events. The concept of career (Hughes 1958) has also been used to depict change. The sociological concept of career again denotes passage through time and events, with a uni-directional aspect to the concept. This directional element is evidenced by the predominant usage of the term to illustrate sequential stages or phases of various forms of work (Hughes 1958: 8–22). Recently, it has been suggested that the concept of career may be too rigid a concept to apply to the long term adaptation of chronic illness and disability (Conrad 1987: 9–10). Conrad (1987) advocates the use of the concept of trajectory by arguing that it:

> . . . may be more appropriate to studies in the experience of illness since it encompasses process and change but does not assume linearity or orderliness (Conrad 1987: 10).

Much sociological research however, has used the concept of career to illustrate process and change in various life domains with respect to disability (Goffman 1961: 32; Locker and Kaufert 1988: 26–7; Gerhardt 1990: 1211–12). In their examination of the impact of changing medical technology on post-polio patients' daily lives, Locker and Kaufert (1988) used the concept of career not only as a passage through time, but as a multidimensional concept. They suggest in the lives of their respondents, technology influences individuals' biophysical functional and psychosocial careers.

The concept of trajectory has also evolved in a manner that suggests it may be used to express the idea of nonlinearity. Strauss and Glaser (1975) have applied the concept of trajectory to chronic illness. The notion of illness trajectory suggests the idea of a nonlinear process. For example, individuals with rheumatoid arthritis or multiple sclerosis will have a nonlinear trajectory punctuated by periods of exacerbation (flare-ups) and remission which are characteristic of these chronic conditions. The notion of illness trajectory encompasses not only the physiological course of the disease but includes the total organisation of work performed by the individual and others and the impact of that work for the individual and others (Strauss *et al* 1982). Again, this suggests that the organisation and impact of work in the care of persons with chronic illness represents a passage through time but one with a fluctuating or nonlinear existence for those with chronic illness and caregivers. Therefore, the concept of trajectory may be used to depict both linear and nonlinear processes.

In this paper, the process of identity reconstruction conceptualised as a pendulum shares with the concepts of trajectory and career that they are shapes or forms to express living with chronic illness or disability. Identity reconstruction as a pendulum, however, differs from these traditional concepts in that it expresses the idea of dual directionality rather than unidirectionality. This feature of the pendulum concept provides an alternative approach to current conceptualisations of life reconstruction after disability.

Methods and data

The paper is derived from data collected on 35 adults living in urban centres of Southern Ontario, who sustained a traumatic spinal cord injury resulting in paralysis to the lower limbs and parts of the trunk (paraplegics). The study group is a snowball sample derived from personal contacts and through advertisements in local newspapers and newsletters. These data were collected by in-depth interviews conducted by the author between November 1988 to September 1989. The interviews, semi-structured in nature and tape recorded, focussed on how individuals reconstructed their lives post injury. Primary areas of concern were reconstruction of labour force participation, community living and the role socio-economic status played in this process. While the issue of identity was not dominant in the formative stages of the research, it became a dominant theme during the early interviews and was subsequently incorporated in an explicit manner for the rest of the interviews.

Twenty-eight men and 7 women were interviewed. This four-to-one ratio of men to women reflects the gender distribution of individuals with spinal cord injuries (Trieschmann 1980; 1988, Maddox 1987: 38). The age at injury ranged from 8 to 52 years, with an average age of 22 years at onset. The majority of respondents had their lesions at the thoracic level of the spine. The current age of respondents was between 22 to 56 years with a mean current age of 32 years. The number of years living with a spinal cord injury ranged between one to 22 years with a mean of 8.9 years. With respect to employment status at the time of the interview, 27 were working full time, five were unemployed (one on long term disability) and three were enrolled in educational programmes. Marital status at the time of the interview was varied; 15 were single (never married); 12 married/cohabiting; 6 separated/divorced and 2 engaged.

All 35 interviews were transcribed from full verbatim responses. Respondents' experiences and accounts were examined from a general symbolic interactionist perspective (Mead 1934, Blumer 1969). A grounded theory method for data analysis was used (Glaser and Strauss 1967, Glaser 1978). In transcribing the interviews 'insight notes' which consisted of ideas, general comments and reactions to the interview data were recorded. This 'memo writing' (Charmaz 1990) assisted in the development of codes and categories of the transcribed text. The Ethnograph Program (Seidel *et al* 1988) was used to assist in the management of these data.

Respondents' accounts are used to illustrate the concepts presented in this paper. Quotations are by respondents who typified the response/concept, but are based upon the dominant themes as mentioned by the majority of participants.

Overview of the pendular shape of identity reconstruction

A description of the pendular reshaping of self among individuals with traumatic spinal cord injuries follows. First, the overall framework will be described. Second, the key features of this framework: the predominant identity views which represent 'outcomes' of identity reconstruction will be detailed. The 'process' element of the pendulum are experiences or situations which shape the identity views. These experiences will be briefly discussed. Last, narrative analysis of two respondents will be presented to illustrate the pendular shape of identity reconstruction.

The pendulum of self refers to a proposed life course of self and identity after the onset of traumatic spinal cord injury (Fig. 1). This model suggests that the emerging self after spinal cord injury swings back and forth like a pendulum between the nondisabled and disabled aspects of self. Between these outer positions on the pendulum, individuals may pass through and experience different degrees of the nondisabled and disabled selves called predominant identity views. These predominant identity views reflect that self which is articulated implicitly or explicitly by the

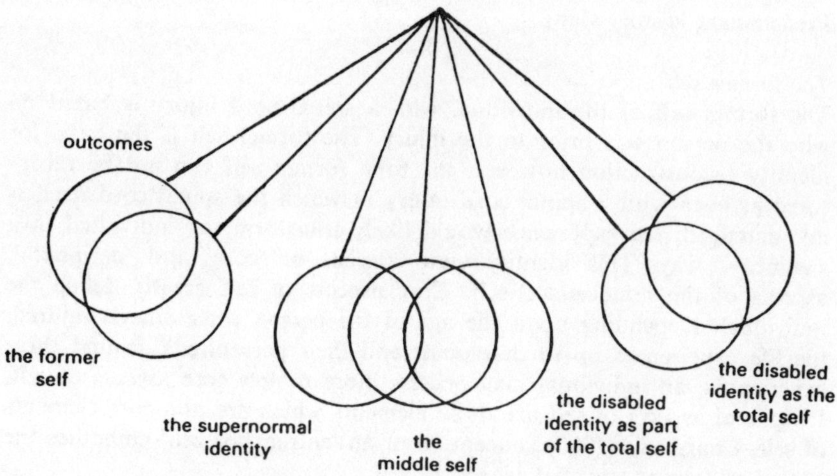

Fig. 1 The pendular reconstruction of self: predominant identity views

individual as the most important self to express over a period of time and/or within a particular situation. There were five predominant identity views emerging from the interviews: *the former self; the supernormal identity; the disabled identity as total self; the disabled identity as an aspect of the total self and the middle self.*

Generally speaking, movement along the pendulum represents a relatively long term process (months or years). Specifically, the usual pendulum shape of movement was from the former self over to the disabled identity as total self, back to the supernormal identity, then to the disabled identity as an aspect of the total self, then moving to the central of the pendulum, the middle self. Individuals, however, may or may not experience all these identities; or a person could be situated at any one of these identities with relatively little movement to any other identity view(s). If individuals reach the middle self, they still carry the other identity views with them. At this point, movement between the identity views continues to reflect a pendular shape as individuals with spinal cord injuries may oscillate between these identity views depending upon the definition of life situations. Movement along the pendulum was influenced by a number of experiences: *loss; sustainment; integration; continuity and development.* These experiences shaped the evolving of self of respondents. Thus the model allows for variability in response over time and situationally.

Predominant identity views

The former self

The former self of the individual with a spinal cord injury is based on who the person was prior to the injury. The former self is the basis for identity reconstruction however, the total former self can not be recaptured as even with a spinal cord injury in which the spinal cord itself is not damaged, the experience would likely transform the individual in a significant way. This identity view consists of 'core' and 'peripheral' aspects of the nondisabled self. Core aspects of self greatly define the individual. Depending upon the age of the person when s/he is injured, the life experiences up to that point and their perceptions around these experiences, an individual may possess more or less core aspects of self. Peripheral aspects of self are those elements which are non-core elements of self. Charmaz's (1987) conception of an 'entrenched self' embodies the notion of core or essential aspects of self:

> These persons hold clear images of their self concepts which they can readily articulate. The entrenched self represents patterns of action, conviction and habits built up over the years. These unchanged patterns had been a source of self respect before illness. After illness, resuming these patterns becomes the person's major objectives. Those who aim for an entrenched self typically know exactly what they wish to do and who they wish to be (Charmaz 1987: 302).

What is problematic is that the majority of individuals who sustain traumatic spinal cord injuries are young adults generally between the ages of 18 to 30 years of age (Trieschmann 1988; Maddox 1987: 38). These individuals may or may not have 'core' aspects to self to use as a basis for action after the spinal cord injury. One respondent, Mr NS, in particular, was injured when he was a teenager remarked:

> *Mr NS*: You know I guess, being young too, being hurt at a young age, did not help. You know, you don't fully mature. If I was older I think the story would have been different.

This particular individual was 16 years old and working at an unskilled trade prior to injury. He spoke about wasting a number of years before getting serious about his life post injury. His 'wasted' years post spinal injury suggests a lack of defined aspects of self upon which to rebuild a valued self.

The disabled identity as total self

The disabled identity as total self is seen by these respondents as mainly a negative identity. It is revealed in primarily two situations: when a respondent treats him/her self as disabled by expecting assistance from others without asking all of the time and/or believing that other people should know what a person with a spinal cord injury can and cannot do. Regarding the first situation, treating oneself as disabled appears to centre around expectations:

> *Mr MK*: When I use to go to school, I expected [others to] let me get a table first because I am in a wheelchair.

Mr MK also remarked about the second way this identity is revealed using an example of a person going to a restaurant with friends and assuming the friends will help carry him/her up to the restaurant. This identity can also be seen in the case of an individual who blames others for bowel and bladder accidents:

> *Mr GS*: People can get really mad about it and blame other people. Like, 'Oh you should not have brought me to this place with this kind of food [that was] going to have this effect on me'.

According to many respondents, the disabled identity as total self is accompanied by variable periods of anger over time. For example, Mrs WD spoke about the initial lack of encouragement to express anger during rehabilitation:

> *Mrs WD*: Well it wasn't until, near the end of my rehab, that I was comfortable enough to tell someone that I am *angry*. I'm not like, all smiling, 'oh this is no big deal, you know its ok; I have a wheelchair, but thats all right.' I was *damn angry*. But there was no one who wanted to hear that? Everybody sort of wanted to hear, 'oh yes, you will be ok, fine, you will be able to manage'.

Zola (1982: 222) believes that the lack of acceptable means to express anger also results in anger turned inward, a form of depression. Mrs WD, at the end of the interview, spoke again of her anger with respect to her feelings about living with a SCI for 14 years:

> *Mrs WD*: I don't think that my feelings have changed much, I am still very angry about the fact that I am disabled for the *rest of my life*. But 10 years ago or even 12 years ago, I, you just have to get on with it. You have two choices. You can get on with your life or you can sit at home and dwell on it. I've just decided to get on with my life. The disability is part of it. I am not happy about it. I am certainly *resentful* about the fact that I can't walk, but that hasn't stopped me from being able to get on with my life.

For Mrs WD and the vast majority of the other respondents, the decision to 'get on with their lives' became a pivotal point in their movement along the pendulum. That anger can arise periodically throughout the remaining life course suggests the continuous impact that the injury has on the lives of these individuals.

The supernormal identity

The supernormal identity is manifested when a respondent engages in activities of an extraordinary nature requiring increased time and energy and/or the person refuses *any* assistance from others. Charmaz (1987) had discovered a similar identity in her analysis of older persons with a variety of progressive disabling conditions. Her supernormal identity refers to a person with a chronic condition who engages in activities that require a level of functioning more demanding than those who are able bodied. Many respondents gave accounts of their supernormal identities in a variety of social situations. Respondents noted they engaged in activities which required more time and energy mainly because of the saliency of the activity to them and to show that they were no worse off than other people.[1]

Engaging in extraordinary activities which were important meant the pursuit of a supernormal identity, reflecting the desire to produce a 'personally valued and socially credited identity in conventional worlds' (Charmaz 1987: 296). Participants in this study discussed experiences to reconstruct personal and socially valued selves as well as to negate 'negative identifying images' (Charmaz 1987: 296). In discussing leisure activities, Mr UO illustrates reconstruction of a valued self:

> *Mr UO*: So I pretty much do what I want. You know to the chagrin of a lot of people. [I ask to who]. To who? Well a lot of people will look around you like, for the last couple of years we have winter vacations down south and people have a look at you and say, 'what is this guy in a wheelchair doing down here?' Like I would just lay on the beach or dive into the pool or do whatever.

In this quote, Mr UO not only rejects negative images by destroying preconceptions, but he knows exactly in what way to do so, based upon the impression he wants to project of himself. He called this 'playing on the edge':

> *Mr UO*: . . . like when I say, 'I'm going horse back riding.' You are doing what? Horseback riding? What are you doing horseback riding? [others say]. Well I say, 'no big deal, I have horses, and I go riding'. And that type of thing. Ah, doing things that other people think I shouldn't be doing. Not that I do them because other people think I shouldn't be, but because I do it. And I want to do it.

These activities, however, are not always defined as positive by others. Another respondent, Mr TE, who has been injured for 11 years spoke about how other people reacted negatively to him engaging in hunting and fishing:

Mr TE: Ah . . . some people have actually come up to me and have told me I am crazy for doing this. They have seen me out hunting out there with the dog, paddling out to a blind (hiding place out on the water) and they actually told me, 'you have got to be crazy to do this'. And like I said, 'I've been doing this for 15 years and you are telling me I'm crazy for doing this, you don't know what you are talking about'. But you know, it just, they see something they are not used to seeing.

He also reflected on the risk taking element of his supernormal identity:

Mr TE: But I pay, like I said, the price to do them. Like I get problems with tendinitis and stuff.

Zola (1982) had also reflected on the consequences of those with disabilities engaging in a supernormal identity during his stay at Het Dorp. He realised that portrayals of persons with disabilities in the film media of the same vein, sent an ominous message that all persons with disabilities should be able to do the same (Zola 1982: 121–2).

The other aspect of the supernormal identity is refusal of assistance from others. The social situation in which this predominant view appears is usually when an individual with a spinal cord injury is getting into their vehicle or going through a door. Another respondent, Mr MK, explains that the 'supercrip' is a person with a spinal cord injury who gets 'totally pissed off' about other people who come by and ask if they can help him/her. Ms EM describes her reaction to offers of help with respect to opening doors and getting into her car:

Ms EM: It depends upon what kind of mood I am in. I am patient and I say, 'no, I am fine'. You know, if I am in a bad mood, I have been known to tell people to f— off! [she laughs]. Which is probably not a very good thing to do, but that is what comes out.

Ms EM's variable response to offers of help is based upon her experience of being offered assistance almost everyday in inappropriate ways:

Ms EM: Just about once a day sort of thing. I will get someone coming up to me at some point. You know at school, I will be going down a hallway and someone will be *miles away* and they will come *running up* to open the door, like you know? I have no problem opening doors on my own and things like that.

It is clear that this identity is one in which individuals with a spinal cord injury engage in over the life course depending upon their definition of various life situations.

The disabled identity as an aspect of the total self

The disabled identity as an aspect of the total self represents one aspect of the person, as opposed to encompassing or nearly encompassing the total self. In other words, respondents considered both their nondisabled and disabled aspects of self, in varying proportions, in the process of life reconstruction. This identity view was frequently manifested in the decisions that respondents made with respect to various life domains (eg decisions around employment). For example, Ms DC, injured since 1980, had worked as a receptionist for a ski wear company after her injury. She left this job to join a bladder research programme which she hoped would increase her bladder capacity. After three years she had to quit due to recurring complications. After further rehabilitation she started to look for work again in 1987. She discussed her limits for work (frequent emptying of the bladder due to her SCI) with respect to her disability as an aspect of her total self that now had to be taken into consideration:

> *Ms DC*: I realized I could not have done half of the stuff I was trying to do. Like receptionist. I would have to go to the bathroom almost every hour in the morning. And you just can't be a receptionist and leave for 10 minutes you know?

Due to a settlement from her accident, Ms DC was able to re-enter the labour force in a business venture which allowed her to organise her work around her paraplegic needs. Another respondent, Mr UO, also illustrates this dual consideration of self (nondisabled and disabled) in making his decision about working in a financial institution versus a health care sales company:

> *Mr UO*: . . . I did not think I would fit into the financial institution so the sales company, I knew I had a lot of contacts with people and with [fiancee] as well working in the industry . . . and as well I thought something that I could get involved with and have a bit more input and see if I could change a few things that I was not happy with in this business.

Mr UO said earlier during this account that he was 'never really that conservative that he could work in a financial institution'. Thus, he illustrates a consideration of his nondisabled self (not being a conservative person) and his disabled self (experience as a consumer with this sales industry). Finally, other respondents spoke about how the disability became a part of their total being. The following account of Mrs WD demonstrates her movement over time to the disabled identity as an aspect of the total self:

> *Mrs WD:* Initially, I sort of felt that I really wasn't a *whole person*. I also felt that I wasn't a *worthy person*. I must have done something *terribly wrong* to have this happen to me in my life. And I have sort of gotten over that and come to terms with that, if it happens, it happens. If you get run over by a bus, it happens. And I feel *good* about myself, I *like myself very much* and the fact that I am disabled, is *just another*

part of my life, I don't like myself any *less* because of it. But I don't like myself *any more* because of it.

Mrs WD suggests in this passage that initially she held the identity view of the disability as the total self, as indicated by her reference to a lack of 'wholeness'. She then speaks about her merging of the disability with her total self. The majority of respondents in this study held this predominant identity view.

The middle self

The middle self is a term coined by Mr MK. In speaking about experiences related to 'treating [him]self as a disabled person (disabled identity as total self)', Mr MK spoke explicitly about his continued adjustment to his spinal cord injury in this next passage, which kindled the idea of the pendulum:

> *Mr MK*: Actually you get to the point where I went to the other extreme. I became so independent that I wanted to do everything myself. I didn't want anyone to help me. You know? And I guess you know, with a lot of disabled people, they all follow the same trends. They all go to one extreme, to another extreme and they bounce back and forth, getting sort of closer and closer to where they should be and finally, hopefully, eventually they get to the middle.

Mr MK expresses the idea of a pendulum when he talks about 'going from one extreme to another extreme and bouncing back and forth' and finally getting to the middle. The middle self, then occurs when a respondent moves closer to the middle of the pendulum. It refers to individuals who act upon both the nondisabled and disabled aspects of self.

The middle self however, incorporates three additional elements. First, the individual with a spinal cord injury understands that s/he is in a wheelchair and this is the way it is and will be. For different respondents, this understanding came at different points in the life reconstructive process. One example was Mr KO who asked to be left alone for three days during his acute care period to figure things out:

> *Mr KO*: In those three days what was left in life. Is this it? Log rolling from side to side in a bed? What about a chair? When are we getting a chair? Would I be strong enough or well enough to be in a chair?

Second, the individual understands there are limitations associated with having a spinal cord injury. One limitation was that many respondents accepted a level of dependency (ie assistance into an inaccessible house) in their lives and did not view it as negative. For example, Mr SS's account of acceptance of dependency in some situations and not others illustrates the pendulum movement around this middle identity view:

Mr SS: Just like I'll let myself get carried into somebody's house where someone else would say, 'I'm going to stay home from Uncle John's because his place is inaccessible,' I'll go to Uncle John's. I'll get carried up the stairs; sometimes I don't. Sometimes it can be frustrating especially if people do not know how to do it and if its a big flight of stairs.

The third element of the middle self is a 'collective disabled consciousness'. This consciousness is illustrated when a respondent considered others with spinal cord injuries or people with other disabilities, in decisions s/he makes with respect to social interaction and everyday life. Individuals may also make comments or reference to persons with disabilities as a distinct and/or as a disadvantaged group similar to others in contemporary North American society. In the following passage, Mr MK describes the 'collective disabled consciousness' of the middle self with respect to the social interaction of assistance into a vehicle:

Mr MK: . . . If someone comes by, wanting to help me, I would tell them, 'thank you very much but I don't need it. I can probably handle it, but I appreciate your help though.' Because who knows? The next guy down the road might not be so lucky. To be able to do it himself. He might get stuck one day. And if I yell at him, the guy here, he will go down the street and he will see the other guy and say, 'oh, well I won't touch you, go ahead, help yourself'. And I don't think that is fair.

In this passage, Mr MK clearly considers his actions and the potential repercussions for other individuals with disabilities.

The other aspect of the collective disabled consciousness is illustrated by Mr GS who describes his personal awakening to the reality that his social situation of being disabled and acquiring assistance is sometimes no different than other segments or groups in society.

Mr GS: I would like to see a more *aware world* for physically disabled people. But I don't want to see an [totally] accessible one. I want to see people being helped into places and helped out and it becomes an accepted thing. . . . When somebody is crossing the street, when you see an older person crossing the street and the cars start to go, somebody runs out and says, 'Stop! This lady is still crossing the street'.

Thus the middle self centres on a mindset that acknowledges and acts upon the nondisabled and disabled aspects of self while incorporating a wider social concern for other persons with disabilities and other segments of society.

This dual consideration of the nondisabled and disabled self in the identity views of the disabled identity as aspect of the total self and the middle self does not mean there is always equal consideration of both aspects all of the time. It means that both aspects of the total self may be taken into consideration, or not, within a given situation, in proportions that are important and specific to the individual and appropriate to the situation at hand. This variable consideration of the nondisabled and disabled aspects of self and the definition of the situation by the individual are central to why identity reconstruction for those with traumatic spinal cord injuries is shaped as a pendulum.

Another respondent, Mr NG typified this movement between identity views. In the following account he spoke about adjusting to wearing a leg bag (to drain urine) around his lower leg:

> *Mr NG*: Its one of the things that I am still embarassed about. Telling people that I have to go around wearing a leg bag. I rather, nah, I am still a little embarassed about that. But now, at first I would probably try to hide the fact, now its, I don't advertise it but I am not shy about it and if you [nondisabled people] don't like it, too bad. I have been at this game too long [laughs].

In the first part of the account, Mr NG vacillated between his former self (embarrassed about the leg bag) and his disabled identity as an aspect of his total self (not embarrassed about the leg bag). In the second part of the account, Mr NG indicates the movement towards not being embarrassed about the leg bag was a long term process.

Experiences as process

Experiences or situations represent 'processes' on the pendulum. Due to the cross-sectional and retrospective nature of these data, the linkage between experiences and identity views can not be viewed in a causal manner. It is suggested that experiences are processes that may influence or shape self. Five 'processes' emerged from the interviews: loss; sustainment; integration; continuity and development of self. These highlight the various contexts involving the nondisabled and disabled aspects of the total self of individuals with traumatic spinal cord injuries.

Loss of the nondisabled self refers to loss of core and peripheral aspects of the nondisabled self of the person prior to the spinal cord injury. It appears that loss of the nondisabled aspects of self may stem from many different experiences, desires and expectations. The greatest amount of loss is experienced just after the onset of injury, notably as body losses. Body losses were related to physical capacities, functional limitations and activity restrictions. Corbin and Strauss (1987: 255–6) discuss the importance of body to conceptions of self as the body performs tasks associated with the various aspects of self. Later loss is experienced through everyday life situations and the continuous acceptance of their injury. Mr NG, injured 12 years ago, epitomises this point:

Mr NG: I think its still tough to deal with. Sometimes it still bothers me. . . . I think that people say you have accepted it for so long, I think you have to continue to accept it everyday.

Other respondents used different phrases to signify that the 'acceptance' of their spinal cord injury was an ongoing dynamic event. They used phrases such as 'slow process of adaptation', 'ongoing learning process' and 'still figuring things out'. These reflections of lived experiences indicate the dynamic nature of identity and why predominant identity views may shift over time and situationally.

Sustaining the nondisabled self refers to maintaining core and/or peripheral aspects of the respondent. Sustainment in this study reflected action taken by the respondent and/or significant others after the onset of injury. Charmaz (1983: 183) has stated that intimates's view of the individual as their former, pre-illness self will sustain and support the individual's self, post injury. Significant others then, sustained the nondisabled self of respondents by maintaining a link between the respondent and their nondisabled world:

Mr GO: My friends would come up on a Friday night and bring a case of beer and sit and drink in the recreation center. Having a good time. Like to sacrifice a Friday night for my friends is a lot. They are into picking up girls every weekend so, to sacrifice that for the hospital kind of makes me feel good.

Integration consists of two components: a process of reclaiming lost aspects of the nondisabled self and an initial process of inclusion of the disabled self. Accounts of integration occurred in many different settings, however the most frequent period of integration was upon discharge from the hospital or rehabilitation centre. The problematic nature of integrating the disabled self was reflected in respondents getting used to the additional concerns and tasks associated with having a spinal cord injury, eg bowel and bladder care. For example, Mr SH who has been living with his spinal cord injury for 19 years, discussed the increased time and energy to deal with the extra concerns. Over time however, the disabled self became more 'accepted' (ie tasks generally became easier to do) and respondents discussed their paraplegic needs as any other need.

Continuity of the nondisabled self refers to the carrying through of core and/or peripheral aspects of the nondisabled self in the life reconstruction process post injury. Continuity is an active process, in that it is generally initiated and carried out by the individual. It is the carrying forward of aspects of the nondisabled self into the life reconstruction process post injury. Continuity then, represents carrying through and acting upon valued aspects of the nondisabled self. The final experience is development of the total self. Development refers to the ongoing 'maturation' of the total self and to the continuing process of inclusion of the disabled self. Development then, involves the nondisabled and disabled selves of the respondent in everyday life. Many respondents spoke of their increase maturing and patience they acquired after their spinal injury.

> *Mr DA*: And I have learned patience that I didn't have before. Ah, in stores, people in a hurry rushing in to get a paper, rushing out again. Getting their evening paper, in a big hurry.

These experiences or 'processes' reflect situational influences on the pendulum of self. These experiences bring to the surface the nondisabled and disabled aspects of self. Also, these experiences or processes illustrate how self is modified through personal and situational definitions.

Case presentations

The discussion of the pendulum shape of identity reconstruction so far has been to illustrate in a segmental manner, the predominant identity views using a variety of respondents. Categorised data however, becomes removed from the individual and the context within which these data emerged. In this section, two cases from different socio-demographic backgrounds have been selected for narrative analysis.

Case Presentation: Mr GS

Mr GS is 31 years old and has been living with his spinal cord injury for 6 years. He is a university graduate who worked in a health care institution as an allied health professional prior to his spinal cord injury. His career plans were directed towards a professional field:

> *Mr GS:* I wanted to pursue a professional career at the time, but I was not quite sure what field. I was working at the time, working in a hospital. On the – ward and I wanted to climb the professional ladder, but I wasn't quite sure what capacity and what sector.

His parents are both working professionals. His interests had changed from organised high school competitive sports to university fine arts which lead to a four year focus on dance (ie modern, ballet) prior to his SCI.

Mr GS was 25 years old when he sustained his SCI in September of 1983. When he was told by his parents of his injury, during the acute stages of his recovery, his sense of loss was immediate and profound:

> *Mr GS:* Well I was really *bummed out* because I was always really active. I used my body a lot. After I stopped playing sports, I got into studying dance. I was a dancer . . . So the body for me was in use *a lot*. And I was pretty bummed out. I thought what does that mean in how I move? Will I be able to feel weightlessness again? Which is what you do when you are dancing and since I didn't know any disabled people, I was getting pretty *cracked* about the whole thing.

At this early stage, Mr GS realised that his SCI would have an impact on a significant core aspect of his former self, his love of dance. He also expressed his sense of shock and general lack of comprehension regarding the overall impact of his injury to his life:

> *Mr GS*: You can't even say that it is a change at that point? Right? You can only say change when you understand or compare. I couldn't even compare because it was too much moment to moment. There was too much shock involved. When someone is in shock they don't understand what change is.

He was however, also aware that for him to understand the implications of this condition, he needed to communicate with other persons with SCI.

Mr GS spent about two weeks in intensive care and was visited by his parents every couple of days. His parents, post acute injury represented to him, a sense of connection with the world he knew and most importantly who he was:

> *Mr GS: Very supportive!* Very supportive. I remember this so well [my name], I opened my eyes and my parents were at the foot of my bed and my mother was crocheting and my father was sitting like he always does with his legs crossed . . . So that was exactly what I wanted to see when I opened my eyes, that my parents were there.

He transferred to a ward for about two months and then was sent to rehabilitation for four months. It was during this time that Mr GS clashed with the rehabilitation staff regarding his 'adjustment'. While he appreciated the physical aspects of rehabilitation, he wanted 'answers to commonsense everyday things'. He wanted someone in a wheelchair to come in and talk to him about 'how to work day to day life'. Mr GS was denied his request and spoke angrily about the situation:

> *Mr GS*: There is a *whole area* that when someone is trying to adjust to something, and when for instance I wanted someone in a wheelchair to come and talk to me. They wouldn't let that happen because of their little professional neuroticism and I felt that hard to take. I was a professional and I said, 'this is not fair. I am paying my bills. I have a right to service.'

In this account, Mr GS illustrates a consideration of his disabled self in his request for learning about day to day life from someone in a wheelchair. Mr GS then displays his core aspects of his former self (allied health professional) in the second half of the account in his argument with the rehabilitation staff. Mr GS did speak to persons with other disabilities on the ward to get the 'inside scoop' regarding various facets of daily life; accessible places to shop, to live; what community agencies to interact with regarding resources. He acknowledges that his previous life experiences assisted in his 'adjustment':

> *Mr GS*: And because of who I was before the accident a lot of that stuff came much easier to me. You take a farm boy, put him in that spot and he knows nothing about how to adjust. I had a lot of professional background, a lot of the community contacts, I was not afraid to ask questions.

Again, Mr GS exhibits aspects of his former self and his prior professional knowledge enables him to take action with respect to his life reconstruction process.

Mr GS did speak to people with other disabilities, because of his desire to learn about his 'adjustment' to his disability. Upon discharge from rehabilitation however, he displays movement back to his nondisabled self (former self) and a clear resistance to his disabled self:

> *Mr GS*: I didn't know how to act with this body. I didn't know how to move with this body. I didn't know how to move with this wheelchair thing. It was like, it had to be a part of me now and I didn't want it to be a part of me now. And I felt very alone, very alone and very sad.

Discharged in March of 1984, Mr GS went on a vacation back home with his best friend over the summer. He spoke in great detail about this vacation: how they drank beer, went canoeing, visited and partied with other university friends. The vacation allowed Mr GS to reclaim some aspects of his nondisabled self by re-establishing important social relations with significant others. These experiences also illustrated the inclusion of the disabled self again into his total self as Mr GS spoke about getting around in rural areas using long leg braces and receiving assistance from his friends. His account cited earlier in the section on the middle identity view, concerning a desire for a more aware world in which people helped others illustrated his collective disabled consciousness at the time of the interview. Mr GS indicated that this developing consciousness began during this vacation period:

> *Mr GS*: And that where I first started to see that was on that trip, you know? And that was ok, I could take it, these were my friends and so it was a very natural integration? It wasn't like strangers were doing a lot of it first for me. Because my first real contact was with my friends and that was ok.

During the fall of 1984, Mr GS went back to his home and joined a number of boards of directors for a variety of voluntary agencies to gain work experience, enrolled in some university courses, played in a wheelchair sport and turned to alternative therapy.

He acknowledges that the merging of his disabled self to his total self was mainly attributed to the time that he spent playing a wheelchair sport and interacting with others who had spinal cord injuries:

> *Mr GS*: I was playing for the ——. And that was *important*. That should never be, that should always be given credit for what can happen around a group, a social group setting.

I asked him specifically what were the benefits of this interaction:

> *Mr GS:* I was accepted by people who were just like me! We were on a trip and we would go into a hotel, they didn't have to ask me if I needed help, they knew what I needed help with. They never went too far or too little.

Mr GS spoke about how his team mates helped him with issues regarding the best means of bladder drainage, how friends and family reacted to their injury, how they went about finding jobs. For Mr GS then, these experiences facilitated inclusion of his disabled self. They were positive experiences that resulted in his growing connection with the disabled community. The following portion of the interview illustrates Mr GS's movement between identity views: his former self; the disabled identity as an aspect of the total self and the middle self over time:

> *Mr GS:* Often with the disabled I found whether it was back then (playing sports) or now (interview), it was the *internal network* and they have got to trust you before they will let you in. [I ask for elaboration]. Well [my name] you are a walkie. You are on the outside (he laughs). They are walkies (points to me), we are gimps, we can say that word to each other for the most part. If you call us that you are like smoked meat! [I ask about the issue of trust]. Its within the circle, there is a certain amount of trust among the disabled community. Even though that fellow disabled person may be a total *ass*——, its like they are a disabled person and they might understand what I have to say just a little bit more.

In the first sentence of this account, Mr GS is speaking from his nondisabled self, his former self, as he refers to the 'disabled' requiring trust from the newly disabled person. When I asked for clarification, Mr GS moved and spoke from his disabled identity as a part of his total self when he referred to himself as disabled (gimp) versus abled bodied (walkie). Mr GS's insider/outsider dicotomy clearly distinguished his identity view (disabled identity as an aspect of the total self) and his reference to a circle or disabled community moves him to speak from the middle self.

Mr GS spent the next year (1986–1987) involved in alternative medicine to maximise his remaining physiological capacity. He spent a year out of the country to increase his ability to walk with long leg braces and canes. His work insurance (long term disability) gave him the financial resources to pursue this course of action. Mr GS's quest to enhance his capacity can be interpreted as engaging in the supernormal identity. The desire to walk initially using increased time and energy with or without the assistance of conventional or nonconventional therapies or devices, was a typical response among many respondents. In addition to the importance of body for physical function, Mr GS expressed his desire to be 'whole' again:

> *Mr GS:* I started to walk with the canes, I walked further. My legs became part of my body again, instead of two things that were just hanging off. I mean I could walk then . . . From a functional point of view, it is important, but from a personal point of view it is just dramatic! Its like getting married! Its like my God, I have got my body back again!

However, Mr GS's growing inclusion of his disabled self moved him out of this supernormal identity view during this period. He realised that he had gone as far as he could with his recovery and that he had come to terms with his SCI and his disabled self (symbolised by the wheelchair):

> *Mr GS:* Like 'Hey [his name] you and this wheelchair better get real friendly because this is life'.

He returned to Ontario and went back to university for a specific programme that would help him in his career choices. During this point in the interview, Mr GS again exhibited movement between identity views in his experiences of returning to university. Mr GS encountered a great deal of inaccessibility at his university and he again expressed frustration about this situation:

> *Mr GS:* I could not get into any of the residences. Can't get into the athletic complex. Can't get into um, to get into the library you have to go through an *intricate* underground maze, from the teaching building, up and down some ramps, special chair lifts, up and down stairs. You got to buzz somebody to come down stairs with the key, it was just *f——ed.* I couldn't get into the business office, couldn't get into the science building. [I asked if these were places he had to go to]. No. These are places that I had a *right to go to!* I paid my student fees, I fought long and hard about this to the dean of students. I even sat on a committee they struck [he swears here]. You should not be getting my student fees because I can't use your services in this university and you are making me pay for it and I can't use it.

In the first part of this account, Mr GS's anger stemmed from his consideration as an individual with a disability (disabled identity as an aspect of self) not having total and reasonable access to a public institution. In the latter half of this account, he speaks more from a middle self as the issue becomes centered on his rights as a student with a disability in which he had to pay full student fees for services he could not use.

Mr GS has gone on to work in the area of nonprofits with a social agency concerned with disability issues. Immediately before the accessibility account, Mr GS's discussed his rationale for returning to university:

> *Mr GS:* So I looked at what my options were, what I wanted to do and I wanted to get back into things that were more business and I knew that I had a strong background in non-profits and I knew that I had a strong background in counselling and I knew that I had a background working in administration. I was looking at the current trends, the centre of our economy was service-oriented, I knew that disabled people were becoming more and more on the forefront. I knew that it would be just a matter of time, before more and more employers saying that we need disabled people and I knew that there were currently laws in the United States, quotas and it was just a matter of time before Canada would come on board with that.

Mr GS's work and related contacts represents his desire for experiences of development or growth of his total or 'future' self:

> *Mr GS:* I really like the stuff that I am doing, its really off the wall, not just about work, I am learning an awful lot about me, about people.

For Mr GS then, his identity reconstruction since his injury represented a pendulum shape, moving into and out of his former self, the supernormal identity, the disabled identity as an aspect of the total self and the middle self. Through his life reconstruction process, he continues to integrate and develop both his nondisabled and disabled aspects of self.

Case presentation: Mr RP

Mr RP is currently 33 years old and has been injured just over a year. He graduated from high school and was very active in many sports, with hockey his main activity. Both of his parents worked in blue collar occupations; his father worked in the construction industry and his mother in a factory. Mr RP entered the construction field where he became a skilled worker in this industry over 12 years (1974–86). During this time, he got married and has two adolescent children.

In 1987, he sustained his spinal cord injury while on the job. Similar to many other respondents, Mr RP knew he had 'broken his back' but was unaware that it involved damage to the spinal cord and its consequences. During rehabilitation, he realised the physical consequences of his injury:

> *Mr RP:* You are obviously depressed as at that time I could not move. I could not transfer myself, could not dress myself, I could not do anything. It was pretty well starting over.

Like other respondents, he was resistant to the inclusion of the newly disabled aspects of self, which in the following account is symbolised by the refusal to use technical aids:

Mr RP: I was trying to dress myself and the occupational therapist had all of these aids but I did not want to use them. I would figure it out myself.

The sudden loss of many aspects of his former self was further reinforced by his awareness of others:

Mr RP: All of the quads (persons with quadraplegia) getting fed, I, I could not handle that at all!

Mr RP continues about his initial feelings during rehabilitation and reveals movement over time to an acceptance of others' disabilities and to a degree his own:

Mr RP: I would just eat [in dining room] and leave. I found that so depressing, but then afterwards near the end of my stay, I was doing quite a bit. I was actually feeding the guys. It did not bother me anymore. I was exposed to it, I guess.

Mr RP's employment status was compatible with that pre-injury, as he remained in the construction field in an alternative capacity. In discussion of his work reconstruction, Mr RP displays a supernormal identity in discussing how he combines brace walking with using his wheelchair for mobility:

Mr RP: I put them [leg braces] underneath my pants and I can put the wheelchair in the trunk [of the car] and then just walk around to the car door [using a walker] and put the walker into the back seat and away I go. [I ask him to continue]. I pull the walker out, get out, walk around, open up the trunk, get out the wheelchair. I have done this a couple of times. I have to work hard. [I ask how long this process takes.] It would take me a good 20 minutes anyways by the time that I have squared around.

In discussing leisure activities, Mr RP again displays his former self and his ambivalence to his disabled self:

Mr RP: Well I use to be very, I use to be very good, baseball. I use to play competitive racquet ball. I just do not think that I would be the same, I would not have the same love for the sport anymore. [I asked why]. I can not get motivated. To do a sport, you have to enjoy it and love what you do and when I played any type of sport, I gave it *150%.* I played hockey and racquet ball, baseball, all on a competitive line. And even though I could probably do it in a wheelchair, whether or not I could accept it, I do not know. I just can not put everything into it and if you can not do that, then I can not see playing.

For Mr RP, the decision not to participate in sports is based upon his reference to his nondisabled aspects of self. It is incompatible for him currently to participate in sports that he had performed in before his injury and he also does not wish to participate in wheelchair sports. Throughout the interview, Mr RP constantly revealed movement mainly between his former self and the supernormal identity. This is not surprising considering Mr RP's reconstruction in various life domains, such as work, accommodation and marital status is generally continuous with his pre-injury life. However, these relative continuities magnify other aspects of life reconstruction which are currently incompatible with his disabled aspects of self, ie participation in sports and being a father to his son:

> *Mr RP:* My son is taking it really hard. We use to do, skiing. He is *really taking this the hardest.*

Mr RP's current plans involve working for another eight years and then, after his family has grown up, he will pursue walking 'in any way possible'. Mr RP acknowledges, however, that he is uncertain how he will feel about his disability in the future:

> *Mr RP:* It would be interesting to interview me in a few years. [I suggest that he would be 'mellow' and he agreed].

It is clear from this statement that Mr RP believes that he will change over time, which indicates movement over time of identity views.

Discussion and conclusions

This paper has described a model of identity reconstruction and transformation among individuals with traumatic spinal cord injuries. The model consists of five predominant identity views which reflects aspects of the nondisabled and disabled self. The shape of the identity reconstruction is of a pendulum, as the 35 respondents in this study moved back and forth between identity views. While I have taken an insider's perspective which focusses on the subjective experiences of living with a disability, my analysis is limited to a sociological view of first person accounts (Conrad 1987: 5). It is also important to remember that the pendulum model was developed using cross-sectional and retrospective data and thus a causal relationship between identity views and experiences can not be established.

The pendulum of self as a model of identity reconstruction, is grounded in the accounts of respondents as they discussed the process of rebuilding their lives. Respondents' accounts of how they reconstructed various aspects of their lives such as labour force participation illustrated how the nondisabled and disabled aspects of self were taken into consideration in everyday life. The pendulum of self addresses the issues of identity reconstruction as a nonlinear pattern; process and outcome; and how disability merges with the nondisabled aspects of self. Each will be discussed in turn.

The nature of identity transformation as dynamic and shifting is depicted in the pendulum of self. The model is constantly in motion as respondents interpret and take action in their world. The fluidity of the model suggest movement between identity views is over a period of time. However movement can conceivably be from moment to moment, situation to situation, or day by day. Both long term and situational movement is grounded in these respondents' accounts and by the interview process itself in which respondents moved back and forth between their nondisabled and disabled aspects of self. This fluidity between predominant identity views means that identity reconstruction is a continuous, evolving dual-directional process and the assumption that people 'adjust' to their disability once and for all is also challenged. The psychological spinal cord literature clearly acknowledges that stage theories of adjustment do not necessarily depict the 'adjustment' to spinal injury and that coping with a spinal cord injury involves a variety of responses (Trieschmann 1988: 43–7). Charmaz's identity hierarchy represents another shape to identity reconstruction among elderly individuals (the largest proportion of her sample was between 40 to 60 years) with progressive deteriorating conditions (eg multiple sclerosis). It is reasonable to assume that there may be other forms or shapes of identity reconstruction for younger individuals with chronic conditions of a relatively stable nature such as traumatic spinal cord injuries. The pendulum shape of identity reconstruction may represent an appropriate depiction of response to disability (identity reconstruction) from spinal cord injury with respect to identity reconstruction. The pendulum of self as a model of identity reconstruction considers both outcomes of identity reconstruction (identity views) and processes or experiences which may shape different aspects of self. Research in the sociology of chronic illness and disability has illuminated various aspects of identity reconstruction as either process or outcome concepts. In this paper, a model of identity reconstruction that considers both elements may increase our understanding of the nature of identity reconstruction and transformation, in a more comprehensive manner. Experiences represent situations or contexts which respondents define and take action upon.

Related to experiences is the assumption that having a disability is inherently and totally negative. These data suggest that this is not always the case. Respondents in this study generally speaking, perceived the identity views as valued positions, the exception perhaps was 'the disabled identity as total self'. This view however, is still an important one as there were accounts expressed by respondents that demonstrated greater or total consideration of the disabled self in specific situations. More specifically, accounts concerning the experience of development and the identity view of the middle self, refute this claim, as many respondents talked about the opportunities to engage in activities that they would not have been able to do before. Others spoke of their own 'maturation' as a person, for example becoming more patient, assertive or considerate of others. Thus, positive experiences may emerge from living with a disability.[2] In the literature, some conceptualisations of identity reconstruction are depicted as downward planes. For example, 'identity hierarchy' (Charmaz 1987) refers to downward movement through the hierarchy with respect to progressive chronic illness. This clearly reflects a differential of value among the identity outcomes she develops in her model.

The pendulum of self also addresses the issue of how inclusive the disability is to the total self concept of the individual. Much research has assumed that the disability is either the most important aspect of the person with a disability and his/her self concept/definition. Fine and Ash (1988: 11–12) argue that a person with a disability is more likely to compare him/herself with others of his/her own gender, age, occupation and other salient social comparison groups. On the other hand, much research has not been explicit in specifically delineating the influence of the disability with respect to identity in their work (Charmaz 1987; Corbin and Strauss 1987). The pendulum of self deals with this dilemma with regards to the consideration of the place of disability in relationship to the total self. The pendulum promotes the variable consideration and merger of the nondisabled and disabled aspects of self to the individuals' total self.

The pendulum of self interrelates a number of concepts to form a grounded middle range substantive theory of identity transformation and reconstruction after traumatic spinal injury (Glaser and Strauss 1967; Glaser 1978). As middle range substantive theory, the generalisability of the findings has to be considered. Conrad (1987: 17–19) believes that the usual form of generalisability (ie can the findings from the study apply to other samples of individuals who are spinal cord injured or other disability) is inappropriate since a random sample is generally not used in most qualitative research. He suggests that an alternative form of generalisability which focusses on the generalisability of concepts be considered. This means how generalisable are the concepts developed in one study to other groups, settings and situations? (Conrad 1990: 1258–9).

It appears that aspects of the pendulum of self are evident in other works on living with a disability and in other substantive areas such as the field of aging. Charmaz's (1983; 1987) concepts of loss[3] and the supernormal identity parallel the concepts in this study. In the field of aging the notion of transformation (Breytsparaak 1984) and continuity in studies of identity among older women (Mac Rae 1990: 257–8) is evident. These examples of generalisability of concepts across substantive areas promotes conceptual strength and increases our understanding of identity transformation in general.

Future research can examine the identity changes using the pendulum model with other disabilities or other situations in which identities may be under assault during unexpected changes, loss and uncertainty, such as the loss of a spouse, recent divorce or losing one's job. Identities may be highly transitory or fluid in these situations, vascillating between identity states. It is this continuous refinement and modifying of the model which will ensure its theoretical and practical relevance with respect to the process of identity reconstruction and transformation.

Address for correspondence:
Dr Karen K. Yoshida,
Department of Rehabilitation, Division of Physical Therapy,
University of Toronto, Toronto, Ontario,
Canada M5T 1W5

Acknowledgments

This study was supported by the National Health Research and Development Program in the form of a National Health and Welfare Ph.D fellowship between 1987–1990, from Health and Welfare Canada. The author also wishes to thank Drs M.J. Kelner, D. Locker, K. Allison and R. Fitzpatrick for their critical review of various drafts of this manuscript.

Notes

1. A colleague who has a SCI, commented on an earlier draft of this paper stating that his supernormal tendencies are not to prove that he is better than others but to prove he is 'not worse off than others'.
2. A colleague spoke about another person who had a disability. This particular individual stated that he did not want to ever be able-bodied again because of what he has learned and experienced with his disability.
3. C. Carpenter's found in her study of individuals with traumatic spinal cord that loss and continuity of the nondisabled self were key concerns. She used an educational learning approach for her study.

References

Anderson, R. and Bury, M. (1988) Introduction. In Anderson, R. and Bury, M. (eds) *Living with Chronic Illness: The Experiences of Patients and Their Families*. London: Unwin Hyman.

Blumer, H. (1969) *Symbolic Interactionism: Perspective and Method*. Englewood Cliffs, New Jersey: Prentice-Hall.

Breytspraak, L. (1984) *The Development of Self in Later Life*. Boston: Little, Brown and Co.

Bury, M. (1982) Chronic illness as biographical disruption, *Sociology of Health and Illness*, 4, 167–82.

Charmaz, K. (1983) Loss of self: a fundamental form of suffering in the chronically ill, *Sociology of Health and Illness*, 5, 168–95.

Charmaz, K. (1987) Struggling for a self: Identity levels of the chronically ill. In Roth, J.P. and Conrad, P. (eds) *Research in the Sociology of Health Care*. Greenwich CT: JAI Press.

Charmaz, K. (1990) Discovering chronic illness: using grounded theory. *Social Science and Medicine*, 30, 1161–72.

Conrad, P. (1987) The experience of illness: recent and new directions in the experience and management of chronic illness. In Roth, J.P. and Conrad, P. (eds) *Research in the Sociology of Health Care*. Greenwich CF: JAI Press.

Conrad, P. (1990) Qualitative research on chronic illness: a commentary on method and conceptual development. *Social Science and Medicine*, 30, 1257–63.

Corbin, J. and Strauss, A.L. (1987) Accompaniments of chronic illness: Changes in body, self, biography and biographical time. In Roth, J.A. and Conrad, P. (eds) *Research in the Sociology of Health and Care*, Greenwich CT: JAI Press.

Corbin, J. and Strauss, A.L. (1988) *Unending Work and Care*, San Francisco. CA: Jossey-Bass Co.

Fine, M. and Ash, A. (1988) Disability beyond stigma: social interaction, discrimination, and activism, *J. Social Issues*, 44, 3–21.

Fontana, A. and Smith, R.W. (1989) Alzheimer's disease victims: The unbecoming of self and the normalization of competence, *Sociological Perspectives*, 32, 35–46.

Gallagher, E.B. (1976) Lines of reconstruction and extension in the Parsonian sociology of illness, *Social Science and Medicine*, 10, 207–18.

Gerhardt, U. (1990) Patients careers in end-stage renal failure, *Social Science and Medicine*, 30, 1211–24.

Glaser, B. and Strauss, A. (1964) *Awareness of Dying*. Chicago: Aldine Pub. Co.

Glaser, B. and Strauss, A.L. (1967) *The Discovery of Grounded Theory: Strategies for Qualitative Research*. Chicago: Aldine Pub. Co.

Glaser, B. (1978) *Theoretical Sensitivity*. Mill Valley CA: Sociology Press.

Goffman, E. (1959) *The Presentation of Self in Everyday Life*. New York: Doubleday.

Goffman, E. (1961) *Asylums: Essays on the Social Situation of Mental Patients and other Inmates*. New York: Anchor (Doubleday).

Goffman, E. (1963) *Stigma: Notes on the Management of Spoiled Identity*. Englewood Cliffs NJ: Prentice-Hall.

Groch, S. (1990) Disability consciousness as common cultural identity. Paper presented at the Annual Meetings of the Society for Disability Studies, Oakland, California.

Hahn, H. (1990) Reformulating a sense of personal identity through the history of disabled people. Paper presented at the Annual Meetings of the Society for Disability, Oakland California.

Hughes, E.C. (1958) *Men at Work*. Glencoe: Free Press.

Locker, D. (1983) *Disability and Disadvantage*. London: Tavistock.

Locker, D. and Kaufert, J. (1988) The breath of life: medical technology and the careers of people with post-respiratory poliomyelitis. *Sociology of Health and Illness*, 10, 23–40.

MacRae, H. (1990) Older women and identity maintenance in later life. *Canadian J. Aging*, 9, 248–67.

Maddox, S. (1987) *Spiral Network*. Spinal Network and Sam Maddox, P.O. Box 4162, Boulder CO. 80306.

Mead, G.H. (1934) *Mind, Self and Society from the Standpoint of a Social Behaviourist*. Chicago: University of Chicago Press.

Orona, C.J. (1990) Temporality and identity loss due to alzheimer's disease. *Social Science and Medicine*, 30, 1247–56.

Seidel, J.V., Kjoiseth, R. and Seymour, E. (1988). *The Ethnograph: a User's Guide* (Version 3.0). Littleton, Colorado: Qualis Research Associates.

Strauss, A.L. (1969) *Mirrors and Masks*. Mill Valley, CA: Sociology Press.

Strauss, A.L., Fagerhaugh, S., Suczek, B. and Wiener, C. (1982) Sentimental work in the technological hospital. *Sociology of Health and Illness*, 4, 254–78.

Strauss, A.L. and Glaser, B.G. (1975) *Chronic Illness and the Quality of Life*. St. Louis, MO: Mosby.

Trieschmann, R.B. (1980) *Spinal Cord Injuries: Psychological, Social and Vocational Rehabilitation*. New York, NY: Pergamon Press.

Trieschmann, R.B. (1988) *Spinal Cord Injuries: Psychological, Social and Vocational Rehabilitation*, 2nd ed. New York, NY: Demos Pub.

Williams, G. (1984) The genesis of chronic illness: narrative reconstruction. *Sociology of Health and Illness*, 6, 175–200.

Zola, I.K. (1982) *Missing Pieces: A Chronicle of Living with a Disability*. Philadelphia: Temple University Press.

[21]

Life Mirrors Work Mirrors Text Mirrors Life . . .*

MARIANNE A. PAGET, *Brandeis University*

This paper is about a series of uncanny coincidences in my life and work. The coincidences are as follows: an article of mine, on the construction of an erroneous medical diagnosis of depression on a woman who was a cancer patient, was performed as theater just at the time I, too, unknowingly had cancer; the cancer was discovered very late and, at the same time, a series of medical errors in my care became clear; I am a medical sociologist and my area of special interest is medical mistakes. I describe my work on medical mistakes and the mistakes in my care and explore the uncanny and the status of error in life as it is lived.

Coincidences are given meaning, shaped by the teller of the tale. In his work on coincidences, Carl Jung (1971) argues that they are fundamental categories of human experience, just as cause or space and time are fundamental categories of experience. Error, too, is fundamental. In my life, error has provided the common thread for a series of uncanny coincidences.

Life . . .

Last year I was involved in the production of an article of mine as theater. I attended rehearsals as often as I could, taking extensive notes on the development of the performance. It was my first opportunity to watch a show go up. All through the months of March, April, and May, I experienced moments of euphoria. I knew I was breaking free of the often pedantic and deadening form for presenting work in the human sciences: the scientific article.

I had wanted to dramatize "On the Work of Talk: Studies in Misunderstandings" (Paget 1983) for a long time. The work is about the construction of an erroneous medical diagnosis of depression on a woman who was a cancer patient. I had written a detailed report, documenting how her diagnosis was misconstrued. When I saw a social science text performed at Northwestern University in January, I began to ask about staging my article. I spoke with Bernard Beck of the Department of Sociology and with Dwight Conquergood of Performance Studies. Beck thought that his daughter Emilie Beck, a student in Performance Studies, might be interested in my work and gave her a copy of my article. She was. She came to me with the first part of a script that I liked very much and we agreed to work together.

The play was called "The Work of Talk" (Paget 1988b). It was a nearly verbatim staging of my article. Early in the preparation of the script, Emilie Beck suggested changing some of the language of my analysis, which was often quite precise and technical. But I did not want to undermine the work's scientific claims in the interest of a more poetic script. I wanted to

* I want to thank Sheila Bienenfeld, Marjorie DeVault, Peter Finkelstein, and Shulamit Reinharz for their helpful suggestions. I also want to thank Teresa Bernardez, George Psathas, and Irving Zola for their strong support of this work.
Editor's note: Marianne Paget died of the cancer she describes here on 22 December 1989. Paget planned this essay to be the first chapter in a book manuscript, "The Text from Life," that she assembled before she died, and that also includes her performance script, letters written during her chemotherapy, and a journal kept during the last weeks of her life. Georgia NeSmith and Marjorie L. DeVault read reviewers' comments and made final edits to the text printed here. Many thanks to them and to Michal McCall, whose comments as a reviewer were particularly helpful to the editors.

preserve the science of the work in the context of the theater. I wanted to do science on stage. That was part of the magic of the performance for me (see Paget 1990).

At the time of the performance, I had what I thought was a back injury that was taking a long time to heal. In January, I saw a physician at the Student Health Service and was told that I was having muscle spasms, presumably from an injured muscle deep in my mid-back. Over the next few months the pain worsened and a regimen of Ibuprofen did not do much good. I had increasing difficulty using my right arm for driving and for carrying packages or books. I returned to the Student Health Center several times because my condition did not improve. (My health insurance plan was connected with the University's Student Health Service.) In April, while in Florida visiting my mother, I saw another physician who told me, once again, that I was having muscle spasms and pain from an injured muscle in my back. Thus, I had a diagnosis, but—as I was to discover too late—the wrong one. In late May, I entered physical therapy and my condition improved greatly, though the back pain was never fully resolved. Eventually, I learned that errors in my diagnosis had jeopardized my life.

Mirrors Work . . .

I am a sociologist and I specialize in the study of mistakes. I was at Northwestern for the year as a Post-Doctoral Fellow in Law and Social Science. My fellowship involved a new direction of research: examining how lawyers talk about medical errors. For some time I had been examining how physicians talk about mistakes. In *The Unity of Mistakes: A Phenomenological Interpretation of Medical Work* (Paget 1988a), for example, I explored accounts of mistakes that physicians made or saw other physicians make. I treated these accounts as texts requiring interpretation. It was as if I had come across documents from another culture, documents that required rendering in the English language. My focus was the physicians' experiences (the subject's experience) of making mistakes in time as time unfolds.

In *The Unity of Mistakes*, I argued that clinical medicine is an error-ridden activity. I mean by *error-ridden activity* that mistakes are an intrinsic feature of medical work, that they cannot be avoided. I do not mean that physicians are at fault in making mistakes, though they, sometimes, are at fault. I mean that their work is intrinsically experimental, uncertain, and prone to error. And I have argued this point of view across works of very different kinds (Paget 1982, 1983, 1988a).

My proposal letter to the Director of the Law and Social Science Program emphasized my work on error and my new research interest in the discourse of negligence. I wanted to examine both how medical mistakes are legally constructed and how the contemporary malpractice insurance crisis is shaping public discourse. The malpractice crisis is seen as an insurance crisis, for example, rather than a crisis in personal injury.

I planned to locate a law firm that specialized in medical and legal disputes about malpractice where I could do field work focusing on negligence as a discourse about personal injury: how cases are processed, how expert testimony is acquired, and how settlements of claims are negotiated and resolved.

In my letter I explained my interest in negligence as follows:

> My interest in negligence has arisen because it is so consistently treated as a problem of a small minority of physicians. Recent reforms in Massachusetts have involved identifying repeated offenders and limiting the value of claims. Yet my sense is that negligence is widespread, not because incompetent physicians practice, though they do, but because error is endemic to the practice of medicine. I have repeatedly argued that medicine is an error-ridden activity. This means that both good and bad physicians commit negligent acts. . . .
>
> A fellowship on negligence, as it is processed legally, will permit me to enlarge my investigation of making mistakes. My most recent work suggests that silence about error produces very spe-

cific kinds of distortions in clinical discourse and thinking. Research on negligence will enable me to address these distortions as they are seen in a legal context. How error is reasoned about in legal disputes and how it is articulated in medical circles are vastly different topics and yet I hope to reveal both as forms of discourse about personal misfortune in patient care.

Because I learned that law firms specialized in defendants' or plaintiffs' work, either one or the other, and because I could not, in good conscience, choose one side or the other, I decided to examine how lawyers talk about medical mistakes in the courtroom. In the courtroom, I could investigate the arguments of both sides. In December and again in April and May, I attended trials at Daley Center in Chicago where lawyers argued the negligence of physicians. The trials were troubling and compelling dramas of mistakes. In the first two trials wrongful death was the issue: the wrongful death of a woman following childbirth and the wrongful death of a woman from breast cancer. The third trial involved brain damage to a baby delivered too late by caesarean section. The jury's award to the first plaintiff, the surviving husband and daughter of a woman who died following childbirth, was $4,600,000. Both the second and third trials were settled prior to a jury verdict. In one instance, the settlement was just under $1 million. In the other, the settlement was sealed by agreement of the participants involved: the parents of a child born brain damaged and the university hospital and physicians involved. I suspected that the settlement was above $5 million. Before the trial began, the plaintiff's attorney had refused a settlement of $2 million.

The courtroom was an extremely rich environment in which to explore error, though, paradoxically, the term mistake was rarely used. I attended each trial for its entire duration, including the selection of the jury, taking extensive notes and acquiring transcripts of trial testimony. I began to explore the image of medicine that was projected in these trials of negligence, the conflicts in the standard of care that invariably appeared in the testimony of expert witnesses, the way authority and expertise were constructed in testimony, and, of course, the juries' verdicts and assessments of damages. I was particularly impressed with the technical and complex arguments surrounding the standard of care. The standard of care is not like a ruler that can be laid down along the flow of events to measure them. It is sharply contested in the courtroom by medical experts.

Mirrors Life . . .

It was while attending the first trial late in December 1987 that I began to experience back pain. Eight months later, I learned that I had cancer. Almost simultaneously, I learned that the errors made in my diagnosis had jeopardized my life. I was told that my condition was incurable.

Friends packed my household and I flew home to Brookline, Massachusetts, to begin treatment at the Dana-Farber Cancer Institute. I struggled with the shock of the diagnosis and with the irony of my situation. I felt very vulnerable.

It was not just that mistakes were made, though they were. It was that so *many* mistakes were made. My Northwestern University physician did not order a chest x-ray in the course of investigating the source of my back pain. The Florida physician, who did order one, misread it as normal. He did not notice the presence of an abnormality in my chest x-ray. Furthermore, he failed to send the x-ray to a radiologist for review. His errors were crucial. Had he seen the abnormality, or had a radiologist seen it, I would have been able to undergo surgery, which would have enhanced the probability of my survival, at least for a time. Both the physician at Northwestern University and I relied on the Florida physician's reading of the x-ray. We continued to assume that the problem was a muscle injury. Soft-tissue injuries take a long time to heal, sometimes longer than broken bones. I entered physical therapy.

Almost four months passed before another x-ray revealed the tumor. By that time, I had several tumors in my liver and other nodules in both lungs.

In a word, my physicians were negligent. I had just begun research on negligence; now I was an example of it.

Mirrors Text . . .

Negligence

Negligence is a particular kind of error. It refers to a violation of the standard of medical care that causes grave injury. In a legal context, expert medical testimony is required to establish the "fact" of negligence.

Because I use terms from everyday life such as "mistake" in my investigations, I am able to follow the way in which these terms are transformed in clinical, legal, and political settings. Often, these terms are stripped of their existential meanings. In the courtroom, for example, the term mistake is, usually, censored when used. It is vague by legal standards since it denotes different and less precise phenomena than negligence.

Interestingly, in the courtroom, negligence is not treated as one kind of error among many, but is, instead, the *only* kind relevant in the courtroom. Although they cause harm, most mistakes in medicine are not negligent mistakes. Because they are not negligent, they are not compensated. They fall, literally, outside the purview of tort law. Just as troubling, in political contexts, medical mistakes are transfigured as insurance claims. They are debated *not* as injuries to patients requiring compensation, but as signs of litigiousness or avarice among plaintiffs and their lawyers. A crisis of injury in an error-ridden activity thus becomes an insurance crisis, a crisis in covering claims.

Phenomenology

My work on error has been phenomenological rather than technical and objectivist. I am not a detached observer attempting to understand objects or things. I am an experiencing subject, methodically attempting to understand other subjects and a subject matter. Furthermore, I live in the same world that I explore. My humanity and my biography enter into my inquiry as does my specialized training.

By a curious trick I never could understand and cannot execute, many sociologists do not live in the world they investigate. They position themselves outside the life-world. There are many dimensions of the alienation from life their "trick" permits. The subject and subject matter become objects of observation, things, or categories to be manipulated, often statistically. The desire to do a particular kind of "science" produces this effect. Desiring a disinterested and unbiased analysis apparently means distancing and denying the self of the sociologist.

The sociologist as an experiencing person is thus ignored. His method takes priority over his life and his social and historical situation. He reports his subject matter through his method and procedures split off from his life. The tendency to produce abstractions remote from everyday life, through a technical language, heightens the self alienation of many sociologists. Research is reported in the third person or, even more startling, concepts and technologies report the research—as if they really could. In the interest of "precision," terms are invented that have no historical dimensions, or terms are stripped of their emotional and historical meanings. The denial of the importance of language in the production of understanding is very crucial in reproducing a technical and inhumane world rather than displaying the technicality of the world that is being analyzed (Smith 1983, 1984).

Phenomenological work involves both the subject's experience and the phenomenologist's experience. Experience means that which is lived through, *Erlebnis*. The subject or subject matter is not an object in the sense of a thing. The subject or subject matter is explored through the subjectivity of the phenomenologist who perceives the subject matter, the phenomena, as a dialectical relation between self understanding and understanding the other. Work in this tradition is reflexive and tacks back and forth between the subject matter and observing the subject matter reflexively.

Writing is a central activity in the production of knowledge in phenomenological sociology (see Paget forthcoming). Writing displays both the subject matter and the scholar of the subject matter. The phenomenologist's presence is crucial. In addition to displaying the self-understanding of the phenomenologist, the process of writing can preserve the poetic and expressive features of life as lived. These features are central to the life-world.

Living in the very society I seek to analyze, taking up issues of this very world in which I live, means that I privilege the world of everyday life. It is, as Alfred Schutz (1962) argued, the paramount reality out of which all other enclaves of meaning are built and to which they all must necessarily return.

Error

Error is fundamental in the life-world. It is part of the ontological inventory of life lived. Perhaps this is one reason why I have not asked "Why did this happen to me?" I have thought rather "Why not me?" Is there any reason why because of my knowledge I might be excluded from the very thing I have explored so closely? Why not me indeed? Error is fundamental in clinical medicine, too, and it is endemic. It is not exceptional and uncommon. I, like everyone else, or rather most everyone else, see physicians about my health. Of course, I feel the irony of my position acutely.

Because I live in the world that I examine, because I take aspects of this world as my field of study, I am, as Manda Cesara (1982) suggests, both an apprentice scholar and apprentice human being. Both my work and I develop in this world which is my field of study. Even now I am using myself and developing as an experiencing subject. Even now my work is developing. This work is a text constructed from my own life and from errors in my life.

Mirrors Life . . .

I have Leiomyosarcoma, a rare smooth muscle cancer that usually appears in the stomach or the uterus. While the primary source of the cancer is unknown, it is presumed to be my lung. Probably an air tube or a large blood vessel (both contain smooth muscle) in my right lung went awry. There are no pain receptors in the lung to report the presence of a tumor. I had no cough. No signal of the problem appeared until the tumor began to press on muscles and ribs deep in my back.

It never occurred to me that I might have cancer, never entered my mind. I was perplexed and annoyed by the pain, but never afraid until late in July when I experienced intense pain, dizziness, and trouble breathing. Then I went to the Student Health Service where I was examined by another physician. Still more mistakes were made. A spine x-ray was ordered rather than a chest x-ray. The orthopedic resident who read the spine x-ray missed the abnormality near my spine.[1] I quickly recovered from this episode. However, one of my friends, who is a physician, suggested that I get a chest x-ray. A few days later I did. Both the lesion and a pleural effusion were visible.

1. The spine x-ray was sent to a radiologist. Eventually he reported an abnormality.

Paradoxically, the errors in my care were aggravated by my very good health. Everyone, including me, was thrown off track by my obvious vitality and high spirits. Aside from the unresolved back pain, I was in very good health. I walked every day along Lake Michigan, usually for at least three miles. I had an excellent diet. Though not a vegetarian, I ate little meat. I meditated. I did Hatha Yoga. I did not smoke (though I once did) and drank very moderately and usually wine. I rarely had a cold or the flu. In fact, I'd had no serious illness in my entire life. Until I became a cancer patient, I had never been hospitalized.

Strangely enough the presence of a tumor in my lung and at my spinal cord jeopardized my practice of yoga. Precisely those areas of my body most central to Hatha Yoga (my breathing and spine) were involved. Off and on during the last year, I have stopped my practice. For six and a half weeks while receiving radiation to my spine and chest, I stopped entirely.

Mirrors Work . . .

To say that my life mirrored my work tells only part of the story. My work on error comes from life and my interest in examining error is connected with its importance in life as it is lived.

Mistakes are not abstract events or numbers, but lived phenomena everyone experiences and must reckon with. A mistake is an incorrect effect of an act, a wrong result. It is known after having been made (there are, of course, rare exceptions in which a mistake is recognized as it is happening and avoided). We use the result to discern the wrongness of what was achieved. Taking the wrong path illustrates this. When someone takes the wrong path, she goes astray; but she only knows that, recognizes it, after already having taken the wrong path. The journey is too long, she does not reach the proper destination. Recognition of error dawns on her. In fact, the archaic meanings of mistake and error refer to taking the wrong path (*Mistaka*) or going astray and wandering about (*Errare*) and are useful for this reason.

The journey of error, the dynamic experience of going wrong, is crucial in understanding medical mistakes. They are rarely simple events like errors in addition. Rather they are complex activities and cognitions that unfold in time.[2]

I have always used "mistake" or "error" rather than more technical terms because these terms come from everyday life. Their meaning can be found in experience as it is lived. In addition, they have a long history and many associations that can be recognized and known in acting in time as it unfolds. That someone is at fault is one association among others of mistake or error. A mistake may provoke blame, or sadness, or regret, or anguish, or self doubt. By contrast, misdiagnosis is a technical term. It does not come from everyday life, but has a specialized realm, the practice of diagnosis and related activities. Misdiagnosis does not have the same psychological associations as mistake. Its associations are to other technical terms like patient management, prognosis, and autopsy. Indeed, in discussing error, the term misdiagnosis may be preferred just because it does not have many experiential meanings. Negligence is both a technical and an experiential term. Its everyday meaning is neglect or carelessness. Its technical meaning, at least in medicine and law, is bad medical practice and suggests culpability. Someone is at fault. In fact, a trial by jury, as I have already suggested, establishes the culpability or innocence of a physician or other malfeasant. In law negligence is a tort, a civil wrong. It does not necessarily mean neglect or carelessness. It means failing to meet a standard of care established in the courtroom.

By using the term mistake or error rather than more abstract and technical terms like negligence, malpractice, misdiagnosis, or mismanagement, I have been trying to preserve a

2. See *The Unity of Mistakes* (Paget 1988) for my analysis of the meaning of mistakes. On mistakes, see also Bosk 1979; Fox 1959; Fox and Swazey 1974; Freidson 1970, 1975; Light 1972; Millman 1977; Stelling and Bucher 1973, and Strauss et al. 1985. See my discussion of their works in chapters two and four of *The Unity of Mistakes*.

connection with the subject's experience in life as lived: your experience and mine, as well as theirs. In fact, the unity of mistakes arises in the recognition of the shared existential experience of error. Everyone makes mistakes and mistakes are inevitable in life as it is lived. I render these common expressions in *The Unity of Mistakes* as follows:

> "Everyone makes mistakes," everyone acts mistakenly in time as it unfolds. The range of mistaken acts is as wide as the realm of human activity, its scale as great or small as the possibilities of human conduct. Everyone lives in time as an unfolding current. Everyone knows what is unspoken. "If I knew then what I know now, if I had it to do all over again, I would have done something else." Everyone knows also the haunting possibility that "I should have known then" what I know now. The time structure of an honest error and a negligent act are identical; so usually is their unintendedness. What is different about a negligent act is that the "should have known then" is not a *should* of the human heart, but an intersubjectively affirmable *should*. But the "should have known then" does not alter the event, the mistake. It marks it as an irretrievable fault of the then of someone's conduct in time and activity.
>
> "Mistakes are inevitable"; mistaken acts are inevitable. Living in time is an unknowing becoming known. What is unspoken about the inevitability of mistakes is the horizon of human conduct. It is a ponderous representation of the unfolding path of our conduct. Mistakes have happened, are happening, and will happen, although they are not willed (Paget 1988a:153-54).

Physicians, like you and I, grapple with the moral quandary of their errors.

Mirrors Text . . .

The Unity of Mistakes

The data I examined in *The Unity of Mistakes* came from a longitudinal study of the training of physicians on which I worked while going through graduate school. Ann G. Olmsted was the primary investigator on the study. She and I interviewed medical students who were in the process of becoming physicians, both in medical school at the end of each year of training, in residency training, and, sometimes, in medical practice. Some 165 individuals were involved. Interviewing students in depth over sometimes six or seven years was an extraordinarily rich and complex experience. I saw, watched, and heard about marked changes in development, interests, commitments, and concerns. The complexity of the training process and the complexity of the development of physicians first provoked my interest in adult development. However, I soon realized that no description of medical work adequately reported what the study's participants were saying about the work of medicine, that is to say, doctoring. I began to focus on how to describe medical work, *not* as a profession, or a science, or an art, or an occupation, or a trade but, dynamically, as an activity, a practice, unfolding in time.[3]

A question about mistakes was on the interview protocol for fourth year students, residents, and practicing physicians. With their replies, I began another kind of description of medical work (as an error-ridden craft) and, simultaneously, another kind of interpretation of mistakes. I called mistakes complex sorrows of action going wrong and examined the experience of being wrong as a distinct experience of being.

> The *being* of being wrong, the nature of the *was* of being wrong, is a place in which any subject dwells in relation to the past. As a subject, as an I among many I's, my understanding of my mistake is different from your understanding of my mistake. My understanding of my mistake, for example, is accessible to me in a way in which it is not accessible to you. Indeed, it is only as accessible to you as you and I allow and desire.
>
> There is always an infinite regress to the story of my mistake but, at some point in time, for all

3. See chapters two and three, Paget 1988.

practical purposes, the story has been told. Its telling resonates with your own experience of the trajectory of acting in time when the character of action has been identified and when it has been understood that we, you and I, are alike in the unfolding of our experience.

The *being* of being wrong, however, is not only about the *I was* of being mistaken. Time winds on, and, in the tomorrows of human conduct, action again unfolds. Speaking again as a human subject, I, like you, will again be mistaken, if I act, and I will continue to dwell in the strange realm of the yesterdays, todays, and tomorrows of my knowledge of my acts.

I suspect, speaking as a human subject, that I can act again only if the blamelessness of my experience of acting can be acknowledged as a human possibility, for I can act tomorrow only in uncertain ways, and sometimes I will be correct and sometimes I will be mistaken (Paget 1988a:150-51).

While listening to participants in the study, I became aware of the problematic status of mistakes in their work—long before I found ways to express the specific nature of the dilemma of their mistakes. Because they work on and with human beings rather than on things or objects, physicians' errors take on special meaning both for them and for their patients.

Error-Work

Mistakes are common, though medical work is not typically thought of as full of error. I am quite used to regarding it that way because I have been, for a number of years, examining medical work (see also Gorowitz and MacIntyre 1976). Anselm Strauss and colleagues (1985) call the production and correction of error in clinical medicine *error-work*. By error-work they mean all the activities that prevent, minimize, define, detect, cover up, or rectify mistakes. Nurses, laboratory technicians, physical therapists, and patients, also, do error-work.

Knowledge that medicine is full of error is not widespread. The reasons for this are complicated. Physicians do not talk freely about errors in their work. They are commonly reticent or silent about them. When they do talk, they frequently prefer technical terms, terms that mask their experience of error. In much the same way, they, also, use technical terms to mask their entire subjectivity. This is a typical feature of masculine and scientific culture. Too, the "idea" of endemic error radically undermines their claim to expertise. Rather, it throws the claim of expertise under new light. *Physicians are "expert" in a work that proceeds by trial and error*. The public is not expert. Physicians are expert in comparison to their patients, who know very little about medical work, though some know a lot about the experience of illness. The experience of illness is not like the diseases physicians treat. Illness and disease are not the same subject matter. The first is experiential; the second is scientific and abstract.

Sociologists, often, have been preoccupied with technical and abstract constructions of their own, concerned with the role of professional knowledge and skills in the modern world, not with the daily practice of professionals. They have too rarely watched medical work up close as a *practice* and practical activity. When they have, sometimes they have engaged in a cynical analysis of the work.

Over the course of my investigations of mistakes, I have talked with many people about error in medicine. Invariably, they tell me about medical mistakes they have suffered. In autobiographical accounts of social scientists—and autobiography is an uncommon impulse in the social sciences—I have found accounts of medical mistakes. For example, Robert Murphy (1987) discusses an "apparently" grave depression, Ann Oakley (1984) recounts a misdiagnosed ectopic pregnancy from which she nearly died, Shulamit Reinharz (1987) explores her painful experience of a miscarriage. In his letters (1979-1989) about his experience with a rare and, usually, deadly cancer, Samuel Kaplan describes a lengthy period in which physicians missed the diagnosis. They failed to biopsy a recurrent skin lesion. Barbara Rosenblum (letters 1985-1988) reports a misdiagnosed breast cancer that eventually led to her death.

Many people are haunted by their sense of being wronged. They have experienced a wrong result. Thus, their sense of mistake is strong. However, a wrong result is not a mistake, though it may be a sign of a mistake. Few of the people I have spoken with have sought to clarify their experience either with their physician or with legal counsel. Little is known about who seeks legal counsel and who does not. Usually, patients think their own experience of error is exceptional and uncommon. The "idea" that error is exceptional and uncommon is persistently reinforced in the cultural life of Americans, in public debates about malpractice, and in the courts where lawyers argue about the exceptional nature of the specific case.

Just before coming to Northwestern University, I had a mammogram that revealed a calcium deposit and led to a biopsy. The biopsy was benign. The mammogram produces a certain percentage of "false positives." Various anomalies in the breast that appear on x-ray and lead to "unnecessary" biopsies are "false positives." "False positive" is one of those technical terms that strips away the experiential connotations of mistake. But how might mistake be used? We would not say that the mammogram was mistaken. The mammogram after all is an x-ray. Should we say that the radiologist is mistaken? She knows that a certain percentage of biopsies will be benign and a certain percentage will be malignant. She does her work, given a set of probabilities. If she is good, and she was, she knows that a "false positive" is preferred over a "false negative." However, some people go undiagnosed, "false negatives." When breast cancer is discovered later, a question of error may arise, and, sometimes, the possibility of negligence. The radiologist may have misread the x-ray, perhaps, or perhaps not.

A good question to ask would be "What are the probabilities that I would experience a medical mistake in the course of medical care?" Rather great, I should say. That it hadn't happened before, though perhaps it had and I wasn't aware of it, I attribute to my very good health. I've rarely had to see physicians about a medical problem. This is not to say that physicians always make mistakes. Rather I mean that error is an intrinsic problem of the diagnostic and therapeutic process.

The Uncanny Naturalized

Jung (1971) calls uncanny coincidences *synchronicity*. He means by the term to identify events that parallel one another and have the same meaning, but no causal connection. That is to say, the coincidence of events with the same meaning does not display a causal sequence.

> Causality is the way we explain the link between two successive events. Synchronicity designates the parallelism of time and meaning between psychic and psychophysical events, which scientific knowledge so far has been unable to reduce to a common principle. The term explains nothing, it simply formulates the occurrence of meaningful coincidences which, in themselves, are chance happenings, but so improbable that we must assume them to be based on some kind of principle, or on some property of the empirical world. (Jung 1971:517-18)

The performance of my work on the construction of an erroneous diagnosis on a woman with cancer did not cause my own cancer, nor did the cancer that I have cause the performance, but they paralleled each other. And the coincidence of the performance and my illness stunned both me and my friends. The performance came first, then the discovery of cancer. Actually the cancer came first, though I did not know about it then. Similarly, my work on error in medicine and the errors in my care as a medical patient did not display a causal chain, though they mirrored each other in ways that seem to me terribly odd and ironic. And, finally, my investigation of negligence, the topic, and negligence in my care coincided. Before my fellowship I had not been particularly interested in negligence as a phenomenon. I was interested in extending my work on error in new ways. And this extension and my own experience of negligence came together quite unexpectedly. These were meaningful coincidental events in my life and work. I did not foresee the parallels. I lived them and saw them later.

Jung felt that naming such phenomena synchronicity explained nothing and he went on to search for an explanatory psychic principle. I shall not follow his argument on extra-sensory perception. Rather, I want to emphasize the importance of synchronicity, the naming of the empirical phenomena. Synchronicity suggests that meaningful events occur and can mirror each other apart from causality. That unexpected, odd, and even tragic events happen without clear causal sequences.

Uncanny coincidences seem unnatural rather than natural phenomena because we tend to disproportionately emphasize causal chains, just as we disattend unexpected and strange juxtapositions. The "uncanny" does not fit our world view. By our world view, I mean a Western and specifically contemporary American world view. Often, we create causal chains and imbue events with causal connections when they do not present themselves that way. We infer unconscious agency, for example, following Freud's discovery of the unconscious. Or, alternatively, we interpret the unexpected and improbable as God's will. Both are causal accounts.

Meaningful coincidences happen quite often. Usually, we dismiss them, actively put them out of mind, because they suggest peculiar conundrums and random disasters. However, I have not done so. Some cultures celebrate unexpected events. Raku glazes, executed by firing ceramic pots in sawdust or wood chips, promote completely uncontrolled effects. The pot's glaze is marked by the fire in unplanned and, often, beautiful ways. That is an essential aspect of the aesthetic of Raku. It values chance. While we do not celebrate and value unexpected and improbable events, we have a term for happy coincidences, serendipity. Mine were disastrous coincidences. We lack a term for them or even a way to talk about them. Bad luck just won't do. Synchronicity is a beginning. Of course, the term should apply to both felicitous and unfortunate parallel events.

Neither do I believe that the events I have outlined occurred randomly, nor do I believe they are so improbable that they cannot be explored. Error is the common thread of these strange juxtapositions.

Reckoning with Error

On the one hand, I have just been emphasizing the way in which coincidences are disattended. On the other hand, I have been calling attention to coincidences and endowing them with meaning. The meaning of these events to me is that they have converged in a crisis with a life-threatening disease, which I am struggling to overcome. I am brought to an encounter with my death through these events, a series of mistakes at many levels. It is not that I am a victim of error or even of chance. There is no simple perpetrator here.

I am the subject of error. I embody it. Even my body has erred.

Cancer is above all a mistake of the body. A cell goes awry in replication, not just once, but several times. It produces a mutation. This mutant reproduces itself again and again. No one seems to know how to stop the unregulated cell growth of mutating cells, least of all me. It is best if they can be cut away, if not, then killed. That is the strategy of scientific medicine.

Strangely, my knowledge of error has helped me deal with the errors in my care. Had I not known about the prevalence of error in medicine I would not have been able to process what has happened to me without bitterness. But I had thought these matters through already, and more than once. I now live out the complex sorrow I have before described.

When I arrived at Dana-Farber and saw my physician, I told him about my work and about what had happened over the last eight months. I had never before discussed my work with a physician treating me. We talked at length. At intervals during the last year, we have discussed the errors in my care again. In his view, the misreading of the chest x-ray harmed me significantly. Though he also believes that I will die from this disease in any case, the Florida physician's mistakes hasten my death.

I have examined the first errant x-ray of my chest and many many x-rays and CAT scans since then. I have talked with friends. I have spoken at length with attorneys both in Illinois and in Florida about my care. In March 1989, a lawyer filed a notice of negligence for me against the Florida physician. In due course the physician was informed of his mistake and shown the chest x-ray. Both he and I were deposed. His insurance company offered to settle out of court. I agreed. I did not file suit in Illinois, though I believe my physician at Northwestern University was negligent. The suit would have been more complicated and difficult to argue from a legal and clinical point of view. More important to me, the physician at Northwestern University recognized his mistakes. At least, I think he did. He knew that he missed the diagnosis because he did not order a chest x-ray until August. He knew that the long delay compromised my life. Oddly, once again, my knowledge of error helped me resolve the issues of negligence in my care, though, sometimes, the process has been very painful.

Error, however, has not been the focus of my concern this last year. Rather cancer has been. And it is cancer that I have fought. I have undergone very arduous chemotherapies and extensive radiation to my spine, 6000 rads, which is all that is allowed. Until recently, my physician and many other physicians, nurses, and technicians who have attended me, have been able to control the cancer.

Strangely too, had I not thought so long about the cancer experience of the patient I examined in "On the Work of Talk," had I not watched the staging of a play in which the terror of cancer was so exquisitely expressed in the whispering of the cast, I would not have been able to describe my own circumstances so plainly. My style has always been to speak out. The performance reinforced my own predisposition.

I believe the production of the performance and my excitement about the production distracted me from my own unresolved back pain. Distraction is not really the right word. Rather, I was so excited by the performance of my work that I rarely thought about the back pain beyond its annoying persistence—my mistake.

When the performance was over I was still so excited that I immediately wrote a paper about the performance called "Performing the Text" and did my own adaptation of the article. In July, when the paper and my script were done, I was still in physical therapy. I waited around Evanston for the problem to resolve itself and, of course, it did not.

Now I write about my life and my work, and my work and my life, and my writing distracts me from the immediacy of my death. My work still excites me. There is so much more to do and say.

References

Bosk, Charles L.
1979 Forgive and Remember: Managing Medical Failure. Chicago: University of Chicago Press.

Cesara, Manda.
1982 Reflections of a Woman Anthropologist: No Hiding Place. New York: Academic Press.

Fox, Renee C.
1959 Experiment Perilous. Glencoe, Ill.: Free Press.

Fox, Renee C., and Judith P. Swazey.
1974 The Courage to Fail: A Social View of Organ Transplants and Dialysis. Chicago: University of Chicago Press.
Freidson, Eliot
1970 The Profession of Medicine: A Study of the Sociology of Applied Knowledge. New York: Dodd, Mead.
1975 Doctoring Together: A Study of Professional Social Control. New York: Elsevier.
Gorowitz, Samuel, and Alasdair MacIntyre.
1976 "Toward a theory of medical fallibility." Journal of Medicine and Philosophy 1:51-71.
Jung, Carl G.
1971 "On synchronicity." The Portable Jung. New York: Viking.
Kaplan, Samuel.
1979-89 Unpublished letters.
Light, Donald W., Jr.
1972 "Psychiatry and suicide: the management of a mistake." American Journal of Sociology 77:821-38.
Millman, Marcia.
1977 The Unkindest Cut: Life in the Backrooms of Medicine. New York: William Morrow.
Murphy, Robert F.
1987 The Body Silent. New York: Henry Holt and Company.
Oakley, Ann.
1984 Taking It Like A Woman. New York: Random House.
Paget, Marianne A.
1982 "Your son is cured now; you may take him home." Culture, Medicine and Psychiatry 6:237-59.
1983 "On the work of talk: studies in misunderstandings." In The Social Organization of Doctor-Patient Communication, ed. Sue Fisher and Alexandra Dundas Todd, 55-74. Washington, D.C.: Center For Applied Linguistics.
1988a The Unity of Mistakes: A Phenomenological Interpretation of Medical Work. Philadelphia: Temple University Press.
1988b "The work of talk." Adapted for performance by Emilie Beck in collaboration with the author. Directed by Emilie Beck. Northwestern University Jones Arts Residential College, The Great Hall. Evanston, Ill., May 14 and 15.
1990 "Performing the text." Journal of Contemporary Ethnography 10:136-55.
Forthcoming " 'Unlearning to not speak.' " Human Studies.
Reinharz, Shulamit
1987 "What's missing in miscarriage?" Journal of Community Psychology 16:84-103.
Rosenblum, Barbara
1985-88 Unpublished letters.
Schutz, Alfred
1962 "On multiple realities." Collected Papers. Vol. I. The Hague: Martinus Nijhoff.
Smith, Dorothy E.
1983 "No one commits suicide: textual analyses of ideological practices." Human Studies 6:309-59.
1984 "Textually mediated social organization." International Social Science Journal 36:59-75.
Stelling, Joan, and Rue Bucher.
1973 "Vocabularies of realism in professional socialization." Social Science and Medicine 7:661-75.
Strauss, Anselm, Shizuko Fagerhaugh, Barbara Suczek, and Carolyn Wiener
1985 Social Organization of Medical Work. Chicago: University of Chicago Press.

Part VII
Alternative Medicine

[22]

Using Alternative Therapies: Marginal Medicine and Central Concerns

Ursula M. Sharma

The legitimacy of alternative medicine is an issue of vital public concern and the growing body of social science research on alternative healing should surely illuminate the political problems involved. I shall begin by reviewing some of the results of this research, and then outline some findings from my own investigations. These suggest that the use of alternative (or complementary) medicine is associated with many other changes in health care practice on the part of individuals and families. Alternative practitioners may be marginal (in a political sense) to the orthodox medical establishment, but the issues which are raised by the use of alternative medicine are central if we are concerned with what patients demand of the health services and how they conceive of health and well-being.

Large scale studies conducted in industrial countries suggest that the usage of alternative medicine is now substantial. The Threshold Foundation study carried out in the UK projected a rate of usage amounting to 5 per cent of the rate of consultation of GPs (Fulder 1984, p. 43). In the Netherlands a study carried out by the Dutch Institute for Preventive Health Care and the Technical and Industrial Organization was directed towards a comparison of opinions and experience of alternative medicine and official medicine; the survey found that 6.9 per cent of the sample of adults had visited one or more natural healer in the past year (Ooijendijk *et al.*, 1981, p. 44). In the absence of prior research the rate of increase in usage of alternative medicine in recent years can only be estimated, and there are problems of comparability between studies, but Fulder is probably correct in predicting a 'UK medical upheaval by the end of the decade' (Fulder, 1984, p. 44).

Who uses alternative medicine? A hypothesis which seems to have informed some research, either explicitly or implicitly, is the idea that users of alternative medicine are possibly marginal *people* as well as users of marginal *medicine*. Much American research seems to address itself to combating the notion that users of unorthodox medicine are likely to be uneducated and illiterate (McGuire, 1988, p. 10, Avina and Schneiderman, 1978). Most studies report that users come from a wide range of backgrounds and suggest no evidence that alternative medicine is the preserve of the 'crank' or hill billy. The Threshold Foundation study suggests that in Britain users of alternative medicine tend to be bunched in the young and middle-aged cohorts and, although coming from a variety of backgrounds, are somewhat more likely to be from the higher status groups (Fulder, 1984, p. 46). Research in Australia and the Netherlands has produced similar findings (Boven *et al.*, 1977, pp. 303 ff; Ooijendijk *et al.*, 1981, p. 19). A number of smaller studies in Europe, Australia and America have found either minor differences in demographic and socio-economic characteristics between samples of users of alternative medicine and control populations (generally a slightly higher proportion of educated or high status patients and a young/middle-aged age profile), or no differences at all (Furnham and Smith, 1988; Kronenfeld and Wasner, 1982; Avina and Schneiderman, 1978; Parker and Tupling, 1976). There is, however, consistent evidence that higher proportions of alternative medicine patients are female (Ooijendijk, Mackenbach and Limberger, 1981, p. 10; Fulder, 1984, p. 46). Are there characteristics of alternative medicine which render it more acceptable or accessible to women, or is it rather that women are more likely to have the kind of health problems which conventional medicine cannot cure?

Why do people use alternative medicine? There can be no doubt that the straightforward answer to this question is simply 'Becaused they have illnesses which conventional medicine has not been able to cure'. A study of patients at the Centre for Alternative Therapies in Southampton indicated that the three complaints for which consultations were most frequently initiated were pain (arthritis, back pain, abdominal pain, headaches), allergies (eczema, urticaria, asthma, rhinitis) and non-specific symptoms such as 'feeling unwell or run down', malaise (Moore *et al.*, 1985). Very similar findings are reported for the Threshold Foundation study (Fulder, 1984, p. 47). The Australian 'Three City' study revealed that problems of the musculo-skeletal system figured most prominently among the complaints for which patients sought alternative healers (Boven *et al.*, 1977, p. 325).

It is not easy to compare data from surveys which rely on the patient's own definition of his/her problem or complaint; respondents use a variety of diagnostic vocabularies which may or may not correspond with those used by conventional doctors or alternative healers. Many alternative systems of healing have their own distinctive nosologies which are not necessarily adopted by their users. Classification by reported symptoms may be more satisfactory but leads to vagueness. 'Malaise', 'feeling unwell', are not very felicitous terms, considered as diagnostic categories. Also if individual forms of therapy are taken separately, there may be wider variation, since some medical systems are suited to (or are peceived as being suited to) particular kinds of complaint (osteopathy and chiropractic for problems of the musculo-skeletal system, for instance). However, the general picture is not at all difficult to grasp. Patients are using unorthodox medicine to deal with conditions (mainly chronic and non-life threatening) for which orthodox medicine can offer symptomatic relief rather than cure. The insistence of the BMA that alternative medicine prove its efficacy through double blind trials of medications or other methods acceptable to orthodox medical science seems therefore oddly irrelevant to these patients' perceptions of their needs. An asthma sufferer who has been unable to obtain more than temporary symptomatic relief from his/her condition under orthodox treatment and is desperate for a permanent cure is unlikely to demand this kind of proof for the efficacy of homoeopathy or acupuncture. He or she is already convinced of the inefficacy of orthodox medicine of his/her disease and has reached a stage of readiness to experiment with other systems. The same is not true of many alternative practitioners as represented through their professional associations or broad groupings like the Research Council for Complementary Medicine or the Confederation of Healing Organisations, some of which are very much concerned with the question of demonstrating the efficacy of alternative medicine in terms acceptable to the scientific establishment.

Social science research can shed little direct light on the question of whether alternative medicine actually works (or at least not in the sense that the medical profession would accept); however, it has a good deal to say on the question of customer satisfaction with the services provided by practitioners. Here again, comparability is a problem, because different studies have used different indicators of satisfaction or have questioned users at different stages of treatment, but the general picture is far from negative. Moore, Phipps and Marcer found that 59 per cent of patients interviewed at a Centre for Alternative Therapies said that they felt better after eight weeks of treatment though only nineteen had completed their treatment at the time (Moore *et al.*, 1985, p. 28). In Australia Parker and Tupling found that of a sample of chiropractic patients 45 per cent reported 'very great' or 'almost total' relief of symptoms, with another 31 per cent stating that they had 'some' relief immediately after treatment. After ten weeks a follow up enquiry indicated that 37 per cent of patients reported total improvement and 32 per cent considerable improvement, 19 per cent some improvement and only 11 per cent no improvement at all (Parker and Tupling, 1976, p. 374). An interesting American study of the perceptions of osteopaths and ordinary physicians in a small town reports a 'cognitive bias in favour of MDs (conventional doctors) but a countervailing pragmatic bias in favour of DOs (osteopaths)' (Riley, 1980, p. 1170). That is, clients had internalized the ideological notion that orthodox medicine has superior efficacy, but in practice expressed satisfaction with unorthodox practitioners whose services they had used to deal with problems the orthodox physicians could not treat. Findings such as these do not, of course, prove that alternative medicine works *better* than conventional medicine (probably most users of orthodox medicine would also be prepared to state that it effects 'some' improvement in their condition if asked) nor does it say anything about whether alternative medicine works according to its own claims or theories. What it does suggest is that levels of patient satisfaction are high enough to ensure that there will be a vigorous demand for the services of alternative healers for the foreseeable future.

I stated earlier that there was a 'simple' answer to the 'straightforward' question as to why people use alternative medicine, and my review of research so far has concentrated on researchers' answers to fairly straightforward questions (Who uses alternative medicine? For what disorders do they seek treatment?). Simple questions, however, are not always the best conceived or most interesting. We may correlate usage of alternative medicine with all kinds of demographic and medical characteristics of sample populations and compare them with control groups in all kinds of respects and still miss some very important dimensions of the demand for services. Can we treat usage of alternative medicine as a 'variable', an isolable piece of behaviour, rather than as a feature of an individual's life situation, perhaps a stage in some wider process of change in health care practice? Are individuals most appropriately taken as the units of study, given that medical sociology has made us aware that individuals frequently take decisions about health care in consultation with household members and kin?

The study which I undertook in 1986 was not designed to compare users of alternative medicine with non-users, but to discover the routes by which patients came to use it. The term 'routes' has a double sense here. It refers both to the particular experiences (ill health, dissatisfaction with NHS) through which the individual arrived at the decision to seek treatment from an alternative practitioner, and also (more literally) the path by which they came to be treated by the particular practitioner selected (the sources of information, referral, etc.). I interviewed thirty people in the Stoke-on-Trent area who had used at least one form of alternative medicine in the past twelve months. The sample was largely obtained by inviting readers of the local newspaper to volunteer their experiences of alternative medicine. We cannot draw any conclusions about the representativeness of such a self selected sample in terms of demographic or socio-economic characteristics, but this was not the purpose of the research.

The interviews were structured to the extent that they covered some standard questions and elicited a corpus of comparable data, but as far as possible I encouraged respondents to deliver this information in the context of their own 'story' of how they had come to use alternative medicine. This left them free to include in their accounts much that I would not have elicited through standardized questions in a set order. For most of the respondents the 'story of how they had come to use alternative medicine' was a narrative with a point, even a moral, which they wished to convey. In many cases the interviewee was describing a process which was by no means complete; the point at which the interviewer encounters the patient cannot be supposed to be the final point in the latter's search for satisfactory health care, and longitudinal studies of individuals (or more appropriately households) will probably be more useful in future.

Using alternative medicine is therefore part of a *process*. While some interviewees could pinpoint predisposing factors in their family background (e.g. usage of herbal medicine by parents, horrific experiences of orthodox medical treatment by a close relative) most took as their starting point their own experience of some chronic disorder and their own subsequent dissatisfaction with the treatment they received for this under the NHS. All had consulted their GP about this illness in the first place and several had seen specialists in connection with diagnosis or treatment. I did not encounter any who had used alternative medicine because they had been brought up to do so, because it was the norm in their ethnic/religious group or for other 'cultural' reasons, apart from one woman whose parents had been ardent adherents of naturopathy, though a larger sample might well identify cases of this kind of usage.

It is important to discuss users' sources of dissatisfaction with orthodox medicine at some length because many of them do not relate straightforwardly to conventional medicine's failure to 'cure' disease so much as to its failure to 'cure' disease on terms that are acceptable to the particular patient. Two individuals did report a conflictual relationship with their GP, but in most cases dissatisfaction was not focused on the perceived incompetence of individual doctors or consultants. The problems with orthodox medicine as offered under the NHS which interviewees mentioned could be grouped as follows.

The claim that conventional medicine fails to get at the 'root cause' of chronic illness or to take a preventative approach, and can therefore only treat the symptoms. For example, a young man suffering from chronic depression had been referred to a psychiatrist and had received anti-depressant drugs which had some temporary effect. But he felt that the basic cause of his state had not been discovered and that therefore he would continue to be liable to periods of depression, a prospect which he did not wish to accept. The experience of acupuncture described by friends who had used it suggested to him that this therapy might effect a long term change in his condition. When he had tried acupuncture it so fascinated him that he decided to train an as acupuncturist himself, and whilst his depression has not entirely ceased to be a problem, the periods of disability are shorter and less frequent.

This is not to say that patients always required a detailed diagnosis or a technical description of what the healer saw as the problem; patients varied very much as to the degree of interest they took in the actual rationale or theory of the forms of healing used. What was more often reported was relief that their dissatisfaction with symptomatic 'cures' had been acknowledged as legitimate and reasonable, and an appreciative sense that the healer was tackling the problem at a more fundamental level that conventional doctors had managed to do.

The fear of drugs which might become habit forming, or the dislike of side effects of particular drugs. Sometimes this took a rather diffuse concern about drugs that are too 'strong' — an imprecise fear of the body being interfered with too drastically. Sometimes there was general anxiety that prolonged or frequent use of drugs would interfere with the body's ability to react to drugs in acute situations, especially with regard to the use of antibiotics for childhood ailments. In other cases the dissatisfaction was based on a very specific experience. For instance, one interviewee's consultant had prescribed drugs for high blood pressure which, she said, made her feel exhausted and weak, 'like an old woman'. When she discovered a herbalist who could treat her she was relieved to be offered medicine which, she said, controlled her condition with no side effects whatsoever. The same interviewee expressed concern over the state of health of her sister who suffered from arthritis and who, she said, had been given ever stronger drugs to control the condition without any real improvement.

The editors of a recent volume on chronic illness point out that, for many patients, living with long term illness involves coping not only with the discomfort or disability caused by the illness itself but also coping with the physical or social demands made by the medical regime prescribed to deal with the illness (Anderson and Bury, 1988, p. 250). Another way of presenting this point might be to say that some patients find the cost of the regime prescribed for an illness outweighs the benefit it confers in terms of increased well-being or ability to live a normal life, and therefore they seek alternative regimes in the hope that their costs will be more acceptable.

Fear or dislike of forms of treatment which are seen as too radical or invasive. A middle-aged woman who suffered from back pain had been offered surgery under the NHS without, however, any guarantee that her condition would be cured. Indeed, she had been told that there was a slight risk that it might become worse. A major operation which did not have any certain outcome seemed to her too drastic a step to take and the risk of a deterioration dismayed her as her work required her to move and lift inmates in an old people's home. She visited a chiropractor at the suggestion of a colleague of her husband and after a fairly lengthy (and at first painful) course of treatment reported an almost complete recovery.

The perceived inability of conventional medicine to cope with the social and experiential aspects of illness. There is now more awareness of the need for personal support in severe or terminal illness, yet even apparently trivial conditions like eczema pose a need for personal support when they are chronic (as patients' self-help groups recognize). The sufferer needs to feel that the healer (of whatever kind) appreciates and does not dismiss the forms of distress or inconvenience which the illness causes. Some interviewees emphasized a desire for practical advice in the day-to-day management of their illness (useful adjustments to diet, suggestions for patterns of rest and exercise, stress management techniques, etc.). It is not by any means the case that all conventional doctors are unable to offer this personal interest and support, nor is it the case that all sufferers found alternative healers willing to provide it. Many healers, however, allow for much longer consultation times than do GPs, especially for a first consultation which may (especially in systems like homoeopathy) involve taking a very detailed case history. A time-consuming form of treatment may be acceptable to the sufferer if s/he feels it is producing some lasting effect.

Dissatisfaction with the kind of relationship between doctor and patient which interviewees feel that conventional medicine requires or presupposes. In many of the interviews, patients communicated a conscious appreciation of the more active role they felt able to play in the management of their illness or the general pursuit of health. Usually this feeling of being in control was described as a by-product of their experiences rather as the goal they had been seeking in the first place. A woman who had suffered from asthma for many years described her encounters with conventional and numerous forms of alternative medicine by saying: 'I am not criticizing other people . . . but I think that very often they go to the doctor and they just accept what the doctor says. I would advise anybody to go to the doctor first, but now I would always use alternative medicine to get a second opinion and treatment if you are not satisfied.' Many took an explicitly consumerist approach; one young man who had recently begun to consult an iridologist and to use herbal medicine described his and his wife's attitude to conventional medicine thus: 'If we need to, then we do go to our GP — we are not totally blinkered. We aim to get the best out of both systems.'

Yet some interviewees recognized that this active, critical and perhaps eclectic approach to health care might be incompatible with the model of the doctor–patient relationship in which the doctor has total responsibility for the treatment and the patient has only to trust and comply. Most interviewees had avoided telling their GPs about any alternative treatment they had received becaused they intended to continue to use the GP's services and did not wish to be seen to violate this model of the GP–patient relationship.

So far I have concentrated on the critical point at which the patient decides for the first time to seek alternative treatment and I have stressed that this decision is compounded of desire for treatment for a specific and (usually) chronic condition and dissatisfaction with the form of treatment received under the NHS, which may not simply relate to conventional medicine's failure to *cure* as much as with failure to cure *on terms acceptable to the patient*. The search for a satisfactory cure for a chronic illness or disorder does not always lead a sufferer directly to the door of an alternative practitioner. Many respondents recounted what can best be described as a programme of self education about their disorder which they had undertaken once they had realized that a quick cure was not likely. One patient had read and assimilated a large number of popular medical books on diet obtained from local bookshops and the public library to inform herself about her dietary allergy before she sought treatment from a herbalist. A woman with chronic asthma had obtained a great deal of information from the popular media, mainly television programmes and women's magazines, before contacting a spiritual healer about whom she had read a magazine article.

Many interviewees described this process of self education as one which changed some of their views on health in general, as well as their views on a specific health problem. A young husband who had suffered from chest problems described how the dietary recommendations of an iridologist caused him and his wife to think more in general about what they ate: 'There has been a lot of information on television and so forth about additives. I started to notice this sort of information more. And I began to talk to Jennifer (a family friend who used the same healer) and I began to wonder whether our diet had always been at fault.' His wife continued: 'It (i.e. the changes in diet which they had made) has improved the quality of our life. We think more about the effects of ageing; one day we shall be at the wrong end of thirty, then forty, then fifty . . . we have been eating wholefoods for two years now, but it is all too easy to abuse your body.'

Most interviewees in the sample, however, described the initial decision to use alternative medicine as prompted by a recommendation to a specific practitioner by a specific member of their network (see Table 9.1). This confirms what many other researchers have found, i.e. that most users come to alternative healing via personal recommendation obtained through informal networks rather than via GPs' referrals or formal channels of information. Table 9.1, however, refers to the *first* experience of alternative medicine, and many patients had used more than one form of alternative medicine, either for the same disease at different times, or more usually, for different diseases. If we include sources of information used for all consultations (not just the first) we find more diverse sources of information, with cultural and political organizations playing a greater part (for example, the Soil Association, vegetarian cookery classes, feminist groups).

Table 9.1 How respondents heard about the 'alternative' healer they used first

Source of information	Number of respondents
'Public' sources:	
Advertisements/Yellow pages	3
GPs' recommendation	1
Local association/organization	1
'Private' sources:	
Friends/acquaintances/colleagues	23
Relatives	2
Total	30

Most patients, however, seemed to have gained the confidence to approach a non-orthodox healer in the first place after hearing some kind of success story about that healer from a relative, friend or colleague, and only used information from more impersonal sources once a personal recommendation had yielded some kind of useful experience. This confirms an observation which practitioners whom I have interviewed have often made, namely that advertisement is hardly an issue. Recommendations circulate by word of mouth and most practitioners interviewed so far have stated that a satisfactory level of clientele can be built up very quickly in this way.

What is striking about the interviewees' stories is that initial usage of one form of alternative medicine is often followed by use of other forms, either serially or simultaneously, for the same or for different illnesses. Some patients had used as many as five types in as many years (see Table 9.2). In only one case was this due to continued failure to obtain any relief. A young man who had a skin condition affecting his scalp and had seen a consultant dermatologist, but without any significant improvement, announced to me his dogged intention of trying as many different forms of medicine in turn until he found one which had some effect. What seemed more common was that some degree of satisfaction (not necessarily total) with the particular form of alternative medicine first sampled led to a more experimental attitude and eventually to trials of other kinds of healing.

Table 9.2 Number of types of alternative medicine used by respondents (either serially or simultaneously)

Types of alternative medicine used:	1	2	3	4	4+	
Number of respondents	9	8	4	7	2	(Total 30)

In many cases this change to a more eclectic approach to health care was one which affected the whole family. This could happen in several ways. In some cases the interviewee had recommended a form of treatment which s/he has used to other members of the family or had used it for children. In other cases the treatment involved the family indirectly insofar as the patient had to observe some regime (usually dietary) which affected the family. A woman who used a particular kind of diet recommended by a herbalist in treating chronic arthritis said that whilst she could not insist that her family eat the diet prescribed for herself, it was convenient to plan meals so that her work was not unnecessarily duplicated. Her family had accepted these changes in family eating patterns, indeed had come to appreciate them. In other cases the regime presented more problems, but only one patient reported downright uncooperative or dismissive attitudes on the part of household members to their usage of alternative medicine. In a few cases patients reported that a spouse or children had regarded their usage of alternative medicine in the light of an eccentric aberration but had not put any obstacles in the way of the interviewee's sticking to the regime prescribed.

When looking at the effects of use of alternative medicine on family health care practices it is important to place these changes in a broader context. Some of the dietary changes and shifts in lifestyle reported by patients as stemming from the recommendations of alternative healers are changes which are being recommended by many other sources of medical authority or information (GPs, popular medicine journals, health promotion campaigns) and are by no means peculiar to alternative medicine 'sub-cultures'. Reduced consumption of animal fats, high fibre diets, regimes of exercise and use of relaxation techniques might be examples. Such changes should be seen as part of more general shifts in thinking about personal and family health care voiced particularly effectively, but not exclusively, by holistic healers.

More significantly, there is little evidence that users of alternative medicine cease entirely to use orthodox medicine, though they may use it less, or for different purposes, or more critically. A sceptical attitude to orthodox medicine did not lead to its abandonment. Usually patients used alternative medicine for specific illnesses or problems and GPs for others. Interviewees had not abandoned the NHS even though dissatisfied with it. In Table 9.3 I have tried to summarize some of the main patterns of usage which I found among the individuals I interviewed. This is not a very satisfactory exercise since it is clear that what we are looking at is a very fluid scene in which many people are in the process of changing the pattern of their 'health seeking behaviour' either as individuals or at the household level, and many of the people I interviewed are likely to change their patterns further in future. But from this table we can see that we do not have to treat users of alternative medicine and users of the health service as two discrete sets of people. Use of alternative medicine generated in a particular situation of illness may continue but alongside orthodox medicine. In some cases initial use of alternative medicine had eventually led to committed devotion to a particular system of alternative medicine to the virtual exclusion of all other systems. This was the case with a farmer who had become convinced of the efficacy of homoeopathy in his twenties, after a severe and painful ear infection. He has, he claimed, never consulted an ordinary doctor since, except once to have a broken arm X-rayed and immobilized, and is an enthusiastic evangelist for homoeopathic treatment.

This degree of exclusive commitment, however, was unusual. Most interviewees could think of occasions during the past twelve months when they had consulted their GP for themselves or for other members of their family, and could envisage other times in the future. Of course, it is possible that users of alternative medicine continue to consult their GPs whilst failing to comply with their prescriptions or instructions for treatment. A study of users of ritual healing groups in America notes that many respondents in the study did consult their doctors about symptoms and might value some aspects of their services (in particular their diagnostic skills) but would reserve the right not to follow the doctor's suggestions for treatment. As the author points out, the very notion of 'compliance' implies a power relationship which some users of alternative medicine have (either explicitly or implicitly) called into question (McGuire, 1988, p. 194).

One very widespread idea which seems to me to be a misconception (at least so far as this country is concerned) is that users of alternative healing are naively attracted by the ideological claims of alternative medicine. Johathan Miller suggested in a recent newspaper article that 'much alternative medicine on offer — acupuncture or homoeo-

Table 9.3 Types of usage of alternative medicine

Conflictual relationship with GP plus occasional or regular use of alternative medicine	2
'Experimental' or eclectic use of alternative medicine	12
Stable and regular use of one form of alternative medicine	9
'Restricted' use of one form of alternative medicine (for a single illness)	7
Total	30

pathy, for example — appeals to soft primitivism', a concept which he defines as 'a belief that there was a time when men were harmonious and happy — the myth of the Golden Age — and possessed with wisdoms we are foolish to ignore and idiotic to forget' (Miller, 1989). Possibly this is so: certainly such ideas are frequently expressed in a variety of quarters. But this would not in itself suffice to explain the increasing use of alternative medicine, which seems related to quite pragmatic objectives such as obtaining a cure for a specific illness or leading a more active and healthy life. Only a very few of the people I interviewed gave explicitly ideological reasons for their initial attraction to alternative medicine, though some, as I have indicated, have altered their way of looking at care of the body and mind as a result of their encounter. So ideological commitment might explain why some people *continue* to use alternative medicine having once used it successfully, insofar as they are convinced by what they learn about it from practitioners, but it would not account for the initial resort to unorthodox medicine itself.

Yet most patients using alternative medicine would seem to be (negatively) dissatisfied with the service offered by orthodox medicine, coming on the whole from its areas of notable failure, rather than (positively) attracted by any alternative world view the former may claim to offer. Two themes recur very frequently in the interviews, and receive widespread mention in the literature on the subject:

1. The demand that the patient's experience and understanding of his or her disease should be acknowledged and treated with respect. Not all interviewees spoke in terms of a more 'equal' relationship with the doctor or healer, but many wanted to be better informed so that they could exercise more control in the management of their illness. Where alternative practitioners took the trouble to explain the rationale of treatment to the patient this was appreciated, and often contrasted with the failure of orthodox doctors to take time to provide information about treatment, or to take account of the patients' experience of his/her illness.

New Directions in the Sociology of Health

2. The demand for what could loosely be called a more 'holistic' approach on the part of doctors. Patients do not always use the term holism, and when they do, they do not always refer to exactly the same thing. However, a recurrent theme in the interviews was the desire that the personal context of illness should be taken into account. The treatment by drugs, which is all that many patients can obtain under the NHS, was often seen as too narrow even where it was 'effective' in terms of sheer relief of symptoms.

The first demand appears to correspond to a feature of the health philosophy of the present Government, namely that the patient should be in a position to 'choose' treatment and to take a high measure of responsibility for his or her own health. Health education is seen very largely in terms of campaigns to modify aspects of life-style which are held to carry risks of ill health. The 'choice' which the patient is to exercise seems at the moment to refer to the choice between private and public medicine or between different private doctors practising orthodox medicine, but the terms of the rhetoric are not dissimilar. The consumer movement, as expressed through journals such as *Which?* and *Self Health*, also implicitly expouses a philosophy of individual responsibility and choice in health matters. All these voices imply the possibility of a demand-led health system, even if they are coming at the idea from different directions. The logic of the free market is that alternative medicine should be allowed to flourish; it will prosper or decline according to the state of demand for its services. Many doctors currently practising orthodox forms of medicine already offer forms of alternative medicine to their patients or take an interest in the holistic health movement. How long will the generally extremely conservative attitude of the medical profession (as expressed officially through the BMA) be able to withstand the effects of a growing market in a political climate dominated by the ethic of the market?

As regards the second demand, the need for a more holistic approach is evidently recognized by many members of the medical profession, even those who are by no means in favour of alternative medicine itself. The British Holistic Medicine Association has many general practitioners among its members and one may find contributions from medical doctors as well as healers and lay people in journals such as *Cadduceus*. Jonathan Miller, in the article already mentioned, admits that the mechanistic model of the human person espoused by modern medicine, and its consequences for treatment, are repulsive to many patients. Many of the patients I interviewed attributed the aspects of NHS treatment which they did not like to the mode of delivery rather than to the system of medicine itself. That is, they recognized that pressures of time and organization make it impossible for doctors to deal with them as whole persons even if they wish to. It is curious that only one of the patients I interviewed had actually obtained orthodox treatment from a private consultant for the condition for which they subsequently sought alternative healing. Perhaps a larger sample would throw light on why some patients consider private medicine such an option and others do not. It has to be remembered that in an area like the one in which I have researched, use of alternative medicine is not necessarily more expensive than use of a private consultant. In fact some of it is remarkably cheap. (At the time of writing £15 for an initial session of three-quarters of an hour to one hour is not unusual for many healers; if one feels better after one or two sessions this may be a cheaper option than visiting a consultant.) So, again, it is difficult to disentangle ideological factors affecting patient's choice of treatment from other more practical considerations.

Use of alternative medicine is still a minority choice, but from what I have said here, it will be clear that it is not a marginal issue. If sociologists are to make a positive contribution to the debate about its legitimacy then they should study it both from the point of view of the patient and that of the practitioner. Alternative medicine is best researched and discussed in the context of concepts such as help/health seeking behaviour or 'treatment strategies'. Though some patients do change their cultural expectations about what doctors or healers should do, or about how illness is caused, as a result of their encounters with alternative medicine, most cannot be said to belong to a separate cultural group; where they express unease over the way in which orthodox medicine delivers its services, they are generally voicing anxieties which they share with many who do not use alternative medicine. Users of alternative medicine are making certain kinds of consumer choice, albeit choices which may have radical consequences for the entire household's lifestyle and habits. As with other patients, their choices derive from the interaction between the nature of their illnesses (chronic, difficult for orthodox medicine to treat) and the nature of their lay referral networks (access to information about specific healers, cultural and political resources).

Alternative medicine therefore is 'marginal' medicine (cf. Wallis and Morley, 1976) only in the obvious sense that it is still used by a minority (albeit a substantial one), and in the political sense that it has limited recognition by the state. Its study has raised issues concerning changes in household health care practice, consumer eclecticism and sources of dissatisfaction with orthodox medicine which should be of central concern to the medical professionals and social scientists alike.

References

ANDERSON, R. and BURY, M. (Eds) (1988) *Living with Chronic Illness*, London, Unwin Hyman.

AVINA, R.L. and SCHNEIDERMAN, L.J. (1978) 'Why Patients Use Homeopathy', *Western Journal of Medicine*, 128, pp. 366–9.

BOVEN, R., LUPTON, G., NAJMAN, J., PAYNE, S., SHEEHAN, M. and WESTON, J. (1977) 'Current Patients of Alternative Healthcare — a Three Cities Study', appendix of a *Report of the Committee of Inquiry into Chiropractice, Osteopathy, Homeopathy and Naturopathy*, Australian Parliamentary Paper no. 102.

FULDER, S. (1984) *The Handbook of Complementary Medicine*, Sevonoaks, Coronet Books.

FURNHAM, A. and SMITH, C. (1988), 'Choosing Alternative Medicine. A comparison of the beliefs of patients using a GP and a homeopath', *Social Science and Medicine*, 26, 7, pp. 685–9.

KRONENFELD, J.J. and WASNER, C. (1982) 'The Use of Unorthodox Therapies and Marginal Practitioners', *Social Science and Medicine*, 16, pp. 1119–25.

MCGUIRE, M.B. (1988) (with assistance of Debra Hunter) *Ritual Healing in Suburban America*, New Brunswick and London, Rutgers University Press.

MILLER, J. (1989) 'Neither fish, fowl nor red herring', *The Independent*, 7 January.

MOORE, J., PHIPPS, K. and MARCER, D. (1985) 'Why do people seek treatment by alternative medicine?', *British Medical Journal*, 290, 5 January, pp. 28–9.

OOIJENDIJK, W.T.M., MACKENBACH, J.P. and LIMBERGER, H.H.B. (1981) *What is Better? An investigation into the use of, and satisfaction with, complementary and official medicine in the Netherlands*, London, Threshold Foundation.

PARKER, G. and TUPLING, H. (1976) 'The Chiropractic Patient: Psychosocial Aspects', *Medical Journal of Australia*, 4, September, pp. 373–9.

RILEY, J.N. (1980) 'Client choices among osteopaths and ordinary physicians in Michigan community', *Social Science and Medicine*, 14B, 2, pp. 111–20.

WALLIS, R. and MORLEY, P. (Eds) (1976) *Marginal Medicine*, London, Peter Owen.

[23]

Caribbean Home Remedies and their Importance for Black Women's Health Care in Britain

Nicki Thorogood

Introduction

This paper looks at the use of bush and other home remedies amongst Afro-Caribbean women in Britain. This seems currently to have received little sociological attention. Rather, there have been analyses of lay beliefs and folk remedies amongst white Britons (Helman, 1984; Blaxter *et al.*,1982; Dunnell and Cartwright, 1972) and of 'cultural' differences in the experience of mental illness (Littlewood and Lipsedge, 1982), or 'guides' for health workers, written with varying degrees of awareness, about differences in the experience of health and health care amongst Britain's ethnic minorities (Mares *et al.*, 1985; Henley, 1979; Fuller and Toon, 1988). There have also been studies of Caribbean folk systems *within* the Caribbean (Kitzinger, 1982; Littlewood, 1988) but seemingly little about whether or how these practices are maintained amongst Afro-Caribbeans in Britain (Morgan, 1988).

The findings in this paper are based on in-depth interviews with thirty-two Afro-Caribbean women living in Hackney. The sample was drawn equally from two age groups (16–30 years and 40–60 years) and two locations (a local Health Centre and by 'word of mouth' in the local community). The research methodology aimed to make visible aspects of the subject's lives as they saw them. In this manner it was hoped to distance this research from assumptions made by other work based on notions of ethnicity and culture. This neglects any consideration of racism — that is, the structural manifestation of power inequalities — and reduces everything to the shortcomings of individuals and their cultures (Pearson, 1986).

The research on which this paper is based (Thorogood, 1988) suggests that this is an area worth considering. For although most of the interviewees felt that 'bush' was very much a thing of their past, certain attitudes and practices remained nevertheless. Further, it is a fascinating and comprehensive system which by its very existence in their past necessarily informs this group's experience of and response to the present. Indeed, I would suggest it plays a considerable part in helping to understand the actions of these people in relation to the medical establishment, whether state or private. This paper aims to conceptualize 'bush' not as an exotic or totally independent system but like other lay systems, as part of a multi-faceted strategy for managing health. It is suggested that the use of 'bush' is rooted in historical experience but can also illustrate contemporary relationships in health care.

Caribbean 'Folk Medicine': Bush and other Home Remedies

Perhaps the best way of understanding how the remedies were (and are) used, and what they are used for is to 'catalogue' those mentioned by the women (Table 10.1). There were three main groups: (a) bush (herbs), (b) proprietary remedies bought from a chemist or shop and (c) home remedies — concoctions made at home that were neither bush nor bought. Several remedies were used for more than one 'complaint', and most 'complaints' had more than one remedy (see also Littlewood, 1988). Several were often mentioned by the same woman. Most of these remedies were those they had used in the West Indies although some were still used in Great Britain. Many women remarked on how their children or grandchildren in this country would not drink the bitter herbs. (Indeed, in general, the women used their GP more and their own remedies less in this country (Thorogood, 1988)).

The remedies listed have been grouped according to the 'complaint' they were used for. There is of necessity some overlap and some areas which are less clear. One of the largest groups by far were 'washouts' and they were taken as diversely as daily or once a year. This inventory shows the wide range of remedies in use as well as the categories of illness which were considered suitable for home treatment. This is not to suggest that they did not use doctors and hospitals — they did; but to suggest that there were constraints upon this use and that these constraints were (and are) structured by race, class and gender.

The list of complaints and remedies often covers three generations and spans two places. The list includes all those self-administered remedies mentioned, whether they referred to children, mothers or grandmothers and whether they were used here or 'home'. However, whilst there were some remedies that belonged specifically to the Caribbean or to Britain, there was a great deal of overlap and many differences were a consequence of the differing times and circumstances rather than a change of attitude. To uncover more about these women's attitudes to, and experience of, bush and home remedies both as children and adults, here and in the West Indies, I shall turn to what they said.

Table 10.1 Bush and other home remedies

Washouts
Cerasee (also called Miraculous Bush)
Camomile tea
Benjamin Herb
Bush tea (herb unspecified)
Senna & Sennakot
Castor Oil
Syrup of figs
Exlax
Epsom Salts
Fynnon Salts
Glauber Salts
Shark Oil
Phsyic
Scotts Emulsion
Liquid of Life (proprietary tonic)

Headaches
Turpentine Bark (cooling poultice)
Cudgil or Bat root (tea & a rub)
Ice Poultice
Limeacol
Laite
Bay rum
'Whizz' (a brand of analgesic)
Aspirin
Panadol

Rashes
Meths

Eczema
Calomine lotion

Skin care
Cocoa butter
Shark liver oil (drunk as tonic)
Soft candle (for babies)
Olive oil (rubbed in to prevent stretch marks during pregnancy)

Tonics
Tree & Bush roots (collected, dried, mashed & boiled, then bottled)
Liquid of Life (proprietary tonic)
Cerasee
Wincarnis or Halls 'tonic wine'
Sarsparilla
Stout & condensed milk & nutmeg
Brandy, milk & water
Guinness
Malt
Vitamins – multivits, Vit. C, Seven Seas
Cod Liver oil
Metatone (proprietary brand)
Complan (proprietary brand)
Nutriment (proprietary brand)
Nu-nu Balsam (spelling uncertain)

Stomach aches
Cerasee
Camomile
Peppermint
Angostura Bitters
Cod Liver oil
Andrews Liver Salts
Blue Bush root (to prevent billiousness from Mangoes)
Boiled orange peel tea

Asthma & bad chests
Ganja (as tea)
Warm Vaseline & Menthol rub
Camphor
'Steam trap' from chemist
Vick
Mucron

Faintness
Limeacol
Smelling salts

Toothache
Vinegar in salt water
Brandy
Teething powder (babies)

Mumps
Warm ash on flannel & tied round cheek

Continued overleaf

Table 10.1 Continued

Scarf tied round cheek
Corn meal poultice
Tobacco leaf poultice

Colds (with no temperature)
Cerasee
Peppermint
Red Bark
Leaf of life
English Plantain
Aniseed
Indian root pills
Honey, lemon & sugar
Lime juice
Coconut oil & garlic (for chest colds)
Ganja (for chest colds)
Salt water gargle (sore throats)

Worms
Worm medicine
Yeast food

Calming down
Limeacol
Bay rum
Ganja tea
Laite
Vinegar in warm water
Cerasee

Period pains
Cerasee
Ginger tea
Anadin (sent from WI at first)
Bush (unspecified)

Whooping Cough
Bush rat

Chicken-pox
Bush rat soup
Jeyes fluid (diluted in bath)

Nourishment
Soup
Beef, Iron & Bone broth
Greens
Orange juice
Sunshine (Vit.D)

Cuts and Grazes
Antiseptic cream
Iodine

Fevers
Thimble Bush with egg whites & brandy
Thimble bible steam bath of field weeds (made with odd number of herbs, e.g. 3, 5, 7)
Quinine (malaria)
Fevergrass
Limeacol (cooling rub)
Laite (cooling rub) (particular to St Lucia)
Bay rum

Jaundice
'Billiousness powder'

Muscle Pains
Bay rum
Limeacol
Sacron (proprietary 'rub')
Deep Heat
Canadian healing oil
Jamaican healing oil
Caribbean healing oil
Soft candle, nutmeg/rum

Measles
Measle Bush (tea & to bathe skin)
Pimento bush
Fever grass root
Tamarind leaf tea (& bath)
Calomine lotion
Parched corn tea (i.e. dried maize)

Table 10.1 Continued

After birth	Benylin (all from chemist) (UK only)
Corn meal porridge	
Metatone	*For children – UK only*
	Phensic
	Junior Aspirin
Coughs	Beechams powders
Linctuses (all from chemist)	Lemsip
Syrups (all from chemist)	Benylin
Ferral compound (all from chemist) (UK only)	Vicks
	Antiseptic

All of the thirty-two women interviewed were familiar with bush and twenty-nine of the women had used it at some point in their lives. The remaining three consisted of one city-born older woman, who perhaps had not had such easy access to bush, and two British-born younger women both of whom had grandmothers in Britain who regularly still used bush. Bush is exactly what it sounds like. The leaves, stalk and sometimes the root of bush is boiled in water with the resulting liquid used as a 'tea' or to bathe with. In the West Indies the appropriate plants are to be found growing in fields as uncultivated bush or in many people's backyards (either planted or wild) along with other vegetables and fruits, the odd chicken or two and maybe even a pig. Thus the leaves can simply be picked and boiled:

> If you are not right back home, you just go out, take of a leaf, boil it, make a tea and you are all right. (Dorothy)

Along with the easily available bush were the proprietary tonics and washouts and some foods mentioned specifically as being used to maintain and promote health. I have grouped them together because they are used in similar ways. All were at least perceived as traditional (either to the family or the Caribbean), were self-administered and were controlled by the interviewee or her mother. No men were mentioned in relation to the decision-making about or administering of appropriate treatment, although Littlewood (1988) notes: 'Men are believed to know more about bush than women, and they treat themselves when working in the bush.' Similarly, Morgan and Watkins (1988) in their study of hypertension note the use of bush remedies amongst their West Indian (*sic*) respondents with no apparent distinction between genders.

The most frequently mentioned bush was Cerasee. Everyone had heard of this and most women had used it, many regularly. It was clearly 'good' for just about anything and was perceived as both preventative and curative. It was frequently mentioned as good for period pains but it was also attributed cleansing and purifying properties which were related to menstruation (Thorogood, 1988). Thus, Ann said:

> A little goes a very long way and it's very good for the blood as well. They say it purifies the blood.

And Pearl, a younger woman, said:

> A form of washout, that cleanses not only your digestive system but it cleanses your womb and everything. Washes you out when you are having trouble with menstruation. It's quite useful. It's good for everything really.

Nevertheless, she doesn't drink it herself and many of the younger women said it was too bitter. Many of the women, both young and old, said they could not get the children to drink it:

> I just couldn't be bothered. It's easier to go to the shop and buy a bottle of linctus and then again, I don't think the children would have drank it because it's bitter. It's very, very bitter. You have to drink a cupful of it and you can imagine . . . these kids take one spoonful of a nasty tasting medicine and they want to spit it out, so definitely I couldn't get them to take a cupful. (Marie)

However, it was still popular amongst older women and the mothers and grandmothers of the younger group.

It was often suggested that there was a 'proper' (i.e. in accordance with the Western 'scientific' medical model) medicinal or health-giving content of these herbal remedies and that they were in some way the 'raw material' of 'much modern medicine'; that is, tablets and 'medicine' (liquid in bottles) (see also Littlewood, 1988). As one older woman said:

> I think that most of those things, because if you get the medicines from the . . . you go to the chemist and buy something sometimes and if you read the contents you will find that a lot of those things are what we used to have. And these health foods and health shops, a lot of these things that they sell are the same things that we used to have to take. (Dorothy)

The cleansing aspect of Cerasee was repeated in many descriptions of home remedies. It is worth now turning to some of the most frequently mentioned categories and considering in more detail how home remedies are used.

Washouts

'Washouts' constituted the most frequently used (and mentioned) remedies as well as the longest list of both herbs and proprietary brands and most of the women (twenty-six) had, at some point during their lives, used a washout regularly. All of the twenty-six who had used washouts had used them regularly in childhood. However, the regularity with which they were given and taken varied enormously. Three older women remembered the whole family being given a dose on August Bank Holiday; four women's (three older and one younger) families had theirs on the first Sunday of the month; two (one older and one younger) had fortnightly doses and four women (two older and two younger) took a washout daily. Others (four older and one younger woman) said they had been given washouts 'occasionally' (although in two cases this still involved the whole family taking them together), and finally some women (one older and four younger) had been given a washout 'when necessary'.

Many women took more than one sort of washout, the most popular combinations including senna, castor oil, salts and 'physic'. The daily doses tended to be either castor oil, salts or syrup of figs and were often combined with a 'tonic' or vitamin supplement such as 'Seven Seas' or Cod Liver Oil. One of the older women recalled having Shark Oil daily. However, washouts taken less frequently tended to consist of more than one thing — e.g. once a month: doses of salts and senna and herb tea (Evelyn); Caster Oil, Epsom salts and camomile tea (Beryl); Senna and Castor oil (Edna); Caster oil and 'physic' every two weeks (Sandra). For two families the August Bank Holiday ritual consisted of taking three types of washout on three consecutive days.

It seems that for the most part life in Britain has changed these habits. Some of the women (five, all older) continue to use washouts, though apparently not very often. Many women said they had stopped as soon as they grew up and their parents stopped forcing them — although this did not always prevent them from forcing their own children! Those that continued abandoned bush from necessity and resorted instead to the more readily available proprietary brands such as Sennakot and Epsom salts. Some women felt washouts were no longer necessary as they had a healthy diet (see below), and others felt that there was no time in this country. This is because after taking a washout it is wise not to go too far away from home for a day or two (hence the Bank Holiday ritual) and as Yvonne says, this is a hard condition to fulfil in this country:

> Because she is with a childminder I don't like the idea of her having diarrhoea and that. If I didn't work Saturday, I'd have the whole weekend and then I could give it to her Saturday and then Sunday we are at home I don't mind. I just try to leave her and give her fresh orange juice or something like that will keep her loose.

In general, those children of the older group who were born in the West Indies, were the most likely to have been given washouts.

Suffice to say here that during the interviews the West Indian diet was generally praised as being 'fresh', 'natural', 'healthy', etc. It is something of a contradiction to find this emphasis on good diet in Britain to some extent compensating for washouts. I suppose that 'fashions' in health care change and it is generally the younger women who talk about diet in this way. As they have said, purgatives no longer fit in with their routine. Neither are children in this country disciplined to take nasty medicine.

What these comments and descriptions show is, I believe, the commonly held view that keeping your 'insides clear' is important whether through washouts or diets. There may be a number of reasons for this. Firstly, taking purgatives and laxatives is a widespread practice. It may also be historically related in that it is more fashionable in some periods than in others. Nevertheless, it seems there is a qualitative difference in attitude between keeping 'regular' or responding to constipation and 'washing your insides out' (although the outcome might be much the same). Washouts, I suggest, indicate different theories and beliefs about the body and ways of treating it and this is consistent with the views of diet outlined above. Central to this set of beliefs is the conceptualization of the body as containing a central passage running from top to bottom, which has to be kept free from 'blockages'. Kitzinger (1982) discusses this, and the possible origins of this type of belief, in her article:

> Jamaican concepts of sickness are composed of two in some ways disparate body cosmologies, one derived from the mediaeval European 'humours' and the other from West African concepts of blockage by objects which whether by sorcery or other means, have obstructed passages so that body substances can no longer flow . . . This is related to the bodily concept in which there is one passage leading between the mouth and the lower orifices, passing through the uterus and the stomach on the way (1982, pp. 198–9).

As the white women in the study to which this research was linked (Gabe and Lipschitz-Phillips, 1982) were regular users of laxatives it would seem likely that their cultural heritage derived from that of mediaeval 'humours'. It is, I suggest, the combination of this and the West African cosmology which leads to the very particular meaning and use of washouts I found amongst Afro-Caribbean women in Britain. Although the women were well aware of the laxative properties of the washouts, there were other elements to it, purifying, cleansing, body maintenance ideas, something like 'Dyno-rod' for humans:

Arlene: . . . it was more like maintenance, just making sure you had it a certain time every week and that was it. Like you have a wash every day, you have that every week or every month.

NT: A kind of washing you inside?

Arlene: Yes, it's not because anything was wrong with you. No it was a regular thing.

Rather more emphasizing the cleaning out aspect was this comment:

> She would give us a regular washout, basically before we went back to school, because she said we ate too much junk at school. I think just once a year. (Joy)

This makes it almost seem like spring cleaning! Stressing the element of purification and cleansing were these remarks:

> Liquid of Life . . . you can buy it in the chemist, it kind of purifies the body or something, it wash all the rubbish away, cleans out the body. (Norma)

and

> Cerasee — that's a form of washout. That cleanses not only your digestive system but it cleanses your womb and everything. (Pearl)

This last comment shows a very clear conception of the linking of internal organs by a central passage. It also seems to me that there are two strands running through these comments, not only that of cleaning or clearing out in a practical sense, but also of cleansing and purifying in a ritualistic way, symbolizing a fresh start, renewal or re-creation, particularly of the reproductive organs.

Tonics

One further kind of internal treatment frequently mentioned, was that of 'tonics'. Some of these were also washouts (Cerasee, Liquid of Life) and therefore cleansing but most were presented as strengthening, 'body building' and nourishing. Tonics were also presented as being a useful pick-me-up:

> I think she (mother) used to take a tonic. Beef, iron and wine, that was it. They used to take it if they feel a bit run down. (Thomasina)

This mixture, therefore, contains 'strength' and 'nourishment' and there were a number of other references to alcohol as tonic.

Alcohol as tonic is implied in Ivy's description of the drink that goes with the steambath for malaria — egg white, brandy and Thimble bible bush; and Marie drank Guinness whilst breast-feeding for nourishment as well as to 'make the baby a little tranquil'. Littlewood (1988) also suggests that alcohol belongs to the hot/cold system, and notes that stout is used to build women up again after childbirth which is seen as purging (and therefore cooling).

The clearest indication of tonic as nourishment was when it was perceived as a direct substitute for food:

> . . . as I said, I've never really felt that down when I was in the West Indies to say I have to take tonics for sickness, you know, or body building or anything. We just normally have the proper meal from day to day and as I said, everything is fresh you know. In my family we never specially had to have tonic to sort of build us up or anything like that. (Ann)

Ann's denial that they needed tonics in her family (since they had proper meals) is contradicted by the detailed description of making tonics that she had given a minute or two earlier:

> Well, we make our own tonics in the West Indies and we more or less make it from roots of trees, certain types of roots that you can get from the bushes, and you get them, dry them, wash them properly and boil that, and then you store that in bottles for a certain amount of time and we use that for tonic and apart from that we have lots of fruits and things and we sort of blend them together, you know.

This is told in a continuous and collective past as if it is commonplace and customary, not only to her family.

Helman (1981) categorizes tranquillizers according to whether they are perceived as 'tonic', 'fuel' or 'food'. The basis for the distinction is made on (a) the level of control over the drug the user feels they have and (b) whether they perceive the drug effect as acting on themselves or (indirectly) on their relationships. Helman also suggests that: '*all* "chemical comforters" — from coffee, alcohol, tobacco and "vitamins" to more powerful psychotropic drugs — can be fitted into this classification' (1981, p. 521).

The descriptions and explanations of 'tonics' amongst these women do fit Helman's category of 'tonic' (episodic, self-administered, acting on the taker) although they are not necessarily reserved for the treatment of illness. Helman (1986, p. 218) adds that prior to the easy availability of psychotropic drugs the symptoms described by 'tonic' users had frequently been treated by patent 'Nerve Tonics', 'Restoratives' and 'Elixirs of Life'. However, the descriptions of 'tonics' given by the women in my sample do not particularly relate to low spirits, loss of vitality, anxiety or tension. They are, it seems, perceived more as a means of 'restoring balance' to 'the system', of providing nourishment and strength, either as an addition or as a means of 'keeping going' (see also Dunnell and Cartwright, 1972; Blaxter and Paterson, 1982). In this sense they are more akin to 'fuel' or 'food', although Helman associated with these categories a loss of personal control and an effect on social relations. These elements are missing from these women's accounts.

This example highlights cultural differences in the experience and perception of illness and therefore the appropriate ways for dealing with it. Whilst it might be possible to fit all 'chemical comforters' into the categories of 'tonic', 'fuel' and 'food', the meanings of these categories is culturally specific. The use of tonics amongst these Afro-Caribbean women was as a source of nourishment, for restoring balance and (occasionally) to keep going and was largely episodic: therefore crossing all three of Helman's categories (see also a discussion of their use of benzodiazapines in Gabe and Thorogood, 1986a). This way of conceptualizing health and illness perhaps has more in common with the Chinese and West African systems described above.

It is interesting to note, however, that there was not very much mention of hot and cold in relation to remedies and none at all in relation to illness. None were referred to as 'hot' or 'cold' as in Chinese or Moslem systems. Again although I never specifically asked about this, I think that if it had been a central feature of their health beliefs it would have surfaced in the classifications and categories in the same way that those about passages and blockages did.

Discussion

How then do bush and other home remedies act as a resource, and what impact do they have on the health behaviour of these women in other domains, e.g. the private and state health services? They act as a resource because they form a body of knowledge about the way the body works and the sources of risks and dangers to it (symbolic and actual) which has grown out of the historical experiences of these women. The way they experience health and illness and the appropriate ways of dealing with this are an expression of their 'culture', their history and their current experience as black women. In this way 'culture' can be reappropriated and seen as part of a dynamic interactive process. Bush and home remedies are completely under the control of the women in my sample (or their mothers) and as such mediate their relationships with both health and illness (structurally experienced) and the institutional health care systems.

What is it that defines an illness as sometimes suitable for treatment by common sense and sometimes worthy of a doctor's attention? It may be that doctor's medicine is sometimes 'unavailable' with the doctor acting as gatekeeper either because surgery hours are short and inconvenient or because he or she (but mostly he) is unwilling to prescribe anything (Stimson and Webb, 1975). Graham suggests that: 'These meetings typically occur at the point where the resources of informal caring have been exhausted' (1984, p. 165). This implies that the same 'illnesses' or at least the same set of symptoms that were once suitably treated at home shift into the public sphere at the point where 'normal' life cannot be maintained (Blaxter and Paterson, 1982). There are also categories of illness which demand instant medical attention (e.g. broken limbs) and are thus clearly outside the common sense boundaries and yet others which may never require a doctor (e.g. colds) (Cornwell, 1984, p. 130). The content of these categories, as we have seen, is not fixed but varies with the social, cultural and historical contexts. The decision to 'see a doctor' is a complex process involving advice, consultation, help and caring from friends and relatives (Friedson, 1961).

Dingwall (1976) also suggests that the 'interests of others may also be taken into account' when deciding whether even to define oneself as ill. This has obvious significance for women and I would further suggest that it is not only family duties and responsibilities (the interests of others) which either prompt or hinder help seeking but also the kind of *treatment* (social and medical) one is given to expect. Clearly, the ascription of illness and subsequent action are socially constructed. Where, when and how treatment is sought will be based on what is available, acceptable and appropriate to the help seeker. Whatever the possible explanations for making the move to seek help from a doctor these will all be structured by the experience of race, class and gender. I suggest 'appropriate treatment' is constructed not only out of historical and cultural knowledge but also by present day experiences.

West Indian women carry out 'routine maintenance' for themselves and their families using bush and home remedies for washouts, tonics, childhood illnesses, minor 'everyday' (Cornwell's 'normal') illness and somewhat more ambivalently, for antenatal care and childbirth. In general, home remedies treat conditions not worthy of a doctor. As we have seen these may be culturally specific as with the older women in this group, some of whom regarded malaria as an everyday complaint to be dealt with at home. The use of bush and other home remedies may also be seen as an extension of women's work within the home. This knowledge and its application is yet another expression of their 'caring' and again constitutes the 'hidden' material base to what appears as emotional labour — tending the sick, routine preventative measures. This is health and illness in the private sphere, learnt and practised by women within the home. Thus, most aspects of health and illness for which bush and home remedies are used are those aspects which would not be considered appropriate to go to the doctor with anyway. In addition to this, there were tales of home remedies succeeding where doctor's medicines had failed, at least as far as the story-teller was concerned.

This might be seen to provide external evidence of the efficacy of home remedies and of the ability of the 'ordinary' people to know better than doctors (Cornwell, 1984, p. 174), particularly on issues of 'normal' illness. It might also be seen as further proof of the remedy being the 'natural', 'unrefined', 'raw' (Levi-Strauss, 1986) form of 'scientific', 'unnatural' doctor's medicine, or at least a constituent of it, particularly in the case of bush (see Dorothy's comments about Cerasee on p. 145. Still further, there are times when home remedies and doctor's medicine are complementary, the former relieving symptoms and 'building up strength' whilst the latter effects a cure.

This no doubt has parallels both in other classes and other cultures. However, the particularity of these women's relation to home treatment has implications for institutional medicine. Bush and home remedies may be seen as constituting an alternative to 'real medicine' as a way of both treating and thinking about 'illness'. When a decision to consult a doctor is made a number of changes take place: a different status is conferred on the 'illness'; control and responsibility, in theory at least, (see Stimson, 1974) shift from the private (women's) to the public (doctor's) sphere; different behavioural rules apply and are legitimated. Consequently a new set of social relations is constructed and with them a new relation to the ideology.

Finally, it is worth noting that the relationship of these women to medicine as a resource was not limited to the state sector. Their experience of the NHS as both workers and patients, again both a consequence and an expression of their class, race and gender positions, informs their reactions and responses to it. This, combined with their historical experience, leads them to take a very consumer-oriented approach towards health care. Equal and appropriate treatment (both medical and personal) cannot be taken for granted but must be sought out (Thorogood, 1989). This view, combined with their realistic appraisal of the politics of NHS finance, means for many of them that private medicine presents a practical alternative. This generally consisted of a paid-for consultation with a GP used in tandem with the NHS. This relationship to private medicine has been considered in detail elsewhere (Thorogood, 1988); however, it is pertinent to note it here. For, as the foregoing more detailed discussion has shown, bush, along with private medicine and the NHS, constitute a range of alternatives in health care available to this group of women. Their use is not discrete and we cannot simply label these practices (both bush and private medicine) as relics of tradition (or 'culture'). It is, I hope, clear that their use by this group of women is an active part of managing their contemporary lives and best understood when analyzed in terms of the women's structural position.

References

BLAXTER, M. and PATERSON, E. (1982) *Mothers and Daughters: a three-generational study of health attitudes and behaviour*, London, HEB.

CORNWELL, J. (1984) *Hard Earned Lives: Accounts of Health and Illness from East London*, London, Tavistock.

DINGWALL, R. (1976) *Aspects of Illness*, London, Martin Robertson.

DUNNELL, K. and CARTWRIGHT, A. (1972) *Medicine Takers, Prescribers and Hoarders*, London, RKP.

FRIEDSON, E. (1961) *Patient's Views of Medical Practice*, New York, Russell Sage Foundation.

FULLER, J.H.S. and TOON, P. (1988) *Medical Practice in a Multi-cultural Society*, Heinemann, London.

GABE, J. and LIPCHITZ-PHILLIPS, S. (1982) 'Evil necessity? The meaning of benzodiazapine use for women patients from one general practice', *Sociology of Health and Illness*, 4, 2, pp. 201–9.

GABE, J. and THOROGOOD, N. (1986a) 'Prescribed drugs and the management of everyday life: the experiences of black and white working class women', *The Sociological Review*, 34, 4, pp. 737–72.

GRAHAM, H. (1984) *Women, Health and the Family*, Brighton, Wheatsheaf.

HELMAN, C. (1981) 'Tonic, Fuel and Food: social and symbolic aspects of the long term use of psychotropic drugs', *Social Science and Medicine*, 15B, 4, pp. 521–33.

HELMAN, C. (1984) 'Feed a cold starve a fever', in BLACK, N., BOSWELL, D., GRAY, A., MURPHY, S. and POPAY, J. *Health and Disease, A Reader*, Milton Keynes, Open University Press.

HELMAN, C. (1986) 'Long term use of psychotropic drugs', in GABE, J. and WILLIAMS, E.P., *op. cit.*

HENLEY, A. (1979) *Asian Patients – In Hospital and at Home*, King Edward's Hospital Fund for London, Tunbridge Wells, Pitman Medical Publishing Company Limited.

KITZINGER, S. (1982) 'The social context of birth', in MACCORMACK, C.P. (Ed.) (1982) *An Ethnography of Fertility and Birth*, London, Academic Press.

LEVI-STRAUSS, C. (1986) *The Raw and the Cooked. Introduction to a Science of Mythology*, Harmondsworth, Peregrine Books, Penguin.

LITTLEWOOD, R. (1988) 'From vice to madness: the semantics of naturalistic and personalistic understandings in Trinidadian local medicine, *Social Science and Medicine*, 27, 2 pp. 129–48.

LITTLEWOOD, R. and LIPSEDGE, M. (1982) *Aliens and Alienists, Ethnic Minorities and Psychiatry*, Harmondsworth, Penguin.

MORGAN, M. and WATKINS, C.J. (1988) 'Managing Hypertension: Beliefs and Responses to medication among cultural groups', *Sociology of Health and Illness*, 10, 4, pp. 561–78.

PEARSON, M. (1986) 'Racist Notions of Ethnicity and Culture in Health Education', in RODMELL, S. and WATT, A. (Eds) *The Politics of Health Education*, London, Tavistock.

STIMSON, G.V. (1974) 'Obeying doctor's orders: a view from the other side', *Social Science and Medicine*, 8, 2, pp. 97–104.

STIMSON, G. and WEBB, B. (1975) *Going to See the Doctor: The Consultation Process in General Practice*, London, RKP.

THOROGOOD, N. (1988) *Health and the management of daily life amongst women of Afro-Caribbean origin living in Hackney*, University of London, unpublished PhD thesis.

THOROGOOD, N. (1989) 'Afro-Caribbean women's experience of the health service', *New Community*, 15, 3.

Keith Bakx

The 'eclipse' of folk medicine in western society

Abstract Folk medicine is generally treated as a residue from pre-scientific times. This article discusses contemporary folk medical practices and locates them firmly in postmodern economy and society. The central theme is that recent transformations in the economy have been paralleled by changes in cultural practices. This is manifest in the increased general awareness of 'green' issues and the rejection of 'modernism' in all its forms including the industrialised therapies of biomedicine which are seen to exacerbate rather than resolve public health problems. It is argued that popular dissatisfaction with biomedicine has increased and that the cultural gap between biomedical practitioners and their patients has become much more visible in recent times. This has contributed greatly to the secular expansion of folk therapies throughout western society. Finally, the article notes the gaps in current research into alternative medical practices and practitioners.

Introduction

That traditional or folk medical systems coexist with and complement biomedicine throughout the so-called Less Developed Countries (LDCs) is well documented. It is estimated that more than half of the world population continues to rely on the offices of non-biomedical practitioners and healers for the treatment of a wide variety of physical and mental illness (Bangotrat and Giesler 1989: 172). It is clear that the relative importance of folk medicine and biomedicine will vary from nation state to nation state and between cultural groups within states. However, the global significance of folk medicine can be gauged by the WHO policy recommendation that this substantial reserve of 'unorthodox' medical personnel should be tapped so as to bring improved primary care to millions of people (WHO 1975: 2).

Sociology of Health & Illness Vol. 13 No. 1 1991 ISSN 0141–9889

Folk is used generically in this article. It subsumes all of those practices which lie outside the 'normal' sphere of operations of orthodox western medical practice. Such 'non-orthodox' practices have been variously described as: quack (Porter 1988), folk (Black 1883), alternative (Vesikukka-Komppa 1982), complementary (Fulder and Munro 1982), fringe (Inglis 1964), natural (Inglis 1980), non-conventional (Council of Europe 1984), and marginal (Wallis and Morley 1976). I use the term 'folk' here unashamedly because it combines two distinct but essentially connected elements: the first is that of culture; the second is that of choice. As this paper will show, medical practices are intimately related to consumer preference patterns that operate within specific cultural milieux.

The persistence of folk medical practices in LDCs has been attributed to a variety of factors. Two main themes emerge. The first concerns the cultural distance between the biomedical fraternity and the local population (Sharpston 1976: 1). Here the barrier lies at the ideological level, ie, resistance from the local community to intrusions into its traditional practices. It is argued that this can be overcome through 'education' or other forms of cultural breakdown. The barriers of the second theme are infrastructural, ie, lack of transport provision (Workneh and Giel 1975: 431), inadequacy of financial resources (Nchinda 1976: 133), and the clustering of biomedical professionals in urban conglomerations (Osuntokun 1975: 423). Here the folk healer is seen to play an interim role. S/he is keeper of the keys to public health until such time as the vacuum of shortage and insufficient outreach of western medicine to the general population has been overcome. It is important to note that neither of these themes touch upon the positive role of traditional or folk practitioners.

In Western society, it is generally assumed that folk practices have more or less died out. The eclipse of folk medicine is put on a par with the decline of religion and the demise of the community. That is to say, it is seen as being inversely proportional to the index of urbanisation or modernisation, themselves 'self evident' measures of the development of capitalism. However, as Ferrarotti (1989 19ff) correctly points out, the 'death of God' or the 'disappearance of religion' is essentially a problem for the orthodox church when faced with declining attendances. What proponents of the secularisation thesis do not take into account is the changing form of religiosity, ie, the types and modes of transition from 'church religion' to 'religion as experience'. The principal point, here, is that religiosity takes a variety of forms and the decline of one form cannot be taken to represent the decline of the whole.

A similar case can be made against the again well documented 'demise of community'. Here, the problem as perceived by Redfield (1942: 297), amongst others, is increasing anomie amongst the population of the urban ghetto caused by the breakdown of traditional communal ties. Again, what is happening is not the death of community per se, but the transition from one form of communal existence to another with a corresponding transformation of cultural and social practices. The postmodern anthropologist could hardly state that an hispanic-speaking block in the barrios of Los Angeles was less of a community, or had less 'community spirit', than an English village of the seventeenth century. An index of the decline of particular institutional practices and cultural values of a given community, rural or urban, is exactly that and nothing more. It is neither an actual measure nor a proxy measure of the decline of all forms of community or association.

Biomedicine itself came of age on the crest of this urban, supposedly secular, wave. Its power base stems from its claim to successful treatment through adherence to scientific orthodoxy and from this vantage point it spent its formative years systematically undermining the knowledge base of other therapeutic systems. Where it failed in this task, it discredited folk practitioners while incorporating their methods. A classic case in point was that of the Mesmerists whose practices were condemned, but later taken over by biomedicine under its 'modern' guise of Hypnotism. Notwithstanding the frequent acceptance by the medical profession of ideas and methods first elaborated by 'unqualified' persons, which is noted in a parliamentary report at the turn of the century (House of Commons 1910: 54), the official biomedical stance was that folk practices were indulged in by two sets of persons, the poor – who didn't know any better – and the rich – who were eccentric (BMA 1909: vii). What is clear is that, despite such an ideological assault and the varying fortunes of particular non-orthodox therapies, western consumers of primary care have voted with their feet and continued to resist biomedicine's monopoly. Folk medicine, like religiosity and community, has been transformed, but not eradicated by the modernist project.

The following discussion will suggest that LDCs do not have the monopoly in medical pluralism. A variety of practices are alive and well in modern Britain. Furthermore, that far from being in its death throes, folk medicine is currently providing a viable and valuable alternative to biomedicine which is itself undergoing a major crisis. This is partly due to the changes in advanced capitalism which is moving from the Fordist to postfordist phase, ie, from an emphasis on production to an emphasis on consumption in which consumer choice dictates the commodity or service profile. From this perspective it will be argued that the current expansion of folk medical practices in Western society is a direct function of the inability of biomedicine to come to terms with the alienation that it has itself induced among the consumers of its own services. To locate the discussion firmly in its context, a brief discussion will first be given concerning changes in contemporary capitalism.

Capitalism after Ford

It is clearly not possible here to provide a detailed analysis of postmodernism, postfordism or poststructuralism as the new epoch has variously come to be known. This has yet to be written. At the risk of over generalisation, recent works have tended to engage themselves in one of two particular aspects of this phenomenon: (a) taxonomies of changes in the economic structure and (b) how these have manifested themselves in new political and cultural forms. The continued engagement with the base-superstructure dichotomy is marked notwithstanding Cutler *et al*'s (1976) devastating critique of this metaphor.

With reference to economic transformations, the new era is frequently characterised in terms of its negation of the former modernist epoch. The latter is identified as being Fordist, ie, mass production, mass consumption, high and growing expenditure on consumer products, producer dominant, little differentiation between commodities reflected in little choice, and with few producers dominating the market (Urry 1989). Postfordism, on the other hand, is characterised by consumer-driven demand based on new forms of credit which creates greater differentiation in purchasing patterns, increased choice with rapid changes in trends, ie, more products with a shorter life, which does not lend itself to mass production. Here, production is undertaken by greater numbers of smaller manufacturing and service companies which can react quickly to such a volatile market (Hall 1989).

Examples taken from the literature include: tourism – from the package holidays of the 1970s and early 80s to individually designed safari-type holidays in the late 80s (Urry 1988); food production – from mass hamburger chains to small specialist restaurants and from mass produced farm products to locally produced 'green' products (Murray 1988); clothing – from mass produced off-the-peg garments to designer wear (Murray 1989). It is obvious that these changes will have a differential effect. Different sections of the public will not have the same access: for example, the growing tide of the unemployed created by the collapse of Fordism itself will be disadvantaged. Pahl's work in Britain points to a polarisation between those households where there is no member in employmoment, ie, totally dependent on state benefits, and those where there are two or more earners (Pahl 1984: 277ff). Similarly, recent works in Europe and the U.S.A. argue that contemporary economic and cultural change has led to the development of an 'underclass' which is outside mainstream social and political life (Murray 1984).

Recent transformations to cultural forms and political practices have also been analysed in terms of their 'difference' to what went on before. As Friedman (1988: 448) points out, Modernism can be defined in terms of a continuous process of accumulation of self in the form of wealth, knowledge and or experience. Here, the realisation of self, just as the realisation of capital, requires control, self-control, which in turn requires the repression of all that is spontaneous: sexuality, pleasure, supersition, fetishism, ie, what is regarded in Freudian terms as primitive. Such self-control channels energy from dissipating itself in primitive desires into culture building, ie, civilisation or modernity.

Postmodernity, in contradistinction, is the combination of nature – libido – and a culture unfettered by modernity – 'sagesse'. It represents a return to both without regressing into traditionalism or primitivism. It is intimately concerned with the restructuring of space through the incorporation of two apparently contradictory trends: globalisation and localisation. It marks the end of Eurocentrism and has brought to the fore the idea of the 'human nation', a decentred global network in which western intellectuals and artists have lost their right to speak for humanity (Jameson 1984: 84–7). Local social and ecological phenomena are valued, not as mere empirical variations which mould local social formations into something more distinctive than the global norm, but because their very recognition offers the possibility of combining culture and nature in such a manner. The local population is transformed from an agentless structure into structureless agents.

Just as the West has become intellectually bankrupt and lost its hegemonic position in world terms, so too have national political and cultural forms. In politics, the changes are manifest in the decline of the mass party and the growth of smaller issue-centred political alliances, eg, Feminists, the Greens, Scottish and Welsh National Parties, Animal Rights Groups, Tenants Associations, and so forth. In cultural terms, it has resulted in a breakdown of the distinction between 'high' and mass/popular culture, a mixing of codes in which pastiche, parody, irony, paradox, and inter-textuality have become the buzz-words of the day. It is represented in the shift from Schoenberg to Cage in music, from Eliot to Ashbery in poetry, from Sartre to Marquez in literature. It is crucial to the current debate concerning the city as a place to live or a place to work.

We are not talking here of a sudden shift, a transformation of all aspects of economy and culture. It is clear that we are witnessing a differential reaction to the excesses of the modernist project by individuals and groups who are repossessing the space that they once delegated to the modernisers. It is in this context that the discussion of the crisis of biomedicine and the resurgence of folk practices will be located. It will be argued that, just as the promises of the 'captains of industry', the scientists, the planners, and other architects of the New Jerusalem were never realised, so too the biomedical 'fraternity' has failed to cure the 'modern' illnesses of the western disease profile as dramatically and effectively as it did, say, 'consumption' earlier this century. Furthermore, the modernist project is perceived as having actually contributed to that poor health profile by creating amongst other things, the industrial city, nuclear pollution, irradiated food, and antibiotic resistant bacteria. In short, modernism, biomedicine included, has become politically and culturally out of 'synch' with a growing section of the population.

Managing the biomedical crisis

In 1986, the British Medical Association established a working party to 'consider the feasibility and possible methods of assessing the value of alternative therapies, whether used alone or to complement other treatments and to report on the evidence to the Board of Science and Education' (BMA 1986: 1). Later that year, the working party published a report entitled 'Alternative Therapy'. Prior to discussing the contents of this report and the extensive criticism that it engendered, it would be useful to look at just what the BMA regards as 'alternative'.

It is used, firstly to describe medical *systems* that are based on beliefs about the nature and causation of disease which are at variance with or antagonistic to current orthodox knowledge. Such systems would include Chiropractice and classical Chinese acupuncture. 'Alternative medicine', here, is equivalent to Wallis and Morley's term 'marginal medicine', ie, that which is not 'orthodox'. The latter can be identified by the existence of a group which displays a high level of consensus as to the causes of and suitable treatments for illness and disease and who are also regarded as the 'approved healers' in that society. In this way, the 'orthodox' sets the parameters for what is 'marginal' or 'alternative', a point which will be returned to later (Fairfoot 1987: 384).

The report also gives 'alternative' a second meaning when it uses it to qualify the word *therapy*. Here, the latter is only regarded as 'alternative' if it is worthy of use as a complement to, or a substitute for, orthodox practices. However, its recognition as such may only come about when claims for its use is 'greatly extended' – presumably only by practitioners working within the biomedical establishment (BMA 1986: 35). It is interesting to note that, while the BMA definition focusses on systems and therapies which originate from outside the biomedical paradigm, the report does not acknowledge that these therapies may be actually administered by practitioners outside that paradigm. It concerns itself with alternative therapies as and when performed by its own members – the 'professionals'. Here, 'alternative' equals 'acceptable' which in turn is not equivalent to therapeutic efficacy. In this report, the BMA sidesteps the thorny issue of the folk practitioners themselves by treating them as if they do not exist, as not worthy of mention.

In this way, the report represents a full-frontal attack on both folk practices and folk practitioners. Such broadsides are rare because they risk disturbing the delicate equilibrium in which the establishment is legitimated by both popular myth and covert legitimation practices. When its 'house is in order', ie, under conditions described by Kuhn (1962) as 'normal science', the BMA holds a 'rational man' stance, that it should be obvious that biomedicine offers the 'only alternative' because it carries the imprimatur of Science. So why did the BMA bother to produce this report, if it is only the ignorant or the eccentric who utilise folk, alternative, marginal, or complementary services? The act of mounting a propaganda campaign against folk therapies and those who practice them raises the very spectre that a viable alternative to orthodox practices might exist. Two possibilities present themselves: either the BMA is concerned that such practices are detrimental to the health of patients and wishes to intervene in the patients' interest; and/or it feels that its hegemonic position is being challenged or usurped.

The style and content of the report suggests that it is less concerned with evaluating the efficacy of folk practices than it is with re-enforcing its own legitimacy as the sole 'Keeper of the Public Health'. Notwithstanding the title of the report – Alternative Therapy – by far the largest section consists of a detailed account of the rise of biomedicine and its 'proven' scientific basis. As Fairfoot (1987: 385) correctly points out, this glowing historical exposition makes no reference to the problems associated with contemporary clinical practice. Given that the working part was unlikely to be ignorant of the latter, it is certainly guilty at least of an error of omission.

Furthermore, the report takes pains to characterise alternative therapies as residues from some pre-modern past. In this, it bears a striking resemblance to a report published by the BMA some eighty years earlier which notes the predeliction of certain sections of British society which 'have their fling against medicine (by taking) a curious pleasure in experimenting with mysterious compounds' (BMA 1909: vii). With reference to the public turning its back on the proven achievements of modern science in general and modern medicine in particular, the later authorised version describes the phenomenon as 'turning back to primitive beliefs and out-moded practices' (BMA 1986: 4). Here the BMA glosses over several crucial factors: firstly, that there has always been a plurality of primary care services in industrial Britain; secondly, that folk medicine may offer something that biomedicine cannot or does not; thirdly, that British society is both politically and culturally diverse and that different subsets of the population may wish to be provided with radically different services. These points will be taken up in the sections that follow.

The publication of the 1986 BMA Report demonstrates the unease with which current folk practices are viewed by the medical establishment. It is apparent that the latter is undergoing a phase of what Kuhn (ibid) calls 'science in crisis' in which conflicting paradigms are competing for hegemony. This is happening at a time when the British establishment has seen the de-professionalisation of a number of its functions. For example, house conveyancing is no longer the exclusive preserve of solicitors. The latter also now compete with barristers for work in the higher courts.

Building societies have begun to provide services which were once within the sole domain of banking institutions. Professionals such as opticians are now allowed to advertise their services by displaying price lists in the windows of their establishments. High street shops are also now in the business of selling over-the-counter prescription spectacles so by-passing the services of the optician altogether.

The Thatcher decade has witnessed an entrenchment of the free market philosophy in which competition becomes an end in itself and the weak go to the wall. The extension of this philosophy from business into the professional sector is well under way. It is clear that the BMA has engaged itself in a zero-sum game with folk practitioners. The stakes are high. If it fails, it will lose its political legitimacy and incur severe economic sanctions. In the light of the above, the BMA report becomes less of a reasoned critique of folk therapies than a political manifesto which seeks to discredit folk practitioners and so maintain its power base.

Medical pluralism in LDCs and the West

The notion of pluralism evolved during the colonial period as a means of systematising the heterogeneous groups of which colonial societies were composed following the imposition of artificial 'nation state' boundaries by the colonial powers. In the early colonial phase, pluralism came to signify the articulation of non-competing groups based on ethnicity and/or religion. That is to say, such groups were regarded as discrete social systems which had their own customs, laws, religion, dress, and frequently their own language. Contact between them took place in the economic arena, ie, in the urban market place, where labour skills and surplus produce were exchanged. This somewhat harmonious version of 'cultural pluralism' is essentially functionalist in its approach, analogous to a biological organism in which each part is separate, but crucial to the operation of the whole.

As colonial societies developed their own bureaucratic elites and bourgeoisie, the concept of pluralism was extended to accommodate an element of competition. Here, political pluralism came to identify systems in which groups from the same cultural or ethno-religious background, but with different economic power bases, competed for political control. This has frequently been characterised as a struggle between 'tradition' and 'modernity', the former being regarded as 'backward', the latter as 'progressive'. That such an ideology developed amongst the bureaucrats and bourgeosie of LDCs is not surprising, given the emphasis on 'modernisation' which was seen as essential if LDCs were to survive the post-colonial period.

However, it is important to note that the classes who stood to gain the most from modernisation were the bureaucracy and the bourgeoisie themselves. One of the principal themes of modernisation is the 'professionalisation' of bureaucratic and other service functions. This involves the creation of a training programme and code of conduct for each profession. More importantly, it entails the segregation of those who are from those who are not deemed suitable for entry into the profession, usually on the basis of educational qualifications. Given that the latter are more likely to be achieved by those living in the urban areas, ie, by the children of the bureaucracy and bourgeoisie, we see that professionalisation is essentially a class struggle which seeks to exclude from its ranks those persons allied to the traditional sector. During such struggles, propaganda campaigns are frequently mounted in which 'traditional' is effectively used as a pejorative and it is in this way that skills which have developed over centuries may be lost to the modernisation project.

It was during the modernisation programme that western medicine was imported into many LDCs. However, as noted earlier, it is restricted in the main to urban centres where the 'modern' elites themselves live. The result is a bi-partite system, medical pluralism, in which traditional therapists are tolerated by the biomedical profession only because they operate in a different cultural and physical space. It would be wrong, however, to assume that the current struggle between folk medicine and biomedicine in contemporary Britain is similarly a conflict between a more archaic traditional sector and a modern sector. To do so would be falling prey to biomedical propaganda, exemplified by the BMA report on alternative medicine, which romanticises such practices as being residual categories of some bygone era. Many current folk practices are contemporaneous with much of biomedical practice. They were developed, not in some pre-modern past, but in the same nineteenth century crucible from which sprang 'science' in general and biomedicine in particular. Because they were founded upon a more holistic approach and frequently practiced by 'lay' persons, they became marginalised, a direct result of the power struggle to professionalise and industrialise medical practice. During this process, the population lost much of its right to self-medication. As George Bernard Shaw (1913) comments in his preface to *The Doctor's Dilemma*, professionalisation is a conspiracy against the laity.

It is important to reiterate that such engagements are more concerned with who shall practice, rather than what those practices should be. While the BMA may cloak its arguments with normative statements concerning the scientificity of those practices engaged in by its members, this conceals the real issue of professional power. If this were not the case, the BMA, as custodian of the professional code, would regulate against non-orthodox therapeutic practice by its members. It is crucial to understand that biomedical orthodoxy is established by convention, not by regulation. As Inglis (1964: 9) points out, once a biomedical practitioner becomes qualified, s/he may practice any form of medicine providing that this does not contravene the law of the land and it conforms with 'professional' standards set by his or her peers. Here, we need to make a distinction between folk therapies and folk practitioners. The former may cross the boundaries between the two paradigms, the latter may not. The BMA document clearly demonstrates that the battle-lines are not being drawn in terms of which therapies are suitable for treating which illnesses or diseases, but over who is going to administer those therapies. We have seen that medical pluralism is just as much a feature of industrial as non-industrial societies. The following sections will analyse the relationship between the opposing paradigms in contemporary Britain and discuss their different cultural and political bases.

Cultural pluralism and primary health care in Britain

In taking such an explicitly combative stand, the BMA has sought to mask the fact that folk medicine, in the very act of competing, may serve as a prop for the ailing biomedical fraternity. It could be argued that folk medicine has functioned in such a way as to support biomedicine by offering a service that biomedicine cannot or does not wish to offer. For example, numerous articles note the lack of time that GPs give to patients, others note that many patients require counselling rather than pills (Crawford: 1980). Folk therapies, because they are time extensive, may provide an environment in which psychological support to the patient through counselling is made available outside of the National Health Service. In effect, alternative medicine here allows biomedicine to function at the level that the latter chooses by filling in the gaps left where biomedicine is not equipped to, or is failing to, fulfill its wider role in the community.

While there is a certain veracity in the above, I would argue that the main strength of folk medicine lies in its role as the provider of real alternatives to mainstream primary care. Here, competition with, rather than support for, biomedicine is the prime mover. I would further argue that the basis of the contemporary expansion of folk therapy, in its many guises, is essentially cultural. I use culture here in its broad sense to include politics. As Stauth and Turner (1988: 509) point out, many sociological and anthropological explanations of culture are elitist. They presuppose, not only a distinction between high and low culture, but also a coherent value system that underpins both. This in turn presupposes a relatively coherent social fabric or community – a mass society with a mass culture. Materialist analyses of mass culture, for example, Marcuse (1964), posit a model in which culture becomes a mere reflection of production. Mass production signifies mass consumption which manifests itself in mass culture. In this way, subordinate groups assimilate the dominant values and practices of the ruling class. Conversely, postmodernist writers, such as Friedman (1988) and Jameson (1985) note the change from mass production and mass consumerism to differential consumer driven demand, ie, from the dictatorship of the production line to the dictatorship of consumer choice. The logic of their argument leads us to believe that the fragmentation of the Fordist production system has been accompanied by a corresponding fragmentation of culture. That is to say, mass culture has eroded into 'cultural egalitarianism' (Jameson 1985: 112).

These two positions are essentially economistic and elitist. They each see the economy as the sole agency in the determination of cultural forms. Closely related to this is their notion of class as the principal locus of differential cultural practices. On the one hand, this fails to take into account the tension between various cultural practices. The existence of mass cultural forms does not necessarily entail their incorporation by the population en masse. On the other hand, the use of 'high' and 'low' in qualifying the word culture lends itself to the exclusion of cultural differentiation which is not based on class position. Cultural diversity, for example, on the basis of gender, age, ethnicity and location, becomes reducible to economic position. I would argue that we are not witnessing a fragmentation of mass culture. It is doubtful that such a phenomenon ever existed in the sense used by these authors. The notion that modernisation or westernisation has led to an homogenised culture within nation states is patently false. It was simply perceived as homogenous because Marxist and liberal alike viewed the entire social system from the vantage point of the economy. What we are really witnessing is an intellectual crisis in which structuralist analyses of culture have been proven inadequate. This is not to suggest that cultural forms and political practices are not currently undergoing a critical transformation. However, I would suggest that the prime mover in this process is not the economy, but the realisation on the part of a whole host of different social groups that the modernist project is bankrupt.

Just as the persistence of traditional therapeutic systems in LDCs has been partially attributed to the cultural distance between the consumers and the biomedical fraternity, so too are western consumers of primary care coming to distance themselves culturally even further from orthodox practitioners, perceived as arch-modernity personified. While no recent data are available on Britain, the process seems to have accelerated over the last decade. It is evidenced by the massive extension of self-medication facilities (eg health food shops, over-the-counter herbal remedies, fitness clinics) and the expansion of alternative practices (eg, aromatherapy, osteopathy and reflexology). It is important to note that self-medication and alternative practices are not new, nor are preventive measures such as keeping fit. What is different is the extent to which they are now practiced and their location within the broader cultural political framework of self-determination, ie, reclaiming control over self and environment.

According to authors such as Glassner (1989), the accelerated pursuit of personal fitness is associated with the arrival at middle-age of the post-war baby boomers. These are now in their forties and encountering signs of their own physical decline. The principal illnesses that this group will exhibit are degenerative rather than infectious which may in some measure be thwarted by preventive measures such as excercise and diet. This has been accompanied by a rise in the general awareness of 'green' issues over the last decade or so which have been differentially taken on board by various groups according to their cultural backgrounds and political persuasions. Environmental pollution is now seen as a major factor in personal health. Thus, we have reached a conjuncture at which a large section of the population has come to reject the modernist cult of consumerism, both in personal and environmental terms. The emergent 'green culture' is just as concerned with the awareness of self as it is of awareness of nature. Within this paradigm, the pollution of self by drugs produced by biomedical industry is equated with the degradation of the environment by those same industries. The rejection of one necessitates the rejection of the other.

Paralleling the phenomenon of cultural distance has been the growth in popular dissatisfaction with biomedical practice itself. On the one hand, biomedicine has become hoisted on the petard of its own propaganda. Its previous spectacular successes in curing disease have not been continued. The prevalence of cancer, heart disease and the common cold bear witness to this. On the other hand, biomedical practices themselves may generate iatrogenic illnesses or discomfort patients in some other way. A popular saying suggests that, while you may feel ill on arrival at the surgery, you will have a disease by the time you leave. A prime example of this was the massive overprescription of tranquillisers and antidepressants to females suffering from ordinary miseries which have their roots in the social environment, rather than in the individual (Gabe and Williams 1986). Another classic case is that of the well publicised effects of the drug thalidomide on fetal development (Henning and Nilsson 1972). Public perception of biomedical failure was also heightened with the closing down of mental institutions and their replacement with what is euphemistically called 'community care' (Goodwin 1989). After a century or more of being educated to leave it to the professionals, the public is now being told that this was all a mistake, that biomedicine is fallible. This has had obvious repercussions for public confidence in biomedical intervention in other fields.

The growth in the number of pressure groups both within and outside of the NHS is also indicative of dissatisfaction with current service provision. These are founded upon the premise that consumer/patient rights should be prioritised over and above clinical expediency (eg, AIMS – Association for the Improvement of Maternity Services, ARM – Association of Radical Midwives). Patient alienation through the over prescription of drugs or impersonal treatment and standardised procedures is a direct outcome of biomedicine's narrow range of explanation and treatment. In the push towards modernity, orthodox practitioners have become constrained by their own world view with the result that the patient has become the object, rather than the subject, of primary health care.

Biomedicine's modernist approach is exemplified in its preference for quantity over quality, for production line methods over cottage industry. During the post-war period, making the professional's working day easier appears to the public as having been placed above patients' needs. This has surfaced in a number of guises. Let us take as an example the case of maternity service provision. During the 1960s and 1970s, much publicity was given to the transformation of maternity units into so-called baby production lines where births were induced so as to occur within office hours. Whilst such practices are now out of favour, largely as a result of consumer pressure, the locus of the struggle has merely moved sideways. The modernist approach to maternity care, exemplified by the Peel Report of 1970, has channelled more and more women into hospital beds for childbirth under the guise of providing the best service possible (Prince and Adams 1987: 5ff; Torres and Reich 1989).

As Annandale (1989) and Benoit (1989) point out, the shift from home to institutional childbirth has led in turn to a change from a vocational approach to midwifery training to a more academic approach resulting in the accelerated transformation of the midwife into an obstetric nurse. Apart from escalating nurse-physician conflict (Chernomas and Chernomas 1989), it has also increased conflict between providers and consumers of maternity services as technology has developed to facilitate the 'management' of the increasing numbers of pregnant women confined to hospital. For example, the arrival of ultrasound scanning techniques has caused great concern that patient safety is being sacrificed for efficient patient management (McNay and Fleming 1984; Scottish Home and Health Dept 1988). Furthermore, many partners of women receiving ultrasound scans have been arbitrarily debarred from being present at the time of the scan, a family event which, according to the Royal College of Obstetricians (1984: 10), encourages maternal and paternal bonding (Winkler and Goodwin 1988).

Vast sums of money have been poured into modernising a medical technology that seems to be solely for the consumption of the medical establishment itself, rather than the patient. Biomedical technological expansion has been vertical, rather than horizontal. Instead of making modern technology more readily available across the board, the effort has been to replace it with an even more modern technology in a few limited fields. This cannot be explained in terms of efficiency as the technological explosion has been accompanied by an increase rather than a reduction in patient waiting lists (Rigge 1990). Certainly it cannot be explained in terms of consumer preference as the patient who has already waited two years for an operation does not really care whether it is undertaken using a scalpel or a thermal lance.

In sum, biomedicine is in danger of losing both its actual and ideological hegemony because: firstly, it has culturally distanced itself from the consumers of its services; secondly, it has failed to match its propaganda promises with real breakthroughs in combatting the diseases created by modernism itself; thirdly, patients have become further alienated by negative physical and psychological experiences at the hands of biomedical practitioners themselves. The following section will discuss the implications of the above for primary care provision and suggest an agenda for future research.

Discussion

The current move in Britain toward privatisation of all services has profound implications for primary care provision. Basically, two main trends can be discerned. Firstly, within the orthodox sector, the division between the public and the private seems to be widening. On the one hand, the NHS is being tied up in a financial straightjacket by Thatcherite policies (RSHG 1987) while, on the other, private medicare funded by insurance plans, eg, BUPA, is expanding apace (Mohan and Woods 1985). Just as with the expansion of parent power in education, which may be moving towards a system of educational vouchers to be used in either the state or private sectors, the scenario presents itself of the issuing of medical vouchers which patients can similary exchange for treatment with the practitioner of their choice. Secondly, the folk sector itself is becoming the site of a major battle. The principal protagonists are those therapeutic systems which want to be seen as more orthodox and those who wish to continue to disassociate themselves from mainstream medicine. Here, being seen as a 'complement' to, rather than as an 'alternative' to, biomedicine is the key issue.

Self help and greater individual choice for the consumer of medical services is obviously a challenge, if not a direct threat, to organised medical authority. The logical continuation of privatisation presents the spectre of folk medicine playing an even greater role in primary health care, if patients are allowed to opt for whichever service they prefer. It is clear that the BMA report on alternative therapies is an attempt to preempt any move towards this. Countering this, moves towards professionalisation of alternative practitioners, such as the recent creation of a CNAA degree course in Osteopathy, will help undermine the argument that folk practitioners are poorly trained. The 'paper chase' may play a crucial role in the decade to come, especially at a time when the European Community is seeking to enact legislation which will restrict licenses to practice to those who hold an approved biomedical qualification and restrict the sale of therapeutic goods, eg, vitamins, to registered pharmacists (Council of Europe 1984).

Obviously, the battle lines are only just being drawn. What we have seen are some preliminary skirmishes prior to the main confrontation, the outcome of which can only be a matter of conjecture. There is nothing intrinsic to primary care that will determine the social nature of that care and we must wait and see whether patient power will match the muscle of the biomedical industrial complex. It is not intended here to engage in a normative discussion regarding the preferability of one primary care paradigm over another. This a matter for individual consumer choice. The expansion of the folk sector may offer a means of providing a plurality of services to suit the needs of a culturally and politically diverse population. It is assumed that folk medicine only reaches a fraction of the population, but this is as yet an unknown.

A MEDLINE computerised bibliographic search revealed 244 articles published between 1984 and 1989 inclusively with 'alternative medicine' as the descriptor. A content analysis of these articles demonstrates the current interests of researchers and what material is available to those seeking information on this subject. The MEDLINE search identified: 59 articles (24 per cent) which gave general descriptions of alternative therapies and their therapeutic and philosophical bases; 47 papers (19 per cent) on the use of alternative therapies in relation to specific diseases, the majority of which (N = 30) were specifically concerned with cancer; 30 (12 per cent) articles which evaluated the efficacy of specific therapies in comparison with biomedical alternatives; 26 (11 per cent) non-evaluative papers on the general 'dangers' of such therapies; 26 (11 per cent) papers on the possible use of folk therapies by nursing and midwifery professionals; 21 (9 per cent) on patient attitudes; 16 (7 per cent) analysed the expansion of the folk sector in terms of contextual economic and political trends; 13 (5 per cent) concerned the use of alternative therapies by biomedical practitioners; and 6 (2 per cent) which discussed the legal implications of using alternative therapies.

While the papers noted above analyse a number of important issues, it is impossible to synthesise a general picture from them because they are isolated studies relating to a variety of economic, political and cultural circumstances. It is this lack of generalisable information that forms the greatest barrier to analyses of the feasibility of alternative practices in relation to national health goals and planning. What is required is a thorough analysis of folk practices, practitioners and their clientele from the therapeutic, economic, cultural and political perspectives. As one of the anonymous referees of this paper quite rightly pointed out, urban health consumers in LDCs oscillate between the 'modern' and 'folk' and 'folk' medical sectors for a variety of reasons. If consumer choice was carried to its logical conclusion, ie, that consumers could choose between all types of healer for all types of condition, this need not necessarily stop at primary care. Of crucial importance are the implications of postmodern forms of health care organisation if this entails a far greater choice for some at the cost of a lower level of service for others. It is ironic that the production-line methods, so essential to the development of biomedicine, were at once both dehumanising and progressive as both rich and poor were lumped together as mere receptacles of disease. If postmodernism fulfils its promise of more humanised medical care systems, will this necessarily entail a return to non-democratic forms of medical practice?

Two final points need to be made. Firstly, the choice of the word 'eclipse', rather than 'demise' or 'disappearance', in the title of this article was deliberate. Eclipses are cyclical and temporary phenomena. Culture is never static, what is unorthodox today may become the orthodoxy of tomorrow. Secondly, if orthodox and folk therapists continue to engage in a battle to capture the hearts, minds and wallets of the consumer, the propaganda war is likely to escalate. Recent innovations in information technology will clearly facilitate this. However, according to Samuel Johnson, a quack is one who proclaims his own medical ability in public places. This poses the question of whether they are all quacks now.

MRC Medical Sociology Unit
6 Lilybank Gardens
Glasgow G12 8QQ

Acknowledgements

My thanks to Sally Macintyre, Charlie Davison and Kate Thomas for their constructive comments on an earlier draft.

References

Alver, Bente (1982) Folk medicine as an open medical system, in Vaskilampi & MacCormack (eds.) *Folk Medicine and Health Culture: Role of Folk Medicine in Modern Health*. Kuopio: Department of Community Health.

Annandale, Ellen (1989) Proletarianisation or restratification of the medical profession? The case of obstetrics, *International Journal of Health Services*, 19, 611–34.

Bangotrat, T. and Gielser, W.M. (1989) Traditional medicine in Bangkok, Thailand, *Geographical Review*, 79, 172–82.

Benoit, Cecilia (1989) The professional socialisation of midwives: balancing art and science, *Sociology of Health and Illness*, 11, 160–80.

Black, William George (1883) *Folk Medicine: A Chapter in the History of Culture.* London: Folklore Society.

British Holistic Medical Association (1986) *Report on the BMA Board of Science Working Party on Alternative Therapy*. London: BHMA.

British Medical Association (1909) *Secret Remedies*. London: BMA.

British Medical Association (1986) *Alternative Therapy*. London: BMA.

Chernomas, R. and Chernomas, W. (1989) Escalation of the nurse-physician conflict: registerd care technologists and the economic crisis, *International Journal of Health Services*, 19, 635–50.

Cooter, R. (ed) (1988) *Studies in the History of Alternative Medicine*. London: MacMillan.

Cooter, R. (1988a) Alternative medicine, alternative cosmology. In Cooter, R. (ed) *Studies in the History of Alternative Medicine*. London: MacMillan.

Coulter, H.L. (1975) *Divided Legacy – A History of the Schism in Medical Thought – Volume 1*. Washington: Wehawken.

Coulter, H.L. (1977) *Divided Legacy – A History of the Schism in Medical Thought – Volume 2*. Washington: Wehawken.

Council of Europe (1984) *Legislation and Administrative Regulations on the Use by Licensed Health Service Personnel of Non-Conventional Methods of Diagnosis and Treatment of Illness*. Strasbourg: Council of Europe.

Crawford, R. (1980) Healthism and the medicalisation of everyday life. *International Journal of Health Services*, 10, 365–88.

Cutler, A., Hindess, B., Hirst, P. and A. Hussain (1976) *Marx's Capital and Capitalism Today*. London: Routledge.

Fairfoot, P. (1987) Alternative therapies: The BMA knows best, *Journal of Social Policy*, 16, 383–90.

Ferrarotti, F. (1989) *The Present State of Sociology in Italy*, London: Sage.

Foster, H. (ed) (1985) *Postmodern Culture*. London: Pluto.

Frankel, S. and G. Lewis (eds) (1988) *A Continuing Trial of Treatment*. Amsterdam: Kluwer.

Friedman, J. (1988) Cultural logics of the global system: A sketch, *Theory, Culture and Society*, 5, 447–60.

Fulder, S. (1984) *The Handbook of Complementary Medicine*. London: Coronet.

Fulder, S. and R. Munro (1982) *The Status of Complementary Medicine in the United Kingdom*. London: Threshold Foundation.

Gabe, J. and Williams, P. (eds) (1986) *Tranquillisers: Social, psychological and clinical perspectives*. London: Tavistock.

Glassner, B. (1989) Fitness and the postmodern self. *Journal of Health and Social Behaviour*, 30, 80–91.

Good, C. (1977) Traditional medicine: An agenda for Medical Geography. *Social Science and Medicine*, 11, 705–13.

Goodwin, S. (1989) Community care for the mentally ill in England and Wales: Myths, assumptions, reality. *Journal of Social Policy*, 18, 27–52.

Hall, S. (1989) The meaning of new times, in Hall, S. and M. Jaques (eds) *New Times: The Changing Face of Politics in the 1990s*. London: Lawrence and Wishart.

Hall, S. and Jaques, M. (eds) (1989) *New Times: The Changing Face of Politics in the 1990s*. London: Lawrence and Wishart.

Hemminki, E. and Kojo-Austin, H. (1989) Problems of multidisciplinary research in health care – The case of birth services. *Acta Sociologica*, 32, 253–60.

Henning, S. and Nilsson, R. (1972) *Thalidomide and the Power of the Drug Companies*. Harmondsworth: Penguin.

House of Commons (1910) *Parliamentary Report as to the Practice of Medicine and Surgery by Unqualified Persons in the United Kingdom*. London.

Illich, Ivan (1975) *Medical Nemesis*. London: Calder and Boyars.

Inglis, Brian (1964) *Fringe Medicine*. London: Faber and Faber.

Inglis, Brian (1980) *Natural Medicine*. London: Fontana.

Jameson, F. (1984) Postmodernism, or the cultural logic of Late Capitalism. *New Left Review*, 146, 53–91.

Jameson, F. (1985) Postmodernism and consumer society, in Foster, H. (ed) *Postmodern Culture*. London: Pluto.

Katz, A. and Levin, L. (1980) Self care is not a solipsistic trap. *International Journal of Health Services*, 10, 329–36.

Kuhn, T. (1962) *The Structure of Scientific Revolutions*, Chicago: University of Chicago Press.

Launso, L. (1989) Integrated medicine – A challenge to the health-care system. *Acta Sociologica*, 32, 237–51.

Lewith, G.T. (1985) *Alternative Therapies: A Guide to Complementary Medicine for the Health Professional*. London: Heinemann.

MacCormack, C. (1981) Health care and the concept of legitimacy. *Social Science and Medicine*, 15, 423–8.

MacCormack, C. (1982) Traditional medicine, folk medicine and alternative medicine, in Vaskilampi and MacCormack (eds) *Folk Medicine and Health Culture: Role of Folk Medicine in Modern Health Care*. Kuopio: Department of Community Health.

Marcuse, H. (1964) *One Dimensional Man*. London: Sphere.

May, J.M. (1977) Medical geography: Its methods and objectives. *Social Science and Medicine*, 11, 715–30.

McNay, M. and Fleming, J. (1984) The safety of diagnostic ultrasound. *British Journal of Hospital Medicine*, July, 35–8.

Mohan, J. and Woods, K.J. (1985) Restructuring health care?: The social geography of public and private health care. *International Journal of Health Services*, 15, 197–215.

Murray, C. (1984) *Losing Ground: American Social Policy, 1950–1980*. New York: Basic Books.

Murray, R. (1988) Life after Henry (Ford). *Marxism Today*, October, 8–13.

Murray, R. (1989) Benetton Britain, in Hall, S. and M. Jaques (eds) *New Times: The Changing Face of Politics in the 1990s*. London: Lawrence and Wishart.

Nchinda, T.C. (1976) Traditional and western medicine in Africa: Collaboration or confrontation? *Tropical Doctor*, July.

Osuntokun, B.O. (1975) The traditional basis of neuropsychiatric practice among the Yorubas of Nigeria. *Tropical and Geographical Medicine*, 27, 422–30.

Pahl, R. (1984) *Divisions of Labour*. Oxford: Blackwell.

Porter, R. (1988) Before the fringe: 'Quackery' and the eighteenth century medical market, in Cooter, R. (ed) *Studies in the History of Alternative Medicine*. London: MacMillan.

Press, I. (1978) Urban folk medicine – A functional overview. *American Anthropologist*, 80, 71–84.

Prince, J. and Adams, M.E. (1987) *The Psychology of Childbirth*. London: Churchill Livingstone.

RSHG (1987) *Facing the Figures: What Really is Happening to the National Health Service?* London: Radical Statistics Health Group.

Redfield, R. (1942) The folk society. *American Journal of Sociology*, 52, 293–308.

Rigge, M. (1990) *Guide to Hospital Waiting Lists – 1990*. London: College of Health.

38 Keith Bakx

Royal College of Obstetricians (1984) *Report of the Working Party on Routine Ultrasound in Pregnancy*. London: RCO.

Scottish Home and Health Department (1988) *Obstetric Ultrasound in Scotland*. Edinburgh: HMSO.

Sharpston, M.J. (1976) Health and human environment. *Finance and Development*, 13, 1.

Shaw, George Bernard (1913) *The Doctor's Dilemma: A Tragedy*. London: Constable.

Stacey, M. (1969) The myth of community studies. *British Journal of Sociology*, 20, 134–47.

Stauth, G. and Turner, B.S. (1988) 'Nostalgia, postmodernism and the critique of mass culture. *Theory, Culture and Society*, 5, 509–26.

Stein, M. (1964) *The Eclipse of Community*. New York: Princeton University Press.

Techatraisak, B. and Gessler, W.M. (1989) Traditional medicine in Bangkok, Thailand. *The Geographical review*, 79, 172–82.

Torrers, A. and Reich, M.R. (1989) The shift from home to institutional childbirth: A comparative study of the United Kingdom and the Netherlands. *International Journal of Health Services*, 19, 405–14.

Urry, J. (1988) Cultural change and contemporary holiday-making. *Theory, Culture and Society*, 5, 35–55.

Urry, J. (1989) The end of organised capitalism, in Hall, S. and M. Jacques (eds) *New Times: The Changing Face of Politics in the 1990s*. London: Lawrence and Wishart.

Vaskilampi, T. and MacCormack, C.P. (eds) (1982) *Folk Medicine and Health Culture: Role of Folk Medicine in Modern Health Care*, Proceedings of the Nordic Research Symposium, 27–28 August, 1981: Kuopio, Finland.

Vesikukka-Komppa, A. (1982) Use of alternative medicine in general practice, in Vaskilampi & MacCormack (eds) *Folk Medicine and Health Culture: Role of Folk Medicine in Modern Health Care* Kuopio: Department of Community Health.

Wallis, R. and Morley, P. (eds) (1976) *Marginal Medicine*. New York: The Free Press.

Warren, S.J. (ed) (1984) *Alternative Medicines: Popular and Policy Perspectives*. London: Tavistock.

Winkler, F. and Goodwin, J. (1988) *Access of Companions to Obstetric Ultrasound Departments*. London: Greater London Association of Community Health Councils.

Workneh, F. and Giel, R. (1975) Medical dilemma: A survey of the healing practice of a coptic priest and an Ethiopian sheik. *Tropical and Geographical Medicine*, 27, 431–39.

World Health Organisation (1975) *Health Manpower Development – Training and Utilization of Traditional Healers and their Collaboration with Health Care Delivery Systems*; 57th Session, Provisional Agenda Item 17, EB57/21, Add. 2, 21, November Geneva: WHO.

World Health Organisation (1978) *Promotion and Development of Traditional Medicine*, Technical Report Series, No. 622, Geneva: WHO.

Deborah C. Glik

The redefinition of the situation: the social construction of spiritual healing experiences

Abstract This paper is based on interviews with 160 persons who were participants in spiritual healing groups in Baltimore between 1981 and 1983. Survey data are used to describe how participants in spiritual healing groups presented their health problems, and how and if these problems were resolved or 'healed' over a six-month period. The majority of respondents claimed some degree of healing, associated mainly with symptom alleviation rather than cure. A process of health problem redefinition occurred among some respondents, that provided better 'fit' with outcome descriptions of healing than original problem formulations. Redefined health problems were often less serious, less medical, more chronic, and more 'emergent' than those initially defined, and respondents who redefined problems were significantly more likely to claim a healing experience. 'Psychologisation' of problems suggest that healing experiences can be conceived as socially constructed events.

Introduction

Religious or spiritual healing beliefs and practices flourish today in Western industrialised societies, a contrast to dominant medical care systems (Frank 1973; Wallis and Morley 1976; Bird and Reimer 1982). A growing literature describes healing belief systems, rituals and practices (Csordas 1983; Easthope 1985; Skultans 1976; Griffith, Mahy and Young 1986; Garrison 1974; Pattison, Lapins and Doerr 1973; Ness 1980; Peacock 1984; McGuire 1988) and their role in New Religious Movements (Fichter 1975; Ellwood 1979; Westley 1983).

The promise of healings of bodily, mental and spiritual ills is of central importance to understand the attraction of persons to groups that practice ritual healing. Thus one approach to the study of healing entails following healing group participants over time to delineate their experiences linked to healing. While some systematic sociological work of this type has been done to depict insiders' views of healing, including works by Kleinman (1980); Sneck (1981); Neitz (1988); Poloma (1984, 1987); and McGuire (1988), few of these studies are prospective. Retrospective accounts of healing and healing testimonials abound, particularly in the popular literature (Levin and Coreil 1986). Such testimonials do not fully delineate processes or impacts that healing events, understood as social phenomenon, have on adherents.

Kleinman and Sung (1979) and Kleinman (1980) have documented prospectively the 'clinical reality' or experience of illness and healing from the healing participants' viewpoint. In studying healing prospectively, Kleinman documented how healing helped persons cope with disease, distress, or unfavourable personal circumstances. Participants' reports of illness and healing, defined within the culturally meaningful symbol systems of Taiwanese shamanistic healing, allowed insiders' views of healing processes to be constructed (Kleinman 1980). However, follow-up data was constrained to a few cases among those initially interviewed.

In a similar fashion, Finkler (1981) studied regular participants of Mexican Spiritualist groups. She found that while some symptoms seemed to clear up with ongoing treatments, adherents tended to deny or minimise distress. In fact there was a general tendency to restructure perceptions about afflictions over time. Similar propensities to realign perceptions of self were noted among Catholic charismatic healing groups in the United States (Csordas 1983).

Data presented here prospectively document the self-descriptions of health problems and their linkage to claims of healing events in the lives of persons active in spiritual healing groups. The rhetoric of healing – i.e., the litanies of success – articulated by persons committed to healing beliefs were compared with changes in health or illness experience. This approach diverges from current attempts to account for an underlying causal aetiology for religious healing experiences. For example, healing experiences have been linked to a placebo effect (Hahn and Kleinman 1983), to suggestion (Frank 1973), to altered states of consciousness (Griffith *et al* 1986), to the 'relaxation' response (Benson and Klipper 1976), and to social support for certain lifestyles (Pattison 1980).

While not discounting the above approaches that ask, 'What is the basis for spiritual or religious healing?,' research questions posed here asked rather, 'What is healed?' and 'How is it experienced?' by those having healing experiences. This approach was seen to be viable for describing healing events from an emic or phenomenological perspective, to indirectly gain insights about the more general question of 'What is healing?'.

Spiritual healing in a mid-Atlantic city

A summary of some characteristics of healing groups observed is presented to contextualise study findings. Spiritual healing in Western culture is a symbolic form of healing, its practice found in groups with wide variations in religious ideologies (Westley 1983; Glik 1988; McGuire 1988). In Baltimore where this research was carried out there was an even distribution between charismatic or pentecostal Christian groups with rigid, biblical doctrines (Sneck 1981) and more liberal or 'humanistic' 'New Age' groups with fluid, syncretic doctrines (Ellwood 1979; Levin and Coreil 1986). In general, Christian Charismatic groups attracted working and middle class adherents while New Age groups attracted middle and upper middle class adherents (Glik 1986, 1988).

Spiritual healing activities generally took place in small groups that coalesced around leaders or healers, persons recognised as having special 'gifts' for healing. The small groups in which most healing activities took place, whether a prayer group in a church basement, a special healing service in a church, or a 'therapeutic touch' session above a health food store, were usually made up of regular participants who had gone through a process of finding and committing themselves to a particular healing group. Groups encouraged social identification and socialisation into group norms and behaviour patterns among participants, who were highly religious and generally committed to healing belief systems espoused (Glik 1990).

Healers in these groups represented heroic role models to participants. Having themselves often gone through suffering, pain, distress or illness and having achieved a modicum of purpose and balance, healers were seen to be 'special.' Healers' spiritual gifts were viewed as causes of their prior hardships, seen as tests of faith or obstacles to be overcome on the way to salvation or enlightenment. Within the context of healing groups these charismatic individuals were outwardly committed to the development of others' attainment of self-realisation, success or healing.

Among groups observed, approaches to health and healing stressed individual choice, the power of mind or faith to heal the body or psyche, reliance on ritualised behaviours to achieve health improvements, and explicit and somewhat traditional norms to gauge personal change. In all the healing groups, participants were primed to expect changes to take place and 'healings' were claimed by members frequently (Ness 1980). Healings legitimated both the role of the healer (Easthope 1985) and provided incentives for the seeker to continue his search for healing. Rather than being a rare event, claims of healings occupied a central role in the ethos of most healing groups.

The large majority of persons studied, claimed some degree of healing and attributed it to their participation and belief in spiritual healing. However, many articulated their experiences in terms of outcomes rather than processes. Data that were collected to provide insights into the sensations and impressions of the healing experience itself were sketchy and will not be reported here. Conversely, the relationships between types of problems cited and healing outcomes reported were more complex than originally anticipated. That is, change in overall health status measured quantitatively was not predictive of whether or not a healing was claimed. On the other hand certain types of problems seemed more amenable to healing claims, and analysis of problems healed provided evidence that adjustments were made in the definition of problems to fit healing claims.

Measures, sample and analysis

Multiple methods of data collection that included both participant observation and survey research were carried out over a two year period (1981–1983). For this analysis, survey data consisted of responses to in-depth open-ended questions about health status, self-reported personal sensations of healing, symptoms of illness, health conditions, explanations of healing, attributions regarding personal health and attributions regarding healing. Interpretation of these findings from survey research are supplemented by data gathered by direct observation of healing groups.

In addition, all respondents filled out standardised health status protocols that were administered at three points in time. These were: 1) an Illness Severity Index; 2) an Index of Subjective Physical Health, based on items from the Spectrum of Physical Health, a widely used self-report symptom checklist (Belloc, Breslow and Hochstim 1971); 3) the Brief Symptom Inventory, a self report inventory of symptoms of psychosocial distress (Derogatis and Melisataros 1983); 4) the Index of General Well-Being, a life satisfaction index (Campbell, Converse and Rogers 1976); and 5) Index of Behavioral Well-Being, a set of items describing adherence to sick or well roles. Alpha reliability for these five Health Status indexes was high, allowing for the use of scores based on summed items for later analyses.

For the purposes of this paper, overall quantitative health status summary scores indicative of quality of life should be considered as background material, the results of which have been reported elsewhere (Glik 1986, 1990 forthcoming). This is because there was no clear-cut or consistent pattern of association between changes in health status, measured quantitatively over time and claims of healing. Lack of a relationship provided the impetus to re-analyse qualitative, in-depth findings and content coded responses of health conditions, illnesses and symptoms derived from these quantitative health status checklists. The latter measures became the focus of this analysis as they better illustrate the relationship between healings claimed and problems resolved in this data set.

Participant observation techniques were used to locate and map healing groups in the Baltimore area. Healing groups were included in the study if they met regularly (weekly or bi-monthly) for the purpose of healing rituals. One hundred and sixty individuals from 23 different healing groups of varying persuasions were recruited for in-depth interviewing. All of the study volunteers were regular participants in weekly or monthly healing rituals. On average, these respondents had been involved in healing for two to three years. Some had been involved more than twenty years, and some less than six months. They were interviewed at three points in time over a six month period. Over the course of the study some (< 10) respondents dropped out of groups or changed from one group to another. However none of these respondents shared an apparent lessening of belief in healing despite changed affiliation.

Data from qualitative open-ended questions were content coded for meaning. Data from quantitative health status questions were used as summary scores or were recoded into specific problem descriptions and more general categories of health conditions. The analysis examined the data for sameness or variability in descriptions of healing experiences or changes in health status attributed to healing among those interviewed.

Who and what was healed

Respondents were mainly between the ages of 35 and 65; 40 per cent were unmarried or divorced, and generally they were white and middle or working class. Women outnumbered men two to one, however, few significant differences between men and women were found on any of the health indicators (Glik 1986). The overall health status of respondents was average for their age range with mainly chronic or stress related conditions reported. Less than seven per cent reported serious or terminal illnesses.

Most respondents initially described more than one health problem. Of the 294 health problems initially described, 114 (40 per cent) could be classified as somatic or psychosomatic, with the most common types of complaints being backaches, chronic pain, arthritis, high blood pressure, headaches, cancer, heart trouble, ulcers and thyroid problems. Eighty-two (28 per cent) psychological problems included symptoms of depression, anxiety, fear or anger. Eleven (3.4 per cent) behavioural problems included smoking, drinking, taking drugs; 10 (3.7 per cent) social problems included divorce, problems with children; 14 (6.7 per cent) situational problems included loss of jobs, lack of money, coping with an elderly parent; 19 (6.4 per cent) moral problems included issues of guilt, responsibility, ethical actions; 39 (13.2 per cent) religious problems included loss of faith, lack of meaning and purpose in life.

Respondents were asked at second and third interviews about the overall degree of healing experienced since the first interview that they attributed to spiritual healing. This question asked about healing in general and hence was not problem-specific. Responses were averaged for the two interviews and represent the overall degree of healing claimed over the course of the study. Thirteen (8.1 per cent) of the respondents claimed that they were 'not at all healed;' 10 (6.3 per cent) claimed they were 'very slightly healed;' 22 (13.7 per cent) claimed they were 'slightly healed;' 44 (27.5 per cent) claimed that they were 'partially healed;' 39 (24.4 per cent) claimed that they were 'almost completely healed;' and 32 (20 per cent) claimed that they were 'completely healed.'

Asking respondents to qualify what problems were healed or not healed, enabled construction of Table 1. Here the degree to which healing occurred was based on whether a specific problem was mentioned as healed or not healed rather than overall healing claimed by a person as documented above. In Table 1 more psychological, physical and religious problems were healed than not healed, whereas the odds for behavioural, social, situational and moral problems were not as favourable.

It should be noted that data in Table 1 are based on self-reports of respondents rather than symptom checklists. In more extensive analyses

Table 1 *Types of Problems Healed* at times 2 and 3 of study (n = 160)*

	Number	*Per cent*
Physical problems	42	26 not healed
	84	53 healed
	34	21 not applicable (no physical problems)
Psychological problems	26	16 not healed
	86	54 healed
	48	30 not applicable (no psychological problems)
Behavioural problems	22	14 not healed
	8	5 healed
	130	81 not applicable (no behavioural problems)
Social problems	17	11 not healed
	16	10 healed
	127	79 not applicable (no social problems)
Situational problems	25	15 not healed
	10	6 healed
	125	78 not applicable (no situational problems)
Moral problems	17	11 not healed
	12	8 healed
	131	82 not applicable (no moral problems)
Religious problems	19	12 not healed
	26	16 healed
	115	72 not applicable (no religious problems)

* Healing scores ranged from 0 (not healed) to 5 (completely healed). In this Table 'Being Healed' encompasses slightly to completely healed.

persons who claimed different degrees of healing and changes in their overall or summary scores on symptoms checklists were compared. For these analyses, change scores were calculated based on before and after measures of summary scores of five Quality of Life measures: Illness, Severity, Physical Well-Being, Life Satisfaction, Psychosocial Distress and Behavioural Well-Being. Using Multivariate Analysis of Variance, degree of change in quality of life scores was compared at different levels of healing. A second analysis used Multivariate Analysis of Co-Variance with repeated measures to assess whether changes over time were significantly different for those who claimed or did not claim healings. None of these analyses demonstrated significant associations between changes in health status and degree of healing claimed. In fact, in these analyses there was little change in health status of respondents generally, an indication that the majority of persons interviewed were well, not ill.[1]

When descriptions of what was healed were content coded it became apparent that healing was often described as a process of symptom alleviation, relief from distress, acceptance of some health or life situation, or adoption of another perspective of one's situation. Examples of quotations from respondents describing their healing experiences are as follows:

> A 61 year old female teacher going through a divorce and dealing with depression and arthritis said, 'Faith and belief has made me accepting of problems. I have been able to fill up with God, and He will not let my problems get to me.'

> A 26 year old female occupational counsellor experiencing difficulties at work remarked that, 'my involvement with healing over the last year provided spiritual inspiration which helped me to make needed changes in my personal and professional life.'

> A 34 year old male real estate broker suffering from stress and lower back pain noted, 'I am now relaxed. I have learned to let go and let God be alive in my body, mind and all my affairs. Life has changed dramatically for the good.'

> A 30 year old female occupational therapy student who was having an 'identity crisis' and marital problems said, 'I used to be very nervous and could not handle stress. Now I am able to deal with everything in a calm and peaceful way. It (healing) has helped me in finding this inner strength that helps me in my everyday living.'

> A 72 year old female retired school teacher with vision and digestive problems claimed, 'I don't feel any one healer has "healed" me, but I feel that the teachings have helped me to heal myself, and accept and live with my conditions.'

> A 47 year old housewife who had heart trouble, angina and a daughter with a serious illness remarked, 'I feel that I shared my problems. I felt warmth and love. My problems became lighter. I felt better and believe it was because of my prayers that I have come this far. Some prayers have been clearly answered.'

> A 73 year old housewife with heart trouble, arthritis and colitis said, 'Peace is found, that is helpful emotionally and physically. I'm a traditional person and I think back to simpler times.'

> A 35 year old female nurse had this description, 'The Lord is healing me on a daily basis. The Lord is the Lord of my life and situations happen daily where the Lord heals the situation. The Lord is a personal God that I know is involved with all aspects of my life.'

The redefinition of the situation

Further analyses of these data revealed another set of findings: a pattern of discrepancy was noted between problems initially presented (Time 1) and those for which healing was claimed (Times 2 and 3). That is, content-coded problems initially defined by respondents did not always match definitions of problems later claimed as healed. Eighty-one respondents (slightly more than half of the sample) defined 128 new problems over the course of the study. Of these 'newly defined' or 'redefined' problems 40 (31 per cent) were physical problems, 43 (33 per cent) were psychological, 6 (5 per cent) were behavioural, 14 (11 per cent) were social, 19 (15 per cent) were situational, 1 (1 per cent) was moral and 5 (4 per cent) were religious.

Further in-depth analysis of redefined problems compared them substantively with initially defined problems and considered how these problems fit into the overall life context of the respondent. Four different dimensions of problem redefinition were identified and are delineated in Table 2. As seen in Table 2, redefined problems were most often less serious, chronic, emergent (i.e., newly articulated but not new) and less medical. Due to the fluid nature of respondents' complaints comprising, for the most part, self-reported somatic, psychosomatic, or psychological symptoms and many having multiple problems, these dimensions are relativistic, i.e., based on differences in degree rather than kind. Following are some examples of cases where problems were redefined:

> A 58 year old male, a printer by profession, initially cited high blood pressure as his major problem. He added in subsequent interviews 'migraine headaches brought on by stress' – a health problem that is chronic, less medical (i.e. more psychological), and in the context of this person's health history 'emergent' and less serious as he had symptoms

Table 2 *Ways Problems Were Redefined (n = 81)*

	Number	Per cent
More serious	18	22
Less serious	60	74
Missing	3	4
Chronic	57	70
Acute	22	27
Missing	2	3
Emergent	61	75
New	18	22
Missing	2	3
More medical	22	27
Less medical	57	70
Missing	2	3

for some time, although infrequently. In this case both the original problem and the redefined problem were partially healed.

A 38 year old Catholic priest, first defined his problems as insomnia and nervousness. As the study progressed he redefined his problems as deep depression and anger caused by conflicts he was having with the church. These problems, while neither more nor less medical than initial problems, were in the context of his life more serious (i.e., more debilitating) but also chronic and emergent. In his case the redefined problems were partially healed.

A 40 year old housewife first described her problems as stomach trouble, i.e., a 'nervous bowel,' that she had suffered from for twenty years. Later she claimed that she had been healed of depression and eczema, two problems that were neither more nor less medical, but less serious in her life context, chronic and 'emergent' – i.e., she had had these symptoms intermittently for some time. In this case all the symptoms reported could be classified as psychosomatic.

An 18 year old gas station attendant initially sought healing for his life situation – i.e., low paying dead-end job and lack of education. In the time frame of the study he was healed of planters warts and skin problems, as well as pain associated with a minor car accident. These problem redefinitions reflect a less common pattern as they were less serious but more acute, new and more medical. This young man's major problem – lack of means to get a better education – was not healed.

A 55 year old housewife complained initially of severe lower back problems. Six months later the problem that was healed was her relationship with her son, a problem whose redefinition was less medical, less serious, chronic and emergent in the context of her life.

Redefinition and healing claims

In describing these cases, it should be recalled that almost half of the respondents did not redefine their problems over the course of the study. No differences were found in a comparison of persons who redefined their problems with those who did not on measures of overall health status, types of problems presented, types of problems healed, or sociodemographic background. Nor did the rate of problem redefinition vary by the length of time the respondent was involved in spiritual healing or by whether the respondents had changed healing group affiliation during the course of the study. Recalling that healing claims were to have been attributed specifically to spiritual healing, one possibility explored was that problem redefinition increased the probability that persons would perceive themselves as healed. Operationalised, this asks if persons who redefined their health problems were more likely to experience healing. Tables 3 and 4 show affirmative evidence for this association as persons who redefined their problems had significantly higher levels of reported healing experiences ($P < .001$) than those who did not. These results lend evidence to the idea that problem redefinition increased the degree or intensity of participants' healing claims. In general, problem redefinition was a gradual rather than a sudden process, also a characteristic of 'being healed.'

Table 3 *Analysis of Variance – Degree of healing claimed by redefinition of the problem at times 2 and 3 (n = 153)*

	Number	*Mean*	*sd*	*F-ratio*
Did not redefine	72	2.7	1.4	
Redefined	81	3.3	1.4	7.6**

*N = 153 due to missing data on redefinition variable
** $P < .01$

One finding of note was that patterns of differences between two major types of healing groups in the Baltimore area, Christian and 'New Age', described previously (Glik 1986, 1988), did not seem to have much influence on data analyses reported here. No significant association was found between type of healing group and types of problems defined, the rate at which problems were redefined, or the degree to which healings were claimed. Lack of association between type of healing group and problem definition and redefinition suggests that these processes occur regardless of ideological, organisational and ritual distinctions.

Table 4 *Analysis of Variance – Degree of healing claimed by status of problem defined*

Status of problem	*Number*	*mean*	*sd*	*F-ratio*
No problem healed	18	.39	.67	37.5***
Old problem healed	72	3.10	1.16	
Redefined problem healed	44	3.22	1.25	
Old + redefined problem healed	26	3.94	1.16	

***P = < .001

Discussion

In this study a prospective research design was used to evaluate how persons regularly involved in spiritual healing groups attribute healing to ongoing personal processes. Using a social constructivist approach, the purpose of this study was to document how persons who engage in a specific social behaviour (healing) construct their 'clinical reality' (Kleinman 1980). The linkage examined here is the relationship between health and healing, subjectively interpreted. Two underlying assumptions were that seeking of relief from illness or distress is a major concern among healing group participants, and that healing is appropriate for the management of illness or distress (Kleinman 1980).

Among respondents, somatic, psychomatic or psychological symptoms were reported more frequently than social, behavioural or other types of symptoms or conditions; a finding common to other studies on non-medical healing (Kleinman 1977; Skultans 1976; Fishman 1979; Finkler 1981). Such problems may not be responsive to conventional medical treatment. Alternatively, persons involved in healing groups may somatise their difficulties (Rosen, Kleinman and Katon 1982). Asked both structured and unstructured questions about health status, respondents did not typically articulate their health problems in terms of religious idioms despite their religiousness (Glik 1988).

The large majority of participants interviewed expressed positive responses to questions concerning healing, even though they were constrained through question phrasing to the time frame of the study. While few persons claimed that their healing had been complete, most cited improvements in some health or life situation. Moreover as in the Kleinman and Sung (1979) and Finkler (1981) studies, for some respondents the underlying conditions tended not to change substantially over the course of the healing process described, although symptoms might be relieved or lessened. These data suggest that among healing group adherents the metaphors of healing and reports of healing experiences apply to a broad spectrum of personal change.

Of interest was the finding that there was a marked trend for symptoms and conditions to be redefined over time among some respondents. Shifts in problem definitions followed identifiable patterns: redefined problems tended to be more diffuse in symptomatology, in origin and in chronicity in persons' lives. Thus redefined problems became 'psychologised' (Helman 1985); moreover, among those who redefined their problems, a greater degree of healing was claimed. This suggests that processes of healing articulated are exogenously triggered events that rely on 'rhetorics' of healing that encourage persons to define and redefine problems within idioms that are appropriate to healing (Csordas 1983). The relatively large sample on which these data are based precluded in-depth monitoring of individuals over time that would have revealed conditions that triggered the initiation of the redefinition process, or how persons who redefined problems are distinct from those who did not: these issues demand further research. Moreover, despite the comprehensiveness of the health status questions in which persons typically listed multiple problems, whether problem redefinition is problem reformulation or problem substitution or both cannot be discerned here. Finally, the degree to which other therapeutic systems were acting on these individuals to influence the 'psychologisation' process was not documented, but for most respondents was probably minimal given their commitment to spiritual healing at the time of the interviews.

Despite these study limitations the quality of healing experiences described and dimensions of 'redefinitions of the situation' and their relationship to healing can be used as evidence that healing events, within the context of spiritual healing groups or belief systems, are social productions or socially constructed events. Among this sample of persons who were committed to the religious worldviews espoused by spiritual healing groups, almost all life events – positive, negative or neutral – were seen to be signs of supernatural or divine intervention, even if outcome descriptions were couched in secular terms and even if those individuals had dropped out of the healing group where they had not been recruited to the study. In this closed system of logic, expectations of healing became self-fulfilling prophecies that caused personal events to be interpreted positively (Kleinman and Sung 1979).

Such findings summon to mind William James (1961) observation that limiting the interpretation of events to the good and positive is a bias of religious belief systems. This teleological cast of thinking, where both the mundane and the extraordinary are invested with sacred meaning and everyday actions become identified with deeper purposes, lies at the very heart of healing belief and practice. Redefinitions in this view occur as part of the ongoing process of identifying and labelling life experiences to fit a noetic worldview. Events or realisations that occur at later points in time compete with or supercede previous concerns, and are themselves proof that 'God works in mysterious ways', a popular phrase among participants who typically believe that the seeker of healing should not be too specific about what is to be healed (McGuire 1982).

Such data is evidence that normative systems of thought and action give spiritual healing its persuasive and therapeutic power for participants. These findings lend support to hypotheses that healing must be understood in terms of treatment of lifestyle (Pattison 1974), the realisation of meaning attributed to a symptom (Bourguignon 1976) or the awakening into a religious worldview (Csordas 1983), rather than the treatment of pathology.

It could be argued that these findings are an artifact of the data collection method, where questions asked over time among respondents committed to healing, forced misrepresentation of the facts about healing and shifting definitions of problems presented. That is, healing claims reported could represent fulfilment of the 'demand hypothesis' in response to the survey questions. Counter arguments rest on the explication of three overlapping aspects of spiritual healing that might predispose persons involved to redefine their situation. These aspects are: the nature of the health problems reported; the nature of spiritual healing processes for individuals involved; and most compellingly, the nature of healing groups as 'therapeutic communities.' The following explications of findings are timed to show how data collected represent valid rather than contrived representations of reality among respondents.

In regards to the problems themselves, many are psychosomatic or somatic problems without clear aetiologies. There is evidence that these types of problems lend themselves easily to shifting symptoms and histories, and processes of negotiation and redefinition (Davis 1986; Helman 1985; Gold 1983; Kleinman 1980). Kleinman and Sung (1979) argue that religious therapies invariably succeed due to the autonomy of illnesses that are not necessarily biomedically defined and that are symptomatically more variable.

Another explication of the findings takes account of the nature of spiritual healing processes. Redefinitions may mirror therapeutic processes of self-discovery or individuation similar to that of psychotherapy. In Csordas' (1983) view, restructuring of problems may reflect a gradual process of socialisation into a religious world view that become redefined as 'spiritual growth' or self-actualisation. In this scenario, problems of which one is aware emerge or recede. Such redefinitions reflect endogenous, psychological or physiological events that are triggered by exogenous actions, that redirect the participants' attention to a new view of self and reality, typically sacred reality (Csordas 1983).

It could be argued that healing is not at all therapeutic and that problem redefinitions are evidence that spiritual healing represents processes of denial, repression, clinging to hope and rationalisation. One counter-argument to this contention is that the literature shows that ritual healing does seem to be effective in the resolution of certain kinds of psychosocial and psychosomatic problems, such as problems in living, the somatisation of stress, problems of adjustment to chronic illness and coping with a disability (Bourguignon 1976; Garrison 1974; Galanter 1980; Kleinman 1980; Ness 1980; Finkler 1985; Glik 1986; Griffith *et al* 1986).

In regard to the influence of the groups themselves, health problem redefinition occurs in secular therapeutic interactions and milieux. For example, according to McKeganey and Bloor (1987) redefinition of a patients' actions in light of particular therapeutic goals and objectives is at the heart of the effectiveness of the 'therapeutic community' for patients recovery (McKeganey and Bloor 1987). Davis (1986) shows how problems of patients of psychotherapy are redefined during interactions with a psychotherapist so that they become more suitable for therapy. Helman (1985) describes a situation where patients and therapists negotiate the redefined aetiology of psychosomatic gastrointestinal and respiratory illnesses to make them more psychological, shifting responsibility to the patient for getting well. Finally, the strength of normative systems of social control in regards to positive self-presentation are suggested by work of Gold (1983) who describes 'impression management' among stroke victims who act well in the therapeutic milieu of rehabilitation centres.

The production of healings provide a focal point for healing group activities and healing events, rather than diagnosis or treatment as in medical care, are the means through which healing group activities are validated and social solidarity maintained. Healing group rituals may push adherents to hasten, manipulate or precipitate 'healing experiences' or 'events,' through the invocation of rhetorics of empowerment or transformation (Csordas 1983; McGuire 1983) through the stimulation of eidetic imagery or altered states of consciousness (Griffith *et al* 1986), or through the use of testimonials (Ness 1980). Such activities may help to create the context for redefinitions of problems that fit group expectations for healing to occur. For example, testimonials provide constant reaffirmation and demonstration of the possibility of problem resolution, and are examples of what is appropriately healed and how healing is experienced by group members (Sneck 1981; Ness 1980). Thus personal accounts of healings experienced within healing groups fit prevailing norms about what can be healed and what cannot: making possible healing events but for a more limited genre of problems (Csordas 1983). A major difference between healing and psychotherapy, medicine, or a 'therapeutic community' is that for the latter problem redefinitions are typically orchestrated or dominated by health professionals. In spiritual healing groups participants play a key role in health problem redefinition.

Conclusions

Empirical studies of religious healing are mainly ethnographic and clinical, and therefore somewhat proscribed in regards to the analysis and description of social characteristics of healing groups and their members. Prospective interview data reported here begin to redress that imbalance. An analysis of qualitative and quantitative data show how variations in social perceptions of health impact on reported outcomes of healing, to build a case that healing experiences are socially constructed events.

A recent critique of social constructivism in medical sociology is that it calls into question underlying medical or psychobiological realities (Bury 1986). Others have argued that this analytic approach reveals important social dimensions of the medical care system (Nicholson and McLaughlin 1987). Adoption of the rhetoric of social constructionism to collect, analyse and interpret data on spiritual healing was neither meant to trivialise the reality of healing or healing events for persons involved, nor to invalidate possible physiological, psychological or sacred dimensions of this complex human activity. Rather the purpose of this exposition was to describe the social dimension of healing, often overlooked in research on the phenomenon. The focus of social constructionism in medical sociology has typically been the socially constructed nature of medically defined realities (Wright and Treacher 1982; Bury 1986; Nicholson and McLaughlin 1987). Within the spiritual healing literature, belief systems and certain symptom complexes are defined as social constructions (Comaroff 1982; McGuire 1988; Csordas 1983) but use of this mode of analysis to document outcome experiences and healing events is less common (Kleinman 1980). The importance of this approach to the study of healing is to understand how clients view their illnesses or life situations, and how they interpret their resolution, transformation or continuation. Thus social contexts influence cognitive representations, which in turn may help persons in such groups 'get well.'

School of Public Health
University of South Carolina
Columbia, USA

Notes

1 These analyses are not reported here in their entirety as they involve a series of complex multivariate analyses that would take time and space to document accurately and would divert attention from the focus of this report – the more significant results from open-ended and qualitative question-asking.

References

Beckford, J. (1985) *Cult Controversies*. London: Tavistock.
Belloc, N. B., Breslow L. and Hochstim J. R. (1971) Measurement of physical health in a general population survey, *American Journal of Epidemiology*. 9, 328–36.
Benson, H. and Klipper, M. Z. (1976) *The Relaxation Response*. Avon Publishers.
Bird, F. and Reimer, B. (1982) Participation rates in new religions and para-religious movements, *Journal for the Scientific Study of Religion*. 21, 1–14.
Bourguignon, E. (1976) The effectiveness of religious healing movements: a review of recent literature, *Transcultural Psychiatry Research Review*. 13, 5–21.
Bury, M. R. (1986) Social constructionism and the development of medical sociology, *Sociology of Health and Illness*. 8, 137–69.
Campbell, A., Converse, P. and Rogers, W. L. (1976) *The Quality of American Life*. New York: Russell Sage Foundation.
Comaroff, J. (1982) Medicine: symbol and ideology. In Wright, P. and Treacher, A. (eds) *The Problem of Medical Knowledge*, Edinburgh: Edinburgh University Press.
Csordas, T. (1983) The rhetoric of transformation in ritual healing, *Culture Medicine and Psychiatry*. 7, 333–75.
Davis, K. (1986) The problem of problem reformulation in psychotherapy, *Sociology of Health and Illness*. 8, 44–74.
Derogatis, L. and Melisateros, N. (1983) The brief symptom inventory: an introductory report, *Psychological Medicine*. 13, 595–605.
Easthope, G. (1985) Three Marginal Healers. in Jones, K. (ed.) *Sickness and Sectarianism*, London: Gower.
Ellwood, R. A. (1979) *Alternative Altars: Unconventional and Eastern Spirituality in America*. Chicago: University of Chicago Press.
Fichter, J. (1975) *The Catholic Cult of the Paraclete*. New York: Sheed and Ward, Inc.
Finkler, K. (1980–81) Non-medical treatments and their outcomes, (Parts 1 & 2) *Culture, Medicine, and Psychiatry*. 4, 271–310, 5, 65–103.
Finkler, K. (1985) The social consequences of wellness: a view of healing outcomes from micro and macro perspectives, *International Journal of Health Services*. 16, 627–42.
Fishman, R. G. (1979) Spiritualism in western New York: a study in ritual healing, *Medical Anthropology*, 3, 1–22.
Foltz, T. (1987) The social construction of reality in para-religious healing groups, *Social Compass*, 34, 397–413.
Freund, P. (1982) *The Civilized Body: Social Domination Control and Health*. Philadelphia: Temple University Press.
Frank, J. (1973) *Persuasion and Healing*. Baltimore: The Johns Hopkins University Press.
Galanter, M. (1980) Psychological induction into the large group: findings from a modern religious sect, *American Journal of Psychiatry*. 137, 1475–579.
Galanter, M. (1984) *Competing Equalities: Law & the Backward Classes in India*. California: University of California Press.
Garrison, V. (1974) Sectarianism and psychosocial adjustment: a controlled

comparison of Puerto Rican pentecostals and catholics. In Zaretzky, I. and Leone, M. (eds.) *Religious Movements in Contemporary America*, Princeton: Princeton University Press.

Glik, D. C. (1986) Psychosocial wellness among spiritual healing adherents, *Social Science and Medicine*. 22, 579–86.

Glik, D. C. (1988) Symbolic, ritual and social dynamics of spiritual healing, *Social Science and Medicine*. 27, 1197–206.

Glik, D. C. (1990) Participation in spiritual healing, religiosity, and mental health, *Sociological Inquiry 60*(2), forthcoming.

Gold, S. J. (1983) Getting well: impression management as stroke rehabilitation, *Qualitative Sociology*. 6, 238–54.

Griffith, E. E. H., Mahy, G. E. and Young J. L. (1986) Psychological benefits of spiritualist baptist 'mourning' II, *American Journal of Psychiatry*, 143, 226–9.

Hahn, R. A. and Kleinman, A. (1983) Biomedical practice and anthropological theory, *American Review of Anthropology*. 12, 313–??.

Helman, C. G. (1985) Psyche, soma and society: the social construction of psychosomatic disorders, *Culture, Medicine and Psychiatry*. 9, 1–26.

James, W. (1961) *The Varieties of Religious Experience*. New York: Collier Press.

Kleinman, A. (1977) Depression, somatization, and the new cross-cultural psychiatry, *Social Science and Medicine*, 11, 3–10.

Kleinman, A. (1980) *Patients and Healers in the Context of Culture*. Berkeley, Calif: University of California Press.

Kleinman, A. and Sung, L. H. (1979) Why do Indigenous Practitioners Successfully Heal?, *Social Science and Medicine* 13 (B), 7–26.

Levin, J. S. and Coreil, J. (1986) 'New age' healing in the U.S., *Social Science and Medicine*. 23, 889–97.

McGuire, M. (1982) *Pentecostal Catholics: Power Charisma and Order in a Religious Movement*. Philadelphia: Temple University Press.

McGuire, M. (1988) *Ritual Healing in Suburban America*. New Brunswick: Rutgers University Press.

McKeganey, N. P. and Bloor, M. J. (1987) Teamwork, information control and therapeutic effectiveness: a tale of two therapeutic communities, *Sociology of Health and Illness* 9, 154–78.

Neitz, M. J. (1987) *Charisma & Community: A Study of Religion in American Culture*. Transaction Books.

Ness, R. C. (1980) The impact of indigenous healing activity – an empirical study of two fundamentalist churches, *Social Science and Medicine*. 14 (B), 167–80.

Nicholson, M. and McLaughlin, C. (1987) Social constructionism and medical sociology: a reply to M. R. Bury, *Sociology of Health and Illness*. 9, 107–26.

Pattison, E. M. (1974) Ideological support for the marginal middle class: faith healing and glossolalia. In Zaretsky, I. and Leon, M. (eds) *Religious Movements in Contemporary America*. Princeton: Princeton University Press.

Pattison, E. M. (1980) Religious youth cults: alternative healing social networks, *Journal of Religion and Health*, 19, 275–86.

Pattison, E. M., Lapins, A. L., and Doerr, H. A. (1973) Faith healing: a study of personality and function, *Journal of Nervous and Mental Disease*, 157, 394–409.

Peacock, J. (1984) Symbolic and psychological anthropology: the case of pentecostal faith healing, *Ethos*, 12, 37–53.

Poloma, M. M. (1984) An empirical assessment of perceptions of healing among assemblies of God members, paper presented to the Society for the Scientific Study of Religion.

Poloma, M. M. (1987) The charismatic movement: is there a new pentecost? In *Social Movements Past and Present Series*. G. K. Hall Publishers.

Rosen, G. A., Kleinman, A. and Katon, W. (1982) Somatization in family practice: a biopsychosocial approach, *The Journal of Family Practice*, 14, 493–502.

Skultans, V. Empathy and Healing. In Landon, J. B. (ed.) *Social Anthropology and Medicine*. New York: Academy Press.

Sneck, W. (1981) *Charismatic Spiritual Gifts: A Phenomenological Analysis*. Washington DC: University Press of America.

Wallis, R. and Morley, P. (1976) *Marginal Medicine*. New York: Free Press.

Westley, F. (1983) *The Complex Forms of the Religious Life: A Durkheimian view of the New Religious Movements*. (AAR Academy Series, 45) Chico, California: Scholar's Press.

Wright, P. and Treacher, A. (eds) *The Problem of Medical Knowledge*. Edinburgh: Edinburgh University Press.

Part VIII
Health Professions and Occupations

[26]

Toward a New Sociology of Medical Education

DONALD W. LIGHT

University of Medicine and Dentistry of New Jersey
Rutgers University

Journal of Health and Social Behavior 1988, Vol. 29 (December):307–322

As the American health care system alters its structure to fit the priorities of institutional buyers, medical schools and academic medical centers are likely to undergo profound change. The time is ripe for a new generation of studies on medical education as a social institution, studies that focus more on organization and power than did the classics. This article outlines the changes taking place and then reviews previous contributions by sociologists of medical education in order to suggest several avenues for future research.

Medical education is on the brink of fundamental change. On one hand, the advances in genetics, microbiology, and other life sciences may alter the curriculum radically and reduce still further the ten years it now takes for doctors to find their knowledge out of date (Friedman and Purcell 1985). Medical education also will have to address the ambivalence created between doctor and patient as physicians become increasingly dependent on technological devices and complicated tests (Arney 1982; Arney and Bergen 1984). On the other hand, the rapid expansion of medical techniques and medical education since the 1960s has become so costly that serious efforts are being made to restrain them (Light and Levine 1988; Starr 1982, pp. 379–449). Under these restraints the practice of medicine has become less attractive, medical students' debts have grown, applications to medical schools have dropped sharply, budgets for medical education are being curtailed for the first time in decades, and a large part of the lay culture is moving toward wellness. At issue is the relationship of medical education as a social institution to the health care system and to the training experience of future physicians who will take care of patients (Light 1986a).

The changing locus of medical education in the matrix of economic, cultural, and organizational forces exhibited by the health care system calls for a new sociology of medical education. This essay attempts to identify the societal changes that are shifting the locus of medical education and then reflects on the "old" sociology of medical education in order to outline future directions. Of particular concern is the need for new conceptual frameworks. As Gallagher and Searle write, "Medical sociology needs to increase its stock of analytic concepts and empirical generalizations in this area" (1989, p. 373). Fox (1989) also asserts that the medical educators have much to learn from commissioning new studies. Like Bloom (1988), I see institutional resistance to change as a major societal problem.

Buyers' Revolt and the New Priorities

About 15 years ago corporate and governmental payers perpetrated a basic shift in power and values by asking what they were getting for their health care dollar and by attempting to stem the rising tide of bills (Havighurst 1986; Leylerle 1984; Light 1988a). Until that time they had been willing to pay for the miracles of postwar medicine and to let the medical profession shape the delivery of services. As described elsewhere (Light 1988a), the institutional result of the professional goals of providing the best clinical medicine to every sick patient and of preserving physicians' autonomy was a system emphasizing specialized technical care, hospital services, local autonomy, private institutions, and pass-through insurance to

* Direct all correspondence to Donald W. Light, Department of Psychiatry, UMDNJ-SOM, 401 Haddon Avenue, Camden, NJ 08103.

pay the bills. No other country has manifested as pure a case of a professionally driven medical system.

At the center of that system stood the medical schools and their clinical institutions, fueling the system with new clinical breakthroughs, developing (with corporations) new medical devices, testing new drugs, serving as the focal points for medical research for society, and training the next generation of physicians on the esoteric problems of a highly selected population of patients. Indeed, much of health care policy emanates from this center with its complex of roles in society (Fox 1986). To a greater degree than in other countries, the organization and financing of medical services in the United States have developed around the priorities of academic medical leaders (Fox 1986; Ludmerer 1985).

The rise of institutional buyers (employers, Medicare, Medicaid) threatens to change this situation (Leyerle 1984; Light and Levine 1988; Starr 1982). One might contrast the ideal type of a provider-driven delivery system with that of a buyer-driven system. Instead of a fragmented system that results from the providers' autonomy, a buyer-driven system emphasizes integrated care and accountability. Instead of emphasizing the best (and professionally most interesting) care, regardless of cost, a buyer-driven system emphasizes prevention, self-care, and primary care. Thousands of corporations have established "wellness" programs to reduce risk factors such as smoking, alcohol and drug consumption, hypertension, high cholesterol, stress, and accidents (Glassner 1988). Aside from Medicare, other institutional buyers do not yet seem to comprehend that the proliferation of specialists produced each year by graduate medical programs—so that physicians in the United States include about 80 percent specialists although only about 20 percent of American medical problems need a specialist's attention—is a source of their frustration at holding down medical expenses (Light 1986b). Costs also are driven up by the relentless proliferation of new medical procedures and technology, the hallmark of academic medical centers. In short, the health care system is shifting so that medical schools and their training institutions find themselves no longer the inspiration and source of advance for a professionally driven system but an impediment and a source of frustration for a buyer-driven system (Light 1986a).

Institutional Values of Medical Education

Underlying this problem is a collection of

FIGURE 1. Dimensions of Change in American Health Care

FROM	*TO*
Provider dominance (a system run and shaped by doctors)	Buyer dominance (an effort to dismantle and reshape the laws, customs, and institutions established by organized medicine to allow buyer choice and competition
Sacred trust in doctors	Distrust of doctors' values, decisions, even competence
Quality assured by medical profession as high (but uneven and unattended)	Quality a major focus of systematic review
"Nonprofit" guild monopoly	Competition for profit (even among nonprofit organizations)
Cottage industry structure	Corporate industry structure
Specialization and subspecialization	Primary care and prevention, with minimal referrals to specialists.
Hospital as the "temple of healing"	Home and office as equal centers of care
Fragmentation of services as a byproduct of preserving physicians' autonomy	Coordination of services to minimize error and reduce unnecessary and inappropriate services and costs (slow in coming)
Payment of costs incurred by doctors' decisions	Fixed prepayment, with demand for a detailed account of decisions and of their efficacy
Cross-subsidization of the poor by the more affluent, of low-tech and service departments by hi-tech departments	Cross-subsidization seen as "cost shifting," a suspect maneuver that imposes hidden charges on buyers

incentives and rewards in medical education as a social institution which are quite different from those sought by institutional buyers. Medical schools and their faculty members are rewarded for obtaining large research grants, developing new clinical techniques, having the results published in refereed journals, and, of course, for growth (Lewis and Sheps 1983; Ludmerer 1985). In themselves these are honorable pursuits which occasionally help prevent illness or improve health, but the collective effect of almost every medical school's striving to emulate the great research centers is to flood the countryside with academically trained specialists who carry a new standard of technical and specialized care to the towns in which they settle.[1] Not only do medical expenses spiral, but far more specialists are produced than are needed to treat esoteric problems in the population. This dislocation, in turn, causes specialized skills to atrophy as physicians treat ordinary problems to fill their calendars (Aiken, Lewis, Craig, Mendenhall, Blendon, and Rogers 1979; Menken 1983; Menken and Sheps 1985).

Surrounding this core of incentives to conduct research and to publish is a complex set of roles that medical schools have assumed over the years. They treat patients, especially very sick patients, and often provide a significant amount of charity care. They conduct clinical research and work on new ways to treat difficult problems. They experiment in new ways of organizing and delivering services. They provide a large number of jobs as a major employer. They help train a wide range of health providers, from technicians to nurses to researchers. One leading academician suggests that we stop using the term "medical school" at all: "There's not a single faculty member who is hired to teach medical students. We should call them 'medical centers' where medical students get trained along with everything else." To a significant degree, all of these functions and activities are shaped (Lewis and Sheps 1983 would say "distorted") by the core values outlined above. Thus the present institutional structure, financing, and culture of academic medicine clash with those of institutional buyers.

The transformation of medical schools into research complexes began after World War II, when the AMA vigorously opposed public funds to pay for medical education but allowed support for research and hospital construction (Starr 1982, pp. 335–78). Research faculty and facilities expanded rapidly, as did hospitals. Postwar health insurance, whose payment schedules were shaped largely by panels of hospital-oriented physicians, emphasized hospital care and technological procedures performed largely by specialists. Ironically, the AMA's stand against governmental support for medical education per se fostered a system that undermined the rank-and-file general practitioners and created new centers of political power such as the Association of American Medical Colleges and speciality societies, which eventually weakened the AMA. It also laid the institutional foundations for the perception that there was a national shortage of physicians by constructing tens of thousands of beds and tripling the size of medical school faculties without a concomitant increase in medical students (Light 1986b, pp. 520–22). The resulting expansion weakened physicians' power in the marketplace.

In its major report on medical education issued in 1984, the Association of American Medical Colleges concluded that teaching medical students "often occupies last place in the competition for faculty time and attention" (AAMC 1984, p. 15). Faculty members are under great pressure to bring in research grants or clinical income; tuition accounts for less than six percent of the budget. Faculty salaries come largely from clinical services and grants, not from university funds; most of the faculty members are on soft money. To a much greater degree than at research universities, nobody is being paid to teach, and the institutional expectations for teaching are much weaker (see Bloom, 1988; Fox 1989, pp. 72–141; Gallagher and Searle 1989). Already it is being suggested that the only way to ensure good medical education may be to cordon it off from the research- and service-driven institution by hiring faculty dedicated solely to teaching "undergraduates" (Ebert and Ginzberg 1988).

It is also important to realize that medical schools are not in control of professional education in the same way as law schools or engineering schools because they do not control postgraduate medical education. This fact is illustrated graphically by recent discussions about shortening the seven to eight-year training program for most doctors either by bringing the residency years under control of the medical schools or by yielding up undergraduates a year earlier to residency programs. This reform, like others, may become tied up in the jurisdictional, institutional, and financial complications that have grown up around medical education (Iglehart 1988).

Countervailing Forces and Institutional Momentum

A number of countervailing forces underlie the basic tension between institutional buyers and academic medical centers. Despite concerted efforts to restrain expenditures, for example, institutional buyers appear to have lost the battle. Medical expenses continue to rise much faster than general inflation even after a decade of wide-ranging efforts to rein them in. It would be more accurate to conclude that the first round of partial and modest measures failed to slow medical expenses, for these efforts focused primarily on hospital care and on modest transfers of costs back to patients (Small 1988). Physicians resisted these initial efforts and drove up outpatient costs at an unprecedented rate. One might depict Round One as "squeezing the balloon": various policies closed in on one part, only for other parts to bulge out. Already a second round is shaping up, which focuses on physicians' practice patterns and payments (e.g. Mitchell, Stason, Calore, Freiman, and Hewes 1987).

Academic medicine, on the other hand, has the support of powerful sociocultural forces. Most citizens, including the executives directing the revolt of institutional buyers, want the best medical treatment for themselves and their loved ones when they become ill (Andersen 1987). As long as patients say, "Do everything you can," an elaborated style of medicine will continue; if a doctor does less than everything, he or she may be sued. For similar reasons, employers who limit benefits or choice may incur their employees' anger. In addition, new laws require that employers provide the same benefits to all employees as to themselves. Thus institutional buyers are constrained from cutting back the comprehensive benefits that have evolved over the decades.[2]

Institutional providers are abetted by the same laws, customs, and institutional arrangements that frustrate institutional buyers of health care. One side's rising cost is the other side's growing income (Reinhardt 1987). Thousands of corporations, including many of the Fortune 500, regard health care as a major area for growth. Several states are pouring taxpayers' dollars into attracting health-related corporations; central to their economic strategy is expanding and upgrading their medical schools as the research nucleus for high-tech health corporations.

Research Implications

The implication for medical sociology is that important research has yet to be conducted on the institutional dynamics and the political economy of medical education. Medical schools and teaching programs need to be analyzed as *a population of organizations* that must adapt to an environment undergoing profound change (Aldrich 1987; Hurley and Kaluzny 1987). Macro studies of medical education would open a new field in medical sociology and would complement the social-psychological tradition in research on medical education.

At the same time, sociologists can offer medical educators much that is unique among the disciplines: no other field offers the rigorous analysis and conceptual tools necessary for understanding *institutional* problems. Psychologists perforce psychologize structural problems; economists do not provide the comparative organizational perspective needed in order to be helpful. It is medical educators' loss that they keep company almost exclusively with these "safe" branches of the social sciences. They may fear that sociologists will be too critical, but sociologists are unlikely to be more severe than "insider" physician-critics such as Ludwig Eichna (1980), David Rogers (1975, 1982), Irving Lewis and Cecil Sheps (1983), Robert Petersdorf (1986), or Robert Ebert (with Ginzberg 1988). Their observations suggest research on the organizational level of internal structure and culture.

Eichna, a full professor, seasoned clinician, and chairman of medicine at "Downstate," decided to go through medical school again in his autumn years and found that "medical-school education is distorted from its primary purpose, care of the patient" (1980, p. 728). Although medicine is a science in which knowledge is growing rapidly. Eichna noted that "medical-school education, influenced by societal pressures for the delivery of medical care, is today permeated by an air of anti-science, even anti-intellectualism. . . . Faculty, especially clinical faculty, abet the students' attitude" (p. 728). He observed a peculiar discrepancy, predating the large increase in clinical services, between all the research that faculty members conduct and the rote-like way in which they teach "undergraduates."

The principal skill used in clinical work, writes Eichna, is problem solving, but students experience little of this. "Fact is king . . . Students detest it, yet by habit they gobble the facts" (p. 729). Moreover, "clinical years continue this nonthinking, requiring only a superficial history, a perfunctory physical examination, a scant analysis, a reflexive listing of all differential possibilities, and then the process of writing for multiple tests for each differential diagnosis" (p. 729). Reflecting on his four years as an undergraduate, Eichna the senior professor makes equally harsh comments about slipping academic standards and the almost total absence of ethics. He recommends a number of changes, mostly in attitudes and values, though much of what he experienced involves structural forces that could benefit from sociological analysis.

David Rogers, formerly professor and then dean of the Johns Hopkins School of Medicine and president of the Robert Wood Johnson Foundation at the time of writing (1982), reports on rap sessions that he held with an entire class of 200 medical students at "a fine medical school." After a hesitant start, "a veritable avalanche" of criticism and anger ensued. "There were blistering testimonials about the poor quality of lectures, about the lack of faculty interest in them as individuals, of dreary never-ending series of quizzes, tests, and other bracings, of insufficient time for study, of the absence of personal contact with faculty, of school unresponsiveness to their needs or their complaints" (p. 11). The small group of students that stayed on after the session were even more frustrated and more angry.

Shaken by what he had heard, and contrasting it with his wonderful experience in medical school during World War II, Rogers started to poll students at other medical schools. The results were equally discouraging. Rogers recommends that medical educators cut teaching hours in the first two years by 40 percent and reserve that time for students to do whatever they want. He believes that as young professionals they will use those "precious decompressing, self-discovery hours" to find what excites them about medicine and to develop a healthier professional outlook for their adult years. This step would help, but again, institutional changes will be needed to address the problems that Rogers identifies.

In their distinctive ways, Lewis and Sheps (1983) and Petersdorf (1986) emphasize that advanced clinical training and academic medical centers (AMCs) focus so closely on specialization and research that they ignore the health needs of the public. The AMCs in effect form a national chain that contains 40 percent of the nation's beds, provides 30 percent of the hospital emergency and outpatient services, and consumes almost 45 percent of all hospital expenditures. Three-quarters of these centers were established in, or have moved to, wealthier metropolitan locations. Although they are considered regional centers (Fox 1986), Lewis and Sheps conclude that they have not shown regional leadership in health problems except for state-of-the-art clinical interventions. Their main "contribution" has been to populate surrounding communities with specialists trained on tertiary-care patients and equipment. Perhaps the most provocative thesis (offered by Lewis and Sheps) is that AMCs should be made publicly accountable for what they do so that they are forced to attend to public health needs.

Ebert and Ginzberg (1988) begin by enumerating basic trends that are reshaping medical practice: the concerted effort of buyers to contain costs, the replacement (when possible) of hospital care with ambulatory care, the substitution (when possible) for physicians by nonphysicians, the active participation of patients and their interest in wellness, the mounting evidence that high-tech interventions prolong life beyond reason, the development of group norms and protocols by which to measure clinical performance, the growth of managed care and gatekeeper roles that monitor referrals, and the widening suspicion that doctors are people who sell their expertise to make money. Academic health centers (AHCs: medical schools and all their affiliated clinical facilities) went off the track, the authors explain, when federal programs provided endless funds for research.

Ebert and Ginzberg are as harsh as the authors before them in describing the artificial, inferior educational program that has ensued. Medical schools, now sandwiched between premed training in college and residencies, "no longer have a clear-cut goal for undergraduate medical education" (p. 20). That mission, they believe, is to train good primary-care physicians. To this end they recommend that medical schools take students after three years of college and organize a four-year curriculum around what is now the two clinical years of medical school and the first two years of graduate medical education, with courses interspersed. The obstacles to this reform presented by accrediting bodies, specialty boards, and AHCs would be considerable (Iglehart 1988).

Again, in this major report on medical education, which is part of a special issue of *Health Affairs* that signals the deep need for reform, the recommendations address only one aspect of medical schools' relationship to the new kind of health care system that is now developing. Sociologists can play a major role in diagnosing the institutional issues and identifying what structural changes are needed.

THE PSYCHOLOGICAL FOCUS OF MEDICAL EDUCATION RESEARCH

Conducting critical studies and comparative organizational research would be a new departure for the sociology of medical education. For decades the field has attended largely to the social psychology and the socialization of students. Granted, a number of the classic studies evaluated educational innovations of the 1950s and 1960s, but the investigators embraced the reforms aimed at comprehensive and more interactive care without analyzing their organizational or political underpinnings (Hammond and Kern 1959; Merton, Reader, and Kendall 1957; Reader and Goss 1967). Sociologically these reforms can be regarded as an overlay or as a large symbolic gesture that medical educators make periodically in response to the depersonalization and fragmentation produced by the underlying high technology and subspecialization (Light 1983, pp. 455–60). Even though the investigators documented how the forces of specialization dealt a fatal wound to the experiments in comprehensive care at Cornell and Colorado, they did not pursue the implications.

The other innovation of that time, giving students clinical exposure in the first years of medical school, survived and inspired a number of variations because it did not threaten the specialty-driven structure of training (Horowitz 1964; Light 1983). The only major reform that has endured is family medicine because it became institutionalized and accredited with its own faculty, departments, and curricula. Nevertheless its legitimacy is questioned constantly by the "regular" departments.

A similar concern for teaching physicians the humanistic, psychosocial, and cultural aspects of patient care lies behind the current emphasis on the humanities. "From the 1950s into the 1980s," writes Renée Fox (1989, p. 100), "American medical schools moved from psychiatry to behavioral science to bioethics to the humanities in their perennial search for a curriculum to more effectively develop students' understanding of emotional, cultural, and social dimensions of human behavior in sickness and health, and foster in them the kinds of humane attitudes and values conducive to this understanding." Yet medical educators, despite their intense concern, do not invite or sponsor studies that would evaluate the results. There is no evidence that seeing patients sooner, or discussing literature makes clinicians more sensitive to their patients. On the contrary, the more recent students of doctor-patient interaction (Fisher 1986; Fisher and Todd 1983; Mishler 1985) continue to document the poor listening skills and the various power plays that have been noted for some time. The problems lie in the structure of training and the culture of clinical work.

Like medical educators, sociologists have focused predominantly on the psychosocial aspects. The sociology of medical education has both benefited from and been restricted by a preoccupation with a limited number of concerns: the "fate of idealism," the development of a professional self-image, training for uncertainty, training for detached concern, coping with too much work, and handling mistakes. Although all of these concerns are important, they constitute only one dimension of medical education as a social phenomenon.

The *Student-Physician* (Merton, Reader, and Kendall 1957) and *Boys in White*

(Becker, Geer, Hughes, and Strauss 1961) may have provided rich insights by talented teams of researchers, but in retrospect it seems remarkable that so many of us spent 20 years debating whether medical students were "boys in white" or "student-physicians" (see Bloom 1979; Fox 1989; Levinson 1967). Few people outside the disciplinary enclave could have cared less, and in the end the debate was found to be somewhat moot. Simpson (1979) came to the reasonable conclusion that the Merton group and the Becker group were studying different variables and that both perspectives on medical education had merit. In one of the best reviews of that work, Fox (1989, pp. 77–79) emphasizes the focus on latent and unconscious themes by the Columbia researchers, in contrast with the focus on manifest learning and student interaction by the Chicago team. Moreover, there was an inherent contradiction in the Becker group's calling situational adjustment "socialization" (Light 1980). Finally, "the Merton-Becker debate is based in part on a false dichotomy, because the power of professionals allows them to construct their work environment so that it is consonant with the beliefs they hold. This situation contrasts with that of nurses, who constantly suffer from being socialized as professionals, but then work as subordinates" (Light 1980, p. 326).

Other social psychological concepts have taken 20 years to mature, such as types of mistakes or types of uncertainty (Bosk 1979; Light 1979b), and their future refinement seems limited. In other words, the sociology of medical education has been preoccupied long enough with a small list of relatively sociopsychological issues. It is time to expand from this body of work, however insightful, to institutional and comparative analysis.

Some Exceptions

A few early studies attended to structural variables. Perhaps the earliest and least known is a report by Patricia Kendall (1961) which came out of the second big study by the Merton group. It compares the impact of both hospital size and degree of academic affiliation on the experience of interns and their attendings. From her national survey, Kendall found that attending physicians at unaffiliated hospitals played a more prominent role in patient care and teaching. Paradoxically, while interns called upon them more (especially in smaller hospitals) and more often used them as standards by which to measure their own work, they were more likely to question the quality of training than interns at affiliated hospitals.

In her comparative study of internships at "University Hospital" and at "Community Hospital," Mumford (1970) found that uncertainty was a legitimate norm as part of the academic culture only at University Hospital. At Community Hospital, interns and others were expected to resolve uncertainties and to get on with their work.[3] To my knowledge, no one has followed this contrast with a comparative analysis of uncertainties and ways of coping in different organizational settings, though Light did this for different specialties (1979b). Mumford also found that only at Community Hospital did the staff show an interest in attending to the psychosocial aspects of patients' problems. Likewise, "gomers" or dull patients were much less of an issue at Community Hospital, even though that hospital admitted a much broader range of patients from the community. Physicians there focused more strongly on responding to the complaints of each patient than on "interesting" medical problems.

Mumford's analysis of how hospital structure generates respect for patients is the missing element in the seemingly endless series of reports by medical educators calling for more sensitive clinicians with better social psychological skills. Ironically, Mumford found academic clinicians themselves and the organization of work in University Hospital at the heart of the problem. A generation later, Mizrahi (1986) still finds that this is the case. Does this observation mean that community hospitals are better places than university hospitals for most physicians to acquire clinical skills and attitudes?

To state the matter more broadly, the structure of a training program—the sequence of experiences, the organization of work, the trainers' background and orientation, the hierarchy of values—constitutes a latent curriculum that affects the residents' clinical habits and perspectives as strongly as the manifest curriculum (Light 1979a, 1980). Certain axes are useful for analyzing or comparing training structures.[4]

The degree to which programs are holistic or segmental and role-diffuse or role-specific affects the relationship between the program and the institutions to which it and the trainee are related. Homogeneity-heterogeneity is another important dimension that refers both to the background or orientation of the training staff and to the degree of diversity within the program at each phase of training. Medical school, for example, usually progresses from extreme homogeneity in the first two years to extreme heterogeneity in the senior years of residency.

Related but somewhat different is the number of role models in a program. The term "role models" refers not so much to the number of staff members as to the degree to which they exemplify the profession and are available or visible for emulation. First-year medical students, for example, complain that the program is very homogeneous but offers few role models.

The degree to which programs are serial or disjunctive is critical to analyzing the socialization experience, as is the degree to which programs are fixed or variable. Certain tonal qualities have organizational components and can make a significant difference" coercive or persuasive, intense or relaxed, positive or negative in focus. Beside these dimensions, one must attend to the program's networks and power relationships with the outside world of professional practice.

Another notable early exception to the usual approach was Bloom's insightful study of power in a medical school (1978). In 1962 Bloom set out to help the faculty and administration understand the sources of tension among the students at "Downstate Medical School." To put it simply, he found that the students wanted practical skills to become good doctors, while the faculty were furiously pursuing research and academic work in order to upgrade what had been the Long Island College of Medicine into a first-rank medical school. Bloom recommended talk, self-study, and decision making among all the faculty members in order to develop common goals. The administration suppressed the report; Bloom inadvertently had exposed the latent power of the dean and the executive council by threatening them with recommendations for democratic decision making. Few if any efforts have been made to follow Bloom's example by analyzing how the power structure in medical schools affects the educational process. This topic will be a particularly rich area for research in the years to come; even though medical schools will not want it, they will benefit most from a professional evaluation of how their power structure affects their programs.

The Prevalence of Suffering

When we move to the level of individual students, we find that suffering is the most pervasive attribute in most sociological studies of medical school, internship, and residency. Sociologists are not known for their bleeding hearts; yet one reads page after page about physicians in training who are exhausted, demoralized, assaulted, insulted, and, finally, skilled at "working the system."[5] In the words of a psychiatric resident at Yale, "The physician who enters into a psychiatric residency has little information available to him concerning the personal price he will pay for his training" (Light 1980, p. 241). Yet in comparison to most residencies, psychiatry has an easy schedule, a light patient load, and a collegial atmosphere. Nevertheless, anxiety is high. The sheer pace of work and the quasi-military hierarchy are two- frequently observed attributes of medical training that help make it a bruising experience. From Becker's medical students in the 1950s (1961) to Miller's interns in the 1960s (1970) to Mizrahi's house staff in the 1980s (1986) to current trainees (Asch and Parker 1988; Letters 1988; McCall 1988), physicians in training are overwhelmed by the volume of material and work.

Little analysis has been performed to discover why the schedule is so exhausting; the answers will be different for medical students than for residents in hard-pressed hospitals. Mizrahi concludes that the key lesson is to get rid of patients: dispense with them as quickly as possible or you will drown. Equally important is the deep-seated tradition of hierarchy: senior residents are arrogant toward new residents, new residents toward interns, interns toward fourth-year students, and ultimately physicians toward patients (Geiger 1975). The economic pressures of cost containment on clinical faculty and the scarcity of "clinical material" will intensify the pressures but may weaken the hierarchy.

Many of these structural features contribute to or intensify the feelings of uncertainty that trainees feel (Light 1979a). They also contain built-in ways in which trainees learn to cope with uncertainties in their work. We now turn to the dynamics of this process.

Toward a Theory of Uncertainty and Its Resolution

Uncertainty stems from two conditions: a perceived lack of definition of the situation and the uselessness of past responses or coping skills. Uncertainty, in turn, is one of two conditions that produce anxiety; the other is a sense of involvement and responsibility in the situation (see Light 1980, pp. 246–56). All of these conditions probably can be found in all types of socialization because they open a person for change; yet medical training programs seem particularly likely to throw students into new situations where they have great responsibility but find their tasks bewildering. Uncertainty resides in structural and cultural contexts and can stem from the number of available options, the fear or reality of external shocks, and the equivocality of the situation.

Renée Fox (1957) captured, through students' journals and observation, the role of uncertainty about what one does not know and what is not known in generating anxiety among medical students. In the clinical years a more complex array of uncertainties arises around diagnosis, treatment plans, relationships among the medical staff involved, and the patient's response (Light 1979b). Yet work must be done; patients must be treated; uncertainties must be resolved.

Situations of anxiety foster strong tendencies toward closure, toward the nearest model that will restore order and calm. People tend first to draw on habits and skills that have worked in the past; this is an important point at which trainees' personalities intersect to shape their emerging professional selves. To the extent that the past repertoire of skills is inadequate, one tends to draw on and in complex ways to introject models of successful coping at hand. Relationships with these models can range from occasions of immense growth to experiences that diminish one's humanity and foster cynicism. Rituals also play an important part in handling uncertainties. Indeed, one could say that rituals arise in conditions of uncertainty and gain importance in proportion to the degree of uncertainty. Foremost among rituals in professional work is technique; trainees tend to "resolve" uncertainties by focusing on technique as an end in itself (Light 1979; Reiser 1978). In the coming years, medical educators will need sociologists to look closely at the structure and the process of these moments of modeling.

Denial and Immunity from Criticism

In medical circles there seems to be a pervasive preoccupation with uncertainty caused by powerful advances in pharmacology, genetics, surgery, and biochemistry (Fox 1980). Yet an emphasis on uncertainty can have its price. Most people can bear only so much uncertainty; too much will lead to its opposite, premature closure. Being open to criticism and learning from it throughout one's career is a principal goal of medical training today; yet medical educators have not confronted the evidence from medical sociologists that the opposite happens.

In their comparative study of residency programs, Bucher and Stelling identify several techniques used to discount criticism, such as disparaging the source, dismissing the issue, or considering the issue a matter of style (1979, pp. 171–73). By the end of the second year, they observed, residents would not accept or learn from criticism. In addition to using these three techniques, residents control uncertainty by focusing on technique as an end rather than a means, gaining autonomy from colleagues so that criticism is not possible, relying on one's clinical experience and accumulated "war stories" as primary sources of validity, and developing "schools" of practice that settle the uncertainty of what to do with ideology. These are all social, not medical rituals or productions (Wuthnow 1987, pp. 148–63). If medical educators want to be serious about the lifelong ability to learn from criticism, they will have to think through the issues systematically with sociologists and psychologists. They also must examine the ways in which the American medical profession makes itself immune from scrutiny and accountability, more so than the British (Payer 1988).

One of the most remarkable patterns observed is denial or some form of amnesia about the suffering experienced during internship and residency, as well as its consequences. Although Mizrahi found that the house staff worked under extraordinary pressure and practiced a deplorable kind of medicine focused on "getting rid of patients," the same doctors looked back a few years later and felt that "although the experience was dehumanizing and took serious tolls on their lives, it was necessary and effective" (1986, p. 162). Having survived the experience is often considered a point of pride and is regarded good for building professional character. Mizrahi adds:

> At almost no time did any members of the sample consider the effects of the context of training on the treatment of the indigent patients they treated and neglected or abused as house officers. They *were*, however, concerned about the treatment of their own patients by housestaff (1986, p. 162).

In addition to examining how uncertainty is handled and how negative aspects of training are denied or even defended (McCue 1985), sociologists have studied the ways in which physicians handle mistakes. In his study of surgical mistakes, Bosk (1979, 1986) found that normative errors were the most serious in residency because they meant that the physician had failed to follow the codes of the profession or the norms of the service on which he or she was being trained. After graduation, however, the same sorts of errors were "disattended" or regarded as matters of "style"; professional discretion and tolerance surrounded them. This finding corroborates Millman's (1976) earlier study of surgeons.

Most telling is Freidson's (1975) study of social control in a model medical group set up to allow continuous surveillance of a physician's work by other members of the group. Yet despite these deliberate and liberal intentions, the physicians used rituals of evasion and "the etiquette of nonconfrontation" even when they observed errors or poor practice procedures. If an objectionable act became a public concern, they closed ranks against the outside world to protect themselves and the reputation of their group. The administration was forced by default to take a greater role than either it or the physicians wanted. This "abdication of the collegium from exercising the effective self-government that it insisted was solely its own legitimate function" (Freidson 1975, p. 239) is the principal reason why external review has become a prevalent feature of medical practice. It seems clear that denial and self-immunization from criticism must undergo profound change as printouts profile clinical decisions not only in training but later in practice. Indeed the question to be researched now may be how physicians respond to volumes of external and seemingly arbitrary review.

Omnipotent Tendencies in Professional Training

Premature closure and a famous article entitled "The Quest for Omnipotence in Professional Training" (Sharaf and Levinson 1964) suggest the need to examine how the structure of residency training fosters tendencies towards omnipotence. I found structural parallels between residency training and the psychodynamic conditions leading to narcissism (Light 1980, pp. 259–77, 297–307). This finding implies that the tendencies of narcissistic personalities would be reinforced by residency training, but the effect of the experience on other personalities is not yet clear.

To state the matter more broadly, there is much work to be done in learning how different kinds of organizational settings foster different kinds of psychological states, such as depressive organizations, schizophrenic organizations, compulsive organizations, grandiose organizations, manic-depressive organizations, and even suicidal organizations (Merry and Brown 1987). Both in training and in their careers, physicians may find themselves in organizations whose culture and structure encourage one or more of these tendencies. Through the latent curriculum of training, through a program's organizational personality, and through the resolutions of anxieties evolve a professional's moral career, the course of values about one's responsibilities, one's perspective on patients, one's priorities in work, and ultimately one's sense of wholeness.

Wilbert Moore (1970), in his overview of professional training, was impressed so strongly by this negative quality that he developed a "punishment theory of socialization." Although this and related theories are incomplete (see Light 1980, p. 316), there are degradation ceremonies (Garfinkel 1956) and parallels to studies of conversion. "The price of this pervasive approach to professional training may be an insensitivity to patient needs, an intolerance of uncertainty, a false and unwarranted sense of conviction, and grandiose behavior that betrays the original mandate of the professions to serve the people" (Light 1980, p. 327). The new development to be researched today is how do physicians respond when they cannot compensate for rituals of degradation by constructing an ego-enhancing practice—because the corporate world of practice has inherently degrading routines. Perhaps someone will soon write about tendencies toward *impotence* in training and practice.

CURRENT TRENDS AND FUTURE RESEARCH

When one considers the findings of past research in the context of the fundamental changes taking place in health care, the implications are disturbing. What happens when uncertainty is so prevalent that even the role models exhibit disequilibrium? In learning detached concern, what happens if one learns that no one is willing to pay for the time it takes to be concerned? How will institutionalized systems of accountability affect autonomy and self-identity? How will training be affected by shorter hospital stays and by the lack of control that characterizes ambulatory settings (Gallagher and Searle 1989, p. 994)?

Structural Strains

Some clues are provided by Mizrahi's (1986) identification of structural strains: between cost containment and the emphasis of academic medicine on using every diagnostic test and trying every treatment that might work; between responsibility for a heavy caseload of patients and the desire to focus on "cases" from which physicians can learn; between the extraordinary benefits of powerful new drugs or procedures and their potential for harm. Mizrahi also notes important limitations under which the house staff work: that the hospital receives persons rejected or released from the rest of the private health care system; that primary and rehabilitative services are neglected in the neighborhood because all resources focus on the one large academic medical center; that the hospital lacks enough beds to serve "the enormous volume of sick patients." On the other hand, perhaps these strains and limitations are not so new; Miller (1970) described similar circumstances at Boston City Hospital in the 1960s. One must be careful to distinguish changes in reality from the intensely felt perceptions of the day. Like Miller (but more so), Mizrahi finds hospital care a combat zone. Resident McGee tells her, "You start regarding them [patients] as they enemy and you really don't care." Resident Edwards says, "They get you before you get them . . . They just destroy you and you don't even want to deal with them."

A major difference, however, is the absence of senior faculty members from clinical teaching. Apparently they feel so much pressure to bring in research grants and/or money from treating patients that they have no time to teach. This is one of several trends that leads Renée Fox to conclude in her current overview that conditions are deteriorating (1989). Other trends include pressures to contain costs, the briefer and shallower experiences received by trainees because patients leave the hospital more quickly, the growing prevalence of very old hospitalized patients who are chronically ill and disabled, the systematic though unintentional downgrading of patient-oriented clinical training, and the demoralization of medical faculty (pp. 99–101).

These and recent developments, such as the increase in AIDS patients at academic centers, the shortage of nurses, and the pressures to increase productivity by altering the division of labor, need to be seen as important subjects for research, where the cool head of an outside investigator can put them into perspective (Aiken and Mullinix 1988; Light 1988). For example, cost containment is not such as unreasonable policy in view of the rapid escalation of expenses, and it may be possible for graduate medical education almost to pay for itself with the billable services that residents provide. What we need to understand are the rhetorics of cost containment and the roles they serve, as well as the ways in which training is affected. To take quite a different example, if patient-oriented clinical training is being downgraded unintentionally, important sociological research is needed in order to discover how the institutions involved produced this trend and what can be done about it.

Research on Socioeconomic Changes

Both sociologists and medical educators could benefit from a resurgence of longitudinal studies of medical education, but these studies should be more comparative and more attentive to structural variables than in the past. From a policy point of view, the basic question is how best to train cohorts of doctors for patient care. The gap between professional training and citizens' health needs might start to close if institutional buyers received or demanded some voice in decision making. A number of new developments are related to this basic element.

First, the site, roles, partners, and patients involved in training are likely to change in the next several years. This fact calls for careful empirical analysis and a rethinking of received truths based on past research and experience. Perhaps the well-trained doctor need not learn on the sickest patients with the most esoteric disorders. Perhaps social, cultural, and psychological factors will attain new importance with ambulatory patients.

Second, the large influx of women into medicine will contribute to these changes in site, roles, and partners, and the changes may alter the tone of professional work. They also may contribute to a greater hierarchy in the profession (with women in the less powerful, more poorly paid positions), which serves the purposes of corporatized health care (Lorber 1984, 1988). This greater internal differentiation will be accompanied by a greater external homogenization as financial supports for working-class candidates of all ethnicities diminish. Medical education once again will reproduce the upper middle class. Sociologists are best equipped to document and analyze medical education as a stratified institution that reproduces class relationships and promotes corporate medicine (Kleinbach 1974; Waitzkin 1983).

Third, the developments noted here mean not only that professional autonomy is threatened but that it may be an archaic way of thinking about what it means to be a professional, a holdover from an earlier and not very relevant image based on the educated gentleman who dispenses his skills to those in need and charges what he thinks appropriate. From a cultural perspective, clinical protocols, medical informatics, and practice profiles limit traditional "autonomy" by building choices into rationalized systems. This situation in turn changes what it means to be a professional, a meaning that also depends on one's organizational locus (Wuthnow 1987, pp. 67, 93).

Fourth, physicians' past ability to act on their socialization by choosing or creating a work life compatible with their professional tastes and values is diminishing. How are graduates responding to the perceived overcrowding of many specialties in medicine and surgery? How do they respond when they obtain only their second- or third-choice specialty? How do differences in the organizational setting of specialities affect the training process? How are physicians with practices altering the organization and nature of their services? What are the various ways in which they respond to having some patients on a fee-for-service basis, some on discount fees, and some on prepaid capitation?

Fifth, we need to follow the lead of Colombotos and Kirchner (1986) in analyzing the interplay between early socialization and professional identity in shaping physicians' approach to their work. Doctors and educators seem to be struggling today for meaning in their work and for a sense of professional commitment. Technology is one source of meaning, around which new kinds of rituals continue to develop (Wuthnow 1987, pp. 90–118). In fact modern medicine, especially in the United States, can be regarded as an increasingly elaborated social ritual against the fear of death. Yet meaning from technology ultimately confronts its own limitations (Garber, Fuchs, and Silverman 1984). Corporatization is another way in which meaning and rituals become institutionalized; yet it too dehumanizes professional work. The professional must fall back on inner resources as the profession's earlier sense of moral authority dissipates.

Finally, the relations between specialization and primary care, between academic medical centers and practitioners in the community, are undergoing stress as the gap widens between the kind of care needed by most of the population and wanted by cost-conscious buyers and the kind of medicine taught by the academic machine. Twenty-five years ago Patricia Kendall (1965) conducted a pioneering study of these relationships; too few sociologists have followed her lead even though the legal, economic, institutional, and network aspects of this nexus are central to the question of how the institutions of medical education relate to society (Light 1986a). Academic medical centers train individuals who become their competition and siphon off good teaching cases as well as revenues (Menken 1983). This situation may lead centers either to incorporate community services in some way, to upstage the competition with still more state-of-the-art services, or both.

In the case of academic centers, these and other strategies have implications for the changing legitimation and identity of the specialties affected. Comparative studies of the networks and the institutional relationships surrounding academic medical centers would be valuable. Likewise their role in the health of the community and in the organization of services needs investigation. Nearly 20 years ago David Mechanic (1971) noted the widening gap between the medical schools' technical orientation and practices in the community. He concluded that it was "inevitable that medical schools will eventually become much more heavily involved in restructuring community patterns of rendering medical care" (1971, p. 530). It would be valuable to analyze the particular ways in which this has happened and how this change has affected the medical training of practitioners.

NOTES

1. Although nearly all medical schools aspire to the research model set by the leaders, the proportion of graduates who become specialists varies directly with the prestige of the medical school. For an early consideration of these matters see Kendall 1971a, Table 16–XVI.
2. For similar reasons, employers who now offer no health benefits are reluctant to begin doing so.
3. Many sociologists today do not know that the quantitative parts of Mumford's book, along with a few other pieces such as Kendall's essay on comparative learning environments (1963), are fragments of a second major research effort by the Columbia team. After completing the massive study of undergraduate education in the 1950s, they realized that medical education did not stop there and obtained funds from the Commonwealth Fund to analyze graduate medical education. It is puzzling that only fragments of each study appeared in print. In view of the talent of the Columbia team, one wonders how much more they might have produced in full reports on both research projects.
4. This selected list is culled from VanMaanen and Schein (1979) and from Light (1980).
5. Sociologists' reputation among medical educators for being critical actually may be based on sympathetic observations about those being trained, which those in charge do not want to hear.

REFERENCES

AAMC (Association of American Medical Colleges). 1984. *Physicians for the Twenty-first Century: The GPEP Report*. Washington, DC: AAMC.

Aiken, L., C. Lewis, J. Craig, R. Mendenhall, R. Blendon, and C. Rogers. 1979. "The Contribution of Specialists to the Delivery of Primary Care: A New Perspective." *New England Journal of Medicine* 300:1363–69.

Aiken, Linda H. and Connie Flynt Mullinix. 1988. "The Nurse Shortage: Myth or Reality?" *New England Journal of Medicine* 317 (10):641–45.

Aldrich, Howard. 1987. "New Paradigms for Old: The Population Perspective's Contribution to Health Services Research." *Medical Care Review* 44(2):257–78.

Andersen, Arthur and Company. 1987. *The Future of Healthcare: Changes and Choices*. Melrose Park, IL: American College of Healthcare Executives.

Arney, William Ray. 1982. *Power and the Profession of Obstetrics*. Chicago: University of Chicago Press.

Arney, William Ray and Bernard J. Bergen. 1984. *Medicine and the Management of Living: Taming the Last Great Beast*. Chicago: University of Chicago Press.

Asch, David A. and Ruth M. Parker. 1988. "The Libby Zion Case: One Step Forward or Two Steps Backward?" *New England Journal of Medicine* 318:771–75.

Becker, Howard S., Blanche Geer, Everett C. Hughes, and Anselm M. Strauss. 1961. *Boys in White: Student Culture in Medical School*. Chicago: University of Chicago Press.

Bloom, Samuel W. 1973. *Power and Dissent in the Medical School*. New York: Free Press.

———. 1979. "Socialization for the Physician's Role: A Review of Some Contributions of Research to Theory." Pp. 3–62 in *Becoming a Physician*, edited by Eileen Shapiro and Leah Lowenstein. Cambridge, MA: Ballinger.

———. 1988. "The Medical School as a Social Organization: The Sources of Resistance to Change." *Journal of Health and Social Behavior* 29(4).

Bosk, Charles A. 1979. *Forgive and Remember*. Chicago: University of Chicago Press.

———. 1986. "Professional Responsibility and Medical Error." Pp. 460–77 in *Applications of Social Science to Clinical Medicine and Health*

Policy, edited by Linda H. Aiken and David Mechanic. New Brunswick, NJ: Rutgers University Press.

Bucher, Rue and Joan G. Stelling. 1977. *Becoming Professional*. Beverly Hills: Sage.

Colombotos, John and Corinne Kirchner. 1986. *Physicians and Social Change*. New York: Oxford.

Ebert, Robert H. and Eli Ginzberg. 1988. "The Reform of Medical Education." *Health Affairs* 7(2):5–38.

Eichna, Ludwig W. 1980. "Medical School Education, 1975–1979." *New England Journal of Medicine* 303(13):727–34.

Fisher, Sue. 1986. *In the Patient's Best Interest: Women and the Politics of Medical Decisions*. New Brunswick, NJ: Rutgers University Press.

Fisher, Sue and Alexandra Todd. 1983. *The Social Organization of Doctor-Patient Communication*. University of Tennessee, Center for Applied Linguistics.

Fox, Daniel M. 1986. *Health Policies, Health Politics: The British and American Experience 1911–1965*. Princeton, NJ: Princeton University Press.

Fox, Renée C. 1957. "Training for Uncertainty." Pp. 207–241 in *The Student-Physician*, edited by R.K. Merton, G.G. Reader, and P.L. Kendall. Cambridge, MA: Harvard University Press.

———. 1980. "The Evolution of Medical Uncertainty," *Milbank Memorial Fund Quarterly/Health and Society* 58(1):1–49.

———. 1989. *The Sociology of Medicine*. Englewood Cliffs, NJ: Prentice-Hall.

Friedman, Charles P. and Elizabeth F. Purcell, eds. 1985. *The New Biology and Medical Education*. New York: Josiah Macy, Jr. Foundation.

Freidson, Eliot. 1975. *Doctoring Together: A Study of Professional Social Control*. New York: Elsevier.

Gallagher, Eugene B. and C. Maureen Searle. Forthcoming. "Content and Context in Health Professional Education." Forthcoming in *Handbook of Medical Sociology*, edited by Howard Freeman and Sol Levine. Englewood Cliffs, NJ: Prentice-Hall.

Garber, Alan M., Victor R. Fuchs, and James F. Silverman. 1984. "Case Mix, Costs, and Outcomes: Differences between Faculty and Community Services in a University Hospital." *New England Journal of Medicine* 310 (19):1231–37.

Garfinkel, Harold. 1956. "Conditions of Successful Degradation Ceremonies." *American Journal of Sociology* 61:420–24.

Geiger, H. Jack. 1975. "The Causes of Dehumanization in Health Care and Prospects for Humanization." Pp. 11–36 in *Humanizing Health Care*, edited by Jan Howard and Anselm Strauss. New York: Wiley.

Glassner, Barry. 1988. *Bodies: Why We Look the Way We Do*. New York.

Hammond, K.R. and F.G. Kern, Jr. 1959. *Teaching Comprehensive Medical Care*. Cambridge, MA: Harvard University Press.

Havighurst, Clark C. 1986. "The Changing Locus of Decision Making in the Health Care Sector." *Journal of Health Politics, Policy and Law* 11 (4):597–735.

Horowitz, M. 1964. *Educating Tomorrow's Doctors*. New York: Appleton-Century-Crofts.

Hurley, Robert E. and Arnold D. Kaluzny. 1987. "Organizational Ecology and Health Services Research: New Answers for Old and New Questions." *Medical Care Review* 44(2):235–56.

Iglehart, John K. 1988. "Medical Schools and the Public Interest: A Conversation with Robert G. Petersdorf." *Health Affairs* 7(2):108–20.

Kendall, Patricia L. 1961. "Impact of Training Programs on the Young Physician's Attitudes and Experiences." *Journal of the American Medical Association* 176:992–97.

———. 1963. "The Learning Environments of Hospitals." Pp. 195–230 in *The Hospital in Modern Society*, edited by E. Freidson. New York: Free Press.

———. 1965. *The Relationship between Medical Educators and Medical Practitioners*. Evanston, IL: Association of American Medical Colleges.

———. 1971a. "Medical Specialization: Trends and Contribution Factors." Chapter 16 in *Psychosocial Aspects of Medical Training*, edited by Robert H. Coombs and Clark E. Vincent. Springfield, IL: Thomas.

———. 1971b. "Consequences of the Trend toward Specialization." Chapter 17 in *Psychosocial Aspects of Medical Training*, edited by Robert H. Coombs and Clark E. Vincent. Springfield, IL: Thomas.

Kleinbach, Grace. 1974. "Social Structure and the Education of Health Personnel." *International Journal of Health Services* 4(2):297–317.

Letters to the Editor. 1988. "Looking at the Training of House Staff." *New England Journal of Medicine* 319:718–22.

Levinson, Daniel J. 1967. "Medical Education and the Theory of Socialization." *Journal of Health and Social Behavior* 8(4):253–64.

Lewis, Irving J. and Cecil G. Sheps. 1983. *The Sick Citadel: The American Academic Medical Center and the Public Interest*. Boston: Odgeschlager, Gunn and Hain.

Leyerle, Betty. 1984. *Moving and Shaking American Medicine*. Westport, CT: Greenwood.

Light, Donald W. 1979a. "Surface Data and Deep Structure: Observing the Organization of Professional Training." *Administrative Science Quarterly* 24(4):310–22.

———. 1979b. "Uncertainty and Control in

Professional Training." *Journal of Health and Social Behavior* 20(4):310–22.

———. 1980. *Becoming Psychiatrists: The Professional Transformation of Self*. New York: Norton.

———. 1983. "Medical and Nursing Education: Surface Behavior and Deep Structure." Pp. 455–78 in *Handbook of Health, Health Care, and the Health Professions*, edited by David Mechanic. New York: Free Press.

———. 1986a. "The Widening Gap between Medical Training and Health Care Needs." *Sociologia Internationalis* 24(1):43–52.

———. 1986b. "Surplus vs. Cost Containment: The Changing Context for Health Providers." Pp. 519–42 in *Applications of Social Science to Clinical Medicine and Health Policy*, edited by Linda Aiken and David Mechanic. New Brunswick, NJ: Rutgers University Press.

———. 1988. "Turf Battles and the Theory of Professional Dominance." Forthcoming in *Research in the Sociology of Health Care*. Vol. 7, edited by Dorothy Wertz. Greenwich, CT: JAI.

———. Forthcoming. "Social Control and the American Health Care System." In *Handbook of Medical Sociology*, Fourth Edition, edited by Howard E. Freeman and Sol Levine. Englewood Cliffs, NJ: Prentice-Hall.

Light, Donald W. and Sol Levine. 1988. "The Changing Character of the Medical Profession." *Milbank Memorial Fund Quarterly* forthcoming.

Lorber, Judith. 1984. *Women Physicians: Careers, Status, and Power*. New York: Tavistock.

———. 1988. "Can the Medical Profession Ever Be a Company of Equals?" Paper delivered at the 1988 ASA meetings, Atlanta, GA.

Ludmerer, Kenneth M. 1985. *Learning To Heal: The Development of American Medical Education*. New York: Basic.

McCall, Timothy B. 1988. "The Impact of Long Working Hours on Resident Physicians." *New England Journal of Medicine* 318:775–78.

McCue, Jack D. 1985. "The Distress of Internship: Causes and Prevention." *New England Journal of Medicine* 312(7):449–52.

Mechanic, David. 1971. "Social Changes Affecting Medical Training and Practice." Chapter 18 in *Psychosocial Aspects of Medical Training*, edited by Robert H. Coombs and Clark E. Vincent. Springfield, IL: Thomas.

Menken, Matthew. 1983. "Consequences of an Oversupply of Medical Specialists: The Case of Neurology." *New England Journal of Medicine* 108:1224–25.

Menken, Matthew and Cecil G. Sheps. 1985. "Consequences of an Oversupply of Specialists: The Case of Neurology." *Journal of the American Medical Association* 253:1926–28.

Merry, Uri and George I. Brown. 1987. *The Neurotic Behavior of Organizations*. New York: Gestalt Institute of Cleveland Press.

Merton, Robert K., George Reader, and Patricia L. Kendall, eds. 1957. *The Student-Physician: Introductory Studies in the Sociology of Medical Education*. Cambridge, MA: Harvard University Press.

Miller, Stephen J. 1970. *Prescription for Leadership*. Chicago: Aldine.

Millman, Marcia. 1976. *The Unkindest Cut: Life in the Backrooms of Medicine*. New York: Morrow.

Mishler, Elliot C. 1985. *The Discourse of Medicine*. Norwood, NJ: Ablex.

Mitchell, Janet B., William B. Stason, Kathleen A. Calore, Marc P. Freiman, and Helene T. Hewes. 1987. "Are Some Surgical Procedures Overpaid?" *Health Affairs* 6(2):121–31.

Mizrahi, Terry. 1986. *Getting Rid of Patients: Contradictions in the Socialization of Physicians*. New Brunswick, NJ: Rutgers University Press.

Moore, Wilbert W. 1970. "Occupational Socialization." Chapter 1 in *Handbook of Socialization Theory*, edited by David Goslin. Chicago: Rand McNally.

Mumford, Emily. 1970. *Interns: From Student to Physician*. Cambridge, MA: Harvard University Press.

Payer, Lynn. 1988. *Medicine and Culture: Varieties in the United States, England, West Germany, and France*. New York: Holt.

Petersdorf, Robert G. 1986. "Medical Schools and Research: Is the Tail Wagging the Dog?" *Daedalus* 106(1):99–118.

Reader, George and Mary E.W. Goss, eds. 1967. *Comprehensive Medical Care and Teaching*. New York: Cornell University Press.

Reinhardt, Uwe E. 1987. "Resource Allocation in Health Care: The Allocation of Lifestyles to Providers." *Milbank Memorial Fund Quarterly* 65(1):153–76.

Reiser, Stanley Joel. 1978. *Medicine and the Reign of Technology*. Cambridge, UK: Cambridge University Press.

Rogers, David E. 1975. "Medical Academe and the Problems of Health Care Provision." *Archives of Internal Medicine* 135:364–69.

———. 1982. "Some Musings on Medical Education: Is It Going Astray?" *Pharos* (Spring):11–14.

Shaiken, Harley. 1986. *Work Transformed: Automation and Labor in the Computer Age*. Lexington, MA: Lexington Books.

Sharaf, Myron R. and Daniel J. Levinson. 1964. "The Quest for Omnipotence in Professional Training." *Psychiatry* 27:125–49.

Simpson, Ida H. 1979. *From Student to Nurse: A Longitudinal Study of Socialization*. Cambridge, UK: Cambridge University Press.

Small, Peter. 1988. "The Health Poll." *Medical Benefits* 5(12)June 30:1–3.

Starr, Paul E. 1982. *The Social Transformation of American Medicine*. New York: Basic.

VanMaanen, John and Edgar H. Schein. 1979. "Toward a Theory of Organizational Socialization." *Organizational Behavior* 1:209–74.

Waitzkin, Howard. 1983. *The Second Sickness: Contradictions of Capitalist Health Care*. New York: Free Press.

Wuthnow, Robert. 1987. *Meaning and Moral Order: Explorations in Cultural Analysis*. Berkeley: University of California Press.

Zuboff, Shoshana. 1988. *In the Age of the Smart Machine*. New York: Basic.

[27]

Learning To Doctor: Reflections on Recent Accounts of the Medical School Years

PETER CONRAD
Brandeis University

Journal of Health and Social Behavior 1988, Vol. 29 (December):323–332

Using recent first-hand accounts by Klass (1987), Konner (1987), LeBaron (1982), and Reilly (1987), this paper examines "insiders' " experiences of medical school. Medical education emphasizes disease, technical procedures, and technological medicine, with scant attention to "caring" aspects of doctoring. Students struggle to learn medicine and to maintain a humanistic or patient-oriented perspective, but the social environment of medical training militates against humanistic doctoring. Toward the end of medical school, students undergo a transformation by adopting the medical-clinical perspective and shifting their identification from patients to doctors. The doctors who maintain a humanistic orientation to medical care appear to be individuals who had developed this orientation before they arrived at medical school. Thus, to increase the number of humanistic physicians, the best strategy may be to alter medical school recruitment and selection policies.

Sociologists have studied medical education in the context of professional socialization at least since the classic works of Becker and Merton and their colleagues (Becker, Geer, Strauss, and Hughes 1961; Merton, Reader, and Kendall 1957). The dilemmas and struggles of medical students to learn their craft and the eventual transformation of students into doctors have become grist for sociological analysis. Most of the available studies are based on data collected through surveys, interviews, and participant observation (Bloom 1973; Broadhead 1982; Coombs 1978; Haas and Shaffir 1987). Although in these cases sociologists have been accorded observer status (Illsley 1975) within the inner sanctums of medical initiation, they remain "outsiders."

In the past two decades enough first-person "insider" accounts of medical education have been published to fill a small bookshelf. From Dr. X's *Intern* (1965) to Samuel Shem's *House of God* (1978) to Michelle Harrison's *A Woman in Residence* (1982), as well as several dozen others (see Stoeckle 1987), young physicians have written about the adventures and tribulations of becoming a doctor. The format of these accounts ranges from fiction to social criticism, but all provide a behind-the-scenes view of medical education. These subjective, insiders' accounts provide a unique resource for understanding medical education from the viewpoint of those who experience it.

In this paper I use four recently published first-person accounts to examine some of the experiences and dilemmas of medical education in the 1980s. I limit myself here to examining the four years of medical school, and focus on the problems and processes of these years.

THE DATA

The four accounts used in this paper are Perri Klass's (1987) *A Not Entirely Benign Procedure*, Melvin Konner's (1987) *Becoming a Doctor*, Charles LeBaron's *(1982) Gentle Vengeance*, and Phillip Reilly's (1987) *To Do No Harm*. Each of these books offers a personal account of the author's experience in

My thanks to Libby Bradshaw, Phil Brown, John Colombotos, Gene Gallagher, Fred Hafferty, Donald Light, and Irving K. Zola for comments on an earlier draft of this paper. The responsibility for the interpretation is, of course, mine. Address correspondence to Department of Sociology, Brandeis University, Waltham, MA 02254.

medical school, although the emphases are different. Klass presents a series of essays written during her four years in medical school; these are not always about medical education per se, but include accounts of her experience with the doctor's role and her reactions to patients. Konner, who has a Ph.D. in anthropology, focuses largely on the third (and key) year of medical school and offers a rich description of personal encounters and experiences. Konner presents a melange of doctors he has encountered, experiences he has had, and patients he has cared for, focusing as much on patients and their problems as on his own medical education. LeBaron describes in detail his experience of the first year of medical school. Reilly articulates his difficulties and triumphs in struggling to learn medicine. He kept a diary like journal during his four years, emphasizing his first encounters (e.g., patient history, pelvic exam, spinal tap) and how much he learned from each patient. These books are more reflective narratives than academic analytic treatises; they are presented without footnotes or references to other works.

These four authors are a self-selected group and are not "typical" medical students. They are self-selected because they chose to chronicle their experiences by writing a book. They are atypical in other ways as well: they attended elite medical schools (Reilly to Yale, the others to Harvard); none went to medical school directly after college; two were in their thirties when they began medical school; two had children before graduating from medical school; two had advanced degrees before entering medical school (Konner a Ph.D. and Reilly a J.D.); and three had published books previously. More than most medical students, these authors were people of "letters," humanists rather than hard scientists. These attributes undoubtedly affected their experience in medical school and the books they produced. At the same time the authors provide us with a special window on medical school, allowing us to see medical education from the viewpoint of reflective "insiders."

When compared to standard sociological data, these accounts have distinct liabilities and at least one important advantage. The liabilities are clear: the data are not collected systematically, they are reports from self-selected "informants," and the authors don't necessarily focus on the most significant sociological issues. Yet these data contain one major advantage over the information collected by sociologists: they are accounts of individuals who had to learn medicine, do doctoring, accept responsibility for patients, and endure sleepless nights. Not even the most committed and most fastidious participant-observer would be required or able to achieve this level of involvement. These are the stories of true insiders.[1] Although insiders have no singular epistemological claim to truth (Merton 1973), in this case their findings align remarkably well with those of sociological outsiders.

As part of their experience as medical students, all four authors recount their impressions of medicine, doctors, and patient care—sometimes in rather critical terms. In this paper I attempt to cull their experience of medical education from their overall experience of medicine. At times this separation is impossible, but I focus as much as is feasible on their experience as medical students *qua* medical students rather than on their observations of medicine and the medical profession.

THE PRECLINICAL YEARS

The first two years of medical school, the so-called preclinical years, are treated with decidedly less attention than the latter two. Klass devotes less than 20 percent of her book to these years, Konner about 10 percent, and Reilly about 30 percent. LeBaron, however, discusses only the first year.

The first year of medical school is devoted largely to the basic sciences and to learning about the normal functioning of the human body. The lecture-based courses in physiology, anatomy, biochemistry, and microbiology are not seen as practical or as uniquely medical in content. The second-year courses such as pathology and immunology, which focus more on disease and medical treatments, are deemed more relevant. Although the courses are generally pass-fail rather than graded, the examinations require a great deal of memorization and rote learning if students are to maintain a respectable rank in their class. Earlier sociologist observers (e.g., Becker et al. 1961) noted that more material is presented than could possibly be learned; thus students develop methods of academic triage and try to ascertain what their instructors really want them to know.

The first material to be jettisoned is information related to the social aspects of medicine.

> "Culture" . . . has a broad meaning for the medical student. It refers to the material that will not have to be memorized for the next test and thus can be safely ignored. Normally, this includes the general theory behind the problem, historical points, social impact, cost factors, direction of future investigations, etc. (LeBaron 1982, p. 49).

Although the courses are meant to give the students a knowledge base for learning clinical medicine, "too many facts are being taught too thoughtlessly in too short a time" (Konner 1987, p. 362), with little time or encouragement for independent analysis.

Labs are an important part of the first two years. The most popular part of the physiology class is a "dog lab," in which students dissect an anesthetized dog which is "destroyed" after the experiment. Klass (1987, p. 32) sees the lab as "toughening" medical students. Not without misgivings, she chooses not to participate in this "prolonged killing of an animal"; she fears it will toughen her in ways she will not like. Some of her fellow students ask her if she is "too sensitive" for dog lab. How will she ever be a doctor and deal with what she must in the hospitals?[2]

One of the most powerful learning experiences in the first year is the student's encounter with cadavers. For several months, in groups of approximately four, medical students meticulously dissect and partially dismember the corpse of a human being. These corpses had been preserved for a year in special solutions, so the skin was leathery and the bodies reeked of formalin. They were the students' first medical encounter with human death; certain "intimacies" were allowed, such as putting one's hand inside a human body or removing internal organs, that were unavailable to most people. For Reilly this first-hand anatomy lesson became the center of his life. As Klass (1987, p. 37) notes:

> For the first time in medical school, I have the sense I am being initiated into a priesthood. This is something that normal people never do.

Though the medical students may name their cadaver and treat it respectfully, at the same time they are beginning an important process in their medical education. As the smell of formalin clings to their clothes and lingers faintly on their fingers for months, the medical students learn not only anatomy but also a certain objectification of the human body, a separation of soma from persona. Lief and Fox (1963) pointed out years ago the significance of the cadaver for the development of the physician's "detached concern." To some extent this depersonalization is an occupational requirement for medical practice, but much of subsequent medical education serves to extend this attitude unnecessarily to living patients.

In the second semester of the second year, as students move closer to clinical care, the workload increases, and so does the anxiety and anticipation. In the context of learning to take histories and do physicals, medical students encounter their first patients. Now that doctoring is becoming real, new anxieties and trepidations arise. The protocol for taking a history probes the intimacies of patients' lives. Reilly (1987, p. 35) experienced discomfort as he interviewed a 50-year-old woman:

> As the questions shifted away from medically safe subjects like pain to more intimate questions about her family, I began to feel extremely uncomfortable, almost as though I were a "peeping Tom." Why should she be asked to unlock the secrets of her family life to me? It could not possibly be relevant to her illness, or could it?

Physical examination can stir up other feelings in medical students. Students tell patients twice their age to get undressed, and then cross conventional barriers of interpersonal space to inspect the intimacies of their bodies. In addition to anxiety about doing it right, students frequently must deal with their own reactions to the patient as well as with discomforting feelings of being invasive. Such feelings are considered extraneous to medical education and are not welcomed by instructors. When Konner (1987, p. 32) confided during a clinical small group meeting that he had examined a very attractive woman and that it had made him uncomfortable, both the instructor and his fellow students looked at him strangely and went on quickly to the next topic. He decided, to his regret, that in the future he would be more cautious about his feelings (see also Smith and Kleinman 1988).

Throughout the preclinical years medical students worked to internalize the vast knowledge that was presented to them. As Klass (1987, p. 29) realized, however, they were learning other aspects of doctoring as well.

> [T]he experience of being socialized into a medical student class was at times disturbing, as was the sense that we were being taught values, though not explicitly, along with basic science and pathophysiology.

Even the students' relationship to time was shifting; they had less control of it. With the increasing workload, LeBaron (1982, p. 79) noticed early in his medical school career that "there's little doubt that we're being trained not to regard any time as a personal preserve."

BEGINNING AN APPRENTICESHIP

In the third year, clinical training begins in earnest. Students go through a series of hospital and clinic rotations or clerkships, each from two weeks to two months long, where they are exposed to medicine in practice and begin to learn the craft of doctoring. These rotations include internal medicine, pediatrics, obstetrics and gynecology, surgery, anesthesiology, neurology, psychiatry, and emergency medicine. Their teachers include clinical faculty ("attendings") and house staff (residents and interns). It is assumed that students will learn more by watching and doing than by reading and studying, but they are also expected to be knowledgeable and well-read regarding each case on each rotation. Because medical students are the newest and most junior members of the medical hierarchy, they must learn from anybody they can. During medical training, individuals on each level of the medical hierarchy learn from those just a year or two farther along. The watchword of clinical training is "See one, do one, teach one." This adage reflects both the emphasis placed on learning procedures (i.e., medical techniques) and the idea that "on-the-job training" typifies advanced stages of medical education. As Klass (1987, p. 55) states, "Clinical medicine has to be learned as an apprenticeship."

The third year is the culmination of medical school. Both Reilly and Konner note that the fourth year, with its emphasis on electives, is anticlimatic after the exposures and struggles of third year. Students spend most of the third year on the wards in teaching hospitals, working long hours. Typically a medical student follows an intern's schedule and is on call every third or fourth night. Students spend much of this year deprived of sleep, trying to master the techniques of medicine. They must learn to take histories, perform various kinds of physical examinations, order and interpret tests, make diagnoses, develop treatment plans, and choose appropriate medications; students also must master techniques like drawing blood, inserting an intravenous line, performing a lumbar puncture, and assisting in surgery. Because they are on the lowest rung of the medical hierarchy, frequently they are saddled with "scut" work such as drawing patients' blood or running to get lab results, which they regard as interfering with their learning.

This learning can be very stressful. Students often find themselves in situations where they simply don't know what to do; or even if they do know what to do, they simply cannot accomplish it. Neophytes can spend 20 minutes trying to find a vein to start an I.V. while pricking the patient continually. Konner (1987, p. 129) describes an experience on his neurology rotation, when he admitted a 50-year-old woman who had experienced headaches and dizziness for a year.

> I was in the medical student's usual sink-or-swim situation. Told nothing about the case, I was expected to interview and examine her and then form hypotheses and suggestions for treatment. I was supposed to pretend to be knowledgeable and wise, or else why would the patient be wasting her time with me?

The anxiety of not knowing anything or not knowing enough is common among medical students.

> It's frightening to feel yourself very ignorant in a setting where sick people are depending on you for care. It's terrifying to learn on patients how to start an I.V. You worry about making a mistake. You worry about hurting someone. On a different

> level, you worry about making a fool of yourself, about looking stupid on rounds (Klass 1987, p. 57).

Strategies for effective "roundsmanship" are survival techniques learned by all medical students. Patient rounds—usually consisting of an attending or an advanced resident going from patient to patient, followed by a gaggle of underling interns and medical students—is intended to be an opportunity for teaching and learning, but frequently is an occasion of severe *angst* for medical students. Medical students often are asked specific questions about disease, diagnosis, treatment, or the latest medical literature. They are expected to answer quickly and correctly. Some people see rounds as a game, whose major goal is to look good in front of whatever colleagues and superiors happen to be present (Reilly 1987, p. 116). Klass (1987, p. 132) contends that "the art of making a good impression no matter what you actually know or don't know" is at the heart of successful roundsmanship. Impression management rather than learning becomes the central feature of rounds. Reilly (1987, p. 117) articulates the rules of roundsmanship for third-year medical students:

> Dress neatly, always carry white unlined three-by-five index cards containing lab results of all patients whom you are following, always look at the house officer who is speaking, ask no less than one but no more than three questions during rounds, never answer a question first unless it is clearly intended for you, never appear to be competing with fellow students, and never challenge a resident's wisdom, especially if you know he or she is wrong and you are right . . . Perhaps the most crucial task is to hone the ability to answer the esoteric questions posed by senior players—not an easy feat. The questions come quickly and without warning, and there is little hope of knowing the correct answer.

Failure at roundsmanship can be a source of great embarrassment. Clinicians are quick to criticize medical students' incompetence (Reilly 1987, p. 84); the terror of being wrong is not outweighed by the ability to think on one's feet. Although it is possible that some learning occurs during rounds, sleep-deprived and stressed medical students spend more energy on preserving face than on absorbing knowledge.

Medical students are acutely aware that they are not doctors; yet in the hospital they are introduced to patients constantly as "young doctors" or "student doctors on the medical team." Although some students probably took comfort in their immediately augmented status, for many, including Reilly (1987, p. 25) and Klass (1987, p. 158), this designation made them feel false and fraudulent. They were not doctors; being called doctors only increased their anxiety about not yet being medically competent or knowledgeable. They were expected, however, to act like doctors and to differentiate themselves from other medical workers. In a poignant incident, Klass (1987, p. 163) and her fellow doctors went to examine a baby who had very dirty, smelly diapers. Klass wanted to change the diapers, but all the other clinicians continued to examine the baby for 40 minutes. It wasn't a question of time or squeamishness, it was dignity: doctors don't change diapers no matter how smelly the examination is.

The clinical years are a confrontation with human tragedy and misfortune. The direct contact with suffering, pain, and death can be emotionally trying. Yet beyond the anxiety and the personal discomfort, the connection and the relations with other human beings and the ability to reduce suffering in patients can be rewarding and exciting. As one clinical professor told students:

> Medicine offers a front row seat on life. For the rest of your days people will bare their souls to you. If you retain the ability to savor this privilege you will all die rich (Reilly 1987, p. 80).

It is the relationships and intimacies with patients that rekindle latent idealism and provide some of the rewards that these students hoped medicine would bring. "The medical students always spend more time with patients than anyone else" (Konner 1987, p. 130); frequently they form special and memorable relationships with individual patients. Reilly (1987, p. 86) "discovers" that physicians learn best from patients, not from books. He writes in detail about Mrs. Landi, a 79-year-old woman with cancer, whom he visited daily for several weeks. Through his care for this woman he discovered the dilemmas of invasive treatment, the difficulties of telling patients the truth, the pathos of dealing with the family, and the intimacies between a caregiver and his dying patient. Konner describes his six-week relationship with Charlotte Kaplan, a 40-year-old woman with inflammatory bowel disease and a severe eating disorder. He began caring for her on his medicine rotation and kept up regular visits even when he moved to the next clinical rotation. He consulted with her regular doctors, fretted about the lack of psychiatric involvement, and, most important, talked with Charlotte and listened to her when no one else did so. He supported her through her postoperative psychotic break, and felt that his presence had made a difference in her care. These student doctors were moved by the all-too-rare occasions when they could truly "care" for patients, although apparently not all were moved in this way. This was much of what they had hoped medicine would be about, and what they struggled to reconcile with reality when they learned otherwise.

HUMANISTIC CARE AND TECHNICAL DOCTORING

Perhaps the most consistent theme that recurred in these accounts was the scarcity of humane and caring encounters between doctors and patients. An "ideology of concern" for patients was voiced on the medical floors—doctors talked about caring for patients and perhaps wanted to do so—but the medical training was set up in a way that discouraged and often prevented such caring (Konner 1987, p. 263).

Doctors' clinical perspectives focused almost entirely on the disease rather than on the illness. Virtually all teaching emphasized the technical aspects of doctoring: diagnosis, treatment, and intervention. Too often this approach caused patients to become the disease: "the lymphoma in Room 304." A fascination with technological intervention pervades medicine, from neonatal intensive care to neurosurgery to cardiac catheterization. These are the frontiers of medicine; techniques such as these carry the greatest prestige in the medical world. They are emphasized by clinical instructors and are seductive to medical students. As Klass (1987, p. 50) comments, "I see all of us, including myself, absorbing the idea that when it comes to tests, technology, interventions, more is better."

Doctors are not taught how to talk to patients. Konner (1987, p. 56) was disturbed at noting that "ignoring patients was normative." During rounds doctors often discussed a patient's case in the patient's presence, and spoke with each other as if he or she were not there. Very little in the medical curriculum focused directly on the "doctor-patient relationship"; clinical instruction about human relations was perfunctory. Reilly (1987, p. 261) captures this truth of medical training: "I was frequently told to 'run down to nuclear medicine' [for test results], but was rarely asked 'to go talk to Mr. Jones.' " Virtually no one cared if a doctor's bedside manner was subpar, although doctors were criticized regularly about other types of incompetence (see Klass 1987, p. 113).

> Far from being embarrassed by brusqueness, residents are more likely to be embarrassed by (and to consider not quite professional) acts and gestures that are other than completely instrumental (Konner 1987, p. 26).

Humane acts not directly affecting medical treatment are all too uncommon in the hospital world.

The situation of the medical student, and later of the house officer, does not lend itself to caring for and about patients. Quite the opposite is the case; the situation often encourages the definition of the patient as an adversary or even as an "enemy." Reilly (1987, p. 226) describes a night when he was exhausted and sleep-deprived:

> At three o'clock in the morning as I stood over [a comatose patient's] bedside starting his I.V. he was an enemy, part of the plot to deprive me of sleep. If he died, I could sleep for another hour. If he lived, I would be up all night.

Students' and house staff's excessive responsibility, overwork (90 to 100 hours a week), sleeplessness, and struggle to master medicine decrease even further the emphasis on humanistic caring. Crude jokes and gallows humor about patients become part of the everyday scene of medicine. Although making fun of patients may release stress, it also sets doctors farther apart from their patients. Reilly (1987, p. 235) describes how house officers made jokes about a patient, although they had not talked to him or told him of his condition:

The way our team, composed of nine

bright, highly educated, caring persons, handled Mr. Garabedian's death also convinced me that something very important was missing from medical training. House officers don't show enough respect for their patients. Two years of 100 hour work-weeks and significant sleep deprivation make new physicians technically proficient but the demands to hone their diagnostic and therapeutic skills leave little time to nurture their compassion.

Of course, there are compassionate and sensitive doctors. Along with the nasty surgeons and arrogant residents they encountered, the medical students came into contact with impressive, empathetic, caring physicians. These were exemplary doctors who cared demonstrably about their patients as persons and who spent time with them and their "illness." They were so uncommon, however, that they became medical heroes. In this world of overwork and technical doctoring, humane encounters with patients are exceptional enough to be worthy for special mention. Konner (1987, pp. 256, 315, 269) was stunned when he heard one doctor actually use the word "tragic" twice about a patient, amazed when he saw a doctor look straight into a patient's eyes and take her hand when speaking to her, and moved the only time he ever saw tears of pity in a physician's eyes.

Today doctors and the medical students they teach are enamored with the technological aspects of medicine. The emphasis in training is overwhelmingly on instrumental rather than interactional patient care. Reilly (1987, p. 261) wonders whether "the power to diagnose and cure has sapped the power to care." The humanistic doctors had to develop their humanistic inclinations before they ever arrived at medical school. There is almost nothing in medical training that encourages compassion, empathy, and "care" for patients; indeed there is a great deal that militates against those qualities. To be a humanistic doctor in our technical world of medicine is to swim against the stream.

A TRANSFORMATION

Medical school is a powerful socializing force. Many students enter training with naive, idealistic views of medicine and leave with a more realistic and cynical outlook. Through the rigor and the tension of medical education, students' beliefs about medical care change as they increasingly adopt the dominant clinical perspective that pervades medicine. Most adopt it readily, while others must be converted; some accept it only uncomfortably; a few resist it actively.

By the final year of medical school, students are more accustomed to the intrusions and intimacies of medicine. As their fund of knowledge and experience grows, they begin to see themselves more comfortably as "doctors." They become acclimated to the discomforts of their apprenticeship and familiar with the pain and suffering of the sick and dying. They have learned how to think like doctors, to accept great responsibility, to cope with medical uncertainties, and, not least, to survive medical training.

The medical student's coming to terms with death may be a critical aspect of his or her transformation. During a six-week rotation Reilly witnessed about a dozen deaths, which had a profound effect on his becoming a doctor.

> I do not completely understand the ways in which these experiences have changed my view of the world. But I am convinced that the period in a student-doctor's training when dying finally becomes palpable constitutes the most significant aspect of his or her metamorphosis (Reilly 1987, p. 228).

Death has taken on a new meaning: medical students are no longer uncomfortable in its presence.

Medical school fundamentally affects one's world view. In the first place, one can never again be a lay person about medicine. One can no longer give personal advice—to friends, relatives and acquaintances—on health and medical matters apart from one's professional self. Subjectively, too, one sees the world differently. Konner, a Verdi aficionado, comments on the film *La Traviata*:

> And the film was more or less wonderful; but the main problem I had was with Violetta's consumption. I could not experience it except as a medical student. I was trying hard to banish medical thoughts, and there I was twisting one of my favorite operas into the perspective of a physician, which I could not abandon even for two hours (1987, p. 297).

The medical-clinical perspective permeates the very tissues of consciousness, forming a new and specific lens for viewing the world. Strongly held convictions, such as the role of midwives in birthing, may be challenged severely and even altered by the medical perspective (Konner 1987). The student's medical innocence has come to an end.

One of the most profound transformations in students is a change in identification. Throughout his training Konner (1987, p. xvi) identified more with patients than with doctors, but by the end of medical school his allegiance had shifted.

> I have been absorbed into the "teamness" of medicine. During my last few months on the wards I tried to be decent to patients, but my bonds, my emotional energy—what psychoanalysts call cathexes—were all with doctors and medical students, and to a lesser extent, nurses. . . . Relations with [patients] should be smooth, cordial, and efficient, but they are certainly not personal (1987, p. 365).

Medical students absorb many of the values of the medical profession along with the biomedical knowledge and techniques. Klass (1987, p. 41) wonders whether she will still be able to become the kind of doctor that attracted her to a medical career.

> But the question is, by the time I finish, will I still remember any of what I originally wanted to be? When I'm through with my training, will I have any way of knowing what kind of doctor I have actually become?

When students complete medical school they are still amateurs at medicine. It is through internship and residency that they complete their apprenticeship and become journeymen. Students typically choose their residency specialties from among the rotations they sampled in the clinical years. Although as students they have little opportunity to ruminate, the residency choice is a consistent background issue during medical school. It is a decision based on personal interests and inclinations, perceived career options and rewards, lifestyle considerations, and intangibles such as relationships with doctors encountered in a specialty. Arguably the most significant decision of the students' medical career, the choice of residency is a branching point that sets them on a path and narrows their field. It marks the end of medical school and the beginning of life as house officer, complete with a new identity, more 100-plus-hour work weeks, increased responsibility, greater expectations by superiors, and the same dilemmas of medical training and caring for patients.

CONCLUSION

In *Gentle Vengeance* LeBaron (1982, p. 58) asks, "What's that hamburger machine that chops up nice kids and turns them into the doctors that I know?" Examining these four accounts gives us some insight into the meat-grinding process. Medical school does an excellent job at imparting medical knowledge and technique, but is inadequate in conveying humane and caring values. There is precious little in medical education that facilitates humanistic medical care. Technological medicine, with its disease orientation, myriad lab tests, complex interventions, and "fix-it" mentality, pays scant attention to teaching about doctor-patient relations. The medical student's life of long hours, sleep deprivation, excessive responsibility, and dealing with unreflective and arrogant superiors inhibits the growth of compassion and empathy. Our medical training system, with its emphasis on facts and technical interventions, produces competent and knowledgeable physicians but not caring doctors.

The accounts reviewed in this paper are all the more compelling because they are written by insiders who have gone through the process. Although outsiders, including sociologists and educators, have been critical of medical education, these accounts by insiders present the perspective of individuals who want to be humane and caring as well as competent and knowledgeable. Granted, these individuals are outliers, students who want to be patient-oriented physicians in the most elite and most specialized of medical settings. Even so, their struggles help us understand more clearly what is amiss in medical education today.

In light of the long-standing debate over whether professional socialization (Merton et al. 1957) or student culture (Becker et al. 1961) is more influential in a doctor's training, these accounts suggest that both perspectives have merit and that a more integrated formulation is in order. Both the structure of medical training and the students' subcultural adaptations may contribute to the experience and outcome of medical education.

If these accounts can be taken as reasonable depictions of medical school in the 1980s, it is striking how little has changed over the years. Even in the light of social and curriculum changes, these accounts corroborate the more analytical sociological fieldwork and research conducted two and three decades ago (Becker et al. 1961; Coombs 1978; Merton et al. 1957). Looking back still further, we find that similar observations were made in 1927 by Harvard physician Francis Weld Peabody in the *Journal of the American Medical Association:*

> The most common criticism made at present by older practitioners is that younger graduates have been taught a great deal about the mechanisms of disease, but very little about the practice of medicine—or, to put it more bluntly, they are too "scientific" and do not know how to take care of patients (Culliton 1984, p. 420).

This comment represents a six-decade series of intermittent but remarkably consistent observations depicting the shortcomings of medical education.

There are sensitive and caring doctors practicing medicine, but I contend that these individuals had a humanistic orientation *before* they came to medical school. Somehow they were able to hold on to their values and to put their caring skills into practice against the odds of medical training.

Repeated calls have been made for reforms in medical education in order to produce more humanistic physicians (Association of American Medical Colleges 1984; Bok 1984), but in view of the nature of medical education in an age of technological medicine it may be very difficult to "create" humanistic and caring doctors.[3] The current curriculum reforms, such as Harvard's "New Pathways" program and the proposals for reducing medical students' and residents' overlong hours, may help (McCall 1988). Another potential mechanism for encouraging humanistic doctoring is changing the reward structure of the medical profession. If the profession recognized and rewarded humanistic interventions equally with technical interventions and gave greater prestige and special attention in medical training to "caring" for patients, it might be able to increase humanistic doctoring.[4]

Even so, the "meat grinder" and the structure of medical organization will be resistant to change. My contention is that short of a yet-uncharted major reform in medical education and practice, the best way to increase the number of sensitive and caring physicians is to recruit and select individuals who already have a well-developed caring, nurturant capacity.[5] These people are most likely to be able to maintain their humane, patient-oriented values in spite of their medical training.

NOTES

1. In the late 1970s I was a "nonparticipant observer" of my wife's medical education. Although I don't draw on these experiences directly, they undoubtedly affected my reading of these books and the argument made in this paper.
2. Klass (1987, p. 33) notes that some women were "particularly vulnerable to this kind of reasoning," and that they had to seize every opportunity to prove they were tough enough and had what it takes to become a doctor. A recent study suggests that as the number of women medical students has increased, sexism in medical school has decreased. The remaining sex discrimination comes from the medical school faculty. Yet because medicine has long been a male-dominated profession, some subtle forms of sexism still remain a part of the medical school culture (Grant 1988; cf. Harrison 1982)
3. I highly recommend Konner's brilliant last chapter to anyone considering reforms of medical education.
4. In the long run, the medical reimbursement system also would have to shift so as to value and reimburse fully a doctor's time for care as well as for procedures.
5. On a practical level, this suggestion implies that if medical schools truly want to produce more humanistic physicians, admissions committees must modify their traditional selection criteria to include indicators of a candidate's compassion, ability to communicate, and orientation toward people and patients. Medical schools may need to look beyond their usual pool of applicants to find students with a background in humanities and social science as well as the conventional premed preparation (cf. Conrad 1986).

REFERENCES

Association of American Medical Colleges. 1984. *Physicians for the Twenty-First Century: The GREP Report: Report of the Panel on the General Professional Education of the Physician and the College Preparation for Medicine*. Washington, DC: Association of American Medical Colleges.

Becker, Howard S., Blanche Geer, Anselm L. Strauss, and Everett C. Hughes. 1961. *Boys in White: Student Culture in Medical School*. Chicago: University of Chicago Press.

Bloom, Samuel W. 1973. *Power and Dissent in Medical School*. New York: Free Press.

Bok, Derek. 1984. "Needed: A New Way to Train Doctors." *Harvard Magazine* 96:32–43, 70–71.

Broadhead, Robert. 1982. *The Private Lives and Professional Identities of Medical Students*. New York: Transaction.

Conrad, Peter. 1986. "The Myth of Cut-Throats among Premedical Students: On the Role of Stereotypes in Justifying Failure and Success." *Journal of Health and Social Behavior* 27:150–60.

Coombs, Robert H. 1978. *Mastering Medicine*. New York: Free Press.

Culliton, Barbara J. 1984. "Medical Education under Fire." *Science* 226:419–20.

Grant, Linda. 1988. "The Gender Climate of Medical School: Perspective of Women and Men Students." *Journal of the American Medical Women's Association* 43:109–19.

Haas, Jack and William Shaffir. 1987. *Becoming Doctors: The Adoption of a Cloak of Competence*. Greenwich, CT: JAI.

Harrison, Michelle. 1982. *A Woman in Residence*. New York: Random House.

Illsley, Raymond. 1975. "Promotion to Observer Status." *Social Science and Medicine* 9:63–75.

Klass, Perri. 1987. *A Not Entirely Benign Procedure: Four Years as a Medical Student*. New York: Putnam.

Konner, Melvin. 1987. *Becoming a Doctor: A Journey of Initiation in Medical School*. New York: Viking.

LeBaron, Charles. 1982. *Gentle Vengeance: An Account of the First Year at Harvard Medical School*. New York: Penguin.

Lief, Harold I. and Renee C. Fox. 1963. "Training for 'Detached Concern' in Medical Students." Pp. 12–35 in *The Psychological Basis of Medical Practice*, edited by H.I. Lief, V. Lief, and N.R. Lief. New York: Harper and Row.

McCall, Timothy B. 1988. "The Impact of Long Working Hours on Resident Physicians." *New England Journal of Medicine* 318:775–79.

Merton, Robert K. 1973. "The Perspectives of Insiders and Outsiders." Pp. 99–136 in *The Sociology of Science*. Chicago: University of Chicago Press.

Merton, Robert K., George G. Reader, and Patricia L. Kendall. 1957. *The Student Physician: Introductory Studies in the Sociology of Medical Education*. Cambridge, MA: Harvard University Press.

Reilly, Phillip. 1987. *To Do No Harm: A Journey through Medical School*. Dover, MA: Auburn House.

Shem, Samuel. 1978. *House of God*. New York: Richard Merek.

Smith, Allen C. III and Sherryl Kleinman. 1988. "Managing Emotions in Medical School: Students' Contacts with the Living and the Dead." Paper presented at the meetings of the American Sociological Association, Atlanta.

Stoeckle, John D. 1987. "Physicians Train and Tell." *Harvard Medical School Alumni Bulletin* 61 (Winter): 9–11.

X, Dr. 1965. *Intern*. New York: Harper and Row.

[28]

Soc. Sci. Med. Vol. 20, No. 2, pp. 133–143, 1985
Printed in Great Britain

0277-9536/85 $3.00 + 0.00
Pergamon Press Ltd

PROFESSIONAL SOCIALIZATION AND SOCIAL CONTROL: FROM MEDICAL STUDENTS TO GENERAL PRACTITIONERS*

ISABELLE BASZANGER

CNRS, Centre d'Etude des Mouvements Sociaux, 54 Boulevard Raspail, 75270 Paris, Cedex 06, France

Abstract—Most American research considers the assimilation of the norms and values of a given profession to be the most important way in which that profession controls the socialization of its future members. This view of social control is based on a problematic pattern of socialization. Using the results of a research into the socialization of general practitioners, a different approach to this problem of social control is suggested that takes into account the specific manner of integration into the university–hospital structures and the ways in which future doctors gain access to the professional world. The hospital with its scientific logic is thus the chief instrument of social control, even though this control is limited by the very nature of the hospital: hospital training only partly controls the application of this scientific knowledge by general practitioners.

The question of social control is at the centre of problems of professional socialization. To study the period of schooling that opens the way to a profession involves asking how the profession sets its boundaries and determines its identity through mechanisms for granting or refusing admission to would-be members. This questioning leads even farther: what means does the professional group use in its attempt to make these members conform to a model that is proposed and shared by the profession? Finally, inquiry about this period of schooling must assess the implementation and effectiveness of these means by taking into account the active roles of those who are to be socialized. Professional socialization, social control and deviance are closely related topics.

Studies of professional socialization have implicitly raised questions about mechanisms for reproducing the profession. The reason for this becomes clear if we recall that among the formal criteria for defining a trade or craft as a profession are education and training. According to Freidson, what distinguishes a profession is "its legitimate, organized autonomy", the fact that

> "professions are *deliberately* granted autonomy, including the exclusive right to determine who can legitimately do its work and how it should be done" [1, p. 72].

By its essence, a profession must define and *control* the education that leads to membership. Therefore, it has an active part in the mechanisms of socialization.

The medical profession has often been considered the archetype of the professions. Questions about professional socialization have crystallized around it. During the mid-1950s in the United States, the concerns of sociologists converged with the interests of the medical profession in training, through a new curriculum, the best possible physicians. The now classical research studies, which came out of this juncture [2,3] started from different theoretical standpoints but elaborated a common approach to basic questions such as: how are students transformed into phsicians? and: how much does the profession control this transformation?

The present article examines the answers given to these questions. After a close look at the model of professional socialization that these studies, beyond their differences, have proposed, the problems raised by it are explicated.

THE ASSIMILATION OF VALUES AS A MECHANISM OF CONTROL?

The functionalist position hypothesizes that schooling is the key moment in professional socialization. Once and for all during this period, the profession takes control over its members by initiating them into their new culture. According to Merton, who develops this hypothesis,

> "The profession of medicine... has its own normative subculture, a body of shared and transmitted ideas, values and standards toward which members of the profession are expected to orient their behaviour. The subculture, then, refers to more than habitual behaviour; its norms codify the values of the profession" [4, p. 71].

These values and norms define the requirements of the physician's role [5]. Since many doctors, during practice, face situations in which they can hardly live up to these requirements, they have had to acquire exactly those values that have been made for regulating their behaviour.

> "... the effective acquisition of these values by medical students is not a matter only of 'medical ethics' which attaches significance to these values in their own right. They can be considered, quite neutrally and without reference to their undoubted ethical status, in terms of their instrumental significance for the effective provision of health care.... They are, presumably, values which serve as effective means to a socially important end... [namely] facilitating sound medical practice.... Medical schools are socially defined as the guardians of these values and norms. The schools have the double function of transmitting to students the cognitive standards of knowledge and skill and the moral standards of values and norms" [4, pp. 76–77].

---

* This article was published in altered form in *Revue fr. Sociol.* **22**, 223–245, 1981. I wish to thank J. D. Reynaud for his helpful comments.

Accordingly, the functionalists investigate how the medical student acquires these norms, which, by definition, enable him to function efficaciously. Merton defines socialization as

"the process through which individuals are inducted into their culture. It involves the acquisition of attitudes and values, of skills and behaviour patterns making up social roles established in the social structure" [4, pp. 40–41].

The student's education is, we might say, certified by his acquirement of an internal balance between paired norms with both of which, as a practitioner, he will hardly be able to comply [6]. This balance places the new doctor squarely within his peers' system of values. The socializing institution thus controls young physicians who 'think, act and feel' [4, p. 7] like members of the profession.

Unlike functionalists, symbolic interactionists deny the possibility of a general theory of the professions, which they consider to be the objects of daily practices [7, 8]. There is no predefined professional role that students must learn to play. The authors of *Boys in White* concentrate upon the educational institution and upon the 'student' status. Medical students are not so much junior professionals as members of a subordinate group who are striving to adapt to and succeed in a very hierarchical organization.

"The young man finds out quite soon that he must learn first to be a medical student; how he will act in the future, when he is a doctor, is not his immediate problem" [3, p. 5].

Like other persons in large organizations, students have to set their 'levels and directions of effort' [3, p. 9] As a group in medical school, they draw up (sometimes covert) strategies in order to graduate. Becker *et al.* show how they develop a subculture that provides them with a degree of autonomy from authoritarian demands. This autonomy is important for the control that the profession exercises over education. What is definitively disproven is that students, passive like modelling clay, let the school socialize them. Their degree of autonomy limits the extent and nature of the profession's control.

"One thing is certain, they never develop exactly as the faculty would wish them to" [9, p. 197].

Although *Boys in White* shows how student autonomy limits professional control, it does not demonstrate how a minimum of social regulation occurs. Of course, the authors do not directly reason in these terms, for socialization is taken to be a situational adjustment students are socialized into the institution or, in the authors' words, 'institutionalized'. To face up to situations after graduation, new adjustments will be necessary. The experiences earned at medical school will be of little use. Here, interactionism runs up against a general difficulty: how to conceive the continuity between these situations? Although interactionists meticulously describe actors' adjustments over time within a given situation, yet time is 'pin-pointed'—it is taken to be the immobile framework of the situation that calls for adjustments. In *Boys in White*, this lapse in continuity opens a gap between present and future.

To account for a minimum of social regulation, the authors of this book implicitly reformulate the problem in terms of the internalization of values. Merton's definition is relativized through the idea of a selective assimilation of the medical culture. As they internalize this culture's key values such as responsibility and clinical experience, students redefine them with respect to their immediate situation. The final word is that professional values, particularly the core value of medical responsibility, are assimilated.

Beyond their differences, functionalists and interactionists admit that the acquirement of values by students is a mechanism of social regulation. Within the present article, a single value—medical responsibility—will be used to discuss this problematic assertion. This discussion will throw light upon the consequent limitations of the hypothetical model of professional socialization. The results of a survey [10] about the socialization of general practitioners, (GPs) will be used to propose another approach to the problem of the control exercised by the profession during the socialization of members-to-be.

According to both of these theoretical approaches, there is a medical culture that has no contact with the 'lay' world. Students have to discover and internalize this culture's key values so that they may, in turn, participate in it. But to what extent do they actually have to learn—discover and assimilate—a value such as responsibility? In the lay world, this value pervades the image of medicine. No studies are needed to prove this. Literature of all sorts, television serials and movies portray medical responsibility in the form of a conflict between the physician as a private person and as a dutiful professional. Of course, his principal duty is to take full care of 'his' patients. Detective novels even go so far as to 'catch' doctors in the act of becoming irresponsible. Many other images could be called to mind that show doctors being crushed under the weight of the responsibilities that they have to assume.

Apparently, medical students do not need to learn this value; rather, they have to learn how to use it within a professional practice. They are confronted with—and socialized through—the way that the profession actually functions. This functioning has more to do with the profession's practices and hierarchy than with its values in themselves. In the passage about pairs of norms, Merton hints at the necessity of learning to redefine a situation:

"For each norm there tends to be at least one coordinate norm, which is, if not inconsistent with the other, at least sufficiently different as to make it difficult for the student and the physician to live up to them both" [4, p. 72].

Medical education teaches students how to blend incompatible norms into a whole that works consonantly. Physicians have apparently learned to balance these pairs of norms, but how is this balance achieved? From norm to coordinate norm is a continuum that makes it possible to explain all shades of attitudes. Beyond its legal and lay implications, is the physician's responsibility so 'dramatic' if anything at all can be justified?

If responsibility is taken to be only a value, a confusion tends to arise between, on the one hand, responsibility in the practical, factual sense of the word (and in this sense, it is not the prerogative of the medical profession alone) and, on the other hand, the way responsibility as a value is used by the profession. Finding out whether students directly assimilate or else redefine such a value would probably not be of much help. As Becker *et al.* suggest, what separates medical students and physicians is not so much the conception of responsibility as their relative positions in a ranking system. These positions on the profession's hierarchical ladder create various possibilities for assuming responsibility.

ANOTHER APPROACH TO SOCIALIZATION: THE CASE OF GENERAL PRACTITIONERS

A problematic model of socialization

Beyond differences, the functionalist and interactionist model of socialization assigns much weight to the period of education. There are, however, three problems with this model. In the first place, it postulates, at the start of the socialization process, a 'lay' student body that has no past, is extrinsic to the medical profession and only exists in opposition to it. Secondly, it also posits a homogeneous but incomplete socializing institution since it leaves out of the picture other - predominant - functions (medical care and research) of the hospital system. As a consequence, the status of students is not analysed in terms of their position within this institution's division of labour. These overlooked functions, in fact, determine a productive role for students within the hospital organization. Finally, this model delineates a unique process limited to a precise period, namely the time of schooling as a sequence of events programmed by the institution. Although, as mentioned, these two dominant theoretical approaches analyse the content of the socialization process differently, both of them make this process and schooling perfectly overlap and, as a result, globally assess socialization without referring either to the actual practice of medicine or to professional integration. Hence, choices determining the nature of this integration are not taken into account. In this model, the outcome of the educational process is a new entity: the physician, or rather the ideal type of physician.

Any attempt to more accurately describe this ideal type runs up against the diversity of real doctors. Nowadays, diversity rather than uniformity characterizes the medical profession. Look at the way the profession is organized so that distinctions are made in terms of both external structural variables (types of practices, forms of payment for services) and internal ones (specialties). Even the specialties are subdivided into professional 'segments' [11] each of which defines for its members components of the physician's role. All this puts the ideal type of physician in its place.

Functionalist and interactionist research has systematically emphasized the homogeneity of this role and the cohesion of its components. The concept of professional socialization has thus been transformed into a model -- an act that has theoretical implications. The principal one is that reality is made not richer but poorer. The coherency of the proposed model presupposes the exclusion of social actors as such. Students come into this model only to be, more or less passively, socialized -- to learn the values of the profession rather than those of professionals. Doctors and professors are only bearers of norms whose attachment to widely different practices is not taken into account. Furthermore, the relationship that brings students and faculty together is not really clarified. The socialization process is isolated from the underlying network of social relations, whether inside or outside the profession. As a result, what had been but a means for dealing with the diversity of social reality is reified.

This set of difficulties led me to bring medical education and professional integration together in order to deal with the processes of socialization. These processes cannot be reduced to the period of schooling that all physicians have had in common. They must be analysed at least up to the point at which both rather definite career choices are made and professional integration has effectively begun. In this article, professional socialization refers less to the process for training professionals than to the mechanisms that lead to exercising a profession. In the case of medicine, these mechanisms involve the student's choice of an academic discipline and, within it, the way that he as a new doctor will actually practise medicine.

Such an analysis entails studying how young physicians set up professional practice. Regardless of the chosen discipline, professional integration can occur in various ways that depend upon the individual's choices, which are the outcome of what can be called a process of professional socialization. Young doctors' career lines have been staked out upon a common field because of the organization both of schooling (universities and hospitals) and of the profession (replacing colleages and setting up practice); but other forces (having to do with previous socialization or participation in extracurricular activities) continually pull upon these lines and reshape this field. This constant interaction of forces from various, sometimes conflictive, sources (such as the faculty, hospitals, professional segments and personal roots) either helps or hinders the student physician on his way toward his first professional practice. Owing to this interaction, career lines running across this field of forces cannot be projected into a single meeting point, at graduation for instance. The socialization processes have many outcomes.

This conception of professional socialization has been applied, herein, to GPs. Before delving into explanations, a few comments are necessary to describe the French medical system, particularly of education.

The 1958 reform of medical education and hospital structures [12] has oriented the whole system around two poles: general medicine and university-related teaching hospitals (*centres hospitalo-universitaires*, hereafter *CHUs*). Whereas CHU doctors are the dominant group in the medical profession, general medicine has been gradually pushed out onto the fringes of the CHUs to the point of becoming a secondary discipline, which is mainly used to sort out or deselect candidates so that specialized services are not overloaded. Although general medicine is principally exercised outside hospitals, all doctors are trained in CHUs.

At the time of the survey [13], medical education

was organized as follows. The first level includes 2 years of undergraduate study in basic sciences. The second level comprises 4 years of which the first is also devoted exclusively to basic sciences but each of the other three, to both lectures in the classroom and clinical training in the CHU. During these 3 years, students are officially *étudiants-hospitaliers*, 'hospital students'. All student physicians go though the same first two levels of education. During a third one-year long level, they undergo, in the CHU, a training period (*stage interné*) that presumably enables them to exercise general medicine. Actually during this seventh year of schooling, they have no clinical responsibilities. Their experiences are much the same as whenever they were hospital students. For this reason, most of those wanting to do general medicine try to learn how to practise it by replacing private practitioners. After this seventh year, students graduate as physicians. Some of them may decide to specialize by obtaining a CES degree (*Certificat d'Etudes Spécialisées*) after, on the average, 4 more years. They have to pass, each year, examinations and, in the last year, a national examination in their specialties.

So far medical education in France does not fundamentally differ from that in other Western countries. There is one noteworthy difference however: specialists can be trained through a second program. Through an extremely competitive examination, the *concours de l'Internat* (not to be confused with internship), the CHUs recruit candidates for training as future staff-members. Only students who have passed the *Internat* may pursue careers in the CHUs and expectantly enter the profession's elite [14]. To sit for this examination, students have to have been admitted to the third year of the second level. In other words, the decision is normally made before the completion of this level common to all medical students. Academic destinies, or fates, differ depending on choices at this point. Stopping our analysis here, before students' careers diverge and before they obtain any professional qualification, would lead us to posit an ideal type of physician.

The way medical education is organized reflects the way the health system is organized: at one end, the CHU elite and, at the other, GPs. This organization incited me to study the socialization of GPs rather than of specialists for several reasons. First of all, a critical phase of student GPs' training takes place outside the CHUs during replacements. Whenever they seek out replacements of practising GPs, their socialization process does not coincide with the period of schooling and is no longer organized by the CHU. Secondly, GPs constitute the category of professionals that the socializing institution does not train for itself. Since general medicine is practised privately as a 'liberal profession' (in other words, by self-employed professionals), GPs as such are seldom present in the hospitals. Students in general medicine hardly have a glimpse at their future role as long as they stay within the CHU. This institution does not directly furnish the GP role with contents.

In spite of being the largest group within the medical profession, GPs, often presented as the profession's unwanted children, have been pushed out onto the fringes of the hospital system. Therefore, understanding how the socializing institution exercises control is essential. Since the hospital system does not need them for its staff, does it not deliberately treat them like rejects from a socialization process that has not been made for them? Or on the contrary but for the same reason, does the profession have other means of controlling their education and training? Not provided by the hospital institution itself, these means might come into play in other places and during other phases.

Loosely structured interviews of GPs at the start of practice seemed to be the most appropriate way to find answers to these questions. The aim was to sketch biographies [15] over a period of more than 10 years. For analysis, I retained 37 interviews with GPs who were setting up or had just set up private practice as well as a few other interviews with GPs who were postponing this act. During interviews, parallels were drawn between events having to do with medical education and those related to extracurricular or background factors. To 'ground' [16] my interpretation in the everyday reality of medical school, I spent a quarter in a Parisian CHU and, particularly, in a service specialized in blood diseases [17]. Phases during the process for socializing GPs were thus discerned and will now be briefly described in relation to questions about control over training.

Medical school years

At the centre of medical education, the CHUs bring together functions of teaching, research and professional practice. They follow an internal logic, or rationality, that does not place teaching at the top of their priorities. Moreover, these other functions make demands on students. The 'hospital student' status is defined, in fact, by a socializing institution that differs significantly from other academic institutions. Because of its specificity, roles can become ambiguous; and conflicts arise. The student status does not necessarily count above all else, for students have a productive role in the CHUs.

This institution provides two formally recognized situations for training: during doctors' rounds with students and during students' duties on wards. GPs vividly recalled these eventful situations during which minimal socialization occurs. The implicit contradiction in the 'hospital student' status is part of these situations. During the rounds, students are reminded that they are 'students'. They remain passive. During ward duty on the contrary, they are active and, in many ways, productive.

Students' activities follow the beat of the ward rounds. There are usually three a week: one by the *chef de clinique*, one by the *agrégé* and one by the *chef de service* [14]. The 'grand round' by the last normally brings together doctors from all ranks. It is part of medical folklore. With their patients' records in hand, students must be ready to answer any and all questions. Wishing to go unnoticed, they usually cluster as far as possible from the *chef*, an act that reflects their objective position in the ranking order. Notwithstanding that they do not receive from these rounds the impression of participating in medical care or in hospital activities, they do thus learn—mainly through watching—various ways to behave toward patients. For instance, they observe how to neutralize patients by disqualifying what they say or how to act toward those who are held blameworthy for their condition (e.g. alcoholism). During rounds, some students come to see how far certain values, including responsibility, exalted in discourse are from the reality of medical practices.

All students are required to spend a given number of hours on duty in the hospital. These hours are scheduled by the wards or by the hospital itself (in admissions or on the emergency ward). Assignments of the latter sort, so-called 'door duty', occur more frequently. Time spent on duty provides an opportunity for training. The student evaluates cases (an act that is not among his daily chores), has the chance to learn technical gestures and manipulations and, often, has firsthand contact with patients (even if during emergencies) in the absence of any intermediary from the medical hierarchy, apart from nurses. Because of the hospital setting, these experiences are not identical to what happens when a patient goes to a GP's private office. Nonetheless ward and door duties are symbolically important for the formation of a professional identity.

For the institution, this student–patient contact carries a risk that the CHU assumes in order to push students to 'take the leap'. Besides, the hospital has the means to make up, the next day, for any mistakes (at least we hope so). Through its hierarchical organization, the socializing institution allows students to play a minimal role. The first role that the student physician tries is that of hospital doctor. The importance of ward and door duty reaches even farther inasmuch as students may assume responsibility in the factual sense of the word. Although time spent on duty is necessary to the running of hospitals, it is also organized to enable students "to acquire a good experience of what must and must not be done in emergencies" [18, p. 11].

A reservation has to be made about control by the profession over this phase of the socialization process. Given the present day conditons under which most of the hours on ward or door duty are spent, the profession does not fully control the earned experiences. Although a student's evaluations and actions during door duty may be contradicted by staff-doctors the next day, he will hear nothing about these criticisms because he will have been assigned for duty on a ward!

Ward or door duty and the rounds are the two high points of socialization within the institution, but the way a student is socialized depends upon his personal adjustments and choices, which the CHU does not necessarily control. Unlike the United States, in the 1950s, the socializing institution in France does not offer students a highly organized program. As mentioned previously, it has established two thresholds where decision must be made, namely whether or not to sit for the *Internat* examination and whether or not to specialize by enrolling in a program for the CES degree. Before one or both of these decisions, which must be made respectively starting in the fifth year or at the end of the sixth year of medical school, students make other choices that characterize their personal adjustments to the hospital system. For instance, they have to choose the wards on which, as hospital students, they want to work. These choices are, of course, restricted within the limits set by academic requirements; but there is room for maneuvering within these limits.

Why is this so? Because the CHUs as university-related hospitals have not been made for the bulk of students. They have developed research and teaching functions, but mainly for members of the medical élite whose careers are grounded, through the *Internat*, within the CHUs themselves. The model of professional integration proposed by this socializing institution emphatically distinguishes between, on one hand, the *internes* who have passed the *Internat* and, on the other, the second- and third-level students in hospital training. Because of this distinction, students have room for drawing up strategies of adaptation more or less independently of the CHU. Lacking clearly defined roles and positions, they have to 'learn' the hospital—how to obtain instruction and what activities to perform. Each student must adapt himself and create his program. In this sense, his socialization within the institution lies in his own hands.

Three types of student adjustments to the hospital system have been constructed out of field work and interviews. Unlike the situational adjustments described by the authors of *Boys in White*, which come out of negotiations between students (or rather a student body) and the faculty, these three types are personal, or individual, implicit means of 'staying above water'. The most frequent way that a student adjusts is to adapt offhandedly, when necessary. This is all the easier inasmuch as hospital students have a position or status in default or for want of anything better having been prepared by the socializing institution. In this first type of adjustment, the student's integration into a hospital service depends upon the reception that he is given. This adjustment is more an effect than a cause of integration. A second type emphasizes the student role to the detriment of any integration. For instance, the student does his job well but unenthusiastically or even refuses 'the least little effort'. Students who are critical of the hospital system often adopt this strategy. Having staked out a place for themselves on its fringes, they are less responsive to hierarchical differences and less sensitive to their own position. A third type of adjustment occurs less often [19]. Using a 'parasitic' tactic, the student makes the most of any opportunities for receiving training or assuming responsibility. He takes his fate into his hands and pushes back the limits that the institution has set on his role.

Although these types of adjustments cannot be expounded herein, attention must be drawn to the value of external factors for explaining them. Among these factors that lie outside the CHUs and beyond their logic, some have to do with the medical profession but not with the socializing institution. For instance, an attraction toward general medicine leads some students to enroll in medical school although they have not been adequately prepared to know how to 'decipher' the hospital system and make room for themselves therein. Attracted to general medicine through the example of (usually distant) relatives or even through childhood experiences with a family doctor, such a student usually adjusts offhandedly to each new situation as it crops up. In fact, most students who adopt the first strategy of adjustment are, in social terms, far removed from medical circles. Another external factor is involvement in nonmedical activities, such as outside jobs, student unions, politics or religious groups. These commitments incline students toward the third type of adjustment. By diversifying the participant's experiences and — unlike his student status — providing him with social 'roots', these activities furnish him with a framework for analysing the reality that he faces as a student. He adapts to — but does not necessarily intend to become part of — the CHU. Accordingly, he tries, for instance, to maximize his learning experiences by taking training in a second-class hospital where he will have more and broader duties. His decision is not motivated by any ambition for a hospital career since he is too 'far' from the best hospital services.

These external factors weigh upon the decision whether or not to become a GP and elucidate for us the choice between two different paths that each student has to make when deciding whether to sit for the *Internat* [20]. If he prepares for this examination, he will scarcely have time for any other activity. External factors carry their full weight here. His decision is often expressed in terms of life-styles, personal interests, family concerns, etc. In short, he chooses 'not to sacrifice his life'. The decision to study for the *Internat* involves more than temporarily or permanently giving up other interesting activities. It is a choice between not only two different paths but two different worlds. Perhaps *vis-à-vis* such an alternative, factors having to do with personal lives and relations carry decisive weight upon whatever choice is made [21]. Integration into these two worlds is at stake. The one world — the medical hierarchy and élite — is more distant. Relations, friends and family make it seem nearer and integration possible for students who choose the path leading to hospital careers. To most interviewed GPs however, nothing was offered as a counterpart for their involvement in activities and groups outside the medical profession. Their decision not to sit for the *Internat* seldom ran up against any obstacle. It was backed by arguments, in common to most students, about rejecting hospital medicine along with its way of dispensing care and, especially, its ranking order. The dead weight of hierarchical relations borne by students tips the scales: the hospital and its doctors serve as a negative model.

The professional élite uses the position or status assigned to hospital students in default as a means of selecting its future members. This selection relies upon students' direct choice 'not to become like them' — like hosital doctors. Thereby, students refuse to adapt to the model of a physician that the socializing institution has made for itself. A first selection — or deselection — takes place. The institution itself performs a second one — an elimination — through the *Internat* examination. This second selection is based more upon what candidates have learned than upon their readiness to adapt to the given model of behaviour.

The first step into the practice of general medicine: replacements

Although replacements are not obligatory, they constitute an informal phase — not organized by the CHUs — in the training of would-be GPs. Students who do not want to specialize usually seek out opportunities for replacing practising GPs. These replacements follow the guidelines laid down by the *Conseil de l'Ordre des Médecins*, a sort of General Medical Council. The frequency of these opportunities argues in favour of an analysis of socialization that connects schooling to the beginning of professional integration. Students may replace GPs on appointed days or every day for up to 3 months. In private offices, pay conditions are, in principle, agreed upon by the two parties. In nonhospital-related clinics or dispensaries, the student substitutes are subject to the conditions that govern all employees.

In the careers of prospective GPs, these replacements are a critical phase that lies outside the socializing institution. Since the CHUs do not, as such, include representatives of general medicine in their ranks, would-be GPs find out, during replacements, what general medicine is like and what its standards are. Most student substitutes have to create, if need be, and test their conceptual framework of general medicine in actual practice. This framework is constructed and reconstructed during replacements. This experience generates choices and leads to adjustments that emphasize certain dimensions in the role of GP that the substitute is trying to construct.

During replacements, students face a new situation — consultations in general medicine — which apparently raises few technical problems. The substitute has at his disposal the GP's files. By going over previously administered treatments, he is initiated to the prescriptions of general medicine. This source of information should not be overestimated since the GP is not there to explain his records, Moreover, the substitute, who seldom sees the sick person a second time, cannot evaluate the efficacy of treatment. Substitutes do not think that hospital pathology, to which they have been accustomed, and pathology in general medicine, which they are discovering, are worlds apart. They have new experiences to acquire, but basically, medical care — diagnosis and therapy — is the same as what they have observed in the CHUs. Replacements are training exercises during which substitutes adapt what they have learned to medical problems that, though new, lie on the same scientific continuum. From this point of view, no gulf separates hospital from general medicine.

Nonetheless, this new situation that substitutes face breaks with the one to which they have been accustomed in the CHUs. Even though the doctor still has a dominant role [22], the underlying social relationship is different. Besides, the student may not know how to handle this position of dominance. In any case, the sick person now has the possibility of imposing some of his own standards. Bargaining, or negotiation, occurs — the student has seldom, if ever, observed this in the CHU. In hospitals, the opinions of medical professionals carry more weight than those of the patients or of nonmedical personnel. Hospitals depend mostly upon a professional network of referrals in order to recruit patients. On the contrary, the private practitioner depends upon clients who choose, in conformity with their 'lay' conceptual framework, their doctor and try to affect the proposed therapy.

"In client-dependent practice, the patient is likely to be in the position of an equal or, at least, of an active participant in the process of diagnosis and management. Being in a relatively early stage of illness and not yet overcome by pain or fear, he always has before him (as the practitioner well knows) the prospect of leaving the office and, instead of coming back, of looking elsewhere for a consultant who uses more familiar notions of illness and treatment" [1, p. 307].

The problem for the substitute is to secure his position in this new social relationship. He might have trouble asserting his authority and professing a professional image. Interactions with clients are decisive, less because they are patients by professional standards than because they are ordinary people who have their own standards, different from those of the profession. Clients affect and even control, in yet another way, how the student substitute settles into this new social relationship.

The student physician uses the replaced doctor in an attempt to more clearly define the role of GP or else to corroborate his tentative definition of it. Because the replaced GP has very little contact with the substitute, the former serves less as a model for the latter than as an absent, positive or negative, reference mark as clients recall the replaced GP's explanations, treatments, prescriptions and habits. Of course, all this happens outside the CHUs, on the fringes of the professional world.

How much does the hospital system control this situation? Might the socializing institution not exercise, through the clients, control over how this social relationship is learned? Significantly, leaders of the medical profession, especially when they address the general public through the mass media, have publicly advocated a 'special dialogue' between 'the' doctor and 'his patient'. This two-sided relationship hardly characterizes doctor–patient contacts in hospitals. There, the patient is under the care of a medical team, not of a single doctor, and the doctor–patient relationship becomes lopsided. The 'special dialogue' refers to a different, practitioner–client, relationship that exists in general medicine. The perpetual propagation of this kind of discourse is neither an accident nor the sign that the deeds of hospital doctors lag behind their words. It is one of the means that the hospital segment of the profession uses in its attempt to control the nature of the relationship between GPs and their clients. In this way, the latter are socialized. By the kind of relationship that a client expects to have with his doctor, he is part of the process for socializing would-be GPs. Obviously, discourse about the special dialogue also aims at consolidating the scientific prestige of hospital medicine in the eyes of the general public and, by ricochet, among GPs.

Although the medical profession indirectly intervenes in this social relationship, it has nothing to say about the content of the GP's role. Every student, during replacements, has to define this role's content. Much of the GP's work is not open to view. It takes place behind closed doors within a closed relationship inside the doctor's office. Much room is left for the GP's individual initiative. He actively 'works up' the client. What the latter brings is raw data that not all doctors process in the same way. For instance, the client, while describing his physical symptoms, might mention problems at work—problems that the physician chooses or refuses to take into consideration during diagnosis. These raw data are variously processed depending upon the value attached to the academic and scientific knowledge that the socializing institution has furnished. Such decisions orient the way that medicine is exercised and the care that is dispensed [23].

These decisions are made under conditions in which students doing replacements must situate themselves in this new, client-dependent relationship. Money is a major dimension thereof. Nearly all interviewed GPs talked about how difficult it was at the start to face up to the resulting interdependency, which they were used to overlooking during hospital training. Owing to this difficulty, some of them even chose to work in clinics or dispensaries where patients do not directly pay the doctor.

What is really at stake, however, in this relationship is *the dequalification of general medicine.* More important than directly paying fees, the client imposes some of his own standards and thus defines the GP's work. For example, he asks his doctor to make a house call simply to renew a prescription. The client partly controls the situation. The content of the GP's workload is up for negotiation.

The hospital system also has means for designating the contents of the GP's job. As medical students in the CHUs see it, this job is on the fringes of medical care. For instance, when a client goes to a doctor's office to obtain a sick leave or vaccination certificate, the GP performs a chore that is peripheral to the tasks that the profession values. As students have observed, these chores are, in hospitals, left up respectively to the administration and to students (or even nurses). Once again, GPs fear lest their job be downgraded.

Facing this situation in which two parties—clients and hospitals—define their role, young GPs react by making career decisions. Different decisions, such as whether to work for fees or for a salary, spring from a single desire: to have control over their own work. Each choice can be a way of resisting this dequalification of general medicine and the downgrading of the general practitioner. The cleavage, recognized by the profession, between private practice for fees and employment on salary is, in fact, not pertinent to understanding young GPs' choices. Some doctors who actively support salaried employment have, given the actual organization of the health system, set up as private, self-employed ('liberal') professionals. They thus feel freer to define their work according to their own standards than if they were on salary. In short, young doctors have started using, to their own ends, this cleavage that the medical profession has interpreted as an alternative between two opposite health or even social systems: 'free vs bureaucratic' medicine. Unaware of GPs' concerns, the profession and, in particular, the socializing institution now seems so distant from the young GPs that it has 'produced'.

THE HOSPITAL SYSTEM AND ITS SCIENTIFIC LOGIC AS A MEANS OF SOCIAL CONTROL

In a way the socializing institution has failed to socialize GPs. Paradoxically, they make up the majority of the medical profession yet have been kept on the fringes of the hospital system. Graduates in general medicine seem to be much the same as they were when they were admitted to medical school. Confronted with various hospital situations during student years, they mainly adjusted offhandedly without changing their other involvements (especially with families and friends); or else in order to 'survive the hospital', they emphasized the student dimension of their role as 'hospital students'. Whenever they adjusted more willfully, their motivations tended to come from factors outside the profession. At first sight, young GPs seem not to have been much socialized by the CHUs. Replacements showed them to what extent their relationship to the medical school system was ambiguous. Experiences acquired during schooling do not enable them to solve the major problem awaiting them, namely the dequalification of general medicine.

There is no systematic relation between, on one hand, adjustments to the hospital (and the strategies underlying them) and, on the other, choices about how to practise medicine. The factors that affect students throughout their school years come from other sources (family, religion, student activism, etc.). This lack of correlation is not due to chance, at least not in the case of GPs. It corresponds to a reality: general medicine is not hospital medicine of a lesser quality. It has specific characteristics, in particular the client relationship, that students do not observe in hospitals.

Medical students do, however, become certified physicians. The socializing institution has successfully socialized GPs. Bedsides the forementioned ward and door duty or the rounds, the medical profession, as a social system, seems to have more durable means of exerting control over members than those used during schooling.

Even more than through imparting key values, the hospital system (along with the profession's elite) perpetuates its domination through its hierarchical organization and legitimating scientific logic. Regardless of student criticisms of the hospital system and of hospital medicine, this institution has an impact upon their careers. Besides serving as a negative model in the choice not to sit for the *Internat* examination, it also marks them in two other ways.

First of all, the hospital, shut off from the outer world, operates according to its own logic and its own internal organization, which leads students to perceive it as 'one big family' with inhouse rules. Daily activities are organized around the requirements of medical care, as stipulated by hospital doctors. In this sense, the hospital is a cozy place that has been made for the doctor rather than the patient. Under pressures that they did not learn how to bear in the CHUs, practising GPs become 'homesick' for this institution.

Secondly, the hospital system marks students for life outside its walls with its image as a place where a scientific logic is expounded. All students receive thoroughgoing education in basic sciences. Instruction tends to present medical problems from a theoretical approach that is fully developed in hospital medicine. Most students serve, at least once, on a ward where such an approach prevails. Even though they ridicule it ('Watch out! This is High Science!'), they nonetheless meet up with an intellectual process that tempts some of them toward the hospital system. The marks left by this meeting come out in students' remarks about being afraid of falling behind after graduation:

"I feel I'm going to go into reverse and regress intellectually, technically and practically. In other words, I'll no longer have, behind me, the whole system pushing me forwards".

As a place where advances in theoretical knowledge are made, the CHUs consolidate their superiority, even in the eyes of GPs who are cut off from them, through their scientific activities and the resulting intellectual prestige. The supremacy of hospital medicine and of its doctors over the whole medical profession is thus legitimated. As a reference mark for all physicians, this scholarship provides operational categories for diagnosing and treating illnesses. It matters little that these categories are criticized by some groups of GPs as being inapplicable in the exercise of general medicine or as being too narrow because they exclude other branches of knowledge, such as psychology.

What is also legitimated through this intellectual prestige is the right of hospital doctors to speak out as leaders of the profession, especially during discussions about health policies. The *Entretiens de Bichat*, a yearly conference that brings hundreds of GPs together at Bichat Hospital in Paris, illustrates this point. As it diffuses information about scientific advances to the lower ranks of the profession, this conference also reminds participants that discoveries are made in the CHUs. Through the mass media, which spend much time reporting on it, this conference also reminds patients and clients of the preeminence of the hospital and of its scientific medicine.

A FRENCH MODEL?

Before leaving the hospital system, students acknowledge this institution's superiority, which is founded upon the value attached to scholarship and upon the status socially assigned to abstract knowledge. GPs have been led to internalize the belief that the hospital segment of the medical profession has a monopoly over theoretical reflection. As GPs, they are excluded from the abstract except insofar as practical, e.g. therapeutic, applications are developed. What characterizes the French medical system is this separation between university-hospital doctors and GPs. The capacity for conceptualization and the stock of knowledge, both measured by the rungs that have been climbed in the professional hierarchy, are used to separate these two groups. Regardless of the latitude they have had in their choices, students, like members of other professional groups in the hospitals, observe how candidates for all positions in the hierarchy are sorted in compliance with a principle that takes knowledge to be a value. They make this observation even if they themselves are not among these candidates. The meaning of this principle is impressed upon them.

Although this research did not adopt a reasoning in terms of the university system, its career channels and selection processes, the question does arise: is the value attached to knowledge, both as a principle for selection and as a means of social control, not distinctive of the French system? In comparison, the American system does not so conspicuously separate hospital doctors from 'the others'. Of course, it also selects its members and places them in a ranking order; but bridges apparently exist between the extreme ends of the hierarchy. Unfortunately, there are no comparative data for assessing how the means of social control are modified as a result of these structural differences.

This distinctive trait of the French system brings to mind what Maurice, Sellier and Silvestre have called the 'principle of the extraction of élites'. Their comparison of companies in France and in West Germany has brought to light interactions between facts of organization and facts of socialization. Unlike in West Germany.

> "the logic of the educational system (and also of occupational training) is, in France, founded upon the principle of the extraction of elites... [In companies] qualified individuals, whether workers or engineers, must rise above the common and thus participate in the elites (which are at the top of every social stratum and socioeconomic category). Every such category produces its own elite stratum following a hierarchical model that this stratum constitutes and reproduces at the same time" [24, p. 223].

Considering all categories of physicians (in hospitals, in general practice or in privately practised specialties) that have been trained by the socializing institution, the French medical system seems to follow this principle. A curriculum in common to all students during the first 6 years of medical school not only determines career orientations but also guarantees the acquisition of the distinctive traits that the majority of physicians have in common [25]. A minimal socialization is achieved. Just as there is a category of white-collars whose occupational success depends upon their degree of integration in their companies, so also there is, in the hospitals, a category of specialists who have managed to adapt to the proposed model of a physician and to the institution's norms. Since the hospital system is not made for students, it is up to them to initiate their own process of socialization with respect both to this institution and to a hierarchy in which they have a place, we might say, through their exclusion. For various reasons, GPs have not accomplished this. The opposition between specialists and generalists can be likened to that between executive and nonexecutive personnel in a company.

Specialists who, until now, have been trained through one of two different channels (the *Internat* and the CES degree) are effectively integrated into the medical hierarchy through what Maurice *et al.* call a "community of socialization". As in companies, this community covers up a fracture within a category, in this case of specialists. Each of the forementioned channels provides its own opportunities for professional integration—into the hospital system through the *Internat* and into private practice through the CES.

CONCLUSION

GPs, in France, are led to position themselves within a ranking order by using the reference marks that the socializing institution (the CHUs) has furnished them during schooling. Once out of the hospital system, they form a peripheral, poorly socialized group that maintains limited relations with the profession's élite. This system that, through successive eliminations or deselections, assigns each person to his position brings to mind Hall's and Freidson's analyses of the organization of the medical profession. Hall [26] describes an inner fraternity of physicians who, at the height of success, controls admission into the community. Those who are admitted have certain—professional as well as social—characteristics and share certain values. Freidson extends this analysis by describing the profession's informal organization into small, homogeneous, exclusive circles. As he declares, "these colleague groups are built up by the mechanisms of patronage and boycott" [1, p. 194].

This comparison should not be made too hastily however. In the first place, Freidson's colleague groups do not fully correspond to specific disciplines. Secondly, the medical profession's formal organization in France definitely separates the private practice from the hospital practice of medicine. The peripheral position internalized by young GPs corresponds to their discipline's position within the profession's formal organization. This fact does not, of course, preclude the establishment of colleague groups upon which physicians' careers depend. What has been described herein is the first stage of socialization. Upon this backdrop, more subtle controls involving narrower segments of the medical profession come into play.

The control exercised by the profession's élite upon the socialization of GPs perhaps runs up against its limit at the very moment of professional integration. Although the intellectual prestige of scientific knowledge in hospitals serves as a means of social and professional control, the very utilization of this knowledge widens the gap between the two ends of the medical hierarchy. The knowledge acquired by GPs is organized in terms of categories having to do with the practice of hospital medicine which, as seen, is not much like that of general medicine. The GP has to find out how to fit what he has learned (in the form in which he has learned it) in with what he observes and experiences. This learning can be used in various ways to diagnose patients' symptoms. Nothing proves that the medical profession controls how this recently acquired academic knowledge is actually used during the exercise of general medicine [27]. The hospital segment of the medical profession sees GPs' patients only when they are referred to hospitals. GPs are relatively free in their decisions to refer patients. Like the students in *Boys in White*, they form a subordinate group; but the fact that they are kept at a distance from the CHUs leaves them room for maneuvering and for redefining their activities. For the profession's dominant strata, these activities are already clearly enough defined: GPs do the initial sorting of patients and serve a psychological support function. Nowadays most GPs do not silently accept this definition. Since 1973, this segment of the profession has formed new associations, in particular the *Société Française de Médecine Générale* and the *Syndicat de la Médecine Générale*.

Who then does set the boundaries between groups within the profession? By pushing GPs ever farther out onto the fringes of the health system, the hospital segment, which is responsible for socializing physicians, runs certain risks. More and more GPs tend to define themselves in terms not of hospital but of general medicine. They thus enlarge the definition of their activities. The base of the hierarchical pyramid is tending toward self-sufficiency.

The National Assembly's adoption in June 1979 of a plan for reforming medical education can be partly interpreted in the light of these tendencies within general medicine. This reform provides for a 2-year 'residency' period for GPs (after the first two levels of medical school that remain in common to all students). During this period that unlike the replacements described herein is to be organized by the CHUs, students will, in principle, have responsibilities during training both in hospitals and with practitioners. These provisions were maintained in a new bill for reforming medical education that was passed in the spring of 1983. Accordingly, the CHUs should keep full control over the education of GPs. Through this additional year of schooling, the CHUs should be able to reduce the distance between themselves and the places where the practice of medicine is learned. They should thus create a closer socializing relationship with students or at least try to be more directly involved whenever GPs begin being integrated into the profession and adjusting to the actual practice of medicine.

REFERENCES

1. Freidson E. *Profession of Medicine, A Study of the Sociology of Applied Knowledge.* Dodd, Mead, New York, 1970. See, in particular, Chap. 4.
2. Merton R., Reader, G. and Kendall P. (Eds) *The Student–Physician, Introductory Studies in the Sociology of Medical Education.* Harvard University Press, Cambridge, MA, 1957.
3. Becker H., Geer B., Hughes E. and Strauss A. *Boys in White, Student Culture in Medical School.* University of Chicago Press, Chicago, 1961.
4. Merton R. Some preliminaries to a sociology of medical education. In *The Student–Physician, Introductory Studies in the Sociology of Medical Education* (Edited by Merton R. *et al.*) pp. 8–80. Harvard University Press, Cambridge, MA, 1957.
5. About this role refer to: Parsons T. Social structure and dynamic process: the case of modern medical practice. In *The Social System.* Free Press, Glencoe, IL, 1951. Pages 428–480 in the 1964 pocketbook edition.
6. R. C. Fox shows how, during medical school, students acquire a 'concerned but not too concerned' attitude and learn to balance an excess of self-confidence with uncertainty. See: Fox R. C. The medical student's training for 'detached concern'. In *The Psychological Basis of Medical Practice* (Edited by Lief H., Lief V. and Lief N.), pp. 12–35. Harper & Row, New York, 1963. See also: Fox R. C. Training for uncertainty. In *The Student–Physician, Introductory Studies in the Sociology of Medical Education* (Edited by Merton R. *et al.*). pp. 207–244. Harvard University Press, Cambridge, MA, 1957.
7. Becker H. The nature of a profession. In *Education for the Professions, 61st Yearbook of the National Society for the Study of Education.* University of Chicago Press, Chicago, 1962.
8. Hughes E. *The Sociological Eye: Selected Papers.* Aldine, Chicago, 1971. Refer, in particular, to the third part.
9. Becker H., Geer B. and Miller S. Medical Education In *Handbook of Medical Education* (Edited by Freeman H., Levine S. and Reader L.) pp. 191–205. Prentice-Hall, Englewood Cliffs, NJ, 1972.
10. Baszanger I. Des généralistes en particulier: une approche biographique des processus de socialisation professionnelle. Doctoral dissertation, presented at the Ecole de Hautes Etudes en Sciences Sociàles, Paris, 1979.
11. See Butcher R. and Strauss A. Profession in process. *Am. J. Sociol.* **46,** 325–334, 1971.
12. Jamous H. *Sociologie de la Décision: La Réforme des Etudes Médicales et des Structures Hospitalières.* CNRS, Paris, 1969.
13. A reorganization, not yet clearly defined, is under way. Two major changes are in the works: more thorough going training for future GPs and unifying the training of specialists.
14. A *concours* is a competitive examination which, under merit system principles, is used to select the highest scoring candidates to fill a preset number of positions. The *concours de l'Internat* is used to recruit students to fill positions as *internes* at the bottom of the CHU ranking system. After 4 years of training, these *internes* (not to be confused with English 'interns'), if they are not appointed as *chefs de clinique*, usually set up private practices in their specialties. Those who manage to stay in the hospital system, specifically in the CHUs, by obtaining this appointments may aspire, over the years, to become *agrégés* or, ultimately, *chefs de service*. English equivalents of these French terms could, at best, be approximate. They have not been given lest the reader be induced in error. The types of education and training provided through the *Internat* and the CES programs are quite different. The student who is preparing for the CES degree receives, in his chosen specialty, advanced theoretical instruction and 'attends' the hospital but has no actual duties there. In contrast, the student who has passed the *Internat*, which tests theoretical knowledge, receives 4 more years of thorough clinical training and, under the supervision of superiors, does much of the daily work in hospital services.
15. About the biographical approach, see: Becker H. S. The life-history in the scientific mosaic. Introduction to Shaw C. *The Jack-Roller: A Delinquent Boy's Own Story*, pp. v–xviii. University of Chicago Press, Chicago, 1966.
16. Obviously, I am referring to the groundwork laid down by Glaser B. and Strauss A. S. *The Discovery of Grounded Theory.* Aldine, Chicago, 1967.
17. For the participant observation method, I am much indebted to R. C. Fox [6] and to the authors of *Boys in White* [3].
18. Meillière D. *La Formation des Médecins.* Editions Lab. Sandoz, Paris, 1975.
19. This discussion concerns only GPs. All medical students can, of course, adjust in these ways. The proportion of all students who adjust in the third way is certainly higher than that of those destined to become GPs. Students who, planning to sit for the *Internat*, strive to be integrated into the hospital system often adjust in a fourth way: they try to be assigned on wards where 'hospital students' are neither wanted nor needed so that they can study full-time for the examination.
20. From the institution's viewpoint, the student who graduates at the end of the normal course of instruction becomes a GP. He has no choice to make other than the initial one namely to enroll in medical school. The interviews, however, show that GPs deliberately decided not to sit for the *Internat*. They did not fail it. From the individual's viewpoint, a positive, voluntary choice is made. It consists in deciding to join a dominated segment of the medical profession. It means staying at the bottom of the hierarchical ladder, which others are climbing. Notwithstanding that the socializing institution does not miss a chance—through words or deeds—to remind students of this, general medicine is not the haven of sloths or flunkers.
21. About the influence of friends, family and close relations, see Hall O. The stages of a medical career *Am. J. Sociol.* **53,** 327–336, 1948.

22. Freidson E. *Professional Dominance, the Social Structure of Medical Care.* Atherton Press, New York, 1970.
23. My thesis (see [10]) proposes four ways GPs define themselves. Each one is the outcome of socialization processes. This typology leads us too far from the problem of social control, the subject of this article. These four definitions (the doctor as a dispenser of medical care, the doctor as a guide, the total doctor of the total person and the community doctor) involve dimensions such as the importance attached to academic knowledge during diagnoses, the self-assigned position in the dispensing of medical care, and the conception of general medicine.
24. Maurice M., Sellier F. and Silvestre J-J. *Production de la Hiérarchie dans l'Entreprise: Recherche d'un Effet Sociétal, Allemagne-France.* LEST, Aix-en-Provence, 1977.
25. "During the competition that ranks students [between the end of primary school and the end of secondary school]... the major distinctive traits, which future workers have in common, are shaped. Post-secondary education... is but the prolongation of this process of stratification beyond the secondary level". Quoted from p. 340 of Maurice M., Sellier F. and Silvestre J-J. La production de la hiérarchie dans l'entreprise: recherche d'un effet sociétal, comparison France-Allemagne. *Revue fr. Sociol.* **20,** 331–336, 1979. Of course, this quotation holds for medical school too.
26. Hall O. Types of mecial careers. *Am. J. Sociol.* **55,** 243–253, 1949.
27. For Hughes, the culmination of the socialization processes occurs whenever professionals bring what they have learned back into interactions with the 'lay' culture. See Hughes E. C. The making of a physician. In *Men and Their Work* pp. 116–130. Free Press, Glencoe, 1958.

[29]

Gender and Medical Socialization

STEVEN C. MARTIN
Albert Einstein College of Medicine

ROBERT M. ARNOLD
University of Pittsburgh

RUTH M. PARKER
Emory University

Journal of Health and Social Behavior 1988, Vol. 29 (December):333–343

Although both gender and professional socialization determine physicians' values, attitudes, and behaviors, the relative importance of each varies. Physicians' career paths demonstrate gender differences: women tend to choose primary care fields and rarely enter surgery, they are paid less and are less likely to be self-employed, and they are underrepresented in positions of authority within medical organizations and in academia. Data on practice style reveal striking similarities in physicians' attitudes toward patient care, knowledge, and clinical behavior, but recent work on physician-patient communication reveals important gender differences. These differences suggest that although medical socialization determines most aspects of practice style, a physician's gender can have an important influence on medical practice.

Sociologists display a growing appreciation for the complexity of interactions that determine professional values, attitudes, and beliefs. Earlier authors tended to emphasize either social background or professional socialization as the primary determinant of professional behavior. Recently, however, scholars have begun to stress that both factors are important, and that they act as *continuous* sources of socialization whose *relative* importance varies over time. In some instances new experiences may supplant or moderate the influence of earlier experiences; in others, prior experience may integrate the impact of new experiences. This conceptual model emphasizes that a dynamic balance between social background and professional socialization determines professional behavior (Bloom 1979; Colombotos and Kirchner 1986).

This analytic framework is well suited for examining physicians. Merton (1957, p. 287) defined socialization as "the process by which people selectively acquire the values and attitudes, the interests, skills, and knowledge—in short, the culture—current in the groups of which they are, or seek to become, a member." Female physicians must respond to the influence of two potent socializing forces; as a result some of their attributes are strikingly similar to those of their male colleagues, whereas others are markedly different. Over time some of these differences attenuate, while others emerge. Effective analysis of the similarities and differences among male and female physicians would require a longitudinal focus on the relative contributions of gender socialization and professional socialization.

Unfortunately, very few studies have adopted this conceptual approach. In the absence of such studies we have elected to

The authors thank Drs. Charles Bosk, John Colombotos, Peter Conrad, Fred Hafferty, Robin Leidner, Diana Long, Regina Morantz-Sanchez, Miriam Sudit, and Sankey Williams for their helpful advice; Julie Nissen for editorial assistance; and Merrilly Calabrese, Amy Laub, and Diane Pecorelli for their secretarial assistance.

Address correspondence to Steven C. Martin, M.D., Department of Epidemiology and Social Medicine, Belfer Bldg., Room 1308, Albert Einstein College of Medicine, 1300 Morris Park Avenue, Bronx, NY 10461.

review data about 1) the career paths and 2) the practice styles of female physicians. We use "career paths" in a broad sense to include specialty choice, practice setting, income, family structure, and professional status. By "practice style" we mean not only physicians' diagnostic and therapeutic approaches but also their behavior in their encounters with patients. These areas reveal important similarities and differences that suggest how gender and medical socialization interact to determine professionals' values, attitudes, and behaviors.

CAREER PATHS OF FEMALE PHYSICIANS

Demographics

Any discussion of gender and medical socialization must begin with the recognition that a fundamental demographic shift has occurred within medicine. In 1960, five percent of all medical school graduates were women, a number that had remained essentially unchanged for 50 years. In the mid-1960s, spurred by the feminist movement and by antidiscrimination legislation, women began to apply to medical school in larger numbers. By 1970 female medical school graduates had risen to 9.2 percent of the total; in 1985 nearly 31 percent of all medical graduates were women (Klepke, Marder, and Silberger 1987).

As medicine has become increasingly attractive to women, its appeal to men has declined. While the percentage of female college graduates applying to medical school increased from 0.8 percent in 1970 to the current rate of 2.3 percent, the percentage of male college graduates applying to medical school dropped from 4.9 percent to 4.2 percent (Klepke et al. 1987). As a result, United States medical schools currently have a smaller total applicant pool that is increasingly female.

The number of actively practicing female physicians reflects this trend. Between 1970 and 1985 the number of active male physicians grew by only 13 percent, while the number of actively practicing female physicians increased 240 percent. Women currently constitute approximately 15 percent of the physician population, a number that will continue to grow in the near future (Klepke et al. 1987).

Specialty Choice and Practice Setting

Female physicians have different career paths from male physicians. Although differences in the specialty choice of male and female residents appear to be decreasing as the number of female physicians increases, distinct patterns of specialty choice still exist. In 1985 nearly 70 percent of female residents, compared to approximately 50 percent of men residents, were training in the primary care fields of family practice, internal medicine, obstetrics-gynecology, pediatrics, and psychiatry. It is still rare for women to enter surgical specialties; only 5 percent of female residents trained in surgery during 1985 (Crowley, Etzel, and Shaw 1987).

In 1985 the specialties with the largest numbers of practicing female physicians were (in descending order) internal medicine, pediatrics, psychiatry, family practice, and obstetrics-gynecology. The large number of female pediatricians and the small number of female surgeons are the key sex differences in specialties among practicing physicians. For male physicians practicing in 1985, surgery was the second most common discipline, following only internal medicine and ahead of family practice, psychiatry, and obstetrics-gynecology (AMA Women in Medicine Project 1987).

Female physicians also choose different practice settings. They are more likely to locate their practices in physician-rich urban areas and disproportionately more likely to become employees rather than going into private practice (Bowman and Gross 1986). In 1986, 50 percent of all female physicians were self-employed, in contrast to nearly 80 percent of male physicians.

The greater demand for primary care practitioners in health maintenance organizations and institutional settings does not fully explain this difference, which is also found in fields with lower percentages of physician employees, such as surgery and obstetrics-gynecology. In every specialty (except anesthesiology), women are less likely to be self-employed than men (AMA Center for Health Policy Research 1987).

Historically, female physicians also have worked fewer weeks per year and fewer hours per week, and have been more likely than their male colleagues to interrupt their careers or to work part time. These differences appear to be declining, however. Recent studies reveal minimal differences between the number of weeks worked per year by male and by female physicians (Frieman and Marder 1984; Silberger, Marder, and Wilke 1987). Although the difference in hours worked per week also has decreased, with women increasing and men decreasing their hours, in 1986 male physicians still averaged 58.2 hours per week, compared to 52.2 hours for female physicians (AMA Center for Health Policy Research 1987).

The average male physician sees 15 percent more patients per week than his female counterpart. Although this difference is due partly to the number of hours worked per week, another major factor is the amount of time spent with individual patients. In a trend that is relatively consistent across specialties, females spent more time with patients, averaging 17 minutes per visit, in contrast to male physicians' average of 13 minutes per visit (U.S. Department of Health and Human Services 1984a).

Status of Female Physicians

Although the number of women in medicine is increasing dramatically and although women are assuming a larger role in patient care, they have not yet achieved equal status in the profession. The income of female physicians is significantly less than their male counterparts'; male physicians average a net yearly income of $118,000 and female physicians average $73,100. Both male physicians' income per hour and their income per visit are significantly higher than female physicians' at all stages of their careers (AMA Center for Health Policy Research 1987). Closer analysis of these figures reveals that these differences in income persist despite controlling for self-employed versus employee status, specialty, age, number of hours worked, and number of patients seen. Three different sophisticated analyses, using income data from 1973, 1977, and 1982 respectively, revealed that between 12 percent and 24 percent of the income difference between male and female physicians remained even after controlling for practice characteristics (Kehrer 1976; Langwell 1982; Ohsfeldt and Culler 1986).

Female physicians also are less likely to hold leadership positions in medical institutions or associations, and are less likely to join the AMA or other medical organizations ("AMA Insights" 1987). In a recent AMA survey, women said that the major reasons they did not join organizations were competing obligations and lack of time (Bowman and Gross 1986). Board certification provides another measure of status in the medical profession. Female physicians are less likely to be board certified; 57 percent of male physicians hold at least one board certification, in contrast to only 38 percent of female physicians. Social factors rather than ability may explain this difference because there are only minimal gender differences in pass rates for the internal medicine, pediatrics, and family practice boards (Brownlee and Butzin 1981; Ellsbury, Schneeweiss, Montano, Gordon, and Duykendall 1987; Norcini, Day, Shea, and Benson 1988).

An alternative measure of the status of female physicians is their position in medical schools. On graduating from medical school, women were more likely than men to choose academic medicine as a career path; this has been true since the 1960s. Even so, women have had greater difficulty than men in achieving promotion and tenure in academia. Data from the Association of American Medical Colleges Faculty Roster System (1987) revealed that among female medical school faculty members first appointed in 1976, 21.7 percent were not on the tenure track, compared to only 15.4 percent of the male academics. Of the full-time academic physicians on the tenure track, 16.6 percent of males had achieved tenure, whereas only 11.5 percent of the women were tenured. Moreover, a study of academic promotion patterns at four United States medical schools showed that at each school the average number of years to promotion for each faculty rank was consistently greater for women (Wallis, Gilder, and Thaler 1981).

The conclusion that women are underrepresented in positions of power is reinforced when one examines the number of women in senior academic administrative positions in medical schools. In the 1975–76 academic year there were no female deans of medical schools; females made up only 3.4 percent of the associate deans and 11.7 percent of the assistant deans. Although the figures have improved somewhat, in the 1986–87 academic year only 1.6 percent of all medical school deans, 9.6 percent of associate deans, and 20 percent of assistant deans were women. In 1987 female chairmen of medical school departments represented less than 5 percent of the chairs in both the basic and the clinical sciences, with a total of 29 in the basic sciences and 44 in the clinical sciences. Conversely, women are overrepresented in the lower echelons of academia (Association of America Medical Colleges 1987).

Family Structure

The family structures of male and female physicians are different. Several studies have revealed that female physicians are less likely to marry and less likely to have children (Callan and Klipstein 1981; Dickstein and Stephenson 1987; Mandelbaum 1978; Ogle, Henry, Durda, and Zivick 1986; Schermerhorn, Colliver, Verhulst, and Schmidt 1986; "Today's Woman, M.D." 1983). These data are particularly interesting because when surveyed at the end of medical school, 85 to 90 percent of both men and women stated that they would like to have children (Heins 1983).

The social roles within marriage also differ markedly for male and for female physicians. Among married physicians, for example, spouses of males were more likely than those of females to stay at home rather than to be employed outside the home. Among physicians without children, 70 percent of physicians' wives were employed outside the home, compared to 95 to 99 percent of physicians' husbands. Once a physician had a child, the numbers differed even more dramatically. The wives of male physicians with children were employed outside the home only 25 percent of the time, in sharp contrast to the unchanged 95 to 99 percent of husbands of female physicians who continued to work outside the home (Ogle et al. 1986).

Domestic responsibilities usually are delegated to women regardless of their occupational status. In one study, 50 percent of the wives of male physicians provided full-time child care; an additional 33 percent provided a major contribution to child care. In contrast, husbands of female physicians were the major source of child care only 0 to 5 percent of the time (Nadelson, Notman, and Lowenstein 1979). In a different study, three-quarters of female physicians surveyed said that they were responsible for housework in their homes. Even when the couple hired help, female physicians typically were expected to arrange day care and household assistance (Heins 1979). Not surprisingly, studies showed that female physicians, even those working over 80 hours per week, spent significantly more time on household chores than did their male counterparts (Landau, Hall, Wartman, and Marlo 1986).

Explaining Career Differences: The Importance of Gender

Although women are increasingly able to join the profession of medicine, their career paths differ from those of their male colleagues. Female physicians are more likely to enter less prestigious primary-care specialties, to work as employees within an organization rather than becoming self-employed, to earn less money, and to hold fewer influential positions in medical schools and other medical organizations. They marry less often and have fewer children than male physicians; within marriages, they shoulder the burden of domestic responsibilities.

Although discrimination cannot be ignored (Lorber 1984), women still must reconcile the imperatives of gender socialization with those of medical socialization. What is the relative importance of each? Gender socialization encourages traditional feminine values. Within medicine the primary care specialties emphasize empathy, nurturing, and communication. Women may be attracted to these fields because they fit better with their self-conception; it may feel more natural to provide primary care. Similarly, women's underrepresentation in authority positions may reflect the fact that in our society women have not been socialized to strive for these positions.

Women's socialization also emphasizes the importance of family life. Because both professional and family life demand significant time commitments, the career paths of female physicians may be explained partly as an effort to cap excessive demands from professional life and to allow for adequate family time. Employee status, seeing fewer patients, and working fewer hours can lessen the encroachment of professional demands on family life. Similarly, remaining single or electing to not have children may lessen the conflict between personal and professional life.

These are not easy decisions. Female medical students (Clark and Reiker 1986; Kris 1985), residents (Butterfield 1988; Elliot and Girard 1986), and practitioners (Ducker 1986) all report greater role stress than their male colleagues. When surveyed, between 30 and 60 percent of female physicians felt that family-career conflicts were important influences on their lives (Callan and Klipstein 1981; Ferrier and Woodward 1982; Nadelson et al. 1979). A survey that asked men and women whether they had changed their career plans because of family influences found that none of the men said they had changed their career plans or behaviors because of family responsibilities, whereas 44 percent of the women stated that they had done so (Nadelson et al. 1979). Other researchers have found that women explicitly sought regular and shorter hours as physicians because of concerns with family life (Dickstein and Stephenson 1987; Ferrier and Woodward 1982). Thus gender socialization is a major influence on the career paths of female physicians.

PRACTICE STYLE

Do Female Doctors Take Care of Patients Differently?

How does the doctor-patient relationship differ, if at all, when the doctor is a woman? If the primary determinant of medical practice is medical socialization, one would expect male and female physicians to have nearly identical practice styles. Conversely, gender differences in practice style are likely to result in part from gender socialization.

Male and female physicians are perceived to have different practice styles. Many health professionals identify female physicians as more interested in interpersonal relationships and better able to listen and empathize with patients. Medical students, for example, reported that they regard female attendings (the faculty doctor with formal clinical responsibility for patients on a given clinical service) as more sensitive, more altruistic, and less egoistic (Scadron, Witte, Axelrod, Greenbeg, Arem, and Meitz 1982). Nurses believe that female physicians are more "humanistic" and have greater "technical" skill in communicating with patients (Stoner 1988). Many physicians also assess women as more humanistic. In a national survey of psychiatric residents, program directors' evaluations suggested that female residents possess superior sensitivity, empathy, and interpersonal perceptivity (Roback, Crowder, and McNeeley 1987). In an analogous study in internal medicine, program directors felt that female residents had more "humanistic attributes" (Norcini et al. 1988).

Patients also perceive female physicians as more humanistic. Shapiro, McGrath, and Anderson (1983) administered the Bem Sex-Role Inventory to male and female patients and asked them to describe the typical male or female doctor. Patients viewed female physicians as androgynous, having both technical and expressive qualities, while they viewed male physicians either as low on both dimensions or as possessing only technical qualities.

Investigators also have examined whether the health care provider's sex influences a patient's satisfaction. Linn, Cope, and Leake (1984) studied the satisfaction of 140 male and 284 female patients with 68 residents (47 male and 21 female) after visits in a general internal medicine clinic. Patients who had seen a female resident reported significantly higher total satisfaction scores than those who had seen a male resident; this finding was true for both male and female patients. Female residents also scored higher on the author's art-of-care scale (a measure of the physician's manner and interpersonal style). Finally, Comstock, Hooper, Goodwin, and Goodwin (1982) studied 150 patients of 15 internal medicine residents (four of whom were female) to analyze the determinants of patient satisfaction. They found that female patients seeing female physicians expressed greater satisfaction with their care than did any other mix of doctors and patients.

These studies of patients' perceptions of female physicians reveal that patients consistently perceive female physicians as more empathic and as better listeners. The fundamental question is whether this perception is based merely on social stereotypes, or whether it is due to distinctive attitudes, knowledge, or behaviors of female physicians.

Physicians' Attitudes toward Patient Care

Upon entering medical school female medical students' attitudes toward patient care differed from male students'. Women were more patient-oriented, had greater interest in patients' emotional problems, and placed higher value on patient contact (Bean and Kitter 1982; Burkett and Kurz 1981; Roos 1977; Walton 1968). As students progressed through medical school, however, it appeared that these gender differences became attenuated (Potts, Katz, and Brandt 1986). Recent studies of students' professional and sociopolitical attitudes confirm these findings. Although freshman women valued the interpersonal, psychosocial, and preventive aspects of the physician's role more highly than did freshman males, these differences attenuated or disappeared among more advanced students (Leserman 1981; Maheux, Defort, and Beland 1988).

Information regarding physicians' rather than students' attitudes toward patients also showed few sex differences (Bernstein and Kane 1981). Male and female physicians responded similarly concerning how they would assess the authenticity, truthfulness, and emotionality of male and female patients (Colameco, Becker, and Simpson 1983). Female physicians' assessment of the type of patients they enjoyed or disliked were no different from male physicians' (Lorber 1984). Finally, residents' self-assessment of their humanistic attitude toward patients did not differ by sex (Linn et al. 1984).

One key exception to this pattern is found in areas related to "women's issues." Female medical students and physicians are more sensitive to issues regarding sex discrimination, contraception, abortion, and appropriate health care for women (Margolis, Greenwood, and Heilbron 1983; Weisman, Nathanson, Teitelbaum, Chase, and King 1986). Such differences in attitude persisted from medical school throughout residency and into practice (Heins 1979; Leichner and Harper 1982; Leserman 1981).

It appears that as students progress through medical school into residency training and practice, sex differences in attitudes toward patient care diminish. Professional socialization tempers the influence of gender socialization. The differences in attitudes that do exist do not appear to be great enough to explain the widespread perception that female physicians practice differently from male physicians.

Physicians' Knowledge

Is there any evidence that male and female physicians emerge from their training with different knowledge? During medical school there appears to be little difference in their academic performance. The rate of academic attrition among female students has never differed significantly from that of their male counterparts (Barondess 1981; Bickel 1988). Although studies reveal that women's performance was slightly lower on standardized tests (National Board examinations, Part I and a school's comprehensive examinations) in the first two years of medical school, scores in the last two years (National Board, Part II) were not significantly different. Furthermore, males and females were equally likely to be selected for a medical school's honor society, and their clinical evaluations during the last two years of school and the first year of residency did not differ (Arnold, Willoughby, Calkins, and Jensen 1981; Harward, Lyons, Porter, and Hunter 1981; Weinberg and Rooney 1973).

Recently, investigators have begun to look more closely at men's and women's performance during residency. The best studies have been conducted by the American Board of Internal Medicine (ABIM); one study compares residents' performance from 1972 through 1982 and a second study compares performance from 1982 through 1986. These studies contain two types of data: the subjective evaluation of residency program directors, using standardized forms, and scores from the written certifying examination. Men consistently received higher scores from residency program evaluators for medical knowledge and technical proficiency, while women received higher marks for humanistic attributes. Women were less likely than men to pass the certifying examination, although this difference has narrowed markedly over the past 15 years. In 1973 only 59 percent of females passed the test (compared to 76% of the males); in 1986, 80 percent of females passed (compared to 86% of the males). The difference between men's and women's mean scores also has narrowed significantly in the last 15 years. In the most recent analysis, gender was found to be a less important explanation of the variance in board certification scores than the applicant's age or the quality of the applicant's medical school or residency (Norcini et al. 1988; Norcini, Fletcher, Quimby, and Shea 1985). Data from other specialties also showed little or no difference in knowledge (Brownlee and Butzin 1981; Ellsbury et al. 1987, Schueneman, Pickleman, and Freeark 1985).

In sum, the differences between male and female physicians' knowledge are small and appear to be narrowing over time. It is doubtful that such small differences are clinically important. The differences between male and female physicians' attitudes and knowledge appear insufficient to explain the widespread perception that male and female physicians practice differently.

Physicians' Behavior

Perhaps the most important research comparing male and female physicians concerns the physician's behavior during clinical encounters. A growing body of data suggests that men and women have similar diagnostic and therapeutic skills; however, there appear to be differences in their communication styles.

Comparisons of gross measures, such as the number of specific treatments ordered or morbidity and mortality rates, revealed few important differences in physicians' diagnostic or therapeutic practices. The National Ambulatory Medical Care Survey, a governmental survey of office visits to approximately 3,000 doctors, revealed no significant differences among the proportions of patients referred to other physicians, seen for drug visits, or admitted to hospitals (U.S. Department of Health and Human Services 1977, 1984a–1984f). Greer and colleagues (1986) found no significant sex differences in the way family practice attendings said they would evaluate common medical problems such as headache or fatigue. Finally, a recent national study of psychiatrists revealed no significant differences between male and female physicians' diagnoses, prescriptions of psychotropic medications, or the frequency with which they hospitalized patients (Fenton, Robinowitz, and Leaf 1987).

One might expect that female physicians would have a better understanding of patients' psychosocial problems. Carol Gilligan's (1982) work highlights the differences in moral reasoning found between men and women. Women more often see moral requirements as arising from the needs of others in the context of particular relationships than as the impartial application of obligations and rights. This "ethic of care" might be expected to make female physicians more sensitive to their patients' needs. Even so, studies have failed to show a significant difference between male and female physicians' appreciation of psychosocial factors during clinical encounters. Bowman and Gehlbach (1980) reviewed 909 patient visits to evaluate whether first-year residents' ability to detect and record psychological, social, and sexual problems depended on the physician's gender. They did not; both female and male residents identified problems in about 40 percent of patients. Similarly, a study analyzing physicians' caring behaviors revealed no difference between male and female physicians (Comstock et al. 1982). A more recent study found no difference between male and female physicians' method of contacting or following up with families after a loved one's death (Toole, Hickam, and Elliot 1985). The perception of women's practice styles as different cannot be explained by differences in diagnostic or therapeutic skills or in attention to psychosocial issues.

A closer analysis of the actual interactions between doctors and patients may explain more clearly why patients have different perceptions of female physicians. New research on physicians' communication which emphasizes medical interviews as a form of discourse (Mishler 1984) provides especially intriguing data.

Female physicians have two conflicting paradigms for the physician-patient interaction. As women in American society, they have been socialized to accept a less directed communication style, especially when interacting with men (Belenky, Clinchy, Goldberger, and Tarule 1986; Thorne and Henley 1975). Women's style of speech typically is characterized by less obtrusiveness; for example, it displays less speech intensity, and more frequent use of hedges and euphemisms. In mixed conversations, men are more likely to interrupt women than vice versa, and women are more likely to allow such interruptions. Men are more likely to decide the topics of conversations and to dominate the turn-taking process. Studies of nonverbal communication show that women are more likely to lower or avert their eyes during conversation with males, to smile, or to allow invasion of their "private space." They are less likely to touch a member of the opposite sex, to stare, or to point (Thorne and Henley 1975).

Physicians in American society are socialized to dominate the doctor-patient interaction. Doctor-patient communication is characterized by physicians using directed questions and emphatic speech to control both the flow and the topics of conversation. Asymmetry in conversational style is emphasized further by the frequency with which physicians ignore patients' questions or refer to patients by their first names. Nonverbal communication shows a similar pattern of control by physicians over patients (Fisher 1983; Fischer and Todd 1987, 1988; Mishler 1984).

How do female physicians integrate these two models of communication? West's (1984, 1985) microanalyses of doctor-patient communications—a study of 21 encounters between residents (17 male and four female) and their patients at a family practice clinic—revealed that male physicians interrupted patients more frequently and used interruptions as a means of exerting control over patients. Female physicians interrupted their patients no more often than they were interrupted. Wasserman and colleagues (1984) videotaped 40 initial health supervision visits to a pediatric clinic in Seattle. Coders found that the four female physicians were more empathic than their five male counterparts, and that increased empathy accounted for mothers' greater satisfaction with female pediatricians. Finally, a study of communication styles of internal medicine residents in New York City noted that female physicians were more egalitarian in their relationships with patients, more responsive to patients' psychosocial issues, and more respectful of their concerns (Greene, Charon, Adelman, and Friedman 1987). The perception that female physicians practice differently from men may result from these differences in communication style.

Although medical socialization seems to dominate most technical aspects of medical care, gender socialization has a larger impact on female physicians' communication style than on males'. The absence of a strong emphasis on patient interviewing during training means that medical socialization is less likely to exert a strong influence on physicians' communication. Because gender socialization strongly influences conversational patterns, gender differences in physicians' communication develop.

CONCLUSION

Physicians' attitudes, values, and behaviors are influenced by diverse sources of socialization. Gender socialization appears to be an especially important influence on the career choices of female physicians. Despite the emphasis in specialization and technology during medical training, female physicians are more likely to enter primary care fields. They also work in job settings that can accommodate better the demands of their family and personal life. In contrast, medical socialization is a more powerful influence on practice style. Technical aspects of medical care show few gender differences. This is not to suggest, however, that medical practice is impervious to gender, a point demonstrated by gender differences in communication style. Future investigations will benefit from an approach which recognizes that both social background and professional socialization are continuous influences whose relative importance varies.

REFERENCES

"AMA Insights." 1987. *Journal of the American Medical Association* 257:2725.

AMA Center for Health Policy Research. 1987. *SMS Report*. Chicago: American Medical Association.

AMA Women in Medicine Project. 1987. *In the Marketplace*. 2nd edition. Chicago: American Medical Association.

Arnold, Louise, T. Lee Willoughby, Virginia Calkins, and Theresa Jensen. 1981. "The Achievement of Men and Women in Medical School." *Journal of American Medical Women's Association* 36:213–21.

Association of American Medical Colleges. 1987. *AAMC Faculty Roster System*. Washington, D.C.: AAMC.

Barondess, Jeremiah A. 1981. "Are Women Different? Some Trends in the Assimilation of

Women in Medicine." *Journal of American Medical Women's Association* 36:95–104.

Bean, B. and L.H. Kitter. 1982. "Helping and Achieving: Cooperation or Competitive Goals for Men and Women in Medical School." *Social Science and Medicine* 16:1377–82.

Belenky, Mary Field, Blyth McVicker Clinchy, Nancy Rule Goldberger, and Jill Mattuck Tarule. 1986. *Women's Way of Knowing: Development of Self, Voice, and Mind*. New York: Basic.

Bernstein, B. and R. Kane. 1981. "Physician Attitudes towards Female Patients." *Medical Care* 19:600–608.

Bickel, Janet. 1988. *Women in Medicine Statistics*. Washington, DC: AAMC.

Bloom, Samuel. 1979. "Socialization for the Physician's Role: A Review of Some Contributions of Research to Theory." Pp. 3–52 in *Becoming a Physician*, edited by Ellen Shapiro and Leah Lowenstein. Cambridge, MA: Ballinger.

Bowman, Marjorie W. and Stephen H. Gehlbach. 1980. "Sex of Physician as a Determinant of Psychosocial Problem Recognition." *Journal of Family Practice* 10:655–59.

Bowman, Marjorie W. and Marcy Lynn Gross. 1986. "Overview of Research on Women in Medicine—Issues for Public Policy Makers." *Public Health Reports* 101:513–21.

Brownlee, Robert C. and Diane W. Butzin. 1981. "Are Women That Different?" *Journal of American Medical Women's Association* 36:378.

Burkett, Gary L. and Dorothy E. Kurz. 1981. "A Comparison of the Professional Values and Career Orientations of Male and Female Medical Students: Some Unintended Consequences of U.S. Public Policy." *Health Policy and Education* 2:33–45.

Butterfield, Paula S. 1988. "The Stress of Residency: A Review of the Literature." *Archives of Internal Medicine* 148:1428–35.

Callan, Clair M. and Eve Klipstein. 1981. "Women Physicians in Connecticut: A Survey." *Connecticut Medicine* 45:494–96.

Clark, J. and P.P. Reiker. 1986. "Gender Differences in Relationships and Stress of Medical and Law Students." *Journal of Medical Education* 61:32–40.

Colameco, Steven, Lauren A. Becker, and Michael Simpson. 1983. "Sex Bias in the Assessment of Patients' Complaints." *Journal of Family Practice* 16:1117–21.

Colombotos, John and Corinne Kirchner. 1986. *Physicians and Social Change*. New York: Oxford University Press.

Comstock, Loretto M., Elizabeth M. Hooper, Jean M. Goodwin, and James S.Z. Goodwin. 1982. "Physician Behaviors That Correlate with Patient Satisfaction." *Journal of Medical Education* 57:105–12.

Crowley, Anne E., Sylvia I. Etzel, and H.A. Shaw. 1987. "Graduate Medical Education in the United States." *JAMA* 258:1031–37.

Dickstein, Leah J. and Judith J. Stephenson. 1987. "A National Survey of Women Physicians in Administrative Roles." *Journal of the American Medical Women's Association* 42:108–11.

Ducker, Dalia G. 1986. "Role Conflict in Women Physicians: A Longitudinal Study." *Journal of American Medical Women's Association* 4:14–16.

Elliot, D.L. and D.E. Girard. 1986. "Gender and the Emotional Impact of Internship." *Journal of the American Medical Women's Association* 41:54–56.

Ellsbury, K., R. Schneeweiss, D.E. Montano, K.C. Gordon, and D. Duykendall. 1987. "Gender Differences and Practice Characteristics of Graduates of Family Medicine Residency." *Journal of Medical Education* 62:895–903.

Fenton, Wayne S., Carolyn B. Robinowitz, and Philip J. Leaf. 1987. "Male and Female Psychiatrists and Their Patients." *American Journal of Psychiatry* 144:358–61.

Ferrier, B.M. and C.A. Woodward. 1982. "Career Choices, Work Patterns and Perceptions of Undergraduate Education of McMaster Medical Graduates: Comparison between Men and Women." *Canadian Medical Association Journal* 126:1411–14.

Fisher, Sue. 1983. *The Social Organization of Doctor-Patient Communication*. Washington, DC: Center for Applied Linguistics.

Fisher, Sue and Alexandra Dundas Todd. 1987. *Discourse in Institutional Authority: Medicine, Education and Law*. Norwood, NJ: Ablex.

———. 1988. *In the Patient's Best Interests: Women in the Politics of Medical Decisions*. New Brunswick, NJ: Rutgers University Press.

Frieman, Marc P. and William D. Marder. 1984. "Changes in Hours Worked by Physicians: 1970–1980." *American Journal of Public Health* 74:348–52.

Gilligan, Carol. 1982. *In a Different Voice: Psychological Theory in Women's Development*. Cambridge, MA: Harvard University Press.

Greene, Michele G., Rita Charon, Ronald Adelman, and Erika Friedmann. 1987. "Language and Behavior of Female and Male Physicians in the Medical Encounter." Unpublished manuscript.

Greer, Steven, Vivian Dickerson, Lawrence J. Schneiderman, Cathie Atkins, and Robert Bass. 1986. "Responses of Male and Female Physicians to Medical Complaints in Male and Female Patients." *Journal of Family Practice* 23:49–53.

Harvard, Donna H., Claudia M. Lyons, Carol Q. Porter, and Rosemary S. Hunter. 1981. "A Comparison of the Performance of Male and

Female Medical Students and Residents." *Journal of Medical Education* 56:853–55.

Heins, Marilyn. 1979. "Career and Life Patterns of Women and Men Physicians." Pp. 217–35 in *Becoming a Physician: Development of Values and Attitudes in Medicine*, edited by Eileen C. Shapiro and Leah M. Lowenstein. Cambridge, MA: Ballinger.

———. 1983. "Medicine and Motherhood." *Journal of the American Medical Association* 249:209–10.

Kehrer, Barbara H. 1976. "Factors Affecting the Incomes of Men and Women Physicians: An Exploratory Analysis." *Journal of Human Resources* 11:526–45.

Klepke, Phillip R., William D. Marder, and Anne B. Silberger. 1987. *The Demographics of Physician Supply: Trends and Projections*. Chicago: American Medical Association.

Kris, K.B. 1985. "Developmental Strains of Female Medical Students." *Journal of the American Medical Association* 40:145–48.

Landau, Carol, Stephanie Hall, Steven A. Wartman, and M.B. Marlo. 1986. "Stress and Social and Family Relationships during the Medical Residency." *Journal of Medical Education* 61:654–60.

Langwell, Kathryn M. 1982. "Factors Affecting the Incomes of Men and Women Physicians: Further Explorations." *Journal of Human Resources* 17:261–75.

Leichner, Pierre and Dan Harper. 1982. "Sex Role Ideology among Physicians." *Canadian Medical Association Journal* 127:380–83.

Leserman, Jane. 1981. *Men and Women in Medical School*. New York: Praeger.

Linn, Lawrence S., Dennis W. Cope, and Barbara Leake. 1984. "The Effect of Gender and Training of Residents on Satisfaction Ratings by Patients." *Journal of Medical Education* 59:964–66.

Lorber, Judith. 1984. *Women Physicians: Careers, Status and Power*. New York: Tavistock.

Maheux, Brigitte, Francine Defort, and Francois Beland. 1988. "Professional and Sociopolitical Attitudes of Medical Students: Gender Differences Reconsidered." *Journal of the American Medical Women's Association* 43:73–76.

Mandelbaum, Dorothy. 1978. *Work, Marriage, and Motherhood—The Career Persistence of Female Physicians*. New York: Praeger.

Margolis, A.J., S. Greenwood, and D. Heilbron. 1983. "Survey of Men and Women Residents Entering United States Obstetric and Gynecology Programs in 1981." *American Journal of Obstetrics and Gynecology* 146:541–46.

Merton, Robert K. 1957. *Social Theory and Social Structure*. Revised edition. Glencoe, IL: Free Press.

Mishler, Elliot G. 1984. *The Discourse of Medicine: Dialectics of Medical Interviews*. Norwood, NJ: Ablex.

Nadelson, Carol C., M.T. Notman, and P. Lowenstein. 1979. "The Practice Patterns, Life Styles, and Stresses of Women and Men Entering Medicine: A Follow-Up Study of Harvard Medical School Graduates from 1967 to 1977." *Journal of the American Medical Association* 34:400–406.

Norcini, John J., Susan C. Day, Judy A. Shea, and John A. Benson. 1988. "Performance of Women on the American Board of Internal Medicine Certifying Examinations, 1983–86." Unpublished paper.

Norcini, John J., Susanne W. Fletcher, Barbara B. Quimby, and Judy A. Shea. 1985. "Performance of Women Candidates on the American Board of Internal Medicine Certifying Examination, 1973–82." *Annals of Internal Medicine* 102:115–18.

Ogle, Karen S., Rebecca C. Henry, Kate Durda and Judith D. Zivick. 1986. "Gender Specific Differences in Family Practice Graduates." *Journal of Family Practice* 23:357–60.

Ohsfeldt, Robert L. and Steven D. Culler. 1986. "Differences in Income between Male and Female Physicians." *Journal of Health Economics* 5:335–46.

Potts, Marilyn K., Barry P. Katz, and Kenneth D. Brandt. 1986. "Sex Differences in Medical Student and Housestaff Attitudes toward the Handicapped." *Journal of American Medical Women's Association* 41:156–60.

Roback, Howard B., Miles K. Crowder, and Judith McNeeley. 1987. "Residency Directors' Perceptions of Gender-Related Differences in the Performance of Psychiatric Residents." *Journal of Medical Education* 62:767–69.

Roos, C. 1977. "Female and Physician: A Sex Role Incongruity." *Journal of Medical Education* 52:345–46.

Scadron, Arlene, Marlis H. Witte, Morris Axelrod, Edward A. Greenberg, Cynthia Arem, and June E.G. Meitz. 1982. "Attitudes towards Women Physicians in Medical Academia." *Journal of the American Medical Association* 247:2803–08.

Schermerhorn, Gerry R., Jerry A. Colliver, Steven J. Verhulst, and Ellen L. Schmidt. 1986. "Factors That Influence Career Patterns of Women Physicians." *Journal of the American Medical Association* 41:74–78.

Scheuneman, A., J. Pickleman, and R.J. Freeark. 1985. "Age, Gender, Lateral Dominance in Prediction of Operative Skill among Several Residents." *Surgery* 98:506–14.

Shapiro, J., E. McGrath, and R.C. Anderson. 1983. "Patients, Medical Students and Physicians' Perception of Male and Female Physicians." *Perception Motor Skills* 56:179–86.

Silberger, Anne B., William D. Marder, and

Richard J. Wilke. 1987. "Practice Characteristics of Male and Female Physicians." *Health Affairs* Winter: 104–109.

Stoner, Martha H. "The Nurse-Physician Relationship: The Effects of the Feminization of Medicine." Unpublished paper.

Thorne, Barrie and Nancy Henley, eds. 1975. *Language and Sex: Differences and Dominance*. Rowley, MA: Newberry House.

"Today's Woman MD." 1983 *Medica Magazine* Fall:40–45.

Toole, Susan W., David H. Hickam, and Diane L. Elliot. 1985. "A Comparison of Men and Women Physicians' Management of Patient Death." *Western Journal of Medicine* 143: 691–93.

U.S. Department of Health and Human Services. 1977. "Characteristics of Visits to Female and Male Physicians: The National Ambulatory Medical Care Survey, United States, 1977." *Vital and Health Statistics* Series 13, 49.

______. 1984a. "The National Ambulatory Medical Care Survey, United States, January 1980–December 1981." *Vital and Health Statistics* Series 13.

______. 1984b. "Patterns of Ambulatory Care in Office Visits to General Surgeons: The National Ambulatory Medical Care Survey, United States, January 1980–December 1981." *Vital and Health Statistics* Series 13, 79.

______. 1984c. "Patterns of Ambulatory Care in Obstetrics and Gynecology: The National Ambulatory Medical Care Survey, United States, January 1980–December 1981." *Vital and Health Statistics* Series 13, 76.

______. 1984d. "Patterns of Ambulatory Care in Pediatrics: The National Ambulatory Medical Care Survey, United States, January 1980–December 1981." *Vital and Health Statistics* Series 13, 75.

______. 1984e. "Patterns of Ambulatory Care in General and Family Practice: The National Ambulatory Medical Care Survey, United States, January 1980–December 1981." *Vital and Health Statistics* Series 13, 73.

______. 1984f. "Patterns of Ambulatory Care in Internal Medicine: The National Ambulatory Medical Care Survey, United States, January 1980–December 1981." *Vital and Health Statistics* Series 13, 80.

Wallis, Lila A., Helena Gilder, and Howard Thaler. 1981. "Advancement of Men and Women in Medical Academia." *Journal of the American Medical Association* 246:2350–53.

Walton, D. 1968. "Sex Differences in Ability and Outlook of Senior Medical Students." *British Journal of Medical Education* 2:156–62.

Wasserman, R.C., T.S. Inui, R.D. Barriatua, W.B. Carter, and P. Lippincott. 1984. "Pediatric Clinicians' Support for Parents Makes a Difference: An Outcome-Based Analysis of Clinical-Parent Interaction." *Pediatrics* 74:1047–53.

Weinberg, Ethel and James F. Rooney. 1973. "The Academic Performance of Women Students in Medical School." *Journal of Medical Education* 48:240–47.

Weisman, Carol S., Constance A. Nathanson, Martha Ann Teitelbaum, Gary A. Chase, and Theodore M. King. 1986. "Abortion Attitudes and Performance among Male and Female Obstetrician-Gynecologists." *Family Planning Perspectives* 18:67–73.

West, Candice. 1984. "When the Doctor is a 'Lady': Power, Status, and Gender in Physician-Patient Encounters." *Symbolic Interaction* 7:87–106.

______. 1985. *Routine Complications*. Bloomington: Indiana University Press.

[30]

The Social Position and Internal Organization of the Medical Profession in the Third World: The Case of Singapore*

STELLA R. QUAH
National University of Singapore

Journal of Health and Social Behavior 1989, Vol. 30 (December):450–466

This paper probes two aspects of the medical profession in Singapore: its structure and its social position. The first section reviews the relevant concepts concerning the structure and the social position of the professions that may be applied to medicine in Singapore. The second section looks into the structure of the medical profession in Singapore from an historical perspective. The third section deals with the internal organization of the medical profession. The fourth section focuses on its social position. The paper concludes with a summary of the main points and a brief comparison of the situation in Singapore with that in other countries.

The questions of knowledge—its definition and boundaries, who possesses it and who does not—are at the core of the analysis of professions everywhere. Forty years ago Moore and Tumin (1949) published a provocative paper on the social functions of ignorance. The ideas presented in that paper remain crucial for understanding the status and the roles of the professions in modern societies. The most relevant of the functions of ignorance identified by Moore and Tumin is "preservative of privileged position." The authors create a dichotomy between ignorance on the part of the outsider or consumer of services and knowledge and secrecy on the part of the professional or service provider (1949, pp. 788–89). Other researchers had identified this phenomenon earlier (Carr-Saunders and Wilson 1933, p. 104), but Moore and Tumin's concept facilitates a more systematic analysis.

Although restrained by the theoretical straitjacket of functionalism, Moore and Tumin managed to apply their ideas on the social functions of ignorance to identify ways in which professionals attempt to augment and maintain their monopoly of specialized knowledge. Two such devices are the use of "specialized and possibly esoteric vocabulary" and "instruments and techniques not intrinsically required for the solution [of the client's problem] but seemingly so" (1949, p. 789). Moreover, professionals must guard their monopoly of knowledge not only from consumers but also from "potential competitors." The most common device for this purpose is "trade secrets and their protection through the control by the professionals themselves of training and thus of access to the privileged positions" (1949, p. 789). The sociological study of the professions has been expanded by innumerable contributions since the time of Moore and Tumin's paper. Yet the concept of the social functions of ignorance remains one of its main underlying premises.

From a more general perspective, it is also useful to consider the conceptual approaches applied to the study of the professions. The three most common are the "process" approach, the "structural-functional" approach, and the "power" approach, all described well by Ritzer (1977). The process approach follows the historical development of an occupation searching for six main characteristics that would "transform" it into a profession or that already have transformed it. These characteristics are 1) full-time engagement in the practice of the occupation; 2) a change of name to sharpen the boundaries of

* Direct correspondence to Stella R. Quah, Ph.D., Department of Sociology, National University of Singapore, Kent Ridge, Singapore 0511, Republic of Singapore

its exclusive domain; 3) the setting up of a national association; 4) the establishment of a training school or its equivalent; 5) a code of ethics; and 6) the seeking of legal and public support and recognition (Ritzer 1977, pp. 46–48).

The structural-functional approach analyzes the "distinctive characteristics" and structure that differentiate professions from other occupations. Six such characteristics are identified by this approach: 1) the possession of, or claim over, a general and systematic body of theory; 2) a norm of autonomy—that is, freedom from external control; 3) a norm of altruism, or the claim of being devoid of self-interest; 4) a norm of authority over clients, or the need for the professional to have the client's trust; 5) a distinctive occupational culture transmitted through socialization of students or recruits; and 6) the recognition of the preceding five characteristics or claims by the law and the community (Ritzer 1977, pp. 48–56).

Unlike the other two approaches, the power approach focuses on two aspects of power, namely "the power needed by an occupation to acquire professional recognition" and "the power such an occupation wields once it has achieved that position" (Ritzer 1977, p. 43). The power approach identifies three main features of such acquisition and retention of professional power: 1) a "margin of indetermination," or the degree to which a task can be routinized; 2) "control over areas of uncertainty"—that is, the consumer's or client's uncertainty regarding the nature and/or possible solution to his problem; and 3) "ideology," or how the professions justify their "privileged status" to expand their power and to deal with internal and external threats (Ritzer 1977, pp. 56–62). Within the context of this approach, power is defined as "the ability of an occupation [or its leaders] to obtain and retain a set of rights and privileges and obligations from social groups that otherwise might not grant them" (Ritzer 1977, p. 56).

An important clarification is in order. Professional expertise per se usually receives social recognition in most modern societies. The high prestige scores given to professional occupations by populations studied in Europe and North America give evidence of such recognition. Yet the power approach deals with something more than the deserved recognition of expertise in a given area of knowledge: A profession is said to have power if it succeeds in overcoming potential resistance from other groups in the community to its expanding influence over aspects of social life *beyond* the boundaries of the profession's expertise. In this connection, one important element common to all three approaches is the recognition of the manipulation of ignorance by the professionals in order to attain or preserve their privileged position. Indeed, such a manipulation is hinted at by three of the six characteristics identified by the process approach: the change of name, the founding of a national association, and the establishment of a training school.

In a more explicit manner, three of the six features identified by the structural-functional approach deal with the manipulation of the client's ignorance: the claim of possession of a systematic body of theory, the norm of autonomy, and the norm of authority over the client. The power approach is more emphatic in this respect. All three of the features identified, but particularly the first two (the margin of indetermination and control over areas of uncertainty), deal directly with the professionals' attempt to contrast their knowledge with the ignorance of outsiders.

Ritzer (1977) proposes an "integrated" approach which would combine features of the process, power, and structural-functional approaches. His approach focuses on three aspects of the analysis of the professions. One aspect is interpreting the characteristics of professions identified by the structural-functional approach not as "real" but either as traits derived from the power that the professions already have or as traits that they do not possess but have been able to convince others that they have (Ritzer 1977, p. 63). Ritzer is not alone in this view. Larson (1977, p. xii) stated that the six characteristics identified by the structural-functional approach "do not tell us what a profession is but only what it pretends to be."

The second aspect of the integrated approach is investigating the structural factors that "greatly reduce" the power of professions. Far from possessing the power that people think they have or that they themselves claim to have, professionals actually depend on the "society's dominant elites" to obtain and retain such power (Ritzer 1977, p. 64). The influence of ideology in determining which occupations are professions, the need for elite or state sponsorship to attain and maintain professional status, and the exaggerated claims of professional attributes and privileges also have been identified by Freidson (1973, 1986) and by Larson (1977), among others. The third and final aspect of the integrated approach is acknowledging that the actual and perceived power of the professions varies not only among different groups in society but also across time and geographical areas (Ritzer 1977, pp. 63–66).

To these three points I would add that the degree of power of the professions also depends on the political and economic structure of the society in question. A decline in the power of the professions, also termed a trend towards "deprofessionalization," has been predicted by several sociologists on the basis of three main changes that they foresee in the economic and political structures of modern societies: 1) a decrease in the level of consumers' ignorance; 2) the consequent demystification of professional activities, and 3) the "proletarianization" of professionals as they become employees of large public and private corporations or institutions and are faced with an increasing demand for democratic accountability (Haug 1973; Oppenheimer 1973; Ritzer 1977, pp. 63–67; Stone 1976). There is no consensus on the premises of "deprofessionalization" and "proletarianization."

The main problem with these premises is the lack of empirical evidence to support them. The current emphasis on high technology as the basis for economic development gives preponderance to the role of professionals. Although the educational level of the man in the street may have increased over the years, the predicted narrowing of the knowledge gap between clients and professionals has not been observed because, among other things, "professionals are producing more esoteric specializations" (Freidson 1986, p. 112). Similarly, although there is a trend among some professionals to become employees in organizations, and although Freidson had suggested earlier that employed professionals may lose control of their work and become "technical workers" under management control (1973), a decade later he is less sure of his prediction. He points out rightly that many professions, at least in the United States, have been "typically employed" and that only the minority of professionals, such as physicians, dentists, and architects, have been traditionally self-employed (1986, pp. 120–22).

More important, Freidson's (1986, pp. 109–33) recent findings suggest that government intervention is a stronger threat to the power of professions than are consumerism, the public's increasing level of education, and most other factors. This point is particularly significant in this discussion because the role of the government features prominently in the development of the medical and other professions in Singapore. As will be shown later, Singapore's data do not support the deprofessionalization premise but do suggest a significant decrease in the level of consumers' ignorance and a corresponding demystification of professional activities.

In addition to the three basic approaches to the study of the professions—the process, structural-functional, and power approaches—and Ritzer's suggestion of the "integrated" approach, another conceptual aspect of interest in this study is the channels of professional influence used by the medical profession in Singapore. In his discussion of the role of professions in American public service, Mosher (1978) states that professional associations are not the only vehicle or even the main vehicle used by professionals to "initiate or modify or veto policy proposals or affect them in their execution" (1978, p. 144). It is important to explore whether the same argument applies to Singapore. The concept of professional influence may help to clarify the role of the medical profession in the modernization of Singapore through its impact on policy formulation and policy implementation. Thus Mosher's five channels of professional influence," summarized below, will serve as another frame of reference in discussing the medical profession in Singapore.

The five channels of professional influence as identified by Mosher (1978, pp. 145–46) are 1) the election or appointment of professionals to high political or judicial office; 2) the effective control or monopoly of the significant managerial and operating positions of administrative agencies by individual professions; 3) the role of professionals who operate within agencies which they do not dominate; 4) the bringing of ideas, modes of thought, and pressures to bear on political, executive, and legislative bodies and on their appropriate committees by professionals through indirect extragovernmental channels such as the mass media, professional associations, and labor unions; and 5) the influence of professionals at one level of government on the operations and policies of another level through, or in alliance with, their professional counterparts at that other level.

This brief overview of relevant conceptual premises identifies some of the important concepts to be probed in the case of the medical profession in Singapore. In summary, regarding the structure and the social position of the medical profession, it is assumed that the features of professions as outlined by the process, structural-functional, power, and integrated approaches are not fully applicable to the medical profession in Singapore. When these characteristics are observed, they do not necessarily occur together, nor do they remain in effect continuously. Even so, I do not agree with Johnson's (1973, p. 285) strong assertion that the professions in the Third World are fundamentally different from their counterparts in developed countries. I hope the evidence from this discussion will shed some light on this issue.

Concerning the channels of professional influence, I assume that in Singapore physicians do exert influence on policy formulation and policy implementation, but more as individuals than as a professional group. Of the five channels identified by Mosher, the two most commonly used are 1) through appointment or election to high political or judicial office and to managerial and executive positions in the public sector, mainly during the past 10 to 15 years, as a result of the political leadership's "search for talent"; and 2) through agencies, both public and private, as consultants. I suggest further that the social and political emphasis on paper qualifications and merit prevalent in Singapore over the past quarter of a century has facilitated access to these various channels by individual professionals, physicians included.

HISTORICAL BACKGROUND

To appreciate the situation of the medical profession in Singapore, one must travel back in time to England. The territory known as Singapore was first taken into the British domain in 1819. Singapore attained self-government in 1959 and independence in 1965. Therefore the historical development of the medical profession in England provides a basis for understanding the situation of the medical profession in the Republic of Singapore today. Indeed, in Singapore and in other British colonies in the nineteenth century, the influence of the British empire took two general forms. One was the "outflow of professional migrants" from England, either as settlers (the pioneers of private enterprise in the professions) or as consultants on contract with the colonial government. The other was the inflow of student from the colonies for professional training in England (Johnson 1973; p. 286). As will be seen later, the latter commenced in Singapore only during the final years of the nineteenth century, whereas the former was practically a permanent feature throughout the colonial period.

Nevertheless, the influence of English professional styles reached British colonies under a set of circumstances that Johnson believes created a unique character in the colonies' professions, including medicine. He argues that a new type of institutionalized occupational control by the state (the British Crown) took place. Johnson labels this control "corporate patronage," in which "it is the client—a powerful, corporate client—which regulates the profession rather than the members of the occupation themselves." This arrangement, of course, is opposite to the idea of professional autonomy. Johnson also asserts that "where corporate patronage prevailed" in the British colonies, the professional ideology involving the principles of autonomy and authority "never developed," even though this ideology of professionalism "was not unimportant" (1973, p. 285).

Johnson's viewpoint is contrary to Larson's (1977) assumption that the modern ideology of professional autonomy developed in England and the United States because the influence of British laissez-faire capitalism was transplanted to the British colonies. The two-way migration of professionals and students between metropolis and colonies, plus the influence of British professional associations, would reinforce such an expectation. Yet Johnson's (1973) findings appear to refute such a development in favor of corporate patronage. The British Crown, it seems, applied the principles of state intervention used in continental Europe to its colonies while allowing a more market-oriented and more flexible development of the professions at home.

Even so, historical accounts of individual professions indicate the presence of state intervention in England through time, albeit applied unevenly among the professions, including medicine. Data from the historical development of medicine in Singapore, in fact, indicate a dual process. Decisive government intervention was present in shaping the structure and the functions of the profession. Yet at the same time, the private sector offered opportunities for the manifestation and strengthening of some or all of the classical characteristics of professions described earlier, including professional ideology. There also existed a complex network of relationships between physicians and the colonial government bureaucracy; this network contributed to the stability and the permanence of the dual development of government intervention and the professional ideology of autonomy, authority over clients, and altruism, among other aspects. Specific examples will illustrate these developments.

In 1815, four years before Sir Stanford Raffles acquired the island of Singapore to incorporate it as a port in the British East Indies trade network, the Apothecaries Act was passed in the British Parliament. This act stressed the need for "regular medical education" to be given to medical practitioners in England in order to protect the health of the community. This was a significant step towards reform of the medical profession because until that time there had been four different groups of practitioners (physicians, surgeons, apothecaries, and druggists) without coordination or "coherent structure" (Carr-Saunders and Wilson 1933, pp. 77–78).

In Singapore, the representative of the British Crown was the East India Company. The Company had set up its Medical Department in Penang (an island to the northwest of what today is Malaysia), which had been under British domain before 1819. It appears that until 1826 the medical needs of the British settlers in the region were met by the Medical Department. The Senior Surgeon had already explored the possibility of training apprentices as assistants; his plan was approved by the Company in 1822 (Lee 1978, pp. 3–4). In 1826 Penang, Malacca, and Singapore were incorporated into the British settlements of Prince of Wales Island, Singapore, and Malacca, or the Straits Settlements for short. Penang was designated as the capital, and the Medical Department kept its headquarters there. This new arrangement prompted an administrative reorganization of the Medical Department to meet new demands. Thus in 1828 the Department included two levels of personnel, the "superior branch" and the "subordinate native branch" of the medical profession. The superior branch was reserved for British practitioners, who occupied the three top administrative positions: Surgeon Major, Surgeon, and Assistant Surgeon. The subordinate medical ranks were open to both British and Eurasians (Lee 1978, pp. 7–9). Only the presence of Eurasians seemed to justify the label "native" for this subordinate level.

In general, the origins of the medical profession in Singapore were marked clearly by state intervention or corporate patronage, to borrow Johnson's (1973) term. The control of access to medical practice was very much in the hands of the British Crown, represented by the Medical Department of the East India Company. It was the Company which introduced the first "Western" physicians to the Malayan archipelago to perform primarily military duties as army surgeons. Later on, by necessity, the service was expanded to include the British civilian population (Lee 1978, p. 3)—more precisely, the "white administrative personnel" in the settlements (Johnson 1973, p. 287). In 1827 the General Hospital, hitherto a combined military and civilian hospital, was declared a separate hospital for civilian patients, including "natives," and required Europeans to pay higher fees than other patients (Lee 1978, pp. 25–26).

The medical needs of the local population were met at that time by an assortment of healing sources, the most common of which were traditional healers in combination with self-prescribed traditional herbal remedies. A few charitable institutions founded by Chinese philanthropists were also available to the indigent. The Thong Chai Medical Institution was one of these; the colonial government provided the land for its building in 1892. Free medical treatment was given "to the poor of all races," using the sinsehs' (Chinese healers') skills in traditional Chinese medicine (Turnbull 1977, pp. 116–17).

At the government level, some medical care was also provided by the Medical Department's subordinate native branch, compromising the Sub-Assistant Surgeon, apothecaries, assistant apothecaries, and apprentices, all of whom could, technically, provide medical care to the population in emergency situations. Yet the personnel in this branch were few and mostly from India—that is, "Eurasians" in addition to Caucasians (Lee 1978, p. 8). The language barrier faced by these assistants when serving the local Chinese or Malay population was observed readily by the Senior Surgeon. He presented to the colonial government his plan for recruiting and training local personnel and for upgrading the branch to "Subordinate Medical Establishment," and received approval in 1853 (Lee 1978, pp. 12–13).

The development of the government's Medical Department throughout the nineteenth century was paralleled by the emergence of opportunities for the creation and expansion of a private sector of medical services. The salaries paid by the East India Company to members of both the higher and the subordinate medical establishment were low, and the conditions of service were poor. Their discontent reached the press; in 1845 a reporter wrote in a local newspaper that "the advantages held out to well-educated Eurasians in the several mercantile houses here render persons of this class perfectly indifferent to remaining in Government employ" (Lee 1978, p. 11).

One year later, one of the apothecaries resigned from government service "and promptly set up private practice and became the principal marine surgeon here and in good practice among the natives" (Lee 1978, p. 11). Low salaries and poor working conditions also led the government physicians to conduct private practices concurrently in order to supplement their income. The government apparently allowed this activity as "compensation" for their low pay. Understandably, this flexibility was detrimental to the quality of medical care provided at the government hospitals. The press criticized this situation strongly in 1869 as "a most pernicious system," stating that doctors "visit the hospitals at stated hours, issue their orders and the apothecary and his apprentice do the rest" (Lee 1978, p. 69).

Because of the poor quality and organization of the government medical services, the setting up of private practice was already common among European physicians who were not in government service and who had perceived a market for their private clinics. One of the earliest signs of this trend towards private practice is a newspaper advertisement published by a British surgeon to this effect in 1834 (Lee 1978, p. 28). A private hospital was already functioning in 1837, but according to Lee's (1978) description, private medical services were more expensive than those in the public hospitals. (Such a cost difference is rather common today.) There were complaints about the high fees charged by the private hospital, but there was also a certain recognition of the physicians' right to charge high fees. This ambivalent feeling was manifested in a local newspaper editorial in 1837: "a charge which is but moderate for an European practitioner in this country may be much more than a sailor's hard-earned pittance can bear" (Lee 1978, p. 29). We must assess with caution the prestige attached to the practice of medicine, as hinted at in this editorial. Why would medicine be perceived as a prestigious occupation in the early years of the colony? The English-language press was addressed to the educated minority, primarily Europeans. At first glance it would appear that the regard for higher education was brought to Singapore by the Europeans and was adopted first by those local groups which had the most contact with the former. Such an assumption, however, would be misleading. In the local population, individuals who possessed healing skills had traditionally been regarded with greater deference than most other gifted or skilled people. More important, among the Chinese, for example, intellectuals or scholars had historically been considered members of the elite in society (Miyazaki 1981; Quah 1989a). In other words, among the Asian immigrants who formed the bulk of the Singapore population in the nineteenth century, there was already a set of values and traditions that assigned high prestige to the practice of healing skills and gave due status recognition to education.

During the period of colonial rule and the intermediate stages before independence, many acts and ordinances were produced to regulate the medical profession. A review of all legislation passed in Singapore from 1866 to 1965 (Srinivasagam 1972, pp. 3–131) reveals that 29 such pieces of legislation were passed or amended. They dealt with matters such as medical education, medical registration, and medicines and advertising. Medical registration, however, was the most widely discussed issue. The discussion began with Ordinance 9 of 1905, which was repealed in 1907 by Ordinance 11. The latter was amended five times between 1907 and 1946, and finally was repealed by Ordinance 23 of 1953; that ordinance itself underwent further amendments before 1965. In the 1953 ordinance, the Medical Council was established as the gatekeeper of the medical profession. The Council consisted of 14 physician members, four of whom represented the government. Another four members represented the universities (the University of Malaya in Kuala Lumpur and the University of Singapore), and the remaining six represented physicians in private practice.

Despite the signs of corporate patronage or state intervention, in the last part of the nineteenth century one may observe already a mild yet significant manifestation of the medical profession's "norm of autonomy," to use Ritzer's term (Ritzer 1977, pp. 50–51)—that is, its efforts to be free from external control. Noting the control that the government could exert over professionals in the colonial civil service, the local English-language press commented in 1870 that physicians were in "an entirely different position" from engineers and accountants. Engineers and accountants in the civil service could not be allowed to conduct private practice, whereas the work of government doctors was "left to their consciences." Following this principle, the press suggested an increase in the government physicians' salaries so that "the allurement of private practice" would be "removed" (Lee 1978, p. 70). If we may assume that the newspapers voiced the general beliefs of the educated population in the colony, these comments convey the community's conviction that the *content* of the medical profession's work should be determined entirely by the doctors themselves.

In fact, by the end of the nineteenth century, as more local young men from well-to-do Baba or Straits Chinese families completed their secondary school education in English, their parents' goal was to send them to England to obtain a degree in medicine or some other profession. Medicine already had attained a high status in their eyes. Lim Boon Keng was one of the first such young men to return to Singapore with a degree in medicine; he promptly became a community leader. Lim was a member of the Legislative Council from 1895 to 1905 in addition to being "founder of the Straits Chinese British Association, member of the Chinese Advisory Board, and first to enroll in Britain's support in the Chinese Volunteer Company in 1901." He founded the Philomathic Society, strengthened Confucian morality in the Chinese community, was co-publisher of the *Straits Chinese Magazine*, and with a medical colleague, Dr. Yin Suat Chuan, "launched a campaign to discourage opium smoking" (Turnbull 1977, pp. 106–17).

Turnbull's (1977) description of the events and people in Singapore at the turn of the century confirms the assumption that individual professionals, in this case physicians, used several channels of influence to assert their status in the colony. Although the higher ranks of the colonial government were restricted to Europeans, young local professionals like Lim Boon Keng

> . . . became leaders in the professions and took their place alongside wealthy merchants as legislative councillors, municipal councillors, and justices of peace. The English-educated professional Asian elite provided a new type of leadership and began a subtle westernizing and modernizing of Singapore society . . . opening the way for the Asian community to assimilate and accept western medicine, the British judicial system and European educational methods (Turnbull 1977, p. 120).

This local intellectual elite was responsible for establishing the medical school in Singapore in 1905. That was a crucial year in the development of the medical profession. The registration of medical practitioners had been legislated earlier in the year, thus serving as an appropriate prelude to the opening of the first medical school.

A brief note on background events is in order here. In 1835 the Madras Medical College was founded. For the rest of the nineteenth century it served as the training center for young Singapore applicants before they were posted to the upper ranks of the Subordinate Branch of the Medical Service. The lowest rank of apprentices had received on-the-job training since 1822, but the results were not satisfactory (Lee 1978, pp. 7–16).

In other words, medical education in Singapore during the nineteenth century was entirely dependent on British facilities either in England or in India. England itself reformed the Oxford University Bachelorship of Medicine only in 1832, and the medical profession there was trying to put its own house in order (Carr-Saunders and Wilson 1933, p. 79). Not until 1905 was the King Edward VII College of Medicine founded; this institution was originally named "the Straits Settlements and Federated Malay States Government Medical School" (Colony of Singapore 1953, p. 22). There was some reluctance on the part of the colonial government to open a medical school. The colonial authorities considered it to be an extremely complex task; when they finally agreed, they hastened to label it "an experiment." In fact, in 1889 the colonial government had attempted to set up a medical school "to train assistant surgeons to treat the natives and to assist the European Medical officers in their routine duties," but only two students applied, and thus the idea was abandoned (Kanagaratnam 1965, p. 20).

This school was to be a higher educational institution for training medical doctors. Its opening was the happy outcome of strong lobbying by the leaders of the Chinese community. They surprised the British authorities with their prompt donation of $87,000 instead of the $71,000 that the government had requested as a precondition to their approval. The money was needed for the medical college's building fund (Turnbull 1977, p. 120). With the opening of the medical college, Singapore and the rest of the Straits Settlements obtained a certain degree of control over the training of their own physicians. The first class of six graduates emerged in 1910 from the original group of 23 first-year medical students (Kanagasuntheram 1965, p. 39). The Licentiate in Medicine and Surgery was recognized by the British General Medical Council in 1916 (Colony of Singapore 1953; Tay 1965, p. 10). The production of medical graduates remained modest until the 1950s, with an average of about 14 graduates per year (Kanagaratnam 1965, p. 22). There were 34 graduates in 1953, and the figures reported by Lim (1965, p. 13) show an annual average of 61 graduates from 1953 to 1965.

As for the power relations between the colony and England, it may be superfluous to say that the Medical College had a certain degree of control. The teaching staff and the curriculum were British; the General Medical Council in London remained the supreme source of professional approval and recognition throughout the colonial period after its creation by the Act of 1858 as the "General Council of Medical Education and Registration of the United Kingdom" (Carr-Saunders and Wilson 1933, pp. 83–84). The teaching staff at first consisted of only part-time practitioners from both the government service and the private sector. Full-time teaching staff was assigned to the College in 1920, when the college was upgraded and was renamed the King Edward VII Medical College (Chen 1965, p. 32; Colbourne 1965, p. 63; Turnbull 1977, p. 120).

From the perspective of power relations between physicians and laymen, physicians controlled medical education in England and consequently in Singapore. The membership of the General Medical Council in England was dominated by physicians. Before 1926 "no layman had ever sat upon the Council"; in 1932 only five of 38 members were Crown appointees. The remainder were appointed by medical corporations, medical schools, and private practitioners (Carr-Saunders and Wilson 1933, p. 84). The path taken by medical education in the colony was determined by the medical profession in Singapore and followed the patterns established in England. This practice continued with increased emphasis as the medical profession consolidated its status in the 1940s and 1950s; to some extent it has remained the norm during the Republic's existence.

The Kind Edward VII Medical College was renamed and upgraded three times, following organizational changes in the English-language university in Singapore. The College became the Faculty of Medicine, including dentistry and pharmacy, and in 1949 was merged with Raffles College (dedicated to arts and sciences subjects) to form the University of Malaya in Singapore. In 1962 the university was renamed the University of Singapore. The latest reorganization and upgrading took place in 1980, when the University of Singapore and Nayang University were merged to form the National University of Singapore. More important, since its inception in 1905, the medical school has been a government institution. It depended on government hospitals for its teaching facilities (Colony of Singapore 1953, pp. 22–23; Tham 1981) until 1985, when the National University Hospital was established on the campus of the National University of Singapore.

Although the teaching of medicine finally was approved by the colonial authorities in 1905, medical research took longer to become established in Singapore. In 1928 a medical research committee was appointed by the British Governor of the Straits Settlements to explore the need for medical research, its scope, and its cost in the Settlements. The committee gave a positive report on the work of the Medical College in Singapore and of the Institute of Medical Research in Kuala Lumpur. Both institutions were staffed with government-appointed physicians and scientists. The committee recommended, however, that the emphasis should be placed on "research applied to Malayan problems," leaving "the field of pure research" to "the laboratories in Europe" (Medical Research Committee 1929, p. 3).

This dependence on British leadership was manifested clearly in the complete reliance on British academic standards and approval of the medical curriculum as well as in the seeking of British recognition for the basic degree of Bachelor of Medicine and Bachelor of Surgery [MBBS] in 1950 and in the establishment of the School of Post-Graduate Medical Studies in 1960. After Singapore achieved independence in 1965, the Medical Faculty's links with England became less conventional. In the 1970s the Faculty took charge of training for the degrees of Master of Medicine and Master of Public Health (Tham 1981; pp. 145–47). In the 1980s it has continued to upgrade the standards of medical education at all levels with the aim of serving as a center of higher medical education for Southeast Asia. In 1988, for example, non-Singaporeans accounted for 70 percent of the physicians enrolled in courses leading to the degrees of Master of Science in Public Health and Master of Science in Community Medicine at the Department of Community, Occupational, and Family Medicine of the Faculty of Medicine. Nevertheless, the ties with the British system still remain; they are represented not only by individual Singaporean physicians' membership in British medical specialty associations or societies but also by the university system of external examiners. Occasionally, however, external examiners have been invited from countries outside the Commonwealth.

As noted in the earlier discussion of the process approach, six key features in the historical development of an occupation would transform it into a profession: full-time practice, a change of name to sharpen the boundaries of its exclusive domain, the setting up of a national association, the establishment of a training school or its equivalent, a code of ethics, and the seeking of legal and public support and recognition (Ritzer 1977, pp. 46–48). In Singapore, medical practice from the beginning was a full-time occupation patterned along the lines of the Hippocratic oath as understood and applied in England. The physicians' control of medical education had been established since 1905, even though medical practitioners did not form a national professional organization until 1959, when the Singapore Medical Association (SMA) was formed.

The SMA, however, was not the first local association of physicians. In 1923 the graduates of the King Edward VII College of Medicine created the Alumni Association; this group was very active as "sponsor and campaigner" for upgrading the College into the University of Malaya. The Alumni Association asked the Colonial Governor to raise the status of the graduates from "assistant surgeons" to medical officers—that is, to a level equal to that of European physicians in the island (Chen 1965, p. 32). Since the 1920s the latter had been organized into the powerful Straits Medical Association. The association supported the Governor's refusal of the Alumni Association's request for upgrading degrees.

In view of its reported activities, the Alumni Association was a de facto professional association for local physicians. On the other hand, some historical accounts (Chen 1965; Gwee 1968) give the impression that the Straits Medical Association was also known as the Malayan Branch of the British Medical Association. This crucial international link gave the Straits Medical Association more legitimacy and status as a professional association than the Alumni Association ever could claim. The superior professional standing of the Straits Medical Association was corroborated by the fact that it served as the immediate predecessor of the current Singapore Medical Association (SMA).

This last change was significant in the historical process of unifying the medical profession in Singapore. Hitherto it had been divided into local and European factions represented by their respective associations. According to Gwee (1968), the British Medical Association gave its full support to the change in name from Straits Medical Association to Singapore Medical Association and transferred the assets of the former to the new SMA. The Alumni Association was not left out completely; it contributed to this historical transformation by converting its own journal into the *Singapore Medical Journal*, the official publication of the SMA. The SMA began its activities with a total membership of 320 (Fong 1982, p. 133). The main objectives of the SMA, established in 1959, remain the same today; these are

> . . . to maintain the honour and interests of the medical profession . . . to foster and preserve the unity and aim of purpose of the medical profession . . . to voice its opinion and to acquaint the Government and other bodies with the policy and attitude of the profession (SMA 1977, p. 1).

From the SMA sprang other affiliated medical societies. Among the first was the Society of General Practitioners, which was established in 1962 with the approval of the SMA (Koh 1982, p. 9). Numerous other societies have been established since then to represent the continuously increasing number of medical specialties in Singapore. All of these societies have served as channels of professional influence within the boundaries established by government intervention.

INTERNAL ORGANIZATION OF THE MEDICAL PROFESSION

The internal organization of the medical profession in Singapore must be understood as the outcome of a balance between government intervention and the traditional desire of the profession to maintain its autonomy. As is standard procedure in all modern nations today, physicians in Singapore must register with the Singapore Medical Council "before they are allowed to practice"; 2,941 medical doctors were registered with the Council in January 1988 (Ministry of Communications and Information 1988, p. 94). This number amounts to about 888 persons per doctor if we consider that the total population in 30 June 1987 was 2,612,800 (Ministry of Communications and Information 1988, p. 3).

The Medical Council serves as the profession's gatekeeper, to use Stone's (1976) term. This body screens entry into the profession and keeps the medical house in order by regulating professional ethics and conduct. The Council shares this function with the Registrar of Medical Practitioners, who is also the Director of Medical Services and Permanent Secretary of the Ministry of Health, as well as an ex-officio member of the Council. Of the other 13 members of the Council, five are appointed directly by the government; two are representatives of the University, one of whom is the Dean of the Faculty of Medicine; and six represent members of the profession at large. The composition of the gatekeeping body illustrates the level of state intervention or patronage; although all the members of the Medical Council are physicians, five represent the government. The presence of university representatives in the gatekeeping body illustrates clearly not only the importance of the professional school in shaping the medical profession, but also, and perhaps more significant, the conviction that the medical profession must have a measure of control over the selection of future medical practitioners.

Thus the medical profession in Singapore is very well organized and represented, although the bodies set up by physicians are indicative of both cohesion and internal differences within the profession. In addition to the Medical Council, which deals with matters of conduct and professional ethics, there is the Academy of Medicine, which concentrates on the scientific and knowledge aspects of the profession. The Singapore Medical Association serves a variety of functions including a role equivalent to that of a trade union, which represents the interests of all medical doctors. Numerous associations of medical specialists represent narrower interests and serve to sharpen the boundary between themselves and general practitioners. The Association of Private Medical Practitioners of Singapore represents the concerns of physicians in the private sector, which differ from those of their counterparts in public service.

Although all these organizations, particularly the Singapore Medical Association (SMA), are active in voicing the profession's position, the scope of their influence and their effectiveness in lobbying are limited. For example, the SMA did not succeed in stopping legislation on abortion, on professional secrecy related to patients' drug addiction, or on the bonding of medical students (Quah 1984, p. 118).

THE SOCIAL POSITION OF THE PROFESSION

A discussion of the social position of physicians in Singapore must involve two interconnected aspects: the community's perception of the prestige of medicine as an occupation and the actual bases for that prestige, particularly income.

A study of social class in Singapore (Quah, Chiew, Ko, and Lee 1989) provides insight into the perceived prestige of medical doctors in the community. Using internationally accepted measures such as the NORC and the United States Census scales (Nam and Powers 1983) to measure occupational prestige in Singapore, the Singapore study found that doctors were ranked at the top. On the NORC scale of occupational prestige, medical doctors received a score of 93 out of a possible 100. Other high-prestige occupations received slightly lower scores; lawyers, 92; engineers, 91; and architects, 88 (Quah, Ko, and Chiew 1989, pp. 461–62).

Singapore is far from unique in the public perception of medicine as the most prestigious occupation. As Table 1 illustrates, a comparison of countries from North and South America, Europe, and Asia, plus Australia, shows clearly that the medical profession is highly prestigious throughout the world. Other high-prestige occupations received consistently lower scores.

Another aspect of occupational prestige is the question of popular consensus. Some occupations may evoke great respect in some sectors of the population but may be regarded less highly by others. This tends to be the case with religious occupations, specifically leaders of various religious groups. The 109 occupations included in the Singapore study were compared in terms of their standard deviations—that is, the level of consensus or agreement in the population concerning the prestige of each occupation. Religious occupations scores were found to have the highest standard deviations, ranging from 1.15 to 1.24. In contrast, the standard deviation for the physicians' prestige score was .64, the third lowest of the 109 occupations studied. The two occupations with lower standard deviations were engineer (SD = .63) and university professor (SD = .61) (Quah 1989b, pp. 366–68). These figures confirm that Singaporeans share a considerable degree of consensus concerning the high prestige of

TABLE 1. Comparison of Occupational Prestige Rankings of Medicine and Other Professions in Selected Countries

	Professions			
Countries	Physician	Lawyer	Engineer	Architect
Singapore (NORC)[a]	93	92	91	88
United States (NORC)[b]	81	75	68	67
United States (SSS)[c]	78	73	70	72
Chile[d]	78	69	77	76
Norway[e]	76	69	68	68
Australia[f]	81	79	75	78
India[g]	76	69	na	na
Indonesia[h]	87	80	82	na
Philippines[i]	79	74	71	na
Thailand[j]	79	61	54	na
Taiwan[k]	79	77	70	na
Japan[l]	73	71	63	na

[a] Quah, Ko, and Chiew (1989, pp. 461–62).
[b] Hauser and Featherman (1977, pp. 320–21).
[c] See Treiman (1977, pp. 293–94). These and the scores that follow for the other countries are Standard Scale Scores (SSS).
[d] Treiman (1977, p. 356).
[e] Treiman (1977, p. 432).
[f] Treiman (1977, p. 332).
[g] Treiman (1977, p. 391).
[h] Treiman (1977, p. 393).
[i] Treiman (1977, p. 436).
[j] Treiman (1977, p. 466).
[k] Treiman (1977, p. 460).
[l] Treiman (1977, p. 406).
na = information not available.

medical doctors in comparison to members of other occupations.

A second relevant aspect of physicians' social position in Singapore is income. As in the case of occupational prestige, it is useful to compare the income of physicians with that of other high-prestige professionals such as lawyers, architects, and engineers.

The annual mean income of medical doctors varies according to years of working experience, like that of most other workers in the labor force. An interesting trend emerges when the annual mean income is seen in terms of the professional's years of experience. Table 2 provides the relevant figures, based on data collected from the 1980 population census. When physicians, lawyers, engineers, and architects are compared, physicians are the top earners only among professionals with fewer than six years of work experience. Among professionals with six or more years of experience, however, lawyers are the top earners, even though the medical profession is slightly higher in social prestige. Medical doctors are the second highest earners among professionals with six to 19 years of work experience, but they fall to third place behind lawyers and architects among the most senior professionals, namely those with 20 or more years of experience.

The data from Table 2 are taken from the 1980 census. Let us look into another, more recent source of data which, although indirect, still provides a relevant perspective. That source is the income of university graduates, published by the National University of Singapore.

As Table 3 shows, fresh medical school graduates earned the lowest average starting salary among the four professions in 1983. The income of new doctors improved in 1986, when they ranked second after new law graduates. Nevertheless, these figures for medical doctors' starting salaries are not far behind the median yearly income of all university graduates in the labor force. The corresponding figures for 1981 and 1986 were $19,716 and $29,298 respectively (as calculated from Ministry of Labour 1987, p. 31).

The main implications of Tables 2 and 3 are 1) that the starting salary of doctors is below the national median salary of university-educated members of the labor force and 2) that although more experienced and better established professionals earn more than fresh graduates, senior lawyers and architects in Singapore tend to have greater earning power than senior physicians. Taken together, these findings suggest that income is not the sole or even the principal reason for the high prestige that the community ascribes to the profession of medicine.

As stated earlier, an important component of physicians' social position is their "channels of influence," the way in which they attempt to attain power and to influence decision making in society. In Singapore, the Singapore Medical Association (SMA) has been active in voicing its members' views and in lobbying for legislative changes, additions, or omissions beneficial to their profession. Government intervention in Singapore, however, restricts the scope of influence and the lobbying effectiveness of professional associations, including the SMA. For example, the SMA did not succeed in stopping legislation that it deemed to be contrary to the medical profession's ideology, such as the legalization of abortion, the overriding of confidentiality concerning drug addicts, and the bonding of medical students.

Referring to this "problem," a former President of SMA lamented that

> . . . there seems to be an unfortunate lack of communication between the government

TABLE 2. Comparison of Annual Mean Income of Medicine and Other Professions by Years of Work Experience, Singapore, 1980 (Singapore Dollars)

Years of Work Experience	Professions			
	Physician	Lawyer	Engineer	Architect
Fewer than 3	$27,503	$18,604	$21,658	$22,717
3 to 5	$32,821	$30,632	$27,234	$28,713
6 to 9	$49,208	$59,348	$35,668	$39,853
10 to 14	$63,999	$75,419	$47,212	$53,126
15 to 19	$75,984	$91,713	$56,480	$73,667
20 or more	$76,685	$166,780	$73,024	$82,883

Source: Quah (1984, p. 86b).

TABLE 3. Comparison of Annual Mean Income of Medicine, Law, Engineering, and Architecture Graduates, Singapore, 1983 and 1986 (Singapore Dollars)

Annual Mean Income	Professions			
	Physician	Lawyer	Engineer	Architect
Total number of graduates				
1983	127	80	139	42
1986	150	160	554	31
Annual mean income				
1983	$19,080	$19,464	$22,392	$21,348
1986	$19,344	$20,796	$19,080	$16,500

Sources: For the 1983 figures see National University of Singapore (1986, pp. 32–34). For the 1986 figures see National University of Singapore (1987, pp. 39–41). The original figures for the monthly mean income were multiplied by 12 to facilitate the comparison with figures in Table 2.

> and the professional organizations . . . This lack of communication and understanding is unfortunate as both government and the medical profession have at heart the interest of the people whom they serve . . . (Lim 1979, p. 38).

Lim gives an accurate description of one side of the story, but in fact the Singapore situation is characterized by a combination of intervention and flexibility on the part of the government. The other side of the story is that despite government intervention, SMA is consulted by policy makers from time to time. As consultants, physicians are asked for their views and suggestions on problems falling within their realm of expertise.

Regarding the use of other channels of influence, studies of the professions in various countries have documented the common tendency among professionals to seek and maintain "proximity to power" (Larson 1977, p. xv). Singapore professionals are no exception, and this tendency is facilitated by the small size of the local talent pool. With a population of only 2.6 million, citizens with professional qualifications have a greater probability of rising to the top than do their counterparts in more populated nations. This probability is enhanced by the prevailing emphasis on merit, as opposed to nepotism or other means of social mobility, and by the political leadership's active recruitment of educated Singaporeans into politics and the civil service. In 1982 the 75 Member of Parliament (MPs) included two physicians; as of 1989 the current 82 members include four. The previous president of the Republic was a highly respected obstetrician; the present head of the Singapore Civil Service and the Permanent Secretary of the Ministry of Health are also medical doctors.

Nevertheless, the presence of physicians in high political or administrative office must be interpreted with caution. We must ask some key questions to test Mosher's (1978) concept of channels of influence. For example, do these high-ranking officials protect the interests of their profession in the course of their work? Are they more likely to yield to their own profession's lobbying than are nonmedical officials or MPs? Anderson and his colleagues (1980) consider this a problem of divided loyalties, specifically the conflict between commitment to one's profession and commitment to one's office. Unfortunately, we lack sufficient data to address these questions here. Yet we must keep in mind that in Singapore, channels of influence are not only taken; they also can be given, facilitated, or withdrawn by the state.

In this respect Singapore's historical and current data tend to support two of the three aspects of Ritzer's (1977) integrated approach. First, the medical profession actually depends on the dominant elites to obtain and retain power. Second, the power of the medical profession varies over time.

Finally, government intervention to curtail the power of physicians is not unique to Singapore. Touhy (1976) sees such intervention as a feature of welfare states that act as watchdogs over the professionals. In fact, specific monitoring programs have been devised in Canada, the United States, and Germany (Freidson 1986; Landsberg 1980; Stone 1976).

CONCLUSION: A COMPARATIVE VIEW

This analysis of the medical profession in Singapore was guided by the features of professions as identified by the process, structural-functional, conflict, and integrated approaches presented in the first section. It has covered the historical development of the profession, highlighting the main aspects of its structure, its internal organization, and its social position.

Most of these characteristics of professions are found in the medical profession in Singapore, where physicians historically have practiced medicine as a full-time occupation. The creation and development of a medical association was originally difficult because of the political, social, and economic conditions of Singapore as a British colony and the corresponding division between local and "European" doctors. Thus the national association underwent several changes both in name and in structure; and the same socioeconomic and political problems were encountered in establishing the medical school. Yet the medical school was set up because of the determination of individual local physicians trained in England and because of the social esteem they received from the local community. This school is now the Faculty of Medicine of the National University of Singapore. In addition, the Singapore Medical Association was born; it is now the umbrella for several medical organizations representing medical specialists. The Singapore Medical Council is the watchdog of medical ethics; the profession has succeeded in obtaining legal and public support and recognition.

Nevertheless, government intervention effectively limits the social power of the medical profession, while the latter is consulted either as a group or as individual physicians in matters pertaining to health policy. Furthermore, medical doctors in Singapore do not differ from their colleagues in other modern nations when they display the norms of autonomy, authority over clients, and altruism as part of their professional ideology. Although the prestige of physicians is high, consumers of medical services are now more highly informed and better educated; thus they are more inclined to judge medical pronouncements and to seek a second or third medical opinion.

Even though the main objective of this paper is the discussion of the Singapore case, the comparative perspective implied throughout the preceding pages may now be presented more explicitly. The historical development of the medical profession in Singapore followed the basic path found in other British colonies, particularly during the nineteenth century. The British Crown exercised strong policy intervention, and British and European physicians were clearly inclined to monopolize medical practice, to the detriment of the development of a strong body of local medical practitioners. The model of medical practice and medical education for the former group was the medical profession in England.

The tradition of policy intervention established by the British colonial government was continued, expanded, and improved by the Republic of Singapore's government after independence. This historical change also marked Singapore's departure from the path of socioeconomic development followed by other former British colonies. As noted in the third section of this paper, legislation monitors the internal organization of the medical profession without preventing physicians from establishing their own associations and professional activities. Singaporean physicians' internal organization emulates that of the medical profession in industrialized countries. This feature is to be expected because the practice of modern medicine in most nations has been ruled by international standards for most of this century. For example, features such as a national medical association, an academy of medicine or its equivalent, a medical code of ethics, and the requirement of international recognition of specialists' training are found in both developed and developing or Third World countries.

Nevertheless, these cross-national similarities cannot overshadow some notable differences. Singapore's rapid pace of economic development, its political structure (based on a pragmatic version of democratic socialism), and the government's policy style (characterized by active intervention) (Quah 1981, 1983) distinguish Singapore from other Third World countries. More important, these characteristics of Singapore's superstructure have a "spillover" effect on the professions, including the medical profession. As a consequence, some differences may be found between the medical profession in Singapore and its counterparts in other developing nations.

To illustrate, a significant difference between the medical profession in the Philippines and in Singapore is that the former enjoys a greater degree of flexibility in managing its own internal organization. It is common for the Filipino medical associations to participate directly in drafting of legislation concerning their own profession (Carino 1973, p. 81). Another notable difference is the serious brain drain faced by Filipino medical services (Carino 1973, p. 82). There are no reliable published figures on the emigration of medical doctors from Singapore, but the ratio of doctors to the population and the annual number of registered doctors indicate a steady increase in the number of medical doctors practicing in Singapore. There were 1,265 persons per doctor in 1978; this ratio improved to 930 persons per doctor in 1986 (Quah 1989c, p. 150). The factors associated with brain drain in any country are complex, and it would be presumptuous to offer reasons for the large number of Filipino physicians leaving their country. Yet in comparing the situation of Singapore with that of the Philippines, we may suggest cautiously two reasons why Singapore does not experience the same high level of physicians' emigrating as the Philippines. One reason may be the higher income and standard of living enjoyed by Singaporeans. The other may be the superior infrastructure of the Singapore health services, which gives physicians access to high-technology medical equipment and facilities in diagnosis, treatment, and research.

In his study of the medical profession in Thailand, Silcock (1977) used the term "indigenised" professional structure. In such situations the government has much less control than in Singapore; codes of ethics are relatively lax; moonlighting is common; brain drain is a serious problem; and national professional associations are not very active or truly representative. Other analysts point out that medical doctors tend to have an aristocratic background and are often found close to the corridors of power, such as the upper ranks of the Thai bureaucracy or the military (Dhiravegin 1975; London 1979). The most noticeable effect of this upper-class background is the large social gap between doctors and most urban poor and rural patients, who form the bulk of the Thai population (Sermsri 1989). There are two key differences between Singapore and Thailand. First, medical doctors in Singapore tend to have a more diverse social class background because of the universal system of education, the emphasis on merit, and subsidized university education, supplemented by grants and scholarships. Second, Singapore does not have the significant rural population and urban poverty belts that characterize many other Third World countries.

Another interesting comparison may be made between Singapore and the People's Republic of China. Although these two countries differ radically in their political systems, communist China and democratic socialist Singapore share a similar level of government commitment to their health care services. This commitment necessarily involves the internal organization and the mode of practice of the medical profession. In China, legislation has succeeded in molding the medical doctors to fit into the dual system of modern and traditional health services (Quah and Li 1989). In contrast, the government in Singapore continues its full support of medical doctors as the only legitimate practitioners of medicine, but permits traditional Chinese physicians to continue their practice under the cloak of business enterprises.

Finally, findings from international comparisons of occupational prestige and social class show that medicine is a highly regarded profession today in most developed and developing countries. According to available information, this attitude has been present in Singapore since it was declared a British territory in 1819. In contrast, Starr's (1982) well-known study of the medical profession in the United States shows that the high prestige of the medical profession in North America is a twentieth-century phenomenon. This difference suggests cultural influences on the perception of medical practitioners. The histories of Asian nations such as China, Japan, and Korea are rich in examples of the social respect and recognition given to individuals who dedicated their lives to studying and practicing medicine. After these nations established contact with the West, that social recognition was expanded to include the practitioners of Western medicine.

This analysis of the medical profession in a Third World country points to the similarities between Singapore and Western nations in the structure of medicine and the social position of physicians. It also calls attention to some of the differences between Singapore and other Third World Asian nations. Further, comparative research must be pursued to enhance our understanding of the structure, role, and contribution of the medical profession in countries with different socioeconomic and political systems.

REFERENCES

Anderson, R.M., R. Perruci, D.E. Schendel, and L.E. Trachman. 1980. *Divided Loyalties: Whistle-Blowing at BART*. West Lafayette, IN: Purdue University Office of Publications.

Carino, Ledivina V. 1973. *The Role of the Professions in Philippine National Development*. Manila: College of Public Administration, University of the Philippines.

Carr-Saunders, Alexander Morris and P.A. Wilson. 1933. *The Professions*. Oxford: Clarendon Press.

Chen, Su Lan. 1965. "Reminiscences." Pp. 31–34 in *Sixty Years of Medical Education: 1905–1965*, edited by Malcolm Stewart Muir and Wong Poi Kwang. Singapore: University of Singapore Medical Society.

Colburne, Michael James. 1965. "Department of Social Medicine and Public Health." Pp. 63–66 in *Sixty Years of Medical Education: 1905–1965*, edited by Malcolm Stewart Muir and Wong Poi Kwang. Singapore: University of Singapore Medical Society.

Colony of Singapore. 1953. *Report of the Committee of Enquiry on Medical Education in Malaya, November-December, 1953*. Singapore: Government Printing Office.

Dhiravegin, Likhit. 1975. "The Power Elite in Thailand. A General Survey with Focus on the Civil Bureaucrats." Pp. 83–102 in *Elites and Development*, edited by Arnold Wehmhoener. Bangkok: Friedrich-Ebert-Stiftung.

Fong, Chan Yoon (ed.) 1982. *Singapore Professional Centre Directory 1981/1982*. Singapore: Singapore Professional Centre.

Freidson, Eliot (ed.). 1973. *The Professions and Their Prospects*. Beverly Hills: Sage.

______. 1986. *Professional Powers*. Chicago: University of Chicago Press.

Gwee, Ah Leng. 1968. "The Singapore Medical Association and the Singapore Medical Journal." Pp. 33–45 in *The First National Medical Convention Souvenir Programme*, edited by the Singapore Medical Association. Singapore: SMA.

Haug, Marie R. 1973. "Deprofessionalisation: An Alternative Hypothesis for the Future." Pp. 195–211 in *Professionalisation and Social Change*, edited by Paul Halmos. Keele, UK: University of Keele.

Hauser, Robert M. and David L. Featherman. 1977. *The Process of Stratification: Trends and Analyses*. New York: Academic Press.

Johnson, Terence. 1973. "Imperialism and the Professions." Pp. 281–310 in *Professionalisation and Social Change*, edited by Paul Halmos. Keele, UK: University of Keele.

Kanagaratnam, K. 1965. "The Early Years of the Medical School." Pp. 20–23 in *Sixty Years of Medical Education: 1905–1965*, edited by Malcolm Stewart Muir and Wong Poi Kwang. Singapore: University of Singapore Medical Society.

Kanagasuntheram, R. 1965. "Department of Anatomy." Pp. 39–40 in *Sixty Years of Medical Education: 1905–1965*, edited by Malcolm Stewart Muir and Wong Poi Kwang. Singapore: University of Singapore Medical Society.

Koh, E.K. 1982. "Early Days of the College." *Singapore Family Physician* 8:8–11.

Landsberg, Henry A. 1980. "The Trend towards Citizen Participation in the Welfare State: Countervailing Power of the Professions." Pp. 228–43 in *Comparative Public Policy and Citizen Participation*, edited by C.R. Foster. New York: Pergamon.

Larson, Magali S. 1977. *The Rise of Professionalism: A Sociological Analysis*. Berkeley: University of California Press.

Lee, Yoon Kiat. 1978. *The Medical History of Early Singapore*. Tokyo: Southeast Asian Medical Information Center.

Lim, Arthur Siew Ming. 1979. "Communication between Government and Professional Organizations." Pp. 36–38 in *Partners in Development*, edited by Fong Chan Yoon. Singapore: Singapore Professional Centre.

Lim, Tay Boh. 1965. "The Role of the University in Medical Education." Pp. 12–14 in *Sixty Years of Medical Education: 1905–1965*, edited by Malcolm Stewart Muir and Wong Poi Kwang. Singapore: University of Singapore Medical Society.

London, Bruce. 1979. "Elites and Class in Thai History: The Comparative Use of Power Elite and Ruling Class Analysis." *Southeast Asian Journal of Social Science* 7:30–59.

Medical Research Committee. 1929. *Proceedings of the Committee Appointed by His Excellency the Governor and High Commissioner to Report on the Question of Medical Research throughout Malaya*. Singapore: Federal Malay State Paper No. 12.

Ministry of Communications and Information. 1988. *Singapore Facts and Pictures, 1988*. Singapore: Information Division, Ministry of Communications and Information.

Ministry of Labour. 1987. *Report on the Labour Force Survey of Singapore, 1986*. Singapore: Research and Statistics Department, Ministry of Labour.

Miyazaki, Ichisada. 1981. *China's Examination Hell*. New Haven: Yale University Press.

Moore, Wilbert E. and Melvin M. Tumin. 1949. "Some Social Functions of Ignorance." *American Sociological Review* 14:787–95.

Mosher, Frederick C. 1978. "Professions in Public Service." *Public Administration Review* 38: 144–50.

Nam. Charles B. and Mary G. Powers. 1983. *The Socioeconomic Approach to Status Measurement*. Houston: Cap and Gown.

National University of Singapore. 1986. *1985 NUS Graduate Employment Survey*. Singapore: Applied Research Corporation.

———. 1987. *1986 NUS Graduate Employment Survey*. Singapore: Applied Research Corporation.

Oppenheimer, M. 1973. "The Proletarianization of the Professionals." Pp. 213–40 in *Professionalisation and Social Change*, edited by Paul Halmos. Keele, UK: University of Keele.

Quah, Stella R. 1981. "Health Policy and Traditional Medicine in Singapore." *Social Science and Medicine* 15A:149–56.

———. 1983. "Social Discipline in Singapore: An Alternative for the Resolution of Social Problems." *Journal of Southeast Asian Studies* 14:266–89.

———. 1984. *Balancing Autonomy and Control: The Case of Professionals in Singapore*. Cambridge: Center for International Studies, Massachusetts Institute of Technology.

———. 1989a. "Education and Social Class in Singapore." Pp. 59–106 in *Social Stratification and Mobility in Singapore*, edited by Stella R. Quah, Chiew Seen Kong, Ko Yiu Chung, and Lee Meng Chee. Singapore: National University of Singapore.

———. 1989b. "The Realities of Social Class." Pp. 360–94 in *Social Stratification and Mobility in Singapore*, edited by Stella R. Quah, Chiew Seen Kong, Ko Yiu Chung, and Lee Meng Chee. Singapore: National University of Singapore.

———. 1989c. "The Best Bargain: Medical Options in Singapore." Pp. 122–159 in *The Triumph of Practicality: Tradition and Modernity in Health Care Utilization in Selected Asian Countries*, edited by Stella R. Quah. Singapore: Institute of Southeast Asian Studies.

Quah, Stella R., Seen Kong Chiew, Yiu Chung Ko, and Meng Chee Lee (eds.). 1989. *Social Stratification and Mobility in Singapore*. Singapore: National University of Singapore.

Quah, Stella R., Yiu Chung Ko, and Seen Kong Chiew. 1989. "Occupational Prestige Scores SOPS and SNORC, Mean, Standard Deviation and Sample Size for 109 Occupations, Singapore, 1983–1984." Pp. 456–63 in *Social Stratification and Mobility in Singapore*, edited by Stella R. Quah, Chiew Seen Kong, Ko Yiu Chung, and Lee Meng Chee. Singapore: National University of Singapore.

Quah, Stella R. and Jing Wei Li, 1989. "Marriage of Convenience: Traditional and Modern Medicine in the People's Republic of China." Pp. 19–42 in *The Triumph of Practicality: Tradition and Modernity in Health Care Utilization in Selected Asian Countries*, edited by Stella R. Quah. Singapore: Institute of Southeast Asian Studies.

Ritzer, George. 1977. *Working, Conflict and Change*. 2nd ed. Englewood Cliffs, NJ: Prentice-Hall.

Sermsri, Santhat. 1989. "Utilization of Traditional and Modern Health Care Services in Thailand." Pp. 160–179 in *The Triumph of Practicality: Tradition and Modernity in Health Care Utilization in Selected Asian Countries*, edited by Stella R. Quah. Singapore: Institute of Southeast Asian Studies.

Silcock, Thomas Henry. 1977. "Thailand: An Indigenous Professional Structure?" in *Professional Structure in Southeast Asia*, edited by Thomas Henry Silcock. Canberra: Australian National University.

SMA (Singapore Medical Association). 1977. *Constitution of the SMA*. Singapore: SMA.

Srinivasagam, Elizabeth et al. (eds.) 1972. *Tables of the Written Laws of the Republic of Singapore, 1819–1971*. Singapore: Malaya Law Review and the University of Singapore.

Starr, Paul E. 1982. *The Social Transformation of American Medicine*. New York: Basic Books.

Stone, Deborah. 1976. "Professionalism and Accountability." *Journal of Health Politics, Policy and Law* 1:33–47.

Tay, T.E. 1965. "The Role of the Medical School in Malaysia." Pp. 10–11 in *Sixty Years of Medical Education: 1905–1965*, edited by Malcolm Steward Muir and Wong Poi Kwang. Singapore: University of Singapore Medical Society.

Tham, Seong Chee. 1981. "Staff and Faculty Development in Singapore." Pp. 137–225 in *Staff and Faculty Development in Southeast Asian Universities*, edited by the Regional Institute of Higher Education. Singapore: Maruzen Asia.

Touhy, C.J. 1976. "Private Government, Property and Professionalism." *Canadian Journal of Political Science* 9:668–81.

Treiman, Donald J. 1977. *Social Stratification in a Comparative Perspective*. New York: Academic Press.

Turnbull, C. Mary. 1977. *A History of Singapore, 1819–1975*. Kuala Lumpur: Oxford University Press.

***STELLA R. QUAH** is a sociologist and senior lecturer in the Department of Sociology, National University of Singapore, Republic of Singapore. In addition to works on the sociology of professions, Dr. Quah has published in medical sociology, social policy, and sociology of the family.*

[31]

Soc. Sci. Med. Vol. 32, No. 9, pp. 1007–1016, 1991
0277-9536/91 $3.00 + 0.00

THE PATIENT'S RIGHT TO INFORMATION IN JAPAN—LEGAL RULES AND DOCTOR'S OPINIONS

HIROYUKI HATTORI,[1] STEPHAN M. SALZBERG,[2] WINSTON P. KIANG,[2] TATSUYA FUJIMIYA,[3] YUTAKA TEJIMA[4] and JUNJI FURUNO[1]

[1]Department Legal Medicine, Yamaguchi University School of Medicine, Ube 755, Japan
[2]Asian Legal Study Program, Faculty of Law, University of British Columbia, Vancouver, B.C., Canada V6T 1Y1
[3]Department of Legal Medicine, Kyoto Prefectural University of Medicine, Kyoto 602, Japan
[4]Faculty of Law, Hiroshima University, Hiroshima 730, Japan

Abstract—A questionnaire survey concerning informed consent was administrated among Japanese physicians in Yamaguchi prefecture. The survey results showed that even though these Japanese physicians are willing to give their patients sufficient information to obtain informed consent, the discretion of the physician to provide information is still prevalent. The survey also revealed that Japanese physicians believe that information regarding the treatment to be administrated should be fully disclosed both in cases when the treatment is still experimental and when it is established among specialists. Finally, the survey showed that despite the liberal attitude of the Japanese physicians toward informed consent, they are reluctant to make medical records accessible to the patients.

It was found that when Japanese physicians were faced with special cases such as prior to administering high-risk diagnostic procedures, prior to disclosing the presence of cancer in their patients, or when faced with patients unwilling to receive treatment, the involvement of the patient's family members in the decision-making process was preferred so as not to aggravate the patient's emotional anxiety. With respect to cancer patients, the survey suggested that many Japanese physicians believe that cancer operations performed without informed consent from the patient should be legal. Finally, the survey concluded that, although the concept of individualized informed consent has been generally accepted among physicians, the involvement of family members in the decision-making process and a conservative attitude toward disclosure of information are still prevalent in Japan.

Key words—informed consent, malpractice, medical record, physician–patient relationship

INTRODUCTION

The Japanese approach to ethical issues in health care has been characterized by the Japanese cultural values of consensus and deference to authority [1]. For example, the late Japanese Emperor Hirohito passed away in early 1989 apparently without ever realizing he had intestinal cancer, thus vividly illustrating the extent to which patients in Japan are deliberately left ignorant of their health condition. Whether the patient be royalty or an ordinary citizen, Japanese doctors still believe disclosure of terminal cancer will cause unnecessary grief [2].

However, with the remarkable development of medical science and technology, philosophical and moral attitudes toward what is considered appropriate medical care or conduct have changed considerably. Issues in medical law and ethics, such as informed consent, have become topics of heated discussion among medical and legal specialists, as well as among the general public. Physicians and lawyers tend to hold widely divergent views on medico-legal issues, and this has contributed to making medical malpractice suits difficult to settle.

In countries such as the United States and West Germany, informed consent has become an essential component in ensuring that patients become knowledgeable participants in choosing health care options. In the American Hospital Association Statement on the Patient's Bill of Rights (1972) [3], the rights of patients are stated explicitly. In Japan, however, the concept of informed consent has not yet been generally accepted by the medical profession. The right of the patient to take part in the decision-making process to a large extent remains ignored.

However certain factors are pressuring traditional attitudes on appropriate medical care or conduct to change. For example, developments in biomedical sciences, such as laboratory medicine and new diagnostic instruments, have caused many physicians to neglect traditional personal contact with their patients. Furthermore, with migration of the younger generation from the rural areas to the cities, local communities have been breaking down. Local physicians have lost the generation-old close ties with patients and their families [4].

Hence, the traditional relationship between physician and patient, which is closely akin to the teacher–student relationship in Japan and involves great deference to the physician's advice and decisions, has thus been rapidly vanishing. For example, even when a physician has conducted a proper medical examination and dispensed appropriate treatment, his patient may complain of less than satisfactory medical service due to the lack of personal rapport between physician and patient. This has led to an increasing number of medical malpractice suits [5]. Many doctors have come to realize that these situations are a necessary risk of practice and, not surprisingly, they have come to adopt a defensive attitude toward patients and treatment. Therefore, to cope with this situation, medical ethics committees have been established in various medical associations and universities. Along with dealing with issues such as organ transplant, brain death and artificial fertilization, the committees examine the increasing trend of medical malpractice claims.

In the present study, a medical, legal and sociological analysis of a questionnaire survey assesses the relationship between physician and patient in the decision-making process regarding medical treatment and the disclosure of information to the patient. This paper first reviews and discusses the relationship between physician and patient. Second, the extent of the information provided to the patient prior to receiving treatment is examined, as well as the accessibility of medical records after treatment. The third section deals with how physicians cope with difficult cases, including the extent to which risks accompanying dangerous medical procedures and the presence of cancer are disclosed. The physicians' response to patients unwilling to receive treatment is also discussed. Finally, this paper attempts to explain the concept and practice of substitute consent, traditionally of great importance in medical care in Japan.

MATERIALS AND METHODS

A questionnaire dealing with medical malpractice issues was prepared with the aid of lawyers, legal scholars and physicians. This questionnaire was prepared based on a previous study conducted in Kyoto in 1984 [6], and consisted of questions encompassing 19 distinct topics including such controversial issues as medical malpractice suits, brain death and artificial fertilization. In situations where court decisions bearing on the issues were available, the language of those decisions was incorporated in the questionnaire statement to which physicians responded. The source of judicial language was not indicated.

The survey was conducted between November 1986 and March 1987. The questionnaire was sent from the Department of Legal Medicine, Yamaguchi University, to physicians and medical students at Yamaguchi University and to hospital staff physicians in Yamaguchi prefecture. Hospitals selected for the survey were Yamaguchi University Hospital and the hospitals located in Yamaguchi prefecture which have exchanges in staff and technology with the university hospital, and which have patient admission facilities. Yamaguchi prefecture is characterized as a rural area, located at the west end of Honshu Island about 1000 km away from Tokyo. The replies were anonymous. Sixty-three percent of the physicians and 80% of the students responded. Composition of the samples is shown in the Table 1. There was no obvious difference between the responses of physicians in the University Hospital and hospital staff physicians. In most cases, responses of medical students also were similar to those of the University physicians and the hospital staff physicians, so, in the discussion, all groups were summed up into one group. For a complete listing of all the questions on the questionnaire, please refer to the Appendix.

Table 1. Composition of the sample

Characteristics	PU	PH	Total
Age			
20–29	60	76	136
30–39	106	193	299
40–49	26	94	120
50–59	10	65	75
60 or older	4	20	24
Specialty area			
Non-surgical (internal medicine, pediatrics, psychiatry dermatology)	61	185	246
Surgical (surgery, orthopediatrics, obstetric-gynecology)	97	232	329
Other	47	31	79

PU, Physicians in University Hosptial.
PH, Physicians in hospital.

In the succeeding sections, the Japanese medical and legal climate surrounding the ethical issues to be investigated in this study will be described as an introduction in order for the reader to understand the results. Then, the results of the questionnaire will be presented, followed by a discussion of the legal rules and prevailing medical attitude on each subject. Concluding remarks were added at the end of each section.

This paper deals only with the questionnaire's findings regarding informed consent.

RESULTS AND DISCUSSION

Informed consent

The concept of informed consent was elaborated in the United States during the first decade of this century [7], and was based upon the right of the patient to be fully and clearly informed before being subjected to medical, and especially surgical treatment. In Japan, emphasis has recently been placed upon informed consent as a central element in the ethical and legal relationship between patient and physician. However, the respect for and perceived authority of doctors in Japan was very strong before the Second World War, and patients fully entrusted doctors with total and final decision-making authority with respect to their own medical treatment. Such an approach was consonant with the prevailing cultural and historical context in Japan. After the war, mainly due to fundamental human rights expressly set forth in the Japanese Constitution and the spread of medical knowledge among citizens, the relationship between patient and doctor and the attitudes of each have changed significantly.

As shown in Table 2, when questioned on their attitude toward informed consent, >55% of the physicians and medical students replied that they would give their patients the necessary information to make an intelligent decision as to what medical care to receive. About 21% of the physicians felt that the decision to inform should depend on the physician, who should use his individual judgement in assessing whether disclosure is advisable.

Table 2. In general, to what extent do you inform the patient of your diagnosis or treatment?

Item	S	PU	PH
(1) The level of explanation by the doctor is up to the doctor's judgement	80 (28.7)	38 (19.2)	91 (21.2)
(2) Information for the patient enabling him to make an informed decision should always be provided	154 (55.2)	117 (59.1)	260 (60.3)
(3) The doctor should inform the patient of all aspects of the diagnosis or treatment	32 (11.5)	36 (18.2)	75 (17.4)
(4) Other answer choices	13 (4.7)	7 (3.5)	5 (1.2)

S, Students.
PU, Physicians in University Hospital.
PH, Physicians in hospital.
Figures in parentheses are percentages.

Legal background of informed consent in Japan

Heavily influenced by German civil law theory, the concept of informed consent in Japan appears in bifurcated form as "Aufklärungspflicht" (physician's duty of disclosure) and "Einstimmung" (patient's consent). As far as legal theory is concerned in Japan, a number of possible sources of the legal duties regarding informed consent with respect to the physician–patient relationship has been identified and discussed by scholars [8, 9]. First, in general, any touching of a person can constitute battery in criminal law unless there has been consent. In the context of medical treatment, the consent of the patient justifies the invasion of his physical integrity, provided that the patient is given a full explanation by his physician. Secondly, the failure to use reasonable care in the conduct of one's activities, resulting in harm to others, constitutes negligence. In an informed consent case, negligence involves not the manner in which the physician performs a medical procedure, diagnoses illness or prescribes medication, etc., but in his making a deficient disclosure to the patient. Third, the arrangement between physican and patient is viewed as a special type of contractual relationship. The contract is usually implied from the actions of the parties and is not expressed in written contractual terms *per se*. The relationship has been interpreted as a kind of 'quasi-mandate', which is one of the enumerated contract types in the Japanese Civil Code concerning an affair other than a juristic act (Art. 656, Japanese Civil Code). Article 645 of the Japanese Civil Code states that on demand of the mandate (in this case, the patient), the mandatory (the physician) must at any time report the condition of business under his management. The mandatory must also report full particulars upon termination of the mandate. Hence, Article 645, which sets forth the 'quasi-mandate' relationship, could thus be considered as one of the legal sources of informed consent.

In most medical malpractice suits, the physician's duty to inform is derived, however, from Article 23 of the Medical Practitioner Act [10]. Article 23 reads:

A physician who diagnoses a patient must prescribe the necessary treatment, and give any other instruction needed for promoting health, either to the patient himself/herself or his/her guardian.

This article is closely related to the physician's duty to give proper instructions for treatment and addresses the physician's advice regarding such matters as drug administration, drinking and exercise, and contraindications for treatment purposes.

Informed consent and malpractice

In the past, most medical malpractice trials involved malpractice with respect to the actual performance of medical examination and treatment. However, ever since Professor Koichi Bai introduced the West German legal concept of informed consent into Japanese academic legal theory in 1970 [11], the number of medical malpractice suits alleging the physician's breach of duty to obtain informed consent has increased steadily. According to the Yamashita report [10], the ratio of the number of suits alleging breach of the duty to obtain informed consent to the total number of malpractice suits exceeded 10%.

In one celebrated case, a young lady was informed by her physician that she had mammary cancer of her right breast and she consented to an operation to remove the breast. However, during the operation, mastopathy was found in the left breast. The physician performed a mastectomy without the patient's consent, believing that the mastopathy had carcinogenic potential. In this case, a Japanese court held for the first time that the operation without consent constituted an illegal physical injury to the patient [10].

Then, in 1981, the Japanese Supreme Court finally discussed informed consent in the context of medical malpractice [12]. A 10 year old boy by chance fell down on the pavement while riding a bicycle and injured his head in the temporal area. A depressed bone fracture was observed. Although an operation was performed to remove the suspected bone fragment from the brain, the boy died of heart failure due to massive brain hemorrhage. The court held that the content of the operation and the risk involved must be explained to the patient or to his or her legal proxy by the attending surgeon. Furthermore, if there exist indefinite factors such as the present symptoms and their etiology, the level of improvement expected by the operation, as well as the exact prognosis and risks if the operation is not performed, then, the physician need not explain the level of assessment in the causative symptom and the preparation to cope with the situation. The medical act taken by the physician includes a series of procedures involving objective assessment and medical judgement of the symptoms and selection of the best available medical treatment. The court also noted that there is always some variability between the appearance of the symptoms and progression of the disease. In light of these facts, this ruling has been interpreted as meaning that the duty of a physician to inform a patient of his condition should be confined to those situations in which the factors involved in a particular condition are to a considerable extent clearly understood, and in which the course and prognosis of the disease are definite.

Generally speaking, a physician's civil liability arises when an obligation to the patient is not fulfilled. In most cases, the same fault may constitute both a breach of contract and the commission of a tort, assuming that the fault is a breach of duty owed to the patient. In Japan, a physician's liability has traditionally been perceived and pursued under the rubric of tort. Under Article 709 of the Japanese Civil Code governing tort liability and jurisprudence thereunder, the plaintiff must prove the requisite factors to establish liability, namely, proof of negligence and causation that the damage resulted from the negligence alleged. However, because medical knowledge is very specialized, it is often very difficult for patients to know in detail the state of their illness and the kind of treatment prescribed by the physicians. It is therefore very onerous for a patient to prove a negligent medical act and the existence of a causal relationship between the act and the alleged injury. In Japan, for reasons related to the patient's limited access to information discussed below, the traditional burden of proof is almost impossible for a patient-plaintiff to meet.

Legal theoreticians have proposed a number of ways to circumvent this difficulty. It has been proposed, for instance, that a physician's liability should be viewed as contractual. According to the Japanese Civil Code (Art. 415), the patient has only to prove a breach of contract to establish the liability of the physician. The courts have also held physicians liable in cases which distinguish between the physician's obligation to produce a particular result as fulfilment of the contract (result obligation), and the physician's obligation to use his best efforts to attain a certain goal (effort obligation). According to the concept of effort obligation, the physician is not liable for unsuccessful results by reason that he followed established medical standards, and, therefore, he used his best efforts.

Ultimately, due to the difficulty of determining the terms of the contract between physician and patient, the burden of proving a breach of contract has proven just as difficult as that needed to prove a tortious medical act [14].

Another approach would shift the burden of proof to the physician or hospital. One possible method for shifting the burden of proof in favor of the patient is to impose a rebuttable presumption of causation, when a "prima facie case" has been made only by the plaintiff. This view states that a causal relationship could be inferred by indirect facts and experiential presumption on this point. In judicial context, as seen in "prima facie case" or presumptive evidence, a fact is presumed to be true and sufficient to sustain a judgement unless the fact is contradicted or rebutted by other evidence. Therefore, the physician must make it clear that what happened did not form an unlawful act on his/her part, but resulted from another cause. Otherwise, the physician should be blamed for a negative medical treatment.

However, if a causal relationship cannot be established, the concept of informed consent has been used as one method to surmount, or at least circumvent the proof problem inherent in a claim, whether in tort or contract, alleging faulty performance of a medical act *per se*. An informed consent approach shifts the focus from the physician's act *per se* to the physician's level of disclosure and failure to attain informed consent [15].

This survey revealed that these Japanese physicians are reluctant to inform the patient of his/her medical condition. Despite the attempt to define informed consent in legal terms, the concept of informed consent seems to have not been prevalent both among legal and medical profession. In some cases, informed consent has been used as a legal technique, for example, to circumvent the difficulty of burden of proof.

The level of disclosure

The level of disclosure to patients has been classified into two categories: the professional standard and the patient-oriented standard. In the United States, during the 1950s and 1960s, the American courts held that the applicable standard of care is measured by what a competent physician, practising in the same capacity, would have disclosed to the patient under the same or similar circumstances—the 'professional standard'. However, due to lack of professional standards and difficulties in obtaining expert witnesses to determine these standards, another standard based on the releasing of as much information as the patient desires—the 'patient-oriented standard'—was established [16].

However, in Japan, no distinctive standard of disclosure has yet been established. It has thus been left to the physicians' judgement as to how much information should be provided to the patient. This approach has been extensively discussed in a series of malpractice suits regarding retinopathy of premature infants caused by hyperoxygen therapy. Because premature infants have difficulty with respiration, hyperoxygen therapy has been used to assist them, but this sometimes has caused an unfortunate side effect called retinopathy (fibrosis).

The next series of questions in our survey involved the level of disclosure by the physician to his/her patient of new medical technology. The questions were based on a series of medical malpractice suits. A new method of treatment using laser therapy had been reported earlier at a medical conference as effective in curing retinopathy. However only two successful cases had been reported at that time [8, 20].

In Table 3 (a), which concerns the level of disclosure physicians chose to communicate with regard to this novel treatment of retinopathy, it is revealed that about half of the physicians surveyed thought that the treatment should be explained to the patient, whereas about 10% of them were of the opinion that disclosure was unnecessary. The rest of the physicians upheld the autonomy of the physicians. They believed that it was up to the physician to decide whether

Table 3. Much discussion concerning the relationship between the level of the disclosure and the treatment involved has been made in the series of medical malpractice suits concerning premature-retinopathy. What do you think of the following points?

(a) The method of treatment is presented at an academic conference, and is under discussion

Item	S	PU	PH
(1) It need not be explained	38 (13.5)	19 (9.4)	35 (8.6)
(2) It should be explained	138 (48.9)	102 (50.5)	197 (48.4)
(3) It depends on the physician's discretion whether it should be explained or not	106 (37.6)	81 (40.1)	175 (43.0)

(b) The method of treatment has been established among specialists, but not undertaken in general practice

Item	S	PU	PH
(1) It need not be explained in principal	20 (7.1)	8 (4.0)	12 (2.9)
(2) It should be explained	186 (66.4)	141 (69.8)	266 (64.9)
(3) It depends on the physician's discretion whether it should be explained or not	72 (25.7)	52 (25.7)	129 (31.5)
(4) Other answer choices	2 (0.7)	1 (0.5)	3 (0.7)

S, Students.
PU, Physicians in University Hospital.
PH, Physicians in hospital.
Figures in parentheses are percentages.

information only available at the experimental stage should be explained to the patient.

In 1974, the Gifu District Court case [17] decided that a doctor using the retinal laser treatment should have explained the treatment to his patient even though the treatment had not been well established as a common means of treatment. Later, on appeal of the same case, the Nagoya High Court held that the minimum duty required of the physician was to practise medicine according to the treatment adopted generally in his or her area of speciality, and that the physician did not have to either explain or carry out the laser therapy which was still experimental at the time [18].

As shown in Table 3 (b), physicians were asked if they would disclose treatment which was not prevalent in general practice but had been established among specialists. Two-thirds of the physicians surveyed thought that the treatment should be explained, whereas only a few thought that the treatment need not be explained. The Kobe District Court held that a physician had the responsibility to let his patient know about the novel laser therapy. The reason for this was that the duty of the physician to explain the treatment was derived, not from the establishment of the efficacy of the treatment among general physicians, but from the existence of a treatment which had been reported to be effective among specialists [19].

Actually speaking it should be understood that, when scientific results are presented at an academic conference, they often contain some speculative factors and are obtained under experimental and restricted conditions. In order to have a therapy introduced into general practice, experiments proving its efficacy and safety should be repeated. Furthermore, the impact of social, financial and geographical factors should be taken into consideration prior to the introduction of this advanced knowledge and technology into general practice. In this regard, a special research team for retinopathy treatment of premature infants, led by the Japanese Ministry of Health and Welfare, published a list of diagnostic criteria in 1975. This list has since been used by the lower courts when considering physicians' liability in this controversial area [20].

In summary, with regard to a novel treatment which is either currently under academic discussion or used primarily by specialists, more than half of the physicians thought such a treatment should be disclosed. However, some physicians still upheld the autonomy of the physician. In a series of malpractice suits in the lower courts concerning premature retinopathy, which became the landmark cases for the level of disclosure, the diagnostic criteria established by the government-led research group were used.

Medical records

Due to the 'closed-door' characteristic of medical care in Japan, the medical record is the only document available for a third party to verify what was undertaken in the medical examination and treatment. When patients are burdened with providing proof for establishing negligence or are suspicious of particular medical practices, they must request that medical records be made available to them.

As shown in Table 4, with regard to a situation where physicians are requested to provide medical records to patients, half of those polled felt their decision would be based on the patient's reason for making the request. About 40% would probably reject such a request, no matter what reason the patient offered. Very few would comply if the patient gave no reason for the expressed desire to see and copy his medical record.

In practice, the right of patients to examine their medical records is often denied. Justice Itoh of the Supreme Court wrote an article concerning this matter and discussed it for the first time in 1974 [21]. According to her view, the contents of obligation in medical actions are very obscure and specialized.

Table 4. How do you cope with a situation where you are requested to provide the medical record of a patient?

Item	S	PU	PH
(1) We meet the request if the patient requests to see and copy the medical record	27 (9.4)	9 (4.4)	21 (5.0)
(2) We make a decision after listening to the reason	161 (56.3)	94 (46.3)	207 (48.9)
(3) We reject the patient's request	94 (32.9)	96 (47.3)	187 (44.2)
(4) Other answer choices	4 (1.4)	4 (2.0)	8 (1.9)

S, Students.
PU, Physicians in University Hospital.
PH, Physicians in hospital.
Figures in parentheses are percentages.

Therefore, article 645 of the Japanese Civil Code calling for the submission of reports on the condition of the business under the mandatory management cannot be applied to medical records.

In Japan, medical records are not the property of the patient—they belong to the doctor (or dentist, hospital, etc.). The Medical Practitioner Act (Art. 24) states that it is the official duty of the practitioner to write a medical record. The medical record serves two purposes. First, it is intended to control medical actions administratively by making doctors justify the appropriateness of the medical treatment they administer. Secondly, the doctors are obliged to submit those records as a memorandum to the government.

In Japan, medical records are principally written by the physicians in German or English, and many abbreviations are often used. Although the use of the POMR (Problem-Oriented Medical Record) method has been recommended in medical schools and in leading hospitals for medical records [22], this practice has not become prevalent among practitioners. Hence, it is extremely difficult not only for a patient, but also for medical experts to read and understand the medical records. Hence, medical records, even if obtainable, are generally not adequate evidentiary material for medical malpractice trials.

Note that, however, once a patient is involved in a medical malpractice trial, and has difficulty in accessing his/her medical records, access can be obtained by the law regarding the preservation of evidence. Under Article 343 of the Japanese Code of Civil Procedure, the court may, if it considers that there exist circumstances that make use of the evidence in question difficult unless examination thereof is made beforehand, conduct examination of evidence upon an appropriate motion.

The results of this study showed that Japanese physicians are reluctant to provide access to medical records. In the legal interpretation, the medical record is conceived of as being not for the patient but for the public purpose. However, if the patient brings suit against the physician, access to the medical record is granted by law.

The involvement of family members in the decision-making process

In the following sections, the role of the family members in the decision-making process and the attainment of informed consent will be examined in the following contexts: in the disclosure of risk, in the disclosure of cancer and in situations where a patient is unwilling to undergo treatment (the 'unwilling patient'). Finally, to summarize the analysis, the unique role of family members in granting substitute consent for the patient will be illustrated.

Disclosure of risk

In Canada and the United States, it is generally accepted that, irrespective of the frequency and severity of the risk, all risks accompanying a particular medical procedure should be revealed to the patient in order to obtain informed consent. In Texas [23] and Hawaii [24], for example, disclosure of risk has been legislated to establish the scope of the risk which the physician must disclose. In Canada, the Supreme Court of Canada [25] has held that, although the circumstances of each particular case must be taken into consideration, the doctor should, without being questioned, disclose any material risks and any special or unusual risks or procedures. The Supreme Court has also held that a mere possibility should be regarded as material and disclosed if its occurrence carries serious consequences, such as paralysis or death.

As shown in Table 5, when questioned on the disclosure of high risk diagnostic procedures, about 55% of the physicians surveyed in Yamaguchi believed that the procedure should be explained to the patient's family members instead of the patient so as not to excessively aggravate the patient's emotional anxiety. About 23% of the physicians replied that they should explain the existence of any risk to the patient directly and if further requested, the incidence and severity of the risk. About 10% of physicians replied that they would always explain the incidence and severity of the risk. Hence the results show that the members of a patient's family play an important role in the disclosure of risk in Japan.

Disclosure of cancer

There is still much controversy among members of the medical profession in Japan as to a physician's responsibility to inform patients on the presence of a life-threatening malignancy or cancer. Some physicians feel that a patient has the right to know and is entitled to an explanation of the nature of his/her disease at an early stage or when the diagnosis has first been confirmed. Others feel that it serves no purpose and might unnecessarily frighten the patient. The majority of physicians have no set rule but adapt their approach to suit the patient's personality, personal situation and ability to comprehend and cope.

Table 5. How do you explain high-risk diagnostic procedures to the patient?

Item	S	PU	PH
(1) We don't explain the risk in order to avoid unnecessary anxiety for the patient	7 (2.4)	2 (1.0)	8 (1.9)
(2) We explain the existence of risk, and if requested by the patient, we explain the incidence and the severity of the risk	66 (22.5)	41 (20.3)	104 (24.2)
(3) We explain the incidence and the severity of the risk, and if the patient seems to be bewildered by the information, the explanation ceases	37 (12.6)	14 (6.9)	30 (7.4)
(4) We explain the incidence and the severity of the risk, and it the patient seems to be bewildered by the information, we explain them to the relatives	170 (58.01)	121 (59.9)	201 (56.0)
(5) We always explain the incidence and the severity of the risk	13 (4.4)	24 (11.9)	47 (10.9)

S, Students.
PU, Physicians in University Hospital.
PH, Physicians in hospital.
Figures in parentheses are percentages.

As shown in Table 6, when questioned on their opinions regarding a case where a physician operates to remove cancerous tissue without informing the patient of the existence of cancer and the physician is sued because there was no consent to the operation, more than half of the physicians surveyed regarded such a suit as ill-founded. Those physicians who viewed such action as a matter of course did not exceed 20%. This result is consistent with that reported in an earlier report by Kanagawa [26], and reflects a characteristic Japanese attitude toward cancer.

In a celebrated case involving tongue cancer [27], a patient was initially diagnosed to have tongue cancer and, despite her doctor's advice, rejected a resection of the tongue. The doctor then explained that she had an ulcer on the tongue without informing her that it was cancerous and proceeded with the partial resection. The Akita District Court held that surgery conducted without the patient's consent was illegal, and the physician was found liable to compensate his patient for damages resulting in her speech impediment.

However, the traditional attitude of the physicians not to disclose cancer has now been called in question and may be changed with the appearance of two landmark cases which introduced two issues: 'Enmei-Rieki' (the benefit of life prolongation) and 'Kitai-Ken' (the right to state of the art) [8]. The benefit-of-life-prolongation principle states that patients should be allowed to enrich their remaining lives. The benefit-of-life-prolongation has been made possible by the development of effective cancer therapy. The right-to-state-of-the-art means that the patients have the right to expect medical examination and treatment at the current level of medical practice. When patients fail to receive such medical examination and treatment from their physicians, as infringement of their rights can arise.

Table 6. An operation for the removal of cancer was undertaken without the patient's informed consent. What do you think of the situation?

Item	S	PU	PH
(1) The operation was illegal	158 (54.5)	112 (56.9)	219 (52.4)
(2) The operation was a matter of course	81 (27.9)	23 (11.7)	69 (16.5)
(3) Other answer choice	51 (17.6)	62 (31.5)	130 (31.1)

S, Students.
PU, Physicians in University Hospital.
PH, Physicians in hospital.
Figures in parentheses are percentages.

Legal claims have also been based on alleged overdisclosure. In one case, a patient argued that the psychological stress caused by the disclosure of cancer had been tortious. The court held that the physician made no effort to protect the-benefit-of-life-prolongation for the patient, although it also decided that informing the patient of cancer is not tortious [28]. Yet, in another case, a plaintiff insisted that if they had been informed of cancer earlier, the patient and the family would have utilized their remaining moments together more dearly. The court held that the interest of the patient produced by earlier information as to the existence of cancer did not warrant protection under law [29]. There is no doubt that, in addition to informed consent, the benefit of life prolongation and the right to current medical treatment will become central issues in the future concerning any discussion on when cancer should be disclosed.

The situation of the unwilling patient

Seriously ill patients rejecting potentially life-saving treatment have created an ethical dilemma for physicians and legal specialists. As shown in Table 7, when the polled physicians were asked what they would do if indispensable life-saving treatments were rejected by the patient, approx. 37% of physicians answered that they would explain the situation to their patient and abide by the patient's decision to accept or reject treatment. About 40% said they would override the patient's wishes and proceed with treatment based on consent obtained from the patient's family.

Such a situation arose in the Oita Local Court in a case involving an adult Jehovah's Witness who had osteosarcoma and yet refused a crucial blood transfusion [30]. The parents of the patient had asked the hospital to make a blood transfusion to the patient despite the patient's refusal. The court considered whether the blood transfusion infringed upon the benefits based on the loss of familial affections called 'Shinzoku-ken'. In Japan, 'Shinzoku-ken' denotes the rights arising from the relationship between the patients and immediate family and is often emphasized. 'Shinzoku-ken' rights are based on the idea that a close bond exists among immediate family members, and that they have the right to enjoy all the

Table 7. If life-saving treatments such as operations or transfusions for children whose parents are Jehovah's Witnesses, etc., are rejected by the patient and/or his or her family, what do you think of the situation?

Item	S	PU	PH
(1) We explain the treatment to the patient, and then if the treatment is rejected, we don't treat the patient	108 (37.0)	71 (34.5)	156 (36.7)
(2) We explain the treatment to the patient, and even if the treatment is rejected, we treat the patient according to standard medical care	31 (10.6)	4 (1.9)	15 (3.5)
(3) We explain the treatment to the patient, and even if the treatment is rejected, we treat the patient with consent of the family members	99 (33.9)	84 (40.8)	178 (41.9)
(4) We explain the treatment to the patient and family members fully, and even if it is rejected by both, we treat the patient	35 (12.0)	26 (12.6)	36 (8.5)
(5) Other answer choices	19 (6.5)	21 (10.2)	40 (9.4)

S, Students.
PU, Physicians in University Hospital.
PH, Physicians in hospital.
Figures in parentheses are percentages.

benefits from that bond. In a provisional disposition, the Oita District Court upheld the right of the adult Jehovah's Witness to refuse the blood transfusion. As well, it was held that the coercion of the transfusion for the Jehovah's Witness was the same as an infringement of the freedom of religion. Hence, the transfusion was not done, and chemotherapy was administered instead.

When a competent adult refuses necessary medical treatment, the following points are generally taken into consideration by the courts:

(1) Has the patient validly and knowingly chosen the course for his life?; and
(2) Is there a compelling state interest which justifies overriding the patient's decision? [31].

There are few circumstances where a state interest is sufficient to override an individual's freedom to act according to his/her religious beliefs. Restricting an adult patient's right to refuse medical treatment is most often based on the welfare of minor children dependent on the patient. In the United States, the court's rationale is that if the patient dies, the children will not be provided for financially or emotionally, and they will become wards of the state. However, in the Japanese case, the involvement of family members in the decision-making process is discussed in terms of 'Shinzoku-ken' instead, and as shown in the questionnaire, this is yet another illustration of how Japanese physicians sometimes prefer to deal with the family members instead of with their patients in order to obtain substitutional consent for the prescribed treatment.

Substitute consent

In general, substitute consent is only acceptable in the West when the patient has given express authority to another person to give or withhold consent on his behalf or when the law invests a person with such power. Most scholarly discussions of substitute consent have been in the context of psychiatrically incompetent patients or emergency conditions. In such contexts, the Japanese form and concept of substitute consent do not differ appreciably from those in the West.

However, in Japan, even in cases where the patient is competent to give his or her individual consent, substitute consent by the family or close relatives is a common practice in order to avoid disturbing the patient emotionally. In the United States, although physicians' rationale for their disclosure behavior was identical, the physicians' attitude toward informing the patient of cancer changed drastically during the period from 1961 to 1977 [32]. Medical doctors in Japan usually inform the family or close relatives of the existence of the cancer, but tell the patient that he has a benign disease. This is a characteristic mode of dealing with such matters in Japan, and while some would argue that it is essentially a deceptive approach, it has customarily been judged acceptable in general practice. In cases of cancer, many Japanese doctors believe that complete information may bring a patient to a state of emotional disturbance and prevent him from making a sound decision. As with most cases, the Japanese tend to favor being indirect, and do not like complete information about a serious condition to be stated explicitly.

Several explanations have attempted to elucidate why substitute consent still prevails in Japan in such cases as disclosure of cancer. First, in the traditional Japanese household (called 'ie'), the authority of the head of the house was strong, and family members were dependent on each other. Despite the modernization and westernization of contemporary Japanese society, this tradition still remains. The Japanese health care system, as Christie W. Kiefer has pointed out in respect to care of the aged, seems to place the responsibility for care on the family [33]. Furthermore, it is characteristic of Japanese culture, generally, that the preservation of harmony and suppression of conflict take priority over individual rights and needs [34]. The notion of 'personhood' or 'self' in Japanese society is quite different from that of the 'individual' in Western society. Accordingly, the individual in most Western societies is conceived to be autonomous, whereas in Japanese society a person is structurally defined in relation to others [35]. These are possible reasons why family members and close friends sometimes make major decisions for an individual.

Secondly, the concept of 'amae' appears to play a major role in substitute consent [36]. The Japanese term 'amae' refers, initially, to the feeling that all normal infants at the breast experience toward their mothers—dependence, the desire to be passively loved, the unwillingness to be separated from the warm mother–child cycle and cast into a world of objective 'reality'. This concept of 'amae' also holds true for adulthood. When the adult patients are faced with difficult and critical situations such as dealing with cancer or high-risk procedures, they are predisposed to depend upon their surrounding family members and friends.

Thirdly, if a family member or friend is threatened with death, the Japanese feel that they should let the patients die in peace (a concept called 'Yasurakani'), without making them go through the agony of knowing their condition [35]. This leads to the practice whereby most of the decisions relating to a patient's medical care are left to the family members and results in the prevalence of substitute consent.

CONCLUSION

This paper has analyzed the results of a survey conducted on a sample of Japanese physicians and medical students concerning patients' access to medical information and patients' rights in the decision-making process. Emphasis has been placed upon the legal and sociological relationship between physician and patient. The legal profession has been active in promoting patients' rights. For example, 'informed consent' before treatment and access to medical records after the treatment have been advocated. In medical malpractice suits several attempts, such as the application of the contract theory between physician and patient and the view of probable causality, have been made to reduce the burden of proof for the patient. However, this survey showed that the Japanese physicians and medical students in this study still uphold their right to use their own discretion in providing their patients with access to medical information. In addition, the survey revealed that more than half of the physicians thought novel information presented at an academic conference level should be provided to the patients. Furthermore, in cases where treatment is experimentally being carried out among specialists, but is not prevalent in general practice, two-thirds of the surveyed physicians were willing to give that information to the patient.

The patient's access to the medical records in Japan is still being denied generally. The survey showed that half of the physicians polled felt their decision to provide medical records would be based on the patient's reason for making the request to examine the medical records, and that 40% of the physicians would probably reject the patient's request for access to the medical records in any event. However, once medical malpractice suits are brought before the courts, the patient can obtain the medical records through the law regarding preservation of evidence.

As for cases concerning cancer, many Japanese physicians believe that operations performed to remove cancerous tissue without the express consent of the patient should be legal, as long as the existence of cancer is disclosed to the family members of the patient. The survey also suggested that family members should still be involved in the decision-making process in sensitive situations, such as in cases of high risk diagnostic procedures and when patients are unwilling to undergo treatment.

Finally, in order to fully understand medical ethics in Japan, one must never ignore the use of substitute consent in the decision-making process for determining medical treatment. From this study, although the concept of informed consent is becoming steadily and increasingly pervasive among the physicians in Japan, it appears that substitute consent given on behalf of an otherwise competent patient is still widely used. It is characterized by the involvement of family members in such decision-making processes as deciding the disclosure of risk, the reporting of cancer, and in cases where treatment is rejected by the patient, and should always be taken into consideration in the discussion of medical ethics in Japan. It appears to be linked to strong and pervasive cultural practices seen in other social relationships.

Acknowledgements—The authors would like to thank the association of civil law and medical law in Kyoto for preparing the questionnaire. We are also grateful to Professors Setsuo Komura and Satoshi Ueki of the Kyoto Prefectural University of Medicine, Dr Nancy Waxler-Morrion of the University of British Columbia, and Yoshiya Wakamatsu especially for their valuable critical comments.

REFERENCES

1. Feldman E. Medical ethics the Japanese way. Hasting Center Report 15 21–24, 1985.
2. Darnton N. *et al.* Whose life is it, anyway? *Newsweek* Jan. 23. p. 61, 1989.
3. Patient's Bill of Rights (American Hospital Association). 1972.
4. Maeda T. Gendai horitsugaku koza, Minpo 6–2 p. 215, Seirinshoin-shinsha Tokyo 1980 (in Japanese).
5. Niimi I. Iryo saiban. In *Nihon no iryo—korekara, Jurist zokan Sogotokushu*, No. 44, pp. 172–177, 1986 (in Japanese).
6. Hattori H. Iryo ni kansuru ishi no ishiki chosa. In *Iryohunso no jirei to soten* (Edited by Komura S. and Ueki S.), pp. 263–276. Kimpodo, Kyoto, 1985 (in Japanese).
7. Schloendorff v Society of New York Hospital. 105 NE92 (NY) 1914.
8. Aeba T. *Iryo jiko no soten*, revised edn, pp. 45–90, Nihonijishinposha, Tokyo, 1987 (in Japanese).
9. Azami T. *Nakai Y Iryo kago nyumon*, pp. 3–48. Seirinshoin-shinsha, Tokyo (in Japanese).
10. Yamashita N. Ishi no setsumei gimu o meguru saikin no tenkai. *Rokkukodai-ronshu* **30**, 96–133 (in Japanese).
11. Bai T. *Iji hogaku e no ayumi*, pp. 3–51. Iwanami-shoten, Tokyo, 1970 (in Japanese).
12. Tokyo District Court. 19/May/1971, Hanreijiho, 660, 62, 1971 (in Japanese).
13. Supreme Court of Japan. 19/June/1981, Hanreijiho, 1011, 54, 1981 (in Japanese).
14. Minpo. In *Yuhikaku-sosho*, Vol. 6, 3rd edn (Edited by Endo *et al.*), pp. 205–214. Yuhikaku, Tokyo, Kyoto 1987 (in Japanese).
15. Machino S. *Kanjya no jiko kettei ken to ho*, pp. 23–24. University of Tokyo Press, Tokyo, 1985 (in Japanese).
16. Appelbaum P. S. *et al. Informed Consent: Legal Theory and Clinical Practice*, pp. 41–47. Oxford University Press, New York, Oxford, 1987.
17. Gifu District Court. 25/March/1974, Hanreijiho, 738, 39, 1974 (in Japanese).
18. Nagoya Higher Court. 2/September/1979, Hanrei Times, 398, 65, 1979 (in Japanese).
19. Kobe District Court. 12/June/1981, Hanreijiho, 1013, 96, 1981 (in Japanese).

20. Noda H. Mijyukuji momakusho no genjyo, Jurist 839, 85–89, 1985 (in Japanese).
21. Itoh K. Shinryo kiroku no imuzyo no toriatsukai no horitsuzyo no toriatsukai o megutte. *Hanrei Times* **302,** 40, 1974 (in Japanese).
22. Aeba A. About the POS (Abstract of the lecture in the Otsu Medical Association) April 1981 (in Japanese).
23. Tex Rev Civ Stat Ann Art 459Di 6.03(a) 6.04(a), (d) (Venon Cum Supp) 1985.
24. Haw Rev Stat 671 3 (b) (Supp) 1984.
25. Reibel v Hughes. 14 CCLT 1980.
26. Kanagawa T. Shinryo ni okeru setsumei to shodaku no zittai. *Jurist* **869,** 50–56, 1986 (in Japanese).
27. Akita District Court. 27/March/1973, Hanreijiho, 718, 98, 1973 (in Japanese).
28. Nagoya District Court. 27/May/1983, Hanreijiho, 1082, 91–109, 1983 (in Japanese).
29. Tokyo Higher Court. 15/March/1983, Hanreijiho, 1072, 105–112, 1983 (in Japanese).
30. Oita District Court. 2/December/1985, Hanreijiho, 1180, 113–115, 1986 (in Japanese).
31. Hirsh H. L. and Phifer H. The interface of medicine, religion, and the law: religious objections to medical treatment. *Med. Law* **4,** 121–139, 1985.
32. Novack D. H. *et al.* Changes in physicians' attitudes toward telling the cancer patient. *JAMA* **241,** 897–900, 1979.
33. Kiefer Christie W. Care of aged in Japan. In *Health, Illness, and Medical Care in Japan: Cultural and Social Dimensions* (Edited by Norbeck E. and Lock M.), pp. 89–109. University of Hawaii Press, Honolulu, 1987.
34. Lock, M. Protests of a good wife and wise mother: medicalization of distress in Japan. In *Health, Illness, and Medical Care in Japan: Cultural and Social Dimensions* (Edited by Norbeck E. and Lock M.), pp. 130–157. University of Hawaii Press, Honolulu, 1987.
35. Ohnuki-Tierney E. My very own illness. In *Illness and Culture in Contemporary Japan: An Anthropological View*, pp. 51–74. Cambridge University Press, Cambridge, 1984.
36. Doi T. *The Anatomy of Dependence*. Kodansha International, Tokyo, 1973.

APPENDIX

The contents of the questionnaire are in the following:

(1) the points which the physicians always ask the patient in the interview
(2) the extent to which physician can get the information concerning the idiosyncracy from the interview
(3) questionnaire paper in case of prophylactic injection
(4) informed consent
(5) the explanation of the risky treatment to the patient
(6) disclosure of the cancer
(7) intensive care
(8) unwillingness to receive the treatment (e.g. Jehovah's Witnesses)
(9) the consent to the surgical operation
(10) the contents of the consent to the surgical operation
(11) the level of explanation and the state of the art in medicine
(12) transfer of the patient to another medical facility
(13) (a) legal and social aspects of medical certificate
(b) legal and social responsibility of the physician when the medical certificate eventually turns out to be wrong
(14) experience of medical malpractice
(15) copy of medical record
(16) brain death
(17) the reason for objecting the brain death
(18) introduction of the advanced technique such as gender selection during pregnancy and artificial fertilization into general practice
(19) the policy in case of the introduction of brain death, euthanasia and organ transplantation into general practice.

[32]

Convergence or Divergence in Third World Medical Education? An Arab Study

EUGENE B. GALLAGHER
University of Kentucky

Journal of Health and Social Behavior 1988, Vol. 29 (December):385–400

Third World societies have adopted Western models of medical education—in curriculum, instructional methods, and implied expectations about the role of the physician. This suggests the "convergence hypothesis." The present study—of a recently established Saudi-Arab medical school—tests and severely challenges that hypothesis. It finds that student aspirations, administration-faculty-student relationships, and the social context for learning were extensively influenced by politico-religious identifications, traditional family and sex-role values, student weakness in the language of instruction, and other extracurricular factors. A full scrutiny of the convergence hypothesis will require studies drawn from other societies cast into a systematic framework for comparison.

Although medical education has been a favored topic in medical sociology for several decades, medical education in non-Western, developing societies has received little attention (Fox 1985). This lack is significant because Third World nations have established many medical schools whose curricula and administrative structure closely resemble those of the West. One report (Kindig and Taylor 1985, p. 3130) shows that Third World nations increased the number of their medical schools by 124 percent between 1955 and 1974, compared with 43 percent for the Western nations. This phenomenon is not only large in scale but also raises a significant sociological question: whether medical education is transformed when it is adopted into non-Western societies.

This question—the primary focus of this paper—fits within the larger question of *cross-national convergence versus divergence* in the development of Third World health care systems, professional organizations, and educational institutions. Do they develop in ways that lessen pre-existing differences from Western prototypes? Do they bear indefinitely the conditioning stamp of distinctive historical forces and cultural roots? Under the influence of political or religious ideologies that reject Western values, do they evolve new structural entities that diverge from Western prototypes? As far as these questions are articulated within medical sociology, the answers have come down mainly on the side of *convergence*. Parsons' typification of the physician role projected that role as a self-contained universal which largely ignored variations in sociocultural context, if only for the sake of theoretical economy. Mechanic (1976) and Field (1973) portray health care systems within total societies in which the health care systems show less variation than the containing society. Their suggestion of convergence is based on the perception that health care systems in all nations exhibit great developmental autonomy and thus have the latitude to resemble increasingly the strongly biomedical, specialist-centered type of system that has come to be the norm in Western industrial societies. Another implication is that the health care system stands in the vanguard of social change and represents a more modern institutional form—one based on the implementation of science—than the traditional kinship, community, and religious institutions. Medi-

* Direct all correspondence to Eugene B. Gallagher, Department of Behavioral Science, University of Kentucky, Lexington, KY 40536-0084. The author wishes to acknowledge the valuable part that Gameel Absood, Akrum Bhatty, John Colombotos, Joan Ferrante, Singaram Naidoo, Saadi Nazhat, and the late Paul Forand played in the formulation of this paper.

cal care can be regarded, in this sense, as a vehicle of modernization.

Similar considerations extend to medical education. Mechanic (1976, p. 27) states: "Medical schools throughout the world tend to emulate those characteristic of modern nations and are part of a worldwide medical community." Behind the broad social mandate that allows medical educators largely to do things their own way is the public and popular expectation, usually translated into government support, that people will benefit from modern medical care and thus from the training of practitioners to provide such care. Medical care and medical education, in Berger, Berger, and Kellner's (1973, p. 139) formulation, are a "sacrament of modernity" in developing societies; they are linked to hopes for deliverance from disease, disability, and early death that are a melancholy part of traditional expectations.

The hypothesis of convergence tends to be supported by an outward examination of Third World medical school curricula, academic organization, qualifying characteristics of faculty and students, and categories of physical plant (teaching hospitals, lecture halls, teaching and research laboratories). Nevertheless, it is possible that elements of an educational system which appear similar to the untutored observer function differently within different socioeconomic and cultural contexts. Consider the physical examination of patients, certainly as basic a feature as any in medical education. In American medical schools, students learn to perform biochemical and bacteriological assays of body fluids in their teaching labs. This exercise links what they learned in their preclinical courses with the practicalities of patient examination, but they are aware that later, in actual practice, they will not be performing such analyses themselves. Instead, the tissues of their future patients will be subject to far more precise, more detailed analysis in automated testing labs. This prospect may impart a make-believe character to their learning. In contrast, much medical care in Third World settings is resource-poor; physical examinations are not conducted with reliance on external resources such as automated testing labs. Thus what doctors learn to do in medical school may have a more realistic quality. In physical examinations they may come to rely more on their own clinical judgment concerning the patient's complaints and symptoms because the medical care system in which they practice is less well endowed.

The foregoing suggests that despite a conventionally standard training regimen, the economic and technological environment of medical care can penetrate into the student's learning psychology and role expectations, with varying implications for their view of their professional future. It also recommends caution in considering the convergence hypothesis—a presumption against inferring convergence too easily on the basis of outwardly similar forms.

This paper contributes to the assessment of the convergence/divergence question in a Third World setting through the case study of an Arab medical school. It examines student-faculty-administration relationships, the cultural dynamics of the learning environment, and medical career commitment. My observations favor divergence, accenting the situations, processes, and forces that make the medical school different from the Western model, while still taking into account the many resemblances to the Western model, particularly at the level of formal organization and curriculum.

SETTING AND METHOD

The data for this study were acquired in the course of the author's academic appointment on the faculty of a Saudi medical school, as a member of the social medicine department.

Following the pattern of medical education common outside the United States, students at the Saudi school are admitted upon completion of their secondary studies rather than after a four-year premedical preparation. The undergraduate curriculum lasts six years: two years of premedical courses including Islamic studies, English, mathematics, physics, biology, and chemistry; two years of preclinical courses including physiology, biochemistry, anatomy, cell biology, social medicine, pathology, and pharmacology; and two years of clinical training that includes clerkships in surgery, internal medicine, pediatrics, radiology, obstetrics, and other medical specialties.

The students in each class were approximately 50 percent male and 50 percent female. About 85 percent came from Saudi Arabia; the remainder came from Gulf nations and North Yemen. All were Arabic speakers and Muslim. They were the products of well-to-do urban families that had benefited from the Kingdom's oil-based prosperity. The education that the medical students received put most of them well above their fathers and far above their mothers in educational attainment.

Although the main purpose of my appointment to the school was to work on curriculum development for social medicine, soon I came to see the value of a sociological study as a supplementary activity of my working environment. Like medical schools everywhere, this school brought into a single organization persons with many different professional, disciplinary, and specialty orientations. Like all Saudi institutions of higher learning, it was anchored in and influenced by its Saudi-Muslim external environment. Further, its participants, particularly the faculty, displayed a remarkable cosmopolitan diversity in ethnic, national, racial, religious, and cultural characteristics.

Studies of undergraduate American and Canadian undergraduate medical education (Becker, Geer, Hughes, and Strauss, 1961; Coombs 1978; Haas and Shaffir 1987; Merton, Reader, and Kendall 1957) stimulated my thinking in regard to substantive issues and methodological approaches. The work of Bucher (1970) and Bloom (1971) also was informative because, unlike the Becker, Merton, Coombs, and Haas-Shaffir studies, it dealt as much with faculty and administration as with students. I wanted the Saudi study to have similar scope. It was clear that in methodology, my study would use primarily ethnographic techniques of participant observation and semistructured interviews, and would resort to institutional records, official memoranda, and other documents issuing from various parts of the medical school. Although the administration was interested in my perceptions as the first sociologist on the faculty, it was not sympathetic to my proposal to conduct a more formal, questionnaire-based study of the school, nor was logistic and research support for such a study available.

I told colleagues and students of my general interests and aim, thus stimulating the flow of information to me. Faculty, administration, and students provided pertinent observations, viewpoints, and insights about teaching and learning processes, organizational dynamics, the impact of the external political culture on the medical school, and other focal sociological topics.

In addition, there were a few opportunities for more systematic data collection. As an assignment in a survey methods course, I asked a fourth-year class to design and administer to themselves a questionnaire on their conceptions of medical practice. At the dean's request, I assisted him in a facultywide survey of "attributes of the ideal medical teacher" for a paper that he presented later at a medical conference.

Despite these facilitations, it was difficult on the whole to assemble objective information beyond what informants proffered to me spontaneously. As noted by the political scientists Braibanti and Al-Farsy (1977, p. 7), "An ethos favorable to data accessibility, objective scholarship, and distribution of publications is not easily or quickly established in any developing country."

Readers may question the use of a Saudi school as an example of Third World medical education because Saudi Arabia is an affluent country and most Third World countries are poor. The 1985 Saudi gross national product per capita stood at $8,850 (*World Development Report* 1987, pp. 202–203); comparable figures for Egypt, Pakistan, and Nigeria respectively were $610, $380, and $800. In addition to a high average, the internal distribution of Saudi wealth is fairly broad after allowance is made for the extremes of affluence found among the 5,000 male members of the Al-Saud ruling family (and their dependents) and for the modest incomes earned by many of the expatriate workers in the Kingdom (estimated variously at 30 to 50 percent of the 12 million inhabitants). In terms of wealth alone, Saudi Arabia falls within the small, exclusive World Bank-denominated category of "high income oil exporters." Yet it is similar to many other Third World societies in regard to other parameters of development, such as levels of industrialization, literacy, and life expectancy (Saudi Arabia males in 1985, 60 years; Egypt, 59; Pakistan, 52; Nigeria, 48).

I would argue further that the privileged, somewhat detached position that medical schools enjoy in Third World societies means that the schools' functional style, development, and organizational problems probably differ less than would be suggested by variations in parameters such as per capita income and life expectancy.

MEDICAL EDUCATION AS A VEHICLE OF MODERNIZATION

Medical education in the West often is regarded as rigidly resistant to change (Ebert 1977; Starr 1982). Frequently it is stated that the reforms of the Flexner era set a basic pattern in the United States which has endured with virtually no change in the ensuing 70 years. Medical education is well designed to incorporate and convey new scientific information while preserving intact its own institutional structure. Although it is close to the research laboratories that are the engines of modern biomedicine, medical education in itself is not seen as malleable, much less as a vehicle of modernization that touches and changes other parts of society.

By contrast, in Third World societies medical education—along with other domains of higher education—is a vehicle of modernization. It removes most students residentially, for the first time in their lives, from the protective confines of a traditional family system. Academically it exposes them to universalistic expectations for learning that is charged with the symbolic modernity of science and technology. It points them occupationally toward a professional career that has little relation to traditional modes of livelihood. Fathers, sons, and brothers can do much for each other in a family business, but medicine is not that kind of business. The responsibilities of patient care bring the physician into contact with sick strangers who ordinarily might be devalued according to prevailing norms of ethnicity and social rank, but the healing ethic learned and practiced in clinical medical education curtails the influence of those norms. The traditional proprieties of relations between the sexes—very strong in Third World societies—are strained when male and female students are exposed to each other, and to faculty and patients, in the diverse situations of medical care. For these reasons medical education is an uprooting experience even for students who originate in the more modernized segments of their society, and it bears the imprint of modernization.

The stresses that medical students undergo, and the personal adjustments they must make, are scarcely acknowledged in formal statements and discourse on admission policy, methods of instruction, and other formal aspects of medical education, but Third World medical educators and administrators are acutely aware of them. The following comments from the medical school dean, taken from my field notes, illustrate this point:

> In connection with his projected survey of student and faculty opinion on "ideal attributes of a medical educator," the dean asked me what sociologists had to say about medical education. He wanted background reading. I gave him an article (Shuval and Adler 1979) on health professional, including medical, education that I thought made for interesting reading—it was lucid to a non-sociologist and representative of current sociological concepts and research approaches.
>
> A week later he called me to discuss the article. I was pleased and surprised to find out that he had digested it thoroughly, but his reaction surprised me. He said that the constant changes in attitude that the students underwent in the course of medical education at the schools in the article (Hadassah and Tel Aviv medical schools in Israel) were the result of a disorganized, uncaring, leaderless environment in which each student had to find his own way. He said that he did not want his medical school to be like that. He said it's the job of the faculty to help the student through the challenge of each stage of medical education—to provide guidance and a coherent intellectual experience, and to protect the student against confusion and overstimulation.
>
> Expanding on his conception of student needs, the dean said that at least 80 percent of his students had a similar background, coming from stable Saudi-Islamic homes that offer great security and comfort—not like the religious and cultural diversity of medical students in North America (where he had gotten a Ph.D. in physiology following his British medical degree). He also mentioned that one of his sons—a 27-year-old unmarried architect—had gotten the idea that he'd like to live on his own (which was unusual for a young man in the Kingdom). He and his wife said, "OK, go ahead," but after two months the son decided that he did not like independent living and moved back home.

The dean's comments stressed the binding, possessive embrace of the Saudi family structure and resonated with other comments I had heard concerning students' adjustment difficulties, such as homesickness. Homesickness occurs on undergraduate campuses in the West, but it is not a theme that emerges in studies of medical education there. Yet it was reported to be fairly common among the younger Saudi medical students and occasionally was a cause of leaving school. Most of the students were separated from their families for the first time upon entering medical school. The younger age of the Saudi medical students, compared with that of students in the United States, accounts somewhat for "away-from-home" adjustment problems, but another factor, alluded to by the dean, is the cohesiveness of the Saudi family system. Other evidence to suggest this factor was the opinion, conveyed to me by the associate dean for admissions, that the Saudi students who had attended well-reputed secondary schools abroad—in Egypt and Pakistan—were in fact no better prepared for medical education than those who had gone to Saudi secondary schools, because they could not concentrate on their studies away from their families.

Sociological studies portray medical education as a training process that, in the end, produces "the doctor" as a standardized product. This general picture also holds true for the Saudi process, but, as the foregoing discussion indicates, Saudi medical education occurs against a background of family and culture that influences the way in which students experience and meet challenges.

The familiar themes in sociological studies of North American medical education—survival, "making it," development of professional identity, formation of student culture, ambivalence in the relationship between students and faculty—are exemplified in the Saudi school, but they are skewed systemically because medical education there is a new phenomenon. The Saudi students, having faced historically unique, puzzling, often stressful situations, can become the carriers of new patterns of relationship and consciousness in the society. Although the very establishment of the medical school and of medical education is a massive stimulus for modernization in a traditional culture, many of my examples of "modernization effects" actually may appear to be better suited to illustrate a contrary effect of divergence (in Berger's terminology, "demodernization") from Western prototypes.

THE MEDICAL SCHOOL AS A STRONGLY ADMINISTERED ENVIRONMENT

I regarded the medical school as a field of social action in which the actors categorized and responded to each other in varying degrees of affinity, solidarity, factionalism, threat, and avoidance. I found that students, administrators, and faculty organized their perceptions, defined themselves, and reacted in terms of four main social categories, as follows (numbers in parentheses are the approximate number of persons in each category):

1. Organizational position: *student*(500)/*administration*(55)/*faculty*(155). Within the faculty category, the following additional distinctions were important: *premedical*(35)/*preclinical* or basic science(75)/*clinical*(45). The students' school class position also was important; each of the six classes was approximately equal in number.
2. Religion: *Muslim*(610)/*non-Muslim*(100)
3. Nationality: *Saudi*(560)/*non-Saudi* or expatriate(150)
4. Gender: *female*(330)/*male*(380)

Of the four categories above, the first—organizational position—is the most basic social axis in earlier studies of Western medical education. It is not a great exaggeration to say that in the Western institution's theory of itself, the participants are there to impart and to receive medical education; their organizational position is vitally important, but their other characteristics are of much less relevance. By contrast, it will be seen that in the Saudi school, organizational position interacts with the other axes (religion, nationality, and gender) to produce configurations that showed clearly the social importance of these "secondary" characteristics.

With the exception of Bloom's and Bucher's work, the earlier studies of Western medical education also paid little attention to the administrative structure of their schools. This approach would be more difficult in the Saudi case: the dean and his administration were not the typically obscure power centers that maintain financial flows, resource access, and administrative infrastructure in Western medical schools. Instead the administration played a salient, assertive role for the following reasons.

First, the school was relatively new, like most Saudi institutions of higher education. Policies and procedures had yet to be refined and consolidated. Officials had not yet worked together long enough to develop smooth routines. For example, although everyone knew that the holidays were approaching, holiday periods were not set officially until two or three weeks in advance; the issuing of exit and re-entry visas for expatriate faculty members required medical school representation to immigration officials, which was hard to regularize into a routine.

Second, high faculty and administration turnover required strong administrative presence to prevent erosion in those procedures that had achieved coherent continuity. Many faculty members left after two or three years; middle- and lower-level administrators circulated frequently between academic employment and the lucrative business opportunities available in the private sector. High turnover in a fledgling institution places a greater burden on administration: fewer precedents can be taken for granted, and more policies must be reset.

Third, the administration not only provided working facilities for faculty members but also served as their landlord in regard to housing and as sponsor for their civil status in Saudi Arabia (making visas possible and providing protection in event of legal or financial difficulties). All faculty members were employed on annual contracts; all faculty members, except for the 10 percent who were Saudi, lived with their accompanying dependents in university-provided housing.

Fourth, the administration's role in facilitating and controlling student life was strong. It was comparable with the role of a high school or middle school principal in the United States, but with the additional condition that the medical school was a residential institution; only a few students commuted from nearby homes. The concept of *in loco parentis* was taken completely for granted, even in regard to the many upper-class students who were married and lived in university-provided married students' quarters. But for their connection with the medical school, most of those students would have lived with the husband's parents under actual rather than proxy parental jurisdiction.

The dean and his administration also saw themselves as the exemplars and protectors of Saudi-Islamic values. The dean's prepotence was suggested by the undercurrent of comment by Muslim faculty members to the effect that attendance for daily prayers at the campus mosque dropped when the dean was away. Participation was voluntary, but the belief prevailed that the dean, a regular participant, took note of their faculty members' presence.

On numerous occasions the dean stated that the maintenance of the values and behavior that the students had learned in their families was as important as any academic attainments. It was the task of the school to aid the students' passage into adult Saudi family and vocational roles.

Beyond observance of well-known Islamic precepts such as prohibition of pork and alcohol, daily prayers, conservative attire (for both males and females), and segregation of females, it was not clear what else might be at risk, but statements by the administration seemed to imply other, more vague dangers from value systems that fostered individualism and philosophical skepticism and promoted the participation of females in public life. The most concentrated source of such risks was the non-Muslim expatriate faculty, recruited from Europe, North America, Australia, and New Zealand.

Though the Western faculty members were not expected to participate in Islamic rites, they were expected to respect the Saudi-Islamic code of values. All expatriate faculty members, both the Western, non-Muslim group and the larger group of Middle Eastern Muslims, were bound by the handbook of regulations for non-Saudis. Article 48 states:

> The contract employee must observe all the present and future laws, regulations, directives and by-laws in effect in the Kingdom. He, together with his dependents and all the members of his family, must respect the prevalent customs, patterns of culture and traditions in the Kingdom. They must not discuss religious matters or discuss politics or interfere with politics.

Like most employee codes, it was not enforced literally, but it created circumspection in the institutional environment.

As a delimited group from whom nothing of religious or civic worth was expected to begin with, the Western, non-Muslim faculty was perhaps less of a cultural threat than the

Muslim faculty members who were not Saudi. The latter had all received university training in the West and thus had been exposed to suspect values, but without the strong identity safeguards that surrounded the Saudis who had done likewise. Most of the Muslim faculty, like the Saudis, were Sunni Muslim, but that was no guarantee that they had the same religious perspective as their Saudi employers; many came from Islamic countries such as Turkey and Egypt, which were more liberal on the extremely sensitive topic of the status of women. The Saudi administrators portrayed themselves as defenders of "Muslim" values, but sometimes they spoke of "Saudi-Muslim" values; although the difference was not defined, the implication of the national label "Saudi" was that only a Saudi national could embody fully those virtues which placed him or her beyond suspicion.

Of great importance was the fact that few of the non-Muslim faculty spoke or read Arabic, whereas Arabic was the mother tongue of all the Muslim faculty members. The language bond gave them social cohesion and enabled them to interact fluidly across categories on the campus. Although all the students and almost all the administrators spoke English—the official language of instruction—the Muslim faculty were in a fair position to serve as culture brokers between the Western faculty on the one hand and the students and administration on the other. This does not mean, however, that the administration regarded the Muslim faculty *en bloc* as culturally trustworthy; rather, particular individuals on the Muslim faculty seemed to be much closer to the administration than others. Some Muslim faculty members were bound indefinitely to their job at the university because they had no other job options, in view of the lack of academic opportunity in their home countries (Egypt, Iran, Lebanon, the West Bank).

Why, one might ask, were expatriate faculty members hired if the host employer feared that they might convey culturally divergent perspectives to an impressionable audience of students?

The answer is that the expatriates were hired for their expertise—their command of knowledge and technique within specialized medical and premedical fields. Very few Saudis were similarly qualified. Virtually no Saudis anywhere had received the doctorate in preclinical subjects, and most of the few Saudis in the Kingdom who were medically qualified (through training abroad) were in private practice. Like other Third World medical schools, this school was committed to a model of excellence that has become the worldwide standard in medical education, whatever the effective range of variation. To approach this standard, the university needed the foreigners, but it needed them more than it wanted them. The Saudi national leadership in the ministries of health and of higher education anticipated that eventually all the Saudi medical schools (and other institutions of higher education) would be staffed fully by home-trained Saudi nationals, but that prospect still lay far in the future.

STUDENT CONSERVATISM AND ADMINISTRATIVE RESPONSE

Although the dean spoke strongly in defense of Islam, others on campus spoke even more strongly. Some orthodox faculty members and students felt that the administration's statements reflected a shallow, nominal commitment, intended merely to provide a bland backdrop to medical education. A few students were particularly outspoken in their convictions. They questioned the protectiveness of the administration toward them when what they perceived as antireligious excesses were permitted to exist. They raised complaints with the administration, which generally acquiesced. The following episodes are illustrative:

- A female student wrote an article in the student newspaper *Avicenna* questioning the need for any non-Muslins on the faculty. She said that whatever their learning and their good intentions in teaching, they did not understand Islam, and their presence undermined Islam's influence.
- Several male students asked that the main (male) library curtain off the windows facing the central campus courtyard so that they would not be able to view female students crossing the yard en route to lab sessions. Although the females always wore the full black cloaks (*aḇbayas*) that were required when they moved off the female campus, the complainants said that the female

students were too much of a distraction from their studies. The library installed curtains in response. The curtains were movable, however, so that students could close or open them according to the sensibilities of whoever was present in the library.

- A male student was offended by several library periodicals—*Smithsonian Magazine, Scientific American*, and *Illustrated London News*—because they contained liquor ads, and by *Psychology Today* because it contained too much about sex. He requested that the library cancel these subscriptions. The librarian canceled everything except *Scientific American:* he kept that magazine because he felt that frequently it contained material of direct relevance to topics that the medical students were studying. He moved it, however, from the open periodical racks to a back room, where it was available only on request. Upon further student complaint, this time to a higher administrative level (the assistant vice-rector for administration), *Scientific American* also was canceled under the assistant vice-rector's signature.
- Several male students refused to take part in off-campus clinical clerkships in Bahrein (outside Saudi Arabia) because they felt that the social atmosphere there was too permissive, with liquor sales and theaters showing "loose" films from the West. This request caused consternation on the Department of Medicine faculty, whose clerkship it was. Some faculty members felt that the clerkship was a vital component of medical training and that no exception could be allowed. When the students petitioned the dean, he said that the decision was up to the department, but he also believed that a substitute requirement should be found for the objecting students. In the end, the decision went in that direction.

None of these incidents pertained to the actual content of medical education as conveyed in texts, lectures, and labs. Although in other times and places Islamic orthodoxy occasionally has opposed the use of laboratory solutions containing alcohol, cadavers for gross anatomy, and (doctrinally) the whole corpus of evolutionary biology as contrary to the creationism of the Quran, there were no reports of student complaint on these points. In general it appears that divergences from Western practice, appearing in the Saudi school as "tensions of modernization," were generated and expressed within the social context of medical education more than within its intellectual-technical content. That is, the pressures and forces that made the medical school diverge from the Western model, emanating from structures and values outside the school, passed over the curriculum in silence. Instead they affected symbolic, psychocultural features of the educational process and, as I will show subsequently, the linking of education to career.

IDENTIFICATION BLOCKAGE AND MODERNIZATION CONFLICTS

It is possible to view medical education as culturally innocuous because it embodies a universal set of facts, principles, and techniques. On this basis a tradition-governed society could embrace it without risking its integrity. Likewise, modern medical care can be accepted as addressing common human infirmities and illnesses, even if it competes sometimes with traditional healing systems that address the same conditions. Such is the view and the hope of the Saudis; they regard medical education and medical care as "technology transfer," analogous to the extensive and successful use that Saudi Arabia has made of Western technology for petroleum production and refining. In this view, Western agents are used as a temporary expedient to launch the enterprise. Likewise, the use of extraterritorial, culturally dubious training sites such as Bahrein is considered temporary. The use of English in teaching (discussed below) also is seen as lasting only until texts and teaching materials in Arabic become available.

Earlier sociological studies of medical education in the West, conducted within a homogeneous cultural matrix, have ignored its context safely. This matrix was a constant to be taken for granted, rather than a variable that required attention and analysis.

Yet these studies also argue strongly that medical education is a complex process, more than a simple human-factors or learning psychology input of technical knowledge. The learning of medicine is colored and propelled by self-concepts that students form of themselves in their present tasks and their anticipations of the future. Medical students undergo transitions in their self-conception. At first they regard themselves as junior scientists who are responsible for mastering the biomedical knowledge dispensed by preclinical faculty. Later they see themselves as clinicians who, though not forsaking scientific method, reshape their role definition to emphasize their attempt to help sick patients. Many students in the preclinical years come to regard their instruction in biochemistry, anatomy, and physiology as an ordeal to be endured and the examinations as obstacles to be traversed en route to learning the essentials of doctoring, which begins in their clerkships. Not even in their clerkships, however, do students acquire much independent scope for clinical judgment and responsibility. Some analysts of the socialization process argue that fledgling doctors learn a mature style of medical practice only when they leave the confines of specialty training and academic medicine altogether—a style structurally free of formally sponsored learning expectations.

The shifting of students' focus and self-conception in the foregoing sequence is stimulated continuously by their reactive identification with the values of successive groups of faculty members. A major leap occurs in the transition from the preclinical to the clinical undergraduate years, from identifying with the value system of biomedical science to identifying with the value system of clinical practice. Whatever the values and enthusiasms among faculty types, the student never lacks models to connect him or her to attainable professional futures.

Identification and role building proceed differently in the Saudi school. It seems that the expatriate faculty, both preclinical and clinical, remain a "foreign object" for the students—admired for their expertise and appreciated for their desire to impart it, but admired and appreciated across a cultural gap. The expatriate faculty members themselves are not a feasible model of what the student might become. Instead, it is the administration—the dean and his corps of associate and assistant deans—who are seen in this light. In a culture where family values and intergenerational ties remain definitionally and sentimentally powerful (to a Saudi youth of either sex, every older male is "uncle" and every older female "aunt"), it is easy for the student to make this identification.

Such an identification is not satisfactory from the standpoint of professional socialization, at least as seen in the Western-based studies. The Saudi student identifies with the administration because it is culturally available—but ostensibly he or she is in training for a professional future, not an administrative one. With blocked identification, the Saudi student might find it inordinately difficult to master medical knowledge; he or she might graduate weak in technical knowledge and skills.

Many faculty members sensed this problem and were concerned about it. They were pleased by the dean's frequently voiced commitment to high academic standards, but the administration sometimes shielded students in ways that seemed to dilute their commitment. The following examples illustrate this point:

- The official working hours of the medical school were 8 a.m. to 4 p.m. In theory a department was free to schedule any of its teaching activities during its allotted periods, but a memo to department chairmen from the vice-dean for academic affairs stated the following:

> I have received repeated complaints from the Chairmen of some Departments and other faculty members that class tests held at 1:00 - 4:00 P.M. disrupt classes in the morning because the students absent themselves to study for such tests. Moreover the students have also complained that this time period is too late in the day, and follows immediately on their lunch, so they feel tired and sleepy.
>
> Your are kindly requested, therefore, to consider holding such class tests first thing in the morning. Your cooperation will be highly appreciated.

In recommending early morning as the best time for examinations, the memo sought to reduce interdepartmental competition for students' attention and energy. It also echoed a presumption widespread in the Middle East—that the afternoon hours are not productive and that one's best work is done early in the day. Offices and businesses in Saudi Arabia and elsewhere in the Middle East currently present a mixed pattern: some are open from 8 a.m. to 12 p.m. and from 5 p.m. to 9 p.m. (the more traditional pattern), and others are open from 9 a.m. to 5 p.m. The memo appeared to cater to students' desire to relax on afternoons when labs were not scheduled. Some faculty members saw in the students' post-lunch sleepiness a bad omen for the kind of schedule they would keep later as doctors.

- All written instructional materials were presented in English; according to policy, all lectures also were to be delivered in English. Many faculty members, however, especially the Anglophones, were distressed that the administration did nothing to prevent the unofficial use of Arabic. It was known that some of the Arabic-speaking faculty—especially those whose English was weak—conducted large portions of their lectures in Arabic, as shown by the following interchange among Anglophone expatriate faculty members:

  Dr. A (biology): You know my office is along the west corridor, next to the biology lecture hall. Some of the lectures carry into my office and I can definitely say that the students are getting material in Arabic. I recently overheard Dr. M. (an Egyptian biology lecturer) give at least 20 minutes of a lecture in Arabic.

  Dr. G (biochemistry): Well, it seems to be a disservice to the students.

  Dr. O (anatomy): It encourages the students who don't understand English to rely on the ones who do, instead of trying harder themselves.

  Dr. S (physics): If they want to be physicians, they are certainly going to need English in the near future, that's very definite. They'll need it to keep up in medicine . . . In my Tuesday and Friday female labs, I have L. K. (Egyptian) as my demonstrator. She consistently speaks English to the girls and requires them to speak English to her. I tell them that it's more important that they speak English than that they understand the physics involved in the experiments. I really believe that.

Problems with language use are rife in many Third World medical schools, where instruction is offered officially in English, French, or other nonindigenous "world" languages. Indigenous languages lack a medical vocabulary and teaching materials suitable to convey the full range of biomedical information. Instructors who are not comfortable in the official language commonly lecture in the indigenous language (if they know it well) and use official-language biomedical terminology as necessary. Students' weakness in the official, nonindigenous language is widespread; thus language itself becomes a burden added to the inherent difficulty of mastering medical knowledge. Tensions regarding Arabic language use are particularly severe because Arabic itself is a major world language (Gallagher 1985).

- Cheating during examinations was felt to be widespread. Noncheating students came forward after examinations and privately told faculty monitors that a lot of cheating occurred through whispering, passing notes, and hiding notes. In recognition of the situation, the vice-dean for academic affairs sent the following memo to chairmen:

  Many students have complained repeatedly that some of their colleagues help each other during class tests. They have before complained directly to some of their teachers regarding this serious problem, without any improvement in the situation.

  You are kindly requested, therefore, to bring this to the information of the faculty members so that monitoring during class tests will be more strict in the future.

Many faculty members felt that the dean's position was too soft. They noted in particular his avoidance of the explicit word "cheat" in the memo. I was told that no student had ever suffered a penalty more severe than a reprimand in the few instances when faculty had lodged and sustained an accusation against a student.

Although student cheating may well be prevalent in many other educational institutions, it had a particular cultural nuance in the Saudi school. The universalistic norms for honesty and individual performance that have come to be accepted (despite many lapses) in Western universities were recognized, but they coexisted with a strong traditional ethic of brother helping brother (or sister helping sister). the stronger helping the weaker. Conversations with students also led me to believe that another element came into play, namely that many students felt the medical school to be culturally alienating. This view implied that dubious behavior—such as cheating—which ordinarily would be condemned was situationally justified here.

Cheating during examinations is a particularly flagrant violation of academic norms. Information came to me suggesting that less flagrant instances also occurred frequently, such as students' copying another student's workbook values during a laboratory exercise, inserting theoretical values obtained from a textbook formula rather than using their own empirically obtained values, or, during dissections, copying textbook-based descriptions of tissues for tissues that in fact were not dissected. Becker et al. note that such behavior at the Kansas medical school they studied was rationalized by students on the basis that it saved their time for more important things (Becker et al. 1961, p. 172). Becker notes that such "cheating is situational: dependent upon faculty perspectives and regulations as students understand them."

The situational basis for ethical lapses was not the same for the Kansas students as for the Saudi students. The Kansas students had a settled culture that enabled them to define certain faculty expectations as a "waste of time"—those that lacked an essential connection with what a physician needs to know. Their orientation was less a desperate grasp for survival than a sophisticated, even if misguided, appraisal of efficient alternatives within a demanding overall situation. For the Saudi students, many of whom were caught in a trap of weak English comprehension, the issue was not efficiency but survival—maintaining a passing average, avoiding faculty criticism and makeup work, and being able to tell their parents that medical school was going well "insha'illah" (as God wills it).

RESTRICTED CAREER COMMITMENT

Applicants to medical schools in the West are scrutinized by admissions boards concerning their academic preparation and their commitment to medicine. Even the best-qualified applicants can scarcely appreciate the many hurdles involved in completing a medical education and in the subsequent practice of medicine. Nevertheless they are caught up in a social process that shapes and sustains their motivation toward learning medicine and then practicing it as a career. The process is a benign concatenation of forces which medical sociologists have studied but which ordinarily is taken for granted by medical educators, administrators, and society at large.

The outcome of the process, however, cannot be taken for granted in Third World societies, where the pull of tradition is still strong, where even the concept of "career" is a still-fragile modern construction, and where traditional motifs skew careers into forms that diverge from Western patterns (Gallagher and Searle 1984).

A survey that I conducted with the fourth-year class (30 female, 24 male respondents) revealed several facets of opinion that reflect distinctive conceptions of medicine. When asked why they wanted to enter medicine, a majority mentioned the idea of service to individual patients, but about 25 percent also mentioned the idea of serving the nation (that is, the Saudi state). This attitude may be connected with the fact that the Saudi students, in a sense, are state employees whose job is to go to medical school. They are not charged for tuition; they also receive free meals, housing, and a monthly cash stipend.

Fifty-four percent *disagreed* with the statement, "It takes more intelligence to be a doctor than to be an airline pilot." This response probably should be taken less as "anti-doctor" than as "pro-pilot"; the pilot's role is more thoroughly technological than the doctor's in a society that reveres technology and has amassed a great deal of it.

Concerning medical expertise, 82 percent agreed with the statement, "A patient should always do just what the doctor says because the doctor knows what is best." The students' response to this extreme statement probably reflects the general cultural predisposition to respect authority.

The physician's role is relatively new in Saudi society, and though it commands great respect, neither this nor any other professional role has been stabilized culturally as representing a new, autonomous order of knowledge and expertise. The traditional sources of authority are exclusively religious and familial.

An important way in which family authority is felt is through its controlling influence in the work life of both males and females—whom they work for and with, and the nature of their work. ("Family" in this sense means one's extended family—parents' siblings, cousins to the second and third degree, and relatives by marriage as well as one's immediate family.) On the basis of his observations at the American University in Beirut, Moracco (1979) writes, "In the Middle East it is expected that young men will carve out their careers through nepotism . . . Ideas that an identity can be found in work, that hard work and frugality should be valued, and that work which helps others is rewarding are not deeply ingrained in the conceptual framework of the Middle-Easterner. The concept of helping others outside of family and close friends . . . is hard to understand. Jobs are arranged for and dispensed through 'wasta'—influence and access to power" (p. 201).

These considerations pose a question: Will the medical students now in training pursue medical careers or will they be absorbed into traditional family occupations? The import of this question loomed large in the minds of the Saudi administrators of the medical school. They anticipated that there would be some falling away from commitment to medicine. Some deplored this prospect as a waste of medical education and a loss to the society; others, taking a broader view, held that even if some students did not become doctors, they would contribute as highly educated people to the advancement of Saudi society.

A further circumstance that argues against career commitment is that many students were channeled into medical school because they were bright, socially mobile young people with good academic records rather than because they were particularly interested in medicine. This channeling effect operated more strongly for the females than for the males because the only careers open to females are medicine and teaching; both are highly prestigious. According to field observation (Papanek 1971, p. 517), the situation is similar in Pakistan: "Medicine and teaching are found to be the most important high prestige occupations for educated women because of the special needs of a female clientele in a sex-segregated system." Nursing in Saudi Arabia is viewed as an essential but socially degrading occupation, to be followed by expatriate females; secretarial or other office work is out of the question because it would involve interaction with nonfamily males.

The play of diversionary nonprofessional forces can be seen in these two events:

- A fourth-year male student asked me, as course coordinator, for permission to accompany his father on a two-week business trip to West Germany. He worked as bookkeeper for his father, who had various businesses including an automobile distributorship. The purpose of the trip was to negotiate contracts for importing auto parts. He promised that he would make up the work he missed. I gave permission, though with reluctance, because he was not a strong student and I felt that he would have difficulty making up the work. I could not help reflecting that this kind of request would be virtually unheard-of in the American and British medical schools I knew. I also learned that similar requests were made occasionally by other students.
- A Saudi faculty member told me that the dean, at a hastily convened meeting of the 12 Saudi faculty members, had told them that several administrative posts would become vacant within the next three months and also that new administrative posts would be created concurrently with the expansion of the school. It was essential, he said, that these posts be filled by Saudis. He described the posts and told the faculty to think it over and come forward with volunteers from among themselves for these posts. He said that he understood well that they might prefer to continue in teaching and patient care, but that the matter was too important for personal predilection to prevail. If there were not enough volunteers, he would proceed to make assignments. (My informant was an ophthalmologist who recently had left that specialty field to become associate dean for library and information services.)

The first event suggests a familial pull away from the professional career, in which the traditional expectation of son helping father intrudes on learning responsibilities. Even here it should be noted that the father's holding an automobile dealership which required travel to Europe is not a traditional form of economic activity; nevertheless it is a form of Arab trading that exemplifies the ways in which older patterns are available to handle new opportunities. Further, the son had a *choice* between going with his father or following the prescribed medical-school schedule of activity. He was not bound by tradition; rather, given a choice, he elected the traditional, family-related alternative. The fact of choice is important; had the student failed to obtain academic leave or had he chosen not to seek it in the first place, he would have remained in school and his father would have managed without his service.

The second episode shows the pull of other, nonfamily exigencies on a professional career line. In this instance the need to maintain Saudi administrative control superverned over career considerations: the Saudis—all of them clinical faculty who had been trained medically abroad—were asked to leave their professional work and to take up administrative duties.

As noted by Berger et al. (1973, pp. 41–62), administrative responsibility in Third World settings is more compatible with traditional modes of social relationship than is science- or technology-based work. The requirements of technology are indifferent to status orders and to generational, gender, and ethnic lines, but such ways of categorizing people can be worked into administrative systems that perpetuate traditional values, though ostensibly they are modern and efficient.

Although the diversion of Saudi faculty from teaching and patient care into administration seems to strike a blow against a professional career, it is important to note that these teachers remained within the medical school. As administrators they maintained an organizational environment where others could teach and practice medicine even if they did not do so themselves.

How does the professional-to-administrator shift affect students' career commitment? The Saudi student was exposed continually to a two-sided image: the expatriate professional expert who was not an administrator, and the Saudi who was an administrator of professionals. It is likely that many of the male medical students, like the medical school administrators, will become the managers of professionals. They will play an ownership and managerial role in the new Saudi medical enterprises, employing expatriate physicians (and other health workers) as the professionals who in turn provide direct services to patients in proprietary clinics and hospitals. Thus the physicians-turned-administrators will retain the imprint of their training, and even without patients to treat they will enjoy much of the esteem accorded to the physician.

To the extent that this projection is borne out by future events, Saudi society will not free itself from dependence on foreign physicians, despite its medical schools. However, if it is able to evolve and control the managerial structure within which foreigners provide medical services, it will maintain cultural hegemony over the educational process.

History provides a counterexample, familiar to Middle Eastern rulers, of the ill effect of relying on foreigners: the Mameluke epoch beginning in thirteenth-century Egypt, when foreign slaves (mamelukes) came to dominate their masters, the Fatimid caliphs. The cultural memory of such events may trigger the nervous absolutism of central governments in Saudi Arabia and other oil-rich states that depend on expatriate labor and professional expertise.

Another, more contemporary example, however, suggests that the Saudis can draw massively on foreign talent while still retaining control of their own house. This example is ARAMCO (Arabian-American Oil Company), the multinational company whose petroleum exploitation and production are virtually the sole basis for contemporary Saudi wealth. In this case the Saudis maintain financial and administrative control; further, a gradually increasing proportion of ARAMCO employees, both in production and administration, are Saudi nationals.

CAREER PROJECTION FOR "LADY DOCTORS"

The contending forces toward and away from career definition and commitment for the female students differ more in degree than in kind from those that face female medical students in Western societies. The claims of family responsibility—being a wife, mother, housekeeper, and hostess—all vie with professional duties for the woman's time, energy, and attention. Many of the Saudi female medical students were married; some of the older ones were mothers as well. (In their pursuit of facilities qualitatively equal to those of the male students, one of the female students' complaints about their library was that it was also used as a nursery because no other space was available.)

Data on the marital status of students, both male and female, was difficult to obtain because it was regarded as private information. It was my impression that most female students who married remained in medical school. Nonetheless some older female students left to get married, whereas the younger students who left did so primarily because of homesickness or academic and English-language difficulty. A Girls' Section dean, who had access to systematic data, reported in an earlier study that "marriage accounts for a withdrawal percentage approaching 16% of all female students enrolled in the fourth year" (Islam 1980, p. 402).

Whatever the similarities in the professional prospects of Saudi and Western female students, there are also important differences, rooted in culture and economics. The following factors bear on the role of the Saudi female physician.

First, because of the tremendous social importance of marriage (for males as well as females), almost every Saudi marries. Fewer females avoid the multiple-role demands of family and profession by remaining single.

Second, those demands are eased significantly by the abundant use of foreign servants as cooks, nannies, chauffeurs, gardeners, and maids, many of whom live in.

Third, the social obligations connected with the extended family (which increase greatly when one marries) and the religious calendar compete with time for professional practice (Altorki 1986). Religious feasts, marriages, condolences, circumcision observances, and social visiting add up to a formidable schedule for women without careers, who presently constitute the great majority; as in the West, expectations are not lowered because a woman has a career. Although the female students were shielded by their student status from the intensive social round, occasionally they sought and received leave from school for major family events. As Saudi daughters they had been socialized well in the protocol and satisfactions of such sociability; rather than viewing it as a forced obligation, many of the female students regretted that school duties separated them from it. Missing the social life was part of the sacrifice of going to school.

Fourth, the professional practice of the Saudi "lady doctor" is conducted entirely with women and children. As in most Third World countries, the same cultural code that restrictively regulates female behavior virtually mandates a large number of female physicians, so that female patients need not be treated by male physicians. The code also implies that female physicians will not treat male patients and, by extension of the female-maternal image, that they will treat children. Although the curriculum for male and for female students was exactly the same, the females probably were drawn more strongly to certain areas, such as reproductive physiology, obstetrics, gynecology, and pediatrics, which they perceived as especially relevant to their future practice. Probably most of the female students will engage in general practice, with emphasis on the medical conditions of women and children.

Female doctors who wish to specialize do not have the same freedom to study abroad that male doctors enjoy because of traditional and official restrictions on independent travel by women. For the foreseeable future, Saudi Arabia will not be able to provide its own specialty training; therefore medical specialists, even in gynecology and obstetrics, will be male rather than female. It is an open question whether Saudi females will prefer to see a less well-trained female physician or a better-trained male specialist. Neither law nor custom prevents a Saudi female patient from consulting a male specialist if she wishes; this is a further example of the unwieldy compromises that arise in the course of modernization in a traditional culture. Ideally, under a separate-but-equal mandate, a female patient should be able to consult a female physician as highly trained as any male; in practice, however, this ideal will be approximated only roughly.

CONCLUSION

Medical education entered Third World societies as an import from the West. This process began during the colonial era, as in Indonesia, India, China, and Egypt, and after the Second World War, as in Nigeria and Saudi Arabia (Brown 1979; Zaidi 1987).

Biomedicine has been accepted in these societies as the knowledge base for the humane technology of modern medical care—a culturally and politically neutral technology that offers no threat to old traditions or emergent national ideologies. Medical education has escaped the hostility and skepticism toward Western social institutions that exist in many Third World societies. More than that, it has been enthusiastically embraced within these societies as evidence of the society's commitment to progress and its capacity to absorb and apply sophisticated science within traditional power and value structures.

From these considerations, I have argued that one should expect a convergence between medical education as found in Third World societies and medical education as found in the West. That is, medical education—like other educational "packages" related to technology—can be imported and implemented without regard to the social fabric of the importing society.

The Saudi-Arab case study I have presented tests the convergence hypothesis. In the Saudi medical college, the cognitive core of biomedical science was the same as that found in the Western model. However, according to my findings, medical education was extensively constrained by family values, bonds of politico-religious solidarity, student and faculty weakness in the language of instruction, and other extracurricular pressures.

In science, a single apt and cogent counterexample can defeat a generalization. One may question whether the Saudi study absolutely defeats the convergence hypothesis—or merely offers a severe challenge to it. In any event, I believe that this sector of the sociology of medical education requires a series of case studies that can create a framework for comparing medical education modes in the variety of cultures and social structures subsumed under the convenient but oversimplifying phrase "Third World." The close comparison of such cases can also deepen our understanding of how medical education works within our own society. When an American medical student, for example, learns lists of terms in anatomy, these terms must at first confront him or her as novel, strange material to be memorized and mastered. How—through what rituals and usages—do they become familiar? What difference does it make if, as in the Saudi school, they were first experienced in an actual foreign language? When we can answer such questions, we can offer, from a sociological standpoint, a more penetrating account of how a student becomes a doctor.

REFERENCES

Altorki, Soraya. 1986. *Women in Saudi Arabia—Ideology and Behavior among the Elite*. New York: Columbia University Press.

Becker, Howard S., Blanche Geer, Everett C. Hughes, and Anselm L. Strauss. 1961. *Boys in White—Student Culture in Medical School*. Chicago: University of Chicago Press.

Berger, Peter, Brigitte Berger, and Hansfried Kellner. 1973. *The Homeless Mind*. New York: Random House.

Bloom, Samuel W. 1971. "The Medical School as a Social System—A Case Study of Faculty-Student Relations." *Milbank Memorial Fund Quarterly* 49 (No. 2, Part 2).

Braibanti, Ralph and Fouad Abdul-salam Al-Farsy. 1977. "Saudi Arabia: A Developmental Perspective." *Journal of South Asian and Middle Eastern Studies* 1(1):3–43.

Brown, E. Richard. 1979. "Exporting Medical Education: Professionalism, Modernization and Imperialism." *Social Science and Medicine* 13A:585–95.

Bucher, Rue. 1970. "Social Process and Power in a Medical School." Pp. 3–48 in *Power in Organizations*, edited by Mayer N. Zald. Nashville: Vanderbilt University Press.

Ebert, Robert. 1977. "Medical Education in the United States." Pp. 171–84 in *Doing Better and Feeling Worse: Health in the United States*, edited by John H. Knowles. (Daedalus, Winter 1977.)

Field, Mark G. 1973. "The Concept of the 'Health System' at the Macrosociological Level." *Social Science and Medicine* 7:763–85.

Fox, Renee C. 1985. "Reflections and Opportunities in the Sociology of Medicine." *Journal of Health and Social Behavior* 26(1):6–14.

Gallagher, Eugene B. 1985. "Medical Education in Saudi Arabia: A Sociological Perspective on Modernization and Language." *Journal of Asian and African Studies* 20(1/2, January and April):1–12.

Gallagher, Eugene B. and C. Maureen Searle. 1984. "Cultural Forces in the Formation of the Saudi Medical Role." *Medical Anthropology* 7(3, Summer):210–21.

Haas, Jack and William Shaffir. 1987. *Becoming Doctors: The Adoption of a Cloak of Competence*. Greenwich, CT: JAI.

Islam, Samira. 1980. "Enrollment and Drop-Out of Saudi Female Medical Students at King Abdulaziz University." Pp. 392–403 in *Proceed-*

ings of the Fourth Saudi Medical Conference. Dammam. Saudi Arabia.

Kindig, David A. and Charles M. Taylor. 1985. "Growth in the International Physician Supply." *Journal of the American Medical Association* 253(21):3129–32.

Mechanic, David. 1976. *The Growth of Bureaucratic Medicine: An Inquiry into the Dynamics of Patient Behavior and Organized Medical Care*. New York: Wiley.

Merton, Robert K., George G. Reader, and Patricia L. Kendall. 1957. *The Student Physician: Introductory Studies in the Sociology of Medical Education*. Cambridge, MA: Harvard University Press.

Moracco, John. 1979. "Arab Countries." Pp. 197–209 in *Guidance and Counseling around the World*, edited by Victor J. Drapela. Washington, DC: International Universities Press.

Papanek, Hanna. 1971. "Purdah in Pakistan: Seclusion and Modern Occupations for Women." *Journal of Marriage and the Family* (August): 517–30.

Shuval, Judith T. and Israel Adler. 1979. "Health Occupations in Israel: Comparative Patterns of Change during Socialization." *Journal of Health and Social Behavior* 20:77–89.

Starr, Paul E. 1982. *The Social Transformation of American Medicine*. New York: Basic Books.

World Development Report. 1987. New York: Oxford University Press.

Zaidi, S. Akbar. 1987. "Undergraduate Medical Education in Underdeveloped Countries: The Case of Pakistan." *Social Science and Medicine* 25(8):911–19.

[33]

Sam Porter

Women in a women's job: the gendered experience of nurses

Abstract The aim of this paper is to examine how the structural influence of gender affects nurses in their working lives. Gender segregation exists both within and between the occupations of medicine and nursing. It is largely founded on the social construction of a skills/caring dichotomy. An analysis of how the gender of nurses and doctors affects their interactions with co-workers reveals that the increasing proportion of female doctors has attenuated power differences between the two occupations. Examination of nurses' attitudes to gender demonstrates that they are very aware of the problem, despite a tendency to accept credentialist justifications of inequality. As a result of this they are becoming more assertive. The issue of sexual stereotyping is addressed and it is noted that popular mythology about sexual relations between doctor and nurses is highly misleading. Privatised aspirations are having a decreasing influence over nurses' working lives. In conclusion, while gender inequality is losing some of its power in nurse-doctor relationships, it is becoming an increasingly significant factor in the relationship between male nurse managers and female workers.

Introduction

Issues of gender have been identified as being of considerable importance in explaining the position of nurses (for example, Mackay 1990). Gender affects nursing in three interconnected ways. Firstly, because nursing is popularly seen as mundane 'women's work', it is devalued (Abbott and Wallace 1990). Secondly, because nursing is situated within a stark sexual division of labour alongside the predominantly male occupation of medicine, gender overdetermines inter-occupational inequalities (Gamarnikow 1978). Thirdly, with the development of a predominantly male managerial elite,

Sociology of Health & Illness Vol. 14 No. 4 1992 ISSN 0141–9889

gender inequalities are increasingly becoming an issue within nursing (Hearn 1982; Carpenter 1977, 1978).

The purpose of this paper is to illuminate, largely through qualitative analysis, how the social structure of gender affects actors within specific social situations, namely two units in a general hospital. Four major substantive areas are addressed: firstly, how gender affects power relations between doctors and nurses; secondly, how gender affects power relations between male and female nurses; thirdly, how nurses interpret issues of gender and finally, how sexual stereotyping affects relations between doctors and nurses.

The sexual division of labour

The most striking difference in the composition of medicine and nursing is gender. Since its rise as an organised profession, medicine has been a predominantly male occupation while nursing has long been regarded as one of the archetypal female occupations. Gamarnikow (1978) has argued that Victorian doctor-nurse-patient relationships could be equated with husband-wife-child relationships. Through their monopoly over diagnosis and prescription, doctors decided who should be a patient and what should be done to them. Nurses were limited, according to Florence Nightingale's precepts, to assisting their medical superiors and to maintaining a hygenic and comfortable environment for their charges who in turn had little knowledge of or authority over what was happening to them. The shadow of these formative role relations remains (Dingwall and McIntosh 1978).

Female disadvantage is not limited to differences between these occupations, it is equally notable within them. Despite recent increases in the number of women entering medical schools, the profession remains firmly in the hands of men (Elston 1977). This is evidenced by vertical segregation within the occupation which means that women occupy proportionately far fewer senior posts than their male counterparts, and also by horizontal segregation. In general surgery for example, less than one per cent of consultants are female. Women tend to be concentrated in specialities such as child and adolescent psychiatry (Oliver and Walford 1991).

Numerically, male entry into nursing has been considerably less significant than female entry into medicine. In 1987, fewer than 10 per cent of nurses in Britain were men (Gaze 1987). The fate of this small male minority has, however, been considerably more auspicious than that of its female counterpart in medicine. Since the introduction of an industrially modelled line management system following the Salmon Report (1966), men have come to dominate the management of both nursing practice and education, to the point where by 1987 they held over 50 per cent of chief nurse and director of nurse education posts in Britain (Gaze 1987). There was an implicit sexism in the Salmon Report; it regarded the 'feminine qualities' of nurses as appropriate to bedside care but as a profound hindrance to efficient administration, in that they encouraged concentration on minutiae at the expense of decisiveness. Salmon saw the direction forward as the promotion of a 'rational', 'masculine' style of management (Carpenter 1978).

It can be seen that gender segregation correlates strongly with both inter- and intra-occupational differentials. The gender inequalities occurring in these two areas can be mutually reinforcing. The successful entry of a male minority into nursing, rather then diluting gender as a major defining factor in occupational differentiation, has exacerbated it by adding male managers to the nurse's burden of male doctors. Conversely, there is some evidence that the increasing entrance of women into medicine is leading to a degree of democratisation in the nurse-doctor relationship (Webster 1985).

Curing versus caring, skill versus sympathy

One of the main themes emerging from the above discussion is that women's second class status both within and between the occupations of nursing and medicine is in part the result of assumptions founded upon a reductionist sociobiological model of gender role differentiation. According to such a model, women, as an extension of their maternal functions, possess expressive, emotional and caring qualities, while men are naturally more instrumental, rational, scientific and decisive. This social construction of the female role has been described by Hearn (1982) as the 'patriarchal feminine'; feminine because it accords to the feminine, 'caring' stereotype; patriarchal because in doing so it reinforces female subordination.

The patriarchal feminine is not simply a descriptive exercise, but involves judgement about the value of various human activities. Those activities which are categorised as being in the male domain are valued more highly than those adjudged appropriate for women (Sayers 1982).

The patriarchal feminine is not, however, the only interpretation open to those who accept 'given' gender differences. An alternative position attaches positive rather than negative evaluations to what are seen as immutable womanly traits. A number of radical feminists (for example de Beauvoir 1983; Firestone 1979) posit biologistic explanations for the sexual division of labour, treating it as a natural, rather than socially generated division (Gamarnikow 1978).

In consonance with such a position, many nursing theorists accept the existence of a skills/caring, male/female dichotomy. This is hardly surprising, given that caring is seen as a core, and indeed unique, attribute of nursing. Defense of the importance of emotional labour is therefore central to the affirmation of nursing's worth (Robinson 1991)[1]. The battleground therefore becomes how the various attributes of nursing and medicine are to be evaluated:

> As long as fields that are stereotypically male, highly technological and illness orientated are held in higher esteem than those that have been stereotypically female, focusing on long-term care, quality of life and health maintenance, there is little reason to foresee major changes in interprofessional relationships . . . (Webster 1985:317).

Claims for occupational equality are based on the assertion that natural female attributes are at least equal to male characteristics and that the 'feminine' tasks performed by nurses are of equal worth to the 'masculine' work of doctors (Gordon 1991). As Salvage puts it, 'Nurses/women should realise that doctors/men have much to learn from them' (1985:171).

Aims and method

Thus far I have examined how gender inequalities influence the structure of medicine and nursing. However, this does not illustrate how these inequalities affect action, nor indeed, how action maintains or transforms structural inequalities. My empirical enquiries were directed to the question of how the social structure of gender inequality influences social action and vice versa.

The empirical material for this paper was gathered over a three month period in 1989, during which I was employed as a staff nurse in a large metropolitan hospital in the north of Ireland. It was hoped that the size and urban location of the hospital would mean that local idiosyncracies would be minimised, thus enhancing the external validity of the research. Being within the British jurisdictional zone, public health provision in this part of Ireland is subsumed within the British National Health Service. Health service structures are similar, though not identical, to those in Britain. For example, implementation of the Griffiths management system has been considerably more tardy here than in the rest of the NHS. When this research was undertaken, the Salmon system of management was extant in the hospital observed.

Most of the information came from the intensive care unit in which I was temporarily employed as a staff nurse. The number of subjects observed, disaggregated for occupation, sex and position were:

	Female	*Male*
Nurses		
Sister/Charge Nurse	4	0
Staff Nurse	22	3
Nursing Auxiliary	4	0
Total	30	3

	Female	Male
Doctors		
Consultant	0	10
Registrar	1	2
Senior House Officer	5	3
Total	6	15

Data were obtained both by participant observation and by informal discussions between myself and the actors involved. The research might be described as quasi-covert in that while I informed my subjects that I was carrying out a project to examine how nurses communicated with other health care occupations, I did not emphasise my interest in the sensitive issues of power and gender.

Initiating talk about gender issues was easy. One factor that helped was my own sex. The fact that I am male had the ironic and useful effect of encouraging female nurses to be extremely frank about their views. Given the latent resentment harboured by many female nurses about what they perceive as the unfair occupational advantages of their male colleagues, the opportunity provided by a male nurse asking them to tell him what they really thought about men in health care was too good to miss.

Working in an intensive care unit facilitated observation. Firstly, six out of the eight beds in the unit were situated in one room. As a consequence, a large proportion of staff activity was easily observable. Secondly, the nature of intensive care nursing, with its high nurse-patient ratio, meant that I had time to observe and record interactions. Nevertheless, pressure of work meant that there were occasions when a considerable period of time elapsed between observation of data and their recording.

Additional data were obtained by a colleague from a general medical ward[2]. The empirical work conducted in this area was guided by the tentative conclusions that emerged from my own data collection, in an attempt to support or falsify them. This was especially important in instances where the numbers involved in the intensive care unit were small. For example, a further five male nurses were observed on the ward. The method of data collection here was solely that of participant observation.

The final source of information for this paper is the most difficult to quantify, but I suspect it was of considerable importance, especially in determination of the direction that the formal research took. This was my seven and a half years of participation in the subject milieu as a clinical nurse.

My method of analysis was based on analytic induction. Questions concerning gender and nursing had emerged from my previous experience as a clinical nurse and from reviewing the literature. These initial questions were:

1) What form did interaction between doctors and nurses take in decision making sequences?[3]

2) Did gender permutations influence the nature of inter- or intra-occupational interaction?
3) Did female nurses utilise the concept of gender in their understanding of their occupational position?
4) How assertive were female nurses with their male co-workers?
5) Was there any basis for the popular stereotyping of nurses' sexual habits?
6) What did nurses think about their stereotype?

Observation of interactions with these questions in mind led to the formulation of tentative answers. These were then tested to ascertain if they could explain the most common forms of interaction. 'Deviant' cases were examined to see if they could be the basis of alternative explanations.

The next step was to test whether my explanations could adequately explain social action occuring in another arena, a general medical ward. Given the variation of divisions of labour between different units, even within a single hospital (Strauss *et al* 1985), I felt it was important to test the generalisability of my conclusions. Because intensive care is in many ways unique as a therapeutic regime, considerable caution needs to be exercised in the extrapolation of results obtained from an ICU[4] to more general claims about the nature of nurse-doctor interactions. Three pertinent specificities of this social situation should be noted. Firstly, the high level of medical intervention that intensive care entails means that there is far more interaction between nurses and doctors in an ICU than in most other units, where a large proportion of care tends to be performed by nurses on their own. Secondly, emphasis on technology reinforces instrumental aspects of care, a factor that might be seen as strengthening medical superordination. Finally, the unit studied was fairly small, which meant that the number of personnel observed was rather low.

The final stage of analysis was an *ex post facto* formal quantification of some of the data. The purpose of this exercise was not to offer strong proofs for my claims. Rather, simple counting techniques were used to strengthen the evidence gained from other methods; to render explicit quantification; and to give a general impression of the data, thus contextualising the extracts of interaction included in the paper (Silverman 1985).

Gender permutations and power

The effects of gender upon nurse-doctor interactions were measured by observing the interactions of four different combinations: male doctors and nurses, female doctors and nurses, female nurses and doctors, male nurses and doctors; and by studying the attitudes of female nurses to their gender roles. The first thing I noted was that the gender of a nurse appeared to have little effect on their interaction with doctors. The male nurses studied were not observed to have any marked increase in authority in relation to doctors as compared to their female counterparts. Indeed the quality of interaction between male nurses and doctors and female nurses and doctors seemed to be identical.

Support for this contention came from counting the number of times male and female nurses were observed to make evaluative comments to doctors in reply to medical requests. While lack of comment by nurses does not necessarily reflect subservience in that silence can mean considered consent, the act of comment is indicative of assertiveness in that it entails an assumption by the nurse that her/his opinion is important.

Table 1 *Occurrences of evaluative verbal responses by staff nurses in reply to doctors' clinical requests by sex of nurse*

	Female per cent	*Male* per cent
Commented to doctor about request	28	22
Complied without comment	72	78
Base	53	36

($X^2 = 0.15$; 1 d.f.; $p < 0.05$)
The association between gender and likelihood of talking back to doctors was not statistically significant

In contrast, the interactions of female doctors with nurses were markedly different from some of their male colleagues. Two instances which occured on the same day illustrate this point. The first involved a male senior house officer who was preparing to perform an aseptic procedure, and who was being assisted by a nurse. His sole verbal communication with the nurse during the entire episode consisted of the demand 'Gloves!'. At the end of the procedure he left the bedside without a word, leaving the nurse to clear up his debris.

The second involved a female SHO who was also performing an aseptic technique. As well as talking to the patient, the doctor also greeted the nurse, engaging in small talk with both nurse and patient throughout the procedure. Her requests were also expressed in a far more polite manner:

Sorry, would you mind opening these gloves for me . . . thanks.

On completing the procedure, she tidied away all her waste rather than leaving the nurse to do it.

This is not to say that all male doctors were as pompous as the one noted above. Indeed, there was considerable variation in the behaviour of male doctors towards nurses. Nor was it the case that there were no exceptions to the rule of sisterly love, as the following interaction between a staff nurse on the medical ward and a newly arrived doctor demonstrates:

> *SN(F)*: Hello, I'm Forename, I staff here. You must be the new JHO.
> *SHO(F)*: Actually, Staff Nurse, I am Doctor Surname and I happen to be a senior house officer.

Nevertheless, it was generally true that most female doctors were considerably more egalitarian than most of their male counterparts.

A quantitative indication of this came from counting the number of times doctors were prepared to tidy up after themselves, rather than leaving debris for nurses to dispose of. While 65 per cent of female doctors observed cleaned up their clinical waste after procedures, the figure was only 36 per cent for male doctors. Even when (male) consultants, who were notably cavalier in their attitude towards procedures, were excluded from the question, the difference remained statistically significant.

The individual variations in behaviour noted are a reminder that while gender may be an important factor in inter-occupational interaction, it is not the only one. Other aspects of status difference have considerable influence. These may be formal prescriptions about occupational roles (Johnson 1972) or reflections of the immediate situational context within which interactions take place (Hughes 1988). These factors can either reinforce or countervail against the influence of gender.

The fact that nurses' gender had far less impact on the quality of inter-occupational interaction than that of doctors probably indicates the power differential that exists between the two groups overall. Being in a weaker occupation means that nurses have less opportunity to engineer the quality of relationships. The inability of males nurses to utilise the advantages of their gender is the result of the ascription to nursing of a position of female subordination. The very factors that afford male nurses intra-occupational advantage work against them in inter-occupational power relations. Conversely, because of their position of authority, doctors have considerable latitude in deciding how they are going to interact with members of other occupations. They have the opportunity to avail themselves of the power that they implicitly possess if they wish to, or to act in a more egalitarian fashion if they do not.

Nurses' attitudes to gender issues

There was a militancy apparent in many nurses concerning doctors' assumptions about their inferior gender and occupational roles. Even when they acceeded to performing 'handmaiden' activities, they often did so with bad grace, as the following incident demonstrates:

> The phone in the doctors' room rang. As all the doctors and nurses on duty were busy with other tasks and unavailable to answer it, a female staff nurse left her tea break to take the call. It was a message for a consultant who was on another phone at the time. The nurse spent

several minutes standing in silence beside the consultant until he had finished his call and then informed him of the content of the other. She then returned to her tea and exclaimed to the other nurses on their break:

SN(F): Nurse, cleaner, secretary, receptionist, that's all they think we are. The old sod didn't even say thank you!

Female nurses were conscious that their gender was a significant factor affecting the status of their occupation, though the value judgements that they attached to this fact differed considerably. A minority (four out of the 19 nurses specifically asked) expressed the view that occupational gender differences were to be explained by men having careers while women simply had jobs until they started a family. These differences in work experiences were seen as reflecting natural differences in the roles of the sexes. These nurses tended to accept their lot with equanimity. Others were considerably more assertive in their attitudes, as the following comment of a ward nurse immediately after an alteraction with a junior house officer demonstrates:

SN(F): If that boy thinks we're little women here at his beck and call, he's going to have to learn the hard way. He's nothing but a wee male chauvinist pig!

Criticism like this was reserved for those male doctors who were openly bombastic or sexist. While nurses were often prepared to explain the position of their own occupation in terms of gender, they rarely applied the same critique to doctors. Sexism was seen as an individual phenomenon of specific doctors rather than an institutional ethos. However, the individualist explanations found in this study may not be entirely representative of nurses' attitudes, as the published opinion of one student nurse demonstrates:

So why do we nurses find ourselves in this [subservient] situation? Nursing is, and always has been, 'women's work' and medicine a man's world (Jones 1987:59)

Female nurses in this study were far more willing to ascribe general categorisations to male nurses. The success of senior male nurses was often put down to their sex. Male nurses in the clinical area, and therefore relatively junior in the nursing hierarchy, were invariably regarded as being on their way to higher things, once again because of their sex. My position as a former clinical nurse now studying at a university meant that I did not escape the brunt of this perception.

While their gender opened up greater career opportunities for male nurses, this did not mean that it gave clinical male nurses any advantage over their female counterparts in the immediate situation that they worked in. Barring an underlying resentment of female nurses about the unfairness of promotional opportunities for men, I found no difference in the attitudes and behaviour of other nurses towards male and female ward nurses of the same grade.

Within the clinical focus of this study, the mechanisms by which men were able to advance themselves within nursing administration were not observed. This is significant, because it means that the generation of male hegemony within nursing management lies outside the doing of nursing. Examination of what these mechanisms are would be a fruitful point of departure for further research.

The persuasiveness of credentialism

It may seem strange that while nurses viewed the position of their own job in terms of gender, they did not extend this outlook to their analysis of the position of medicine. After all, the positions of the two occupations are inextricably linked, and the brute fact of gender segregation appears to be obvious. However, the difference in attitude of female nurses to male nurses and to male doctors may be due to a difference in familiarity that they have about the processes of occupational advancement.

Because of a high degree of occupational segregation, nurses do not have a great deal of knowledge about how occupational advancement operates for doctors. They are confronted by doctors as people already possessing enabling qualifications and legal licence. These entitlements to occupational superiority are portrayed as being the unproblematic and exclusive result of a meritocratic process. It is hardly surprising, therefore, that nurses find it difficult to form a generalised gendered critique of the position of their medical counterparts[5]. This is testament to the justificatory power of credentialism in the maintenance of occupational closure (Berlant 1975).

Because nurses have had direct experience of the conditions pertaining in the processes of occupational advancement within their own occupation, they take a more cynical attitude towards them. Often either they, or someone they know, has been passed over in favour of a male colleague. This familiarity means that gender bias can less easily be hidden by the guise of functionalist justifications such as educational or experiential differentials.

Increasing assertiveness

While most nurses accepted that the position of doctors was largely due to their accrued credentials, this did not mean that they necessarily saw doctoring as a more important facet of health care than the activities that nurses were involved in. A number of nurses expressed their belief in the importance of nursing care in the promotion of health. The debate about the relative merits of technological intervention and human kindness was illustrated by a brief altercation between a junior doctor and a senior staff nurse:

> *JHO(M)*: Anyone can do a nurse's job, but there's not many people that can do what I can do.
> *SN(F)*: Oh yea? You wouldn't know how to care for your own granny if you had to. There's more to helping people than sticking needles in them, you know.

This interaction is interesting both because it indicates the positive evaluation many nurses put upon the caring role of nursing and as an example of the degree of assertiveness of nurses in their relationships with medical colleagues. The emphasis that nursing theorists such as Salvage (1985) place upon the autonomy and importance of nursing actions has gained acceptance by at least a segment of clinical nurses.

This assertiveness was also displayed in more formal interactions with doctors. I noted many instances where nurses were prepared to challenge medical orders, and indeed, their challenges were often successful, as this instance of a junior house officer requesting a female staff nurse to alter the feeding regime of a patient demonstrates:

> *JHO(M)*: Mrs Surname should be eating by now. Can you start her on a soft diet?
> *SN(F)*: Well, she's still very nauseated. I think she could stay on fluids for a while longer.
> *JHO(M)*: That's fine, we'll leave her until tomorrow and see if she's up to it then.

It can be seen that nurses do not act in an unreflexively subordinate way towards their medical colleagues (Porter 1991). While nursing input into decision making in instances like the above does not enjoy official sanction, in that the doctor still has the legally grounded option to ignore the nurse's input, the fact that it occurs, and occurs frequently, may indicate a changing relationship between these occupations.

In the 1960s, Stein (1967) developed the idea of the 'doctor-nurse game' to characterise the nature of inter-occupational interaction. Stein argued that while nurses were ostensibly deferent to doctors, their deference masked a considerable input into health care decision making. The doctor-nurse game involved nurses making implicit recommendations through the use of statements about the condition of a patient. This masquerade enabled doctors to utilise nurses' knowledge while maintaining the pretence of their own omniscience.

In a study of interaction in a casualty department in 1980, Hughes (1988) noted that while the doctor-nurse game was still played, in certain circumstances nurses were quite prepared to be openly assertive with their medical colleagues.

In the present study, nurses' open assertiveness, rather than being dependent upon specific enabling situational circumstances, appears to have become a more generalised phenomenon.

The impression that there has been an alteration in the relationship between doctors and nurses since the 1960s is reinforced by Stein in his recent reassessment of the doctor-nurse game:

> The 1967 game was an intricate interaction carefully developed over time in which both players were willing participants. What is happening now is that one of the players (the nurse) has unilaterally decided to stop playing the game and instead is consciously and actively attempting to change . . . how nurses relate to other health professionals (Stein *et al* 1990: 547).

However, the extent of nursing's autonomy should not be exaggerated. Davies (1977) has argued that the occupational strategies that informed nursing during the Nightingale era, which included deference to doctors, remain influential. In addition, not all efforts to increase the independence of nursing have been entirely successful. Despite the introduction of a formalised procedure of diagnosis, prescription and evaluation known as the nursing process, nursing has not, as yet, successfully attained effective diagnostic autonomy (Porter 1991)[6]. This is of significance if one accepts Johnson's (1972) contention that control over diagnosis is the key to inter-occupational authority.

Sexual stereotyping

The final aspect I wish to deal with is that of sexual stereotyping. This entails the image of nurses as being sexually permissive, most notably with young male doctors. These stereotypes are important because, if they bear any relation to real life, it is obvious that gender inequalities will be considerably overdetermined by sexual attitudes.

Muff (1982) has argued that the sexual stereotyping that nurses are subjected to is the result of myths generated by a male fear of the feminine other. However, while Muff's psychoanalytic approach demonstrates the depth of these attitudes, it tends towards an ahistorical and immutable conception of mythical stereotypes. Kalisch and Kalisch (1982a,b,c) have argued that this particular portrayal of nurses is an historically recent phenomenon. Up until the 1960s, media portrayal of nurses was largely that of chaste young women. During the era of sexual 'liberation' this altered radically, with nurses being increasingly portrayed as promiscuous playthings of their medical colleagues.

Kalisch and Kalisch do not speculate as to why this may be so. However, if it is accepted that the images of nurses reflect the images of women in general, a pattern can be identified. Sexual liberalisation was a double-edged sword. While it allowed for greater personal freedom, it also brought into starker relief the subordination of women through their sexual roles. If male power and supremacy is expressed through sexuality (Millett 1972), then openness about sex will exacerbate its significance for male domination. In eras when sex is repressed, the domestic, caring roles of women are more prominent aspects of justificatory ideologies for their oppression. Thus the image of nurses prior to the 1960s was often one of altruistic angels.

Because of the nature of their work, which involves intimate contact with bodies, and indeed with unpleasant bodily functions and dysfunctions, nurses seem to be singled out more than most female occupational groups as the butt of sexual stereotyping. The fear of the other is exacerbated by the other's intrusion into physical aspects of life which are normally closely guarded secrets. Consequently, the mythical stereotypes employed are all the more grotesque. Nurses' intrusions into the bodies of others are countered by the demeaning of nurses' own bodies.

Despite the ubiquity of images in popular culture which portray nurses as the sexual chattels of their medical colleagues, I found no empirical evidence to suggest that the hospital units studied were simmering fleshpots whose primary purpose was to facilitate the libidinous proclivities of young doctors. While occasional instances of sexual innuendo and mild flirtation were noted, these were of a fairly innocuous nature. No evidence of intimate relationships between doctors and nurses was discovered, although it has to be admitted that by their very nature such interactions would tend to be discreetly handled by those involved. Analysis of the company nurses reported keeping on evenings out showed that the people they socialised with were rarely medical personnel. Indeed, only twice did nurses inform me that they had been in the company of doctors, and even then it had been in the context of group outings. While it would be overstating the case to say that intimate contacts between male doctors and female nurses never occur, it does seem that the myths about nurses' sexual behaviour are exactly that – myths.

It is hardly surprising that nurses find this state of affairs particularly galling. The level of their resentment was displayed in a discussion about a grossly sexist portrayal of nurses in a daily newspaper. The conversation was concluded with the following comment on the writer of the piece by a young staff nurse:

> *SN(F)*: I just wish that one day that bastard becomes sick and I get to nurse him. I tell you, he'll never have another sexual thought in his life by the time I've finished with him.

The influence of lateral 'female' roles

Paradoxically, given that the fixation with the sexuality of nurses appears to be a relatively recent phenomenon, it appears that the dearth of romantic involvement between doctors and nurses that now pertains was not always the case. A significant proportion of senior doctors were married to nurses or former nurses. The lack of interest shown by younger doctors in their nursing colleagues seems to be partially the result of the large influx of women into medicine. With the progressive equalising of the gender ratio, male doctors have an increasing opportunity to develop personal relationships with their peers. A number of doctor-doctor personal relationships were noted in the study.

There may also be a change in the way nurses view the prospect of doctors as future partners. Earlier studies of nursing almost universally identified an ambivalence on the part of nurses towards their occupation (Davis and Oleson 1963, Dingwall 1977, Simpson 1979, Weitzman 1982). These writers, whose ideological bent ranges from interactionism and phenomenology, to functionalism and feminism, all seem to agree that occupational commitment was comprised by lateral female roles and the prospect of family life and motherhood. If nurses gave their private ambitions precedence over their career aspirations, then seeking a high status partner from the medical profession would seem a feasible tactic.

Contrary to the conclusions of previous studies, which posited that, because of their gender, nurses rarely regarded their employment as a career, I would argue that for many nurses this is no longer the case. While I have already noted that a minority of nurses in my study continued to regard their work as an interval before the adoption of the domestic role, most were quite definite that they were in the occupation for reasons to do with the occupation itself, whether this was simply to earn a wage, or because of the satisfaction that being in a 'caring profession' brings. Moreover, a number of nurses (nine out of the 19 with whom it was discussed) explicitly stated that, notwithstanding their desire to marry, they saw their job as a career which they expected to follow throughout their working lives.

Male doctors' attentions towards female doctors rather than nurses caused amusement rather than resentment in the female nurses observed. This was evidenced by nurses' reactions to several emotional imbroglios between female and male doctors which occurred on the medical ward where more junior medical personnel worked. Their attitude was summed up by one rather cynical staff nurse:

SN(F): It's great fun watching them break each other's hearts!

With the increasing perception of nursing as a career in itself, the instrumental motivation of using it to find a marriage partner has become, if not completely defunct, at least increasingly anachronistic.

Conclusion: one step forward and one step back

In conclusion, it can be seen that gender remains one of the most important factors in nurses' experience. Its effect, however, may be changing over time. I would contend that these changes reflect general trends in the position of women in our society. If the subordination of nurses in the Nightingale era was an extension of the overtly oppressed situation that women found themselves in at that time, the rather more convoluted and mutable nature of nurses' relations with doctors that pertain today reflect the gradual alteration of the position of women as a whole. We should be cautious, however, about seeing this process as a uniform, if exceedingly gradual, march towards gender equality.

Certainly, there were a number of aspects identified in this study that indicated that change was taking place in this direction. Most notable of these was the refusal of many nurses to acquiesce without objection to the subordinate position that some doctors expected them to take. These actions were predicated upon an increasingly positive self-evaluation of nurses about their role as female workers. The fact that the ideology of feminism is alive and well on hospital wards can only augur well for future developments in the position of nurses. In addition, the increasing proportion of female doctors seems to be leading to an attenuation of gender as a factor in nurse-doctor power relations.

On the other hand, the increase in male authority within nursing over the last quarter of a century must be taken into account. While female nurses are certainly aware of this process, to date little has been done to tackle it. Indeed, the indications are that nursing will increasingly become an occupation divided between male managers and female ward workers. Following the Griffiths report (1983) into NHS management, the Salmon system has been abandoned, with lines of authority exclusive to nurses being replaced by a flexible, generic system of management. While I am unaware of any quantitative measurements of the effects of Griffiths on the gender ratio, there is good reason to suppose that, if anything, gender imbalance will be exacerbated because nurse managers will now have to compete for their positions with managers from predominantly male occupations such as medicine and private business.

There is bitter irony in the fact that at a time when the problems of gender in relation to doctors are being at least partially resolved, the issue has reappeared with just as much vigour in a different locus. Because of its increasing salience, the problem of male domination within nursing indicates a need for further analysis.[7]

Department of Sociology and Social Policy,
The Queen's University of Belfast

Acknowledgements

I would like to thank Eithne McLaughlin, Steven Yearley and the paper's referees for their helpful comments on earlier drafts of this article.

Notes

1 While nursing theorists tend to concentrate on the expressive, 'feminine' aptitudes of nurses, this identification is by no means unproblematic in that it does not take into account the manual nature of the job (Symonds 1991).
2 Observation of interactions on the general medical ward were carried out by Sandra Ryan. I would like to record my appreciation for her significant contribution to this paper.
3 I have discussed this question in a previous paper (Porter 1991).
4 The abbreviations used in this paper denote the following:
ICU: Intensive Care Unit
SN: Staff nurse.
JHO: Junior house officer.
SHO: Senior house officer.
(F): Female.
(M): Male
5 This facet of social interaction has been noted by Bhaskar, who observes that while society is a skilled accomplishment of active agents, 'the social world may be opaque to the social agents upon whose activity it depends . . .' (1989:4). One of the aspects of this opacity is the existence of what he calls 'unacknowledged conditions'. It would seem that the role gender plays in the occupational advancement of medicine is at least partially unacknowledged by nurses.
6 It is possible to frame this problem in terms of structuration theory. Giddens (1976) argues that the processes of structuration involve an interplay of meanings, norms and power. It might be observed that while the meanings and norms involved in inter-occupational relations between nursing and medicine have significantly altered, formal power has not because it is embedded in the relatively immutable structure of state sanctioned legality.
7 This article is based on a paper given to the 1991 annual conference of the Sociological Association of Ireland, 19–21 April, Termonfeckin, Co. Louth.

References

Abbott, P. and Wallace, C. (1990) The sociology of the caring professions: an introduction. In Abbott, P. and Wallace, C. (eds.) *The Sociology of the Caring Professions*. London: Falmer.

de Beauvoir, S. (1983) *The Second Sex*. Harmondsworth: Penguin.

Berlant, J.L. (1975) *Profession and Monopoly*. Berkley, Cal.: University of California Press.

Bhaskar, R. (1989) *Reclaiming Reality: A Critical Introduction to Contemporary Philosophy*. London: Verso.
Carpenter, M. (1977) The new managerialism and professionalism in nursing. In Stacey, M. *et al* (eds.) *Health and the Division of Labour*. London: Croom Helm.
Carpenter, M. (1978) Managerialism and the division of labour in nursing. In Dingwall, R. and McIntosh, J. (eds.) *Readings in the Sociology of Nursing*. Edinburgh: Churchill Livingstone.
Davies, C. (1977) Continuities in the development of hospital nursing in Britain, *Journal of Advanced Nursing*, 2, 479–93.
Davis, F. and Olsen, V.L. (1963) Initiation into a woman's profession: identity problems in the status transition of coed to student nurse, *Sociometry*, 26,89–101.
Dingwall, R. (1977) *The Social Organization of Health Visitor Training*. London: Croom Helm.
Dingwall, R. and McIntosh, J. (eds.) (1978) *Readings in the Sociology of Nursing*. Edinburgh: Churchill Livingstone.
Elston, A.M. (1977) Women in the medical profession: whose problem? In Stacey, M. *et al* (eds.) *Health and the Division of Labour*. London: Croom Helm.
Firestone, S. (1979) *The Dialectic of Sex: The Case for Feminist Revolution*. London: The Women's Press.
Gamarnikow, E. (1978) Sexual division of labour: the case of nursing. In Kuhn, A. and Wolpe, A. (eds.) *Feminism and Materialism*. London: Routledge and Kegan Paul.
Gaze, H. (1987) Men in nursing, *Nursing Times*, 83, 25–7.
Giddens, A. (1976) *New Rules of Sociological Method*. London: Hutchinson.
Gordon, S. (1991) Fear of caring: the feminist paradox. *American Journal of Nursing*. February, 44–8.
Griffiths, R. (1983) *Enquiry into NHS Management*. London: Department of Health and Social Services.
Hearn, J. (1982) Notes on patriarchy, professionalization and the semi-professions, *Sociology*, 16, 184–202.
Hughes, D. (1988) When nurse knows best: some aspects of nurse/doctor interaction in a casualty department, *Sociology of Health and Illness*, 10, 1–22.
Johnson, T.J. (1972) *Professions and Power*. London: Macmillan.
Jones, C. (1987) Handmaiden mentality, *Nursing Times*, 83, 59.
Kalisch, P.A. and Kalisch, B.J. (1982a) Nurses on prime-time television, *American Journal of Nursing*. February, 265–70.
Kalisch, P.A. and Kalisch, B.J. (1982b) The image of the nurse in motion pictures, *American Journal of Nursing*. April, 605–11.
Kalisch, P. A. and Kalisch, B.J. (1982c) The image of nurses in novels, *American Journal of Nursing*. August, 1220–4.
Mackay, L. (1990) Nursing: just another job?. In Abbott, P. and Wallace, C. (eds.) *The Sociology of the Caring Professions*. London: Falmer.
Millett, K. (1971) *Sexual Politics*. London: Sphere.
Muff, J. (1982) Handmaiden, battle-ax, whore: an exploration into the fantasies, myths, and stereotypes about nurses. In Muff, J. (ed.) *Socialization, Sexism and Stereotyping: Women's Issues in Nursing*. Prospect Heights, Ill.: Waveland.
Oliver, D.and Walford, D. (1991) Chairpersons of the Working Party on Women

Doctors and their Careers, *Women Doctors and their Careers*. London: Department of Health.

Porter, S. (1991) A participant observation study of power relations between nurses and doctors in a general hospital, *Journal of Advanced Nursing*, 16,728–35.

Robinson, J. (1991) Working with doctors: educational conditioning, *Nursing Times*, 87, 28–31.

Salmon, B. (1966) *Report of the Committee on Senior Nursing Staff Structure*. London: HMSO.

Salvage, J. (1985) *The Politics of Nursing*. London: Heinemann.

Sayers, J. (1982) *Biological Politics: Feminist and Anti-Feminist Perspectives*. London: Tavistock.

Silverman, D. (1985) *Qualitative Methodology and Sociology*. Aldershot: Gower.

Simpson, I.H. (1979) *From Student to Nurse: A Longitudinal Study of Socialization*. Cambridge: Cambridge University Press.

Stein, L. (1967) The doctor-nurse game, *Archives of General Psychiatry*, 16, 699–703.

Stein, L., Watts, D.T., Howell, T. (1990) The doctor-nurse game revisited, *New England Journal of Medicine*. 322, 546–9.

Strauss, A., Fagerhaugh, S., Suczec, B. and Weiner, C. (1985) *The Social Organization of Medical Work*. Chicago, University of Chicago Press.

Symonds, A. (1991) Angels and interfering busybodies: the social construction of two occupations, *Sociology of Health and Illness*, 13, 247–64.

Webster, D. (1985) Medical students' views of the role of the nurse, *Nursing Research*, 34, 313–17.

Weitzman, L.J. (1982) Sex-role socialization, in Muff, J. (ed.) *Socialization, Sexism and Stereotyping: Women's Issues in Nursing*. Prospect Heights, Ill.: Waveland.

Part IX
Hospitals

[34]

PAYING THE HOSPITAL: AMERICAN PROBLEMS AND FOREIGN SOLUTIONS

William A. Glaser

Hospital financing in the United States suffers from many problems. Many persons lack access because they lack third-party coverage. Among those covered, benefits vary, and persons receive unequal services. Costs are high and are uncontrolled. The hospital is burdened by complicated relations with many payers. In order to cover their costs and earn extra cash, hospitals overcharge the more generous third parties, and recriminations result. All other developed countries have either statutory health insurance, national health services, or full public financing of privately managed hospitals. Whatever the financing method, all countries avoid the problems prevailing in the United States. All citizens are covered, all have access, and hospitals reject no one for financial reasons. All citizens have equal benefits and receive the same basic services. Regulation by government and negotiations with health insurance carriers guarantee the hospital's operating costs to service its catchment area adequately, but also prevent the hospital from installing excessive equipment and excessive staff. Each hospital is paid by all-payer standard rates, administration of reimbursement is simple, and shifting of costs among payers is both unnecessary and administratively impossible. Costs are contained by the total management of the system, not by fragmented efforts by separate insurance carriers. Considerable strategic thinking by government, the providers, and other interest groups sets guidelines for spending levels every year to meet the country's clinical needs but also to stay within its fiscal capacity. Capital investment for new treatments depends on government grants and evaluation of needs.

The methods of financing hospitals create a number of problems in the United States:

- Many persons lack any insurance coverage and cannot get access. If they are accepted for inpatient or outpatient care, they may have to go to the less desirable or more distant establishments.
- Even if they are covered by insurance, persons have some benefits but not others.
- Costs are high and cannot be controlled.
- Patients with good insurance coverage are overcharged.
- The system is complicated and baffles patients, physicians, and government officials. Patients rarely understand their coverage and risk denials when they seek care. Confusion and disputes are common.

International Journal of Health Services, Volume 21, Number 3, Pages 389–399, 1991

- Expensive services proliferate across the country. Hospitals duplicate services rather than cooperate.

The individual hospital itself experiences many problems from the U.S. financing system:

- It cannot predict its patient flow, revenue, capital investment, and survival. If its obligations exceed its revenue, it can go bankrupt.
- It experiences bad debts, particularly in the emergency room and outpatient department.
- It must deal with many payers with different allowances and rules. Administrative complexity and administrative costs are high.
- It must shift costs furtively from one payer to another, in order to make up its budget.

FOREIGN FINANCING SYSTEMS

Every country has had difficulties in its hospital sector—at first in expanding access and improving services, and recently in controlling costs. Every other developed country has solved the problems that beset the United States. This article briefly describes the principal methods. A complete summary of the European, Canadian, and U.S. experiences appears elsewhere (1).

All other developed countries cover their populations by universal and obligatory systems. Several countries—France, Germany, Holland, Belgium, and others—have "national health insurance." All persons are required to enroll in health insurance carriers. Social security payroll taxes on employers and on subscribers are channeled into each subscriber's carrier. The carriers, hospitals, and physicians remain private and self-governing, as they were before the system was enacted. Government's role is limited to a few regulatory functions and to adding some cash. Subscribers and their dependents choose physicians and hospitals freely, and their insurance carriers pay the claims (2).

A few countries—Great Britain, Sweden, Italy, Spain, and the countries of Eastern Europe—have "national health services." Government takes over hospitals and employs the physicians. Financing is part of the general budget of the national or provincial government. All citizens of the country are eligible for full benefits (3).

Canada has a hybrid arrangement that is neither insurance nor a health service. Government pays hospital and physician claims from its general budget. Hospitals and physicians remain private. All citizens receive full benefits (4).

THE PUBLIC'S ACCESS AND BENEFITS

Under all the foregoing systems, all citizens are completely covered for basic hospital care. In countries with statutory health insurance, coverage started with industrial workers and miners; it was expanded to other occupations, to the self-employed, to pensioners, and to the unemployed in successive amendments to the law; and now it is nearly universal in every country. The present coverage is shown in Table 1. The only groups not covered by obligatory insurance are the best-paid managers, entrepreneurs,

Table 1

Extent and forms of insurance coverage, Western Europe[a]

Basic coverage	France	West Germany	Holland[b]	Belgium	Switzerland
Sickness funds					
Obligatory by law	98%	77%	51%	98%	25%
Voluntary	—	12%	19%	1%	71%
Private insurance companies	1.5%	9%	30%	1%	2%
Not insured	0.5%	2%	0.1%	0+%	2%
Total	100%	100%	100%	100%	100%
Total population in millions	53	61	14	10	6.4

[a]Source: reference 2.

[b]Before 1990, 19 percent of the Dutch population were nonobligatory members of the sickness funds and 30 percent were nonobligatory subscribers to the private carriers. Since 1990, all are required to join a third party of their choice.

and professionals—all of whom buy private insurance. In countries with national health services and in Canada, every inhabitant was covered in full when the scheme went into effect.

Both the obligatory insurance and the private health insurance for the elite cover basic inpatient clinical care—housing and ward service, food, nursing, clinical care by physicians, and so on. Since almost no one arrives at the hospital without coverage, the European and Canadian hospitals experience almost none of the bad debts that are a prominent problem in the United States.

All citizens are guaranteed primary care under the parts of the European and Canadian programs covering physician services, and nearly every citizen has a private physician in office practice. Therefore, few patients come to the hospital in a deteriorated emergency situation because they had lacked previous ambulatory services. For example, the critical maternal and neonatal conditions that burden U.S. hospitals are rare in other developed countries, even where, as in England and France, there are low-income and minority groups at risk.

Since all citizens are covered and are paid for in full, all are welcomed in every hospital. Hospitals are not identified with only poor or only rich clienteles. Municipally owned hospitals have an overwhelmingly poor or minority clientele in the United States, but they have a diversified patient census abroad. Because the basic benefits are the same for all persons, all receive the same basic services in the mainstream hospitals. Since these are free countries, the rich can buy private insurance to cover supplementary benefits in the mainstream hospitals (such as a private room or personal attention by the medical chief of service), or to cover care in the few elite private clinics. But the basic medical care of the privately insured is no different. Because of the absence of financial barriers and because generous inpatient benefits make unnecessary the extramural treatment of surgical cases, utilization and bed occupancy are higher in several (not all) European countries than in the United States. Table 2 shows the proportion of each population that is hospitalized during one year. One would then expect Europe to spend

Table 2

Utilization of inpatient service, Western Europe and North America[a]

	Percentage of population hospitalized (1987)	Bed-days per person in population (1986)
National health service		
United Kingdom	14.7	2.1
Sweden	20.0	4.4
Italy	15.0	1.6
National health insurance		
West Germany	21.1	3.5
France	21.2	3.3
The Netherlands	11.0	3.8
Belgium	14.6	2.8
Switzerland	13.2	3.0
Canada	14.5	2.0
United States	14.7	1.7

[a]Source: Poullier, J. P. Health care expenditure and other data. *Health Care Financing Rev.*, Annu. Suppl., 1989, Tables 20, 21.

more than the United States on hospital care, but—as I will show later in this article—it does not.

COVERING THE HOSPITAL'S COSTS

All foreign financing systems intend to pay each hospital's unique cost for its particular patient load. In national health insurance, a neutral regulator examines the hospital's past costs, past utilization, and prospective budget for the next year. The local office of the insurance carrier gives its opinion about the hospital's past performance and future needs. The regulator then approves the prospective budget, often after cutting certain lines that seem excessive upon close scrutiny. The prospective rate then is used for all claims during the next year: the total hospital budget is divided among the health insurance carriers according to their admissions and is paid in installments (in France, under global budgeting), or it is made up by per diems from the insurance carriers according to their subscribers' inpatient days (in Holland, Germany, Switzerland, and elsewhere) (1, pp. 84–108, 121–146).

In countries with national health services (such as Great Britain and Sweden) and in Canada, government decides what the hospital needs and pays it in full from the annual government budget. In theory, government should be pledged to cover each hospital's unique costs in full. But, if government budgets are squeezed, government may pay the hospital less than the minima preferred by its managers. During the early years of public financing, the hospital managers negotiate their prospective budgets with the Ministries of Health, and the Ministries try to cover cost over-runs. But eventually the Treasury imposes stricter discipline on the Ministries, the latter can provide no more than a fixed annual limit to each hospital, and the hospital managers learn to operate within the grant (1, pp. 164–196).

The standard reimbursement rate governs all payers: every country but the United States has an "all-payer" system. A hospital "loses" on expensive cases and "gains" on others, but it covers its costs overall. For each insurance carrier, volume is so high and case mix is so varied that the case load averages out. The method is simple and standardized, and therefore both hospital and carrier minimize administrative costs. The hospital has neither the need nor the opportunity to overcharge some carriers on the grounds that other carriers underpay. The financial juggling ("cost-shifting") and recriminations that dominate U.S. hospital reimbursement are absent abroad (5).

No country uses a fixed rate for each type of case across all hospitals, as in diagnosis related groups (DRGs) in the United States. The goal abroad is to cover each hospital's unique costs: a prospective budget that will fulfill its needs is approved in advance by regulators or by negotiators; the global grants or per diems are calculated to cover costs during the next year without profits or losses. If government and the insurance carriers deem a hospital essential for a community, its costs are covered and it is protected from the bankruptcy that might result from fluctuations in admissions. In contrast, DRG payments for each admission in a rural U.S. hospital leave rural establishments in financial trouble, because of their low occupancy. Rural interest groups then press Congress to manipulate the reimbursement formulas.

Because of the break-even method of reimbursement and because of close monitoring of clinical performance and finances by regulators and by the health insurance carriers, European and Canadian hospitals have no opportunity to underserve and pocket the cash.

COST CONTAINMENT

The costs of acute hospital care absorb about half of nearly every country's total health care spending. Because of the aging of populations, greater service intensity, and more complex technology, hospital costs everywhere can grow without limit. But all countries with national health insurance and national health services must control hospital costs: those with insurance must halt the steady increase in payroll taxes and in government subsidies; those with national health services must reduce the budget deficits that afflict all their governments; leaders in health believe that money must be transferred from secondary and tertiary care into primary and long-term care.

Government does not dictate limits in countries with national health insurance, since the carriers are autonomous, the hospitals are private and municipal, and the system is supposed to remain independent. But government must be the watchdog, lest hospital spending exceed the economic capacity of society, lest payroll taxes become excessive, and lest the insurance carriers become insolvent. Guidelines about prudent increases in hospital operating reimbursement ("expenditure targets") emerge every year from consultations among government ministries, the health insurance carriers, the hospital association, other health provider associations, employers' associations, the trade unions, and other interest groups. These guidelines are enforced by the reimbursement decisions by rate regulators and by the insurance carriers.

National health services contain costs over hospitals, because the national government's budget officers and legislature require the Ministry of Health to operate within the available money ("expenditure caps"). The level of spending depends on the decisions of the democratic political process: some countries (such as Sweden) make hospital care the center of their health services and consistently spend more tax money on hospitals than do others (like Britain and Eastern European countries); spending is tight in periods of government austerity and generous at other times. Hospital managers learn to appeal to the electorate to avoid serious cuts.

Levels of spending and rates of increase are shown in Table 3. During the 1970s every country had a cost explosion in hospital finance. All countries with organized methods of cost containment now have lower levels of spending than the United States. U.S. hospital spending regularly increases each year at twice (or more than) the rate of inflation. (Switzerland too now limits hospital costs, but they appear to rise relative to inflation, only because its basic inflation rate is low). Other developed countries spend less on hospitals than does the United States, despite the similarities in the health needs of their populations, the use of identical clinical methods, and the similarities in quality and clinical outcome. And other developed countries spend less on hospitals, despite their higher inpatient admissions and larger number of beds.

The United States spends more on hospital operations for several reasons. First, the United States employs more people in hospitals than any other developed country (Table 4). The American visitor to any foreign hospital immediately notices the lower levels of staffing and the more efficient work pace. The technically advanced European and Canadian hospitals have more personnel than the less complex establishments, but each type uses—and wastes—fewer people than its U.S. counterpart. Similar overstaffing and higher costs appear when the United States is compared with Europe in many other organizational and economic sectors. During scrutiny of the hospital's prospective budget, rate regulators (as in France and in Holland) and negotiators (such as the sickness funds in Germany) insist that the hospital not carry unnecessary employees. Under strict global budgeting, the government grants long ago squeezed hospitals so that they have long been forced to operate with the fewest number of employees (as in Canada and Sweden) or with low wages (as in Great Britain).

Another crucial cause of the higher U.S. hospital costs is the U.S. method of adopting and financing new buildings and new equipment. U.S. hospitals compete to install them, and the financing system compels payers to cover high capital costs. New technology proliferates despite duplications. All other countries limit expensive installations. I will explain the difference later in this article.

Another cause of the higher U.S. hospital costs is administrative overhead. Every U.S. hospital must maintain a large claims department because there are so many third parties and self-payers, each payer with different rates and allowances. Often the same patient is covered by several payers with different procedures. In contrast, hospital reimbursement in every other country is standardized across payers and is simple. Every U.S. hospital must maintain a large and growing staff to deal with the burden of "managed care," that is, the communication with payers for approval before hospitalization, concurrent review, and retrospective evaluation of necessary service after discharge. Every payer has its own "managed care" procedures, so the hospital must answer different forms with different requirements. In contrast, utilization review in every other country is standardized across payers and is simple. U.S. hospitals must maintain extensive documentation, partly to create a list of patient charges for billing some payers

Table 3

Effects of predominant method of hospital rate control on hospital operating costs, Western Europe and North America[a,b]

System for controlling hospital costs	Percentage of GDP spent on all health care (1987)	Percentage of GDP spent on all hospitals (1987)	Per capita expenditure on all hospitals, U.S. dollars (1987)[c]	Average percentage annual increase in total hospital spending (1980–87)	Average annual increase relative to rise in GDP price deflator (1980–87)
Global budgeting					
United Kingdom					
NHS	6.1	3.0	353	7.2	1.3
Canada	8.6	4.4	754	10.4	1.9
Sweden	9.0	6.3	874	9.3	1.3
Rate regulation					
France	8.6	3.9	500	10.9	1.4
Netherlands	8.5	4.8	592	3.6	1.6
Negotiations					
West Germany	8.2	4.8	422	5.2	1.9
Mixed					
Switzerland	7.7	3.6	736	7.5	2.2
Belgium	7.2	2.4	296	8.1	1.7
United States	11.2	5.3	969	9.9	2.2

[a]Sources: Calculated from Poullier, J. P. Health care expenditure and other data. *Health Care Financing Rev.*, Annu. Suppl., 1989, Tables 1, 3, 61; *OECD Monthly Economic Indicators*, 1987, Table 32.

[b]Gross domestic product (GDP) = GNP + [income in the domestic market accruing to foreigners abroad] − [income accruing to domestic residents arising from investment abroad].

[c]Purchasing power parities against the U.S. dollar (1.00 in 1987) were British pound = 0.60, Canadian dollar = 1.23, Swedish krona = 8.65, German deutsche mark = 2.47, French franc = 7.45, Dutch guilder = 2.41, Belgian franc = 44.7, Swiss franc = 2.42.

and partly to protect staff against lawsuits. In contrast, European and Canadian hospitals rarely bill charges and rarely are sued. U.S. hospitals have legal costs that are small or nonexistent abroad. Cost figures have never been isolated for hospital administration in Europe, Canada, and the United States, but the American visitor can easily see the smaller scale abroad.

Another reason for the higher U.S. hospital costs is the weaker method of cost containment in the United States. Americans boast of their "managed care" methods, but these are unique to each payer, the hospital is invited to shift costs from each payer to others with weaker bargaining power, and the numerous arrangements may increase rather than reduce total costs. Europe and Canada now manage their hospital sectors in order to contain costs, but the U.S. system is unmanaged as a whole. Even when one of the states tries to regulate all hospital rates (as in New Jersey, New York, and Maryland) or when a large U.S. payer tries to negotiate prospective budgets with all hospitals (as in Blue Cross), the methods are implemented more permissively than are rate regulation and rate negotiation in Europe (1, pp. 109–115, 146–157; 6).

Table 4

Employment in health, Western Europe and North America, 1985[a]

System for controlling hospital costs	All health employees per 1,000 population	Hospital personnel, per occupied bed
Global budgeting		
United Kingdom NHS	2.16	2.40
Canada	2.34	2.13
Sweden	3.94	1.85
Rate regulation		
France	2.21	1.37
Netherlands	2.26	1.55
Negotiations		
West Germany	2.31	1.21
Mixed		
Switzerland	2.69	1.67
Belgium	1.70	1.11
United States	2.57	2.75

[a]Source: Calculated from Poullier, J. P. Health care expenditure and other data. *Health Care Financing Rev.*, Annu. Suppl., 1989, Tables 26, 45, 61.

CAPITAL INVESTMENT

Once, in all countries, new buildings and equipment were paid for by the charitable organizations that owned the hospitals. Now in most countries with national health insurance, in all countries with national health services, and in Canada, hospitals depend primarily on grants from government budgets. This method prevents the proliferation of advanced and expensive technical services across the country. The services are concentrated in a few major centers—often the teaching hospitals—with expert staffs and high utilization. If a new method is perfected and becomes an essential part of modern practice, such as diagnostic imaging, it is then allowed to spread throughout the country, still with government grants.

The U.S. method is rare abroad: the medical staff of any hospital presses for the new and expensive program, the hospital borrows money in the bond market to buy the equipment and reconstruct the building, the hospital raises its rates and forces payers to help pay off the debt, and all physicians with admitting privileges are encouraged to utilize (and overutilize) the new service. The scenario demonstrates how competition can increase rather than reduce the costs of the system. If the hospital does not buy the new equipment and improve the building, its physicians will hospitalize their patients elsewhere, the hospital will lose admissions, and it will go bankrupt. Every hospital must install the expensive new program in order to protect its market. The hospital encourages greater use to earn revenue to service the debt; physicians can earn many new and high fees; and greater numbers of patients are drawn in. Services are duplicated (7).

The only limits on the U.S. self-financing system are the prudence of hospital boards, the caution of state and local bond-issuing agencies that help nonprofit hospitals obtain tax-free financing, and the capacity of the bond market. The U.S. system lacks planners and central grantors to channel new programs to places of proven need and high utilization, to prevent wasteful duplication. Besides adding unregulated acquisition and interest costs to health care, the method contributes to the expensive staffing of U.S. hospitals. Every new program adds well-paid technicians and secretaries. Because of the large and nearly uncontrolled domestic market, the U.S. medical equipment industry during the 1980s dominated the world. U.S. firms had between 40 and 65 percent of the world's total shares in medical electronics, surgical equipment, cardiac pacemakers, and many other lines (8). This windfall for the U.S. economy may soon diminish; German, French, and Japanese medical equipment companies have learned to sell in their regulated but large markets and are beginning to win shares of the U.S. market.

A few countries (Holland and Switzerland) once used the method whereby hospitals made their own investment decisions, could borrow without restriction, and amortized debt with higher rates charged to payers. But the method caused cost explosions during the 1970s and now is controlled by facilities planning and by strict regulation of operating budgets.

If a new method becomes a recognized part of medical practice and the physicians wish to use it, countries with national health insurance try to expand installations to keep pace with demand. Once a clinical method is recognized, the insurance laws make it an entitlement of all patients needing it in the judgment of the physicians. In the case of temporary shortages of capacity, the insurance carriers send the patients to neighboring countries, and the waiting lists soon clear. Cost containment methods are intended to make the system efficient without underservicing.

Strict government budget limits in countries with national health services may result in shortages and waiting lists for certain expensive programs, such as open-heart surgery, cancer treatment, neonatal care, and others. Cost containment with exclusively public money can result in temporary underservicing and in priorities for those most needing care. Because the health service is a government program, the mass media, opposition political parties, and interest groups seeking more money (particularly the medical association) denounce the government-of-the-day for mismanaging and underfunding health care. After a political uproar, the Parliament appropriates more money to expand the particular facilities and to reduce the waiting lists. The controversy always revolves around one set of benefits and invariably overlooks the harmony and prompt access in all other health programs.

THE NEED FOR TRUE REFORM

In the United States, reforming hospital finance has been talked about for 20 years. Several devices have been introduced that have shifted rather than solved the problem. The much touted replacement of Medicare's retrospective cost reimbursement by "prospective reimbursement" did not adopt true "prospective reimbursement," since the individual hospital still does not know its allowable costs and revenue in advance. The endless discussion of Medicare reforms conceals the fact that Medicare supplies only part of every hospital's revenue, that most operating reimbursement and capital come from sources unaffected by Medicare reforms. The publicized DRG system still does not make reimbursement understandable and predictable: the payers and state regulatory program groupings that use DRGs employ different groupings, cost weights, and financial values. In order to avoid low DRG prices, hospitals shift much work to outpatient departments with different payment allowances and with greater clinical risks. Cost shifting is more pronounced than ever, exacerbated by "managed care" on behalf of a few payers. New methods of controlling admissions and service intensity increase administrative costs and disputes as market-efficient insurance spreads, coverage diminishes, and hospitals' bad debts increase. As state governments are forced by Washington to add Medicaid benefits for some groups, they conserve their budgets by avoiding other possible beneficiaries. More tinkering will yield only more—not less—trouble.

The experience of all other developed countries demonstrates that a stable and effective hospital sector requires a comprehensive health-financing system. It would go beyond reform of hospital reimbursement alone. The United States cannot remedy the troubles of its hospitals without mending its ways. Universal statutory health insurance would cover the entire population, levying payroll taxes on all employees, on their employers, and on the self-employed, thereby distributing the burden widely and raising enough revenue. Full public financing of the British and Canadian type is unlikely to be enacted by Congress, but health insurance of the European type—preserving the insurance carriers as fiscal intermediaries and limiting government—is more realistic politically (2).

Machinery for making decisions and settling conflicts of interest is fundamental to harmonious reimbursement. A mix of public regulation and payer–hospital negotiation would be necessary to evaluate each hospital's past performance and prospective budget. Human judgment and discussion would replace the U.S. mirage of automatic financial formulas. The decision-making machinery would make the decisions, and the parties would not run to Congress and to the law courts for changes.

Hospitals would be guaranteed their costs to serve the clinical needs of their catchment areas, instead of the present tumult from fears of bankruptcy. Reimbursement rules would be standardized and all-payer units would be adopted, thereby eliminating the present cost-shifting and administrative complexity. Hospitals could concentrate on their clinical missions.

A system of health finance would be created. The system would negotiate a consensus over clinical needs, investment priorities, and expenditure targets. The system would contain costs. The United States would no longer be distracted by constant turmoil in hospital finance.

REFERENCES

1. Glaser, W. A. *Paying the Hospital*. Jossey-Bass, San Francisco, 1987.
2. Glaser, W. A. *Health Insurance in Practice*. Jossey-Bass, San Francisco, 1991.
3. Sidel, V. W., and Sidel, R. *A Healthy State*, Ed. 2. Pantheon Books, New York, 1983.
4. Crichton, A., Hsu, D., and Tsang, S. *Canada's Health Care System*. Canadian Hospital Association, Ottawa, 1990.
5. Glaser, W. A. Juggling multiple payers. *Inquiry* 21: 178–188, 1984.
6. Glaser, W. A. Hospital rate regulation—American and foreign comparisons. *J. Health Polit. Policy Law*. 8: 702–731, 1984.

7. Robinson, J. C., and Luft, H. S. Competition and the cost of hospital care. *JAMA* 257: 3241–3245, 1987.
8. Moreau, J.-G., and Bimont, P. L'industrie du matériel biomédical. *Rev. Fr. Aff. Soc.* 34(4): 191–204, 1980.

Direct reprint requests to:

Dr. William A. Glaser
Graduate School of Management
The New School for Social Research
66 Fifth Avenue
New York, NY 10011

Part X
Health Care Delivery and Social Change

Simon J. Williams, Michael Calnan, Sarah L. Cant and Joanne Coyle

All change in the NHS? Implications of the NHS reforms for primary care prevention

Abstract: The paper provides a review of the implications of the recent NHS reforms – i.e. the *Griffiths Report* (1983), *Promoting Better Health* (1987), *Working for Patients* (1989) and the new GP contract (1990) – for primary care prevention. Three major themes are identified as the *leitmotivs* running through these reforms: first, the introduction of *general management* into the NHS; secondly, the introduction of *market principles* into the NHS, and; thirdly, the increasing emphasis upon *health promotion and disease prevention*. The first section of the paper offers a critical review of the Government's health promotion strategy, one in which, it is argued, the primary care sector will play a central role. Hence, taking the issue of primary care prevention as a case-study, the paper then proceeds to discuss the implications of these recent reforms (i.e. managerialism and market principles) for primary care prevention at a number of different levels: namely, for FHSAs, DHAs, GPs, nurses, and consumers. The final section of the paper considers the potential impact of these reforms for the *professional autonomy* of GPs and nurses, particularly in relation to the proletarianisation and deprofessionalisation theses. The paper concludes with a theoretical discussion and interpretation of the themes and issues raised within the course of the paper.

Introduction

Underlying the recent NHS reforms (e.g. *Working for Patients* and the new GP contract) are certain dominant themes. First, there has been the introduction of general management within the NHS and secondly, the ushering in of market principles. Also detectable is an increasing empha-

Sociology of Health & Illness Vol. 15 No. 1 1993 ISSN 0141–9889

sis upon health promotion and disease prevention within the NHS, a central part of which involves the primary care sector. In short, it is clear that one of the key aims of these recent NHS changes is to usher in a new era of preventive activity, particularly in the primary care sector, within a much more tightly managed, efficient and competitive NHS.

As mentioned above, a central part of this health promotion strategy is focused upon the primary care sector. Hence, taking the theme of primary care prevention as a case-study, this paper attempts to examine and discuss the implications of these recent NHS reforms (i.e. general management and market principles) for the various actors and agencies within the primary care sector. Certainly, the central role which the primary care sector will play in the Government's health promotion drive makes this a topic ripe for consideration and discussion. For example, how will the introduction of general management and market principles affect the various actors and agencies within the primary care sector?; what are their implications for primary care prevention?; and what implications do they have for the professional autonomy of those who work within the primary care sector? These are some of the issues we wish to consider within the course of this paper. However, before doing so, a critical discussion of the recent (re)emergence of health promotion and disease prevention on the political agenda may provide a useful backdrop to the discussion which follows.

Health promotion and disease prevention in the 1990s: a critical appraisal

Published in November 1987, *Promoting Better Health: The Governments Programme for Improving Primary Health Care* signified a major turning point regarding not only the issue of prevention, but also the place and function of primary health care within the NHS. This document contained a number of key proposals for improving primary care and, as the title suggests, placed the issue of prevention firmly back upon the political agenda. As it stated: '. . . the next big challenge for the NHS, and one especially for primary care, is to shift the emphasis from an illness service to a health service offering help to prevent disease and disability.'

The subsequent Government reforms of the NHS have carried this policy forward and reflect a growing recognition of, and commitment to, the importance of health promotion and disease. In particular, the new GP contract, administered by the FHSA, now specifically includes health promotion and disease prevention as part of the GPs terms of service requirements. It also makes provision for the additional remuneration of health promotion clinics, for training in health promotion, and for the employment of a much wider range of ancillary staff who could become involved in health promotion and disease prevention within the primary care sector.

Under the new GP contract a fee is paid for checking the height, weight, blood pressure and urine of newly registered patients. In addition, all patients between the ages of 16 and 74 who have not consulted a doctor within the past three years will be invited for a check-up. Also, reimbursement is provided via the FHSA for the provision of more structured health promotion clinics such as well person, blood pressure, smoking and dietary clinics. While doubts have been expressed about the take up rate of the non-consulters and the benefits of urine testing for the presence of glucose, overall this should increase the number of patients receiving health education and screening.

Clearly the factors underpinning the recent emphasis upon health promotion and disease prevention are complex, difficult to determine, and perhaps even contradictory. However, in addition to pressure from the medical profession, particularly a series of reports published in the early 1980s by the Royal College of General Practitioners (Calnan 1990), the following factors seem important. First, the issue of prevention, at least as it is currently being marketed, may resonate with the wider political and ideological stance of the Government. That is to say, an ideology which emphasises self-reliance and individual responsibility in all walks of life, including health, together with the 'rolling back of the frontiers of the state'. Secondly, the issue of prevention may be perceived politically as a 'vote catcher'. Certainly there is an underlying assumption within the health promotion initiative that the public actually want and value such service provision. In this sense Klein (1989) may be wrong in arguing that there is 'no political constituency' for prevention. Thirdly, given the fact that the major causes of morbidity and mortality within the UK are not only very costly but also, to a large extent, preventable (e.g. lung cancer, CHD, stroke etc.), part of the reason may be economic in nature. In short, prevention, in the long-term at least, may offer one potential means of cost containment within the NHS. This economic argument is perhaps less convincing than the others as some have argued that prevention will not necessarily be less costly in the long-run as people may live longer to be ill more often. Moreover, the benefits and pay-offs of prevention are to be had in the future (Klein 1989) whilst governments have a tendency to think in the shorter-term.

Finally, the emergence of prevention on the political agenda may also reflect and resonate with the previously mentioned themes of the NHS reforms; namely, managerialism and the market place. That is to say, the specification of health promotion activities and disease prevention targets (c.f. the recent Green Paper [1991] and White Paper [1992] on *The Health of the Nation*) may readily fit in with the managerial and market place imperatives of effective and efficient health service provision, the attainment of quantifiable targets and outcome measures, cost-containment and the introduction of performance related pay. Of course, regarding this final point, there lurks the obvious danger of making the various strands of these reforms seem part of some grandiose overall plan which may not, in reality, exist. Rather, the health care policy arena is perhaps more accurately characterised as being one where policy changes are often unconnected and divergent in their implications (Harrison, Hunter and Pollitt 1990). In short, whilst it remains possible that the various strands of the reforms identified within this paper are indeed connected and possess a collective logic, in reality the situation is likely to be quite the reverse (i.e. individualistically formulated policies which are unconnected and possess no overall collective logic).

As mentioned earlier, it is clear that a central plank of current Government policy and thinking concerning health promotion and disease prevention emphasises a move towards the primary health care team; that is to say, a GP-led model primarily based upon screening for individual risk-factors and health and life-style advice, either opportunistically or within the more structured setting of the health promotion clinic. In addition to the above mentioned series of reports published in the early 1980s by the *Royal College of General Practitioners* (Calnan 1991), the origin of this particular focus upon the primary health care sector, according to the policy documents, stems from the unique access which GPs have to the population. Indeed, some 99 per cent of the population are registered with a GP and, on average, consult their doctor four times a year. As *Promoting Better Health* (1987:13) states:

> Through their regular contacts with families and patients, family doctors and other members of the primary health care team such as health visitors, community nurses and practice nurses are well placed to promote good health and to prevent ill-health by giving advice on life-style, by providing screening for certain conditions for example high blood pressure and by improving take-up of vaccination and immunisation.

According to Beattie (1991), such an approach may be described as 'top-down' or prescriptive, whereby professionals attempt to shape and modify individual behaviour through health education and persuasion – what Beattie (1991) terms a 'health persuasion model'. Yet, as a number of commentators have argued, this represents a rather restricted approach towards health promotion and disease prevention; one which emphasises a 'medical model' of screening and detection of 'at-risk' patients as well as the necessity of producing quantifiable results. This may mean having to spend more time on medically rather than socially oriented problems.

Indeed, as Beattie (1991) points out, there are a range of other options which might be considered, some of which focus upon the individual and involve the professional, and others which are targeted at populations or communities. Thus, in contrast to this individualistic emphasis, an alternative 'top-down' model is premised upon a broader, more collective, type of approach – what Beattie (1991) terms 'legislative action' for health. Certainly the emergence of the recent Government Green Paper (1991) and White Paper (1992) on *The Health of the Nation* signifies both an acknowledgement of, and a move towards, this broader based type of approach. Indeed, the emphasis is upon shared responsibility for health promotion and disease prevention across a broad range of government departments and other agencies both inside and outside the NHS. Hence, not only do the NHS and the Department of Health (DoH) have key roles to play, but so too do the Departments of Environment, Energy, Transport, Education, Employment, Trade and Industry, Social Security, the Treasury, Home Office, Ministry of Agriculture Fisheries and Food, the Health and Safety Commission and Executive, together with local authorities, the voluntary sector, employers and employees' organisations etc.

However, as we argued in a recent review article (Williams, Calnan and Cant 1991), whilst the recent Green Paper (1991) – and since the time of that article, the subsequent Government White Paper (1992) – is to be welcomed, representing as it does a significant advance in Government thinking on public health issues, it tends to be rather too long on description and analysis and too short on action. Hence strategic targets for health (e.g. 30 per cent reduction in CHD and stroke mortality below age 65 by the year 2000, and reducing smoking to 22 per cent in males and 21 per cent in females by the year 2000) are stressed at the expense of effective means for achieving them. Moreover, despite this collective orientation, a strong emphasis still remains within the document upon the former model and the role of individual life-styles and behaviour. Finally, the Government's cavalier handling of the persistent and growing inequalities in health which exist in England today, and its side-stepping of the thorny issue of poverty – surely one of *the* major public health challenges of the 1990s – represent major shortcomings of the document. Although the subsequent Government White Paper – which focuses upon five key areas (i.e. heart disease and strokes, cancers, mental illness, sexual health and accidents), and four 'risk factor targets' (i.e. smoking, diet and nutrition, blood pressure and HIV/AIDS) – does represent a step forward in terms of specifying how it proposes to 'make the strategy work', criticism is still likely to centre on its handling of at least two key issues: firstly, the effects on health of social inequalities and poverty, and secondly, tobacco advertising. For example, concerning the latter issue, senior chest and respiratory consultants reacted immediately to what they saw as the Governments 'negative stance' on smoking, claiming that: 'As far as smoking is concerned this is a blank paper not a White Paper' (Guardian, July 9th 1992:6).

In contrast to these two 'top-down' models, an alternative option involves both the professional and client in a more negotiated relationship. In this model individual clients are invited to engage in active reflection and review their lifestyles and the scope for change – what

Beattie (1991) terms a 'personal counselling for health' model. Such an approach draws upon a more 'holistic' model of health, where counsellor and client are in a more symmetrical relationship, although responsibility still rests with the individual. Clearly, if doctors and nurses are to engage in such a counselling role there may need to be a change in the structure of their traditional relationships with patients, and their use of a broader perspective on health.

Finally, another negotiated but collective type of model concerns what Beattie (1991) terms the 'community development' for health approach. This characterises the cluster of interventions in which groups of people band together to take joint action on health related issues.

Beattie's (1990) conceptual grid serves the heuristic purpose of helping highlight the broad range and scope of health promotion and disease prevention options available. Moreover, it also offers the possibility of conceptually locating and clarifying current Government policies within this area. As we have argued, current Government policy tends to focus predominantly upon the first two of these models – i.e. top-down individualistic health persuasion and, more recently, a new emphasis in the Green and White Papers upon a more collective approach which, not only stresses the key role of the NHS, but also the necessity of shared responsibility and legislative action for health. Of course, the extent to which the proposals and targets contained in this document represent merely a rhetorical manoeuvre by the Government, or instead become transformed into concrete action across a number of agencies and tangible health gains for the population as a whole, remains to be seen; only time will tell.

Clearly, there is scope for the Government to take a more interventionist role aimed at social as well as individual change. Indeed, there is a strong argument for developing a more coherent national policy at a number of different levels. Thus, a combination of regulations, fiscal policies and education may provide the necessary environment for effective action. For example, a coherent smoking control policy might involve a package measure including large increases in the price of cigarettes, legislative controls over tobacco advertising, as well as education campaigns. Some of these have, of course, been suggested by the Labour Party in their recent health promotion document *The Better Way to a Healthy Britain* (1991), although any coherent policy should also recognise the costs as well as the benefits of different policy options and attempt to find solutions for dealing with these problems (e.g. the social costs of inducing guilt and anxiety amongst those groups whose circumstances are such that a change in smoking habits is very difficult). Similarly, there is a need to develop a far more coherent policy for food and health, one which involves influencing production as well as consumption. Again there are a range of policy options such as the increased education of providers, professionals and consumers; replacements for hazardous foods; differential pricing systems for healthy and harmful foods; provision of healthy foods in institutions run by the government and local authorities, and regulations to encourage the production of leaner meats (Williams, Calnan and Cant 1991; Calnan 1991). Once again, some of these options have been adopted in the Labour Party document. However, there needs to be a rigorous evaluation of these food health policy options as has been carried out in the areas of smoking and alcohol control (Maynard and Tether 1989; Godfrey and Robinson 1990).

Having offered a critical review, drawing upon the social science literature, of the current health promotion initiative – an initiative in which, as we have argued, the primary care sector plays a major role – it is to a more detailed consideration of the implications of what we have identified as the other two major themes of the recent NHS reforms (i.e. general management and market principles) for the various actors and agencies engaged in primary care prevention that the paper now turns.

Managerialism

The bold step of introducing general management principles into the NHS dates back to the Griffiths Report of 1983. As Strong and Robinson (1990) note, mere administration was to be abolished and in its place came managerialism. Essentially, Griffiths defined general management as: '. . . the responsibility, drawn together in one person, at different levels of the organisation, for planning, implementation and control of performance' (1983:11). According to Griffiths, a managerial approach involved the planning of policy and the setting of targets, managing and facilitating the implementation of policy and monitoring performance. The objective was to attain a much more informed and determined approach towards budgetary controls, and within the NHS, this meant a stricter control over both professional and manual labour costs and performance (Cox 1990).

The subsequent proposals contained in the 1989 White Paper *Working for Patients* built upon the implementation of the Griffiths Reforms, and further shifted the 'frontier of control' clearly and explicitly in favour of managers (Hunter 1991). Yet, as Burns (1981 cited in Hunter 1991) suggests, there exists a fundamental tension between, on the one hand, the *collaborative system* which characterises the organisation of health services and, on the other hand, *managerialism*, which stresses formal accountability and monitoring. According to Burns managerialism is founded upon *distrust*, whilst, in contrast, collaboration is founded upon *trust*. It is in this sense that Burns expresses concern that the imposition of managerialism upon what is fundamentally a collaborative health care system, may well prove destructive.

In considering the primary care sector, perhaps one of the major changes has been the fact that GPs, who historically have been relatively free from state intervention, are now managerially accountable to an entirely 'new beast'; namely, the Family Health Services Authority (FHSAs), who are the successors, of those former 'managerial eunuchs' (Klein 1987), the old FPCs. Indeed, it is in relation to the FHSA, GP and (community) nursing interface that this managerialism within the primary care sector will have its greatest impact.

It was *Promoting Better Health: The Government's Programme for Improving Primary Health Care* (1987), which conferred upon Family Practitioner Committees (FPCs, now FHSAs) an 'extended' and 'strengthened' managerial and planning role. Central objectives for the FPCs and the Family Health Services (FHS) contained within this document were to be as follows:

1 Making services more responsive to the identified needs of consumers.
2 Giving consumers the widest possible choice in obtaining high quality primary health care services.
3 Raising standards of care.
4 Promoting health and preventing illness.
5 Improving value for money.
6 Enabling clearer priorities to be set for FHS in relation to the rest of the NHS.

The subsequent reforms specified within *Working for Patients* (1989) extended the new managerial role of FHSAs envisaged in *Promoting Better Health* (1987) and the new GP contract. In all this it is clear that, as the recent report *FHSAs: Today's and Tomorrow's Priorities* (1991) states, 1990 was possibly one of the most challenging times in the history of the family health services. Key changes have included the introduction of general management into the FHS; the reconstitution of the Authority; the implementation of the new GP contract; the integration of general practice within the wider NHS framework; the transfer of accountability from the Department of Health to Regional Health Authorities; and the challenge to the existing medicine/management interface within the FHS.

In all these respects, collaboration with DHAs will be crucial. Obstacles and barriers to effective collaboration in the past have included some of the following: difficulties understanding each other's roles and responsibilities – FPCs having traditionally been regarded merely as administrative 'pay and rations' bodies; the differing salary, administrative and staffing structures within DHAs and FPCs; the lack of staff and resources with which to fulfil their new roles and the need to restructure and retrain; and, finally, a lack of co-terminosity between DHAs and FPCs – one third of FPCs having to work with three or more DHAs (Allsop and May 1986).

Certainly the transformation from 'Committee' to 'Authority' status is more than just a semantic exercise. FHSAs should now perceive themselves as independent authorities in their own right just like DHAs and RHAs, and should act and be treated accordingly as equal partners. Moreover, the fact that FHSAs are now accountable to Regions and through them to the Management Executive, lays the foundations both for greater organisational integration and for the development of a more corporate approach to the planning of primary health care services.

Indeed, concerning the issue of collaboration, there are at least four possible models or scenarios concerning the place and function of health promotion services within the new NHS structures. In the first model, the health promotion/education unit becomes a part of the Department of Public Health Medicine and assumes largely a purchasing function. In the second model, health promotion may become a provider unit contracted to by DHAs and other agencies such as the FHSA for health promotion advice and services. The third model is one of multiple health promotion provider units servicing different organisations – one for the DHA, one for the FHSA, one for Local Authority etc. Finally, the most futuristic model, is one of health promotion units and community units moving across to FHSA/Primary Health Care Authorities (PHCAs). This latter model would certainly represent a significant further enhancement of the FHSAs managerial role, particularly with respect to health promotion. Certainly it is clear that the logic of the NHS reforms are pushing towards the eventual merger of DHAs and FHSAs as single purchasing authorities within the internal market *vis-a-vis* the GP fund-holders. In the short-term, however, it is likely that health promotion activity will continue to be split or spread across both DHAs and FHSAs, and that DHAs with a strong public health function and health promotion strategy will be loathe to relinquish this to the FHSAs.

However, irrespective of which one of these models finally prevails – and this is likely to be quite variable across the country – the managerial tasks now facing FHSAs with respect to health promotion within the primary care sector include the following:

1 Implementing and monitoring the new GP contract.
2 Managing the ancillary staff scheme: including the targeting of the cash-limited ancillary staff budget; the need to collaborate with DHAs over the employment and deployment of community nursing services.
3 The development of practice premises: clearly the bedrock of the health promotion initiative within the primary care sector is founded upon adequate practice premises, especially as primary health care teams expand.
4 Providing advice, support and encouragement to primary health care teams in developing their health promotion services and activities (e.g. via the appointment of health promotion facilitators, interfacing DHA and FHSA health promotion support services etc.).

52 Simon J. Williams Michael Calnan, Sarah L. Cant and Joanne Coyle

5 Collaborating with DHAs and other agencies over the training of primary health care teams in health promotion and disease prevention techniques.
6 Approving, setting standards and monitoring the quality of health promotion clinics and activities (e.g. drawing up ideal clinic guidelines and/or risk assessment protocols etc.).
7 Needs assessment and information technology: including the collection of epidemiological data with which to plan services; collaborating and sharing information with DHAs; helping GPs in the production of their annual reports and using this data for planning purposes; conducting consumer satisfaction surveys; and, finally, encouraging and supporting the development of information technology with general practice.
8 Supporting family practitioners in developing high quality 'consumer responsive services' tailored to local need and establish 'consumer feed-back groups' who input into the planning process.

Whilst DHA health promotion responsibilities include:

1 Collecting, interpreting and analysing information regarding the health and needs of their resident population.
2 Agreeing priorities for targeting effective health service interventions.
3 Working with the local community to 'promote and maintain health'.
4 Collaboration with other agencies over the development of joint health promotion strategies and policies – including FHSAs on primary care and local authorities regarding wider public health issues.
5 Making specific recommendations for the achievement of health outcome objectives.

Of course, for GPs the main thrust of new managerialism has come through their relationship with the FHSAs. In short, GPs, for the first time in their history, have become managerially accountable to the new FHSAs. Certainly, it is a good example of the introduction of the Griffiths managerial principles into primary care although the actual managerial role of the FHSAs is still unclear. However, in addition to their increased administrative role, there appear to be at least two other main areas in which this new managerialism will have an impact upon GPs and the primary health care team.

First, a major element of the managerial revolution within primary care concerns the role of the new GP fund-holders. GP fund-holders will receive their budgets directly from the RHA and will be able to contract for services within the new internal market on behalf of their practice populations – unconstrained by the placing of DHA contracts. This may also include a broad range of health promotion staff and services (e.g. health promotion staff and services, dieticians, cardiologists, psychologists etc.). It seems likely that services such a health promotion and disease prevention will prove to be particularly lucrative and attractive options for these GP fund-holders to provide, whilst services for the chronically sick and disabled – who will represent a drain on the fund-holders budgets – will prove to be less so. Moreover, the increased management role involved in becoming a fund-holding general practice may detract from the quality of the doctor-patient relationship. However, the increased scope of general practitioners to fund activities which they choose may lead to better quality preventive care with adequate support at least in some practice. In this respect, activities such as blood pressure testing should be facilitated by the abolition of restrictions on the range and numbers of staff that may attract reimbursement. Thus, general practitioners may in future be able to employ the greater numbers of staff and the greater variety of staff, for instance a dietician, that a properly supported programme will require. Yet as Sacks and Marsden (1989) point out, the employment of such staff may not be as financially lucrative (i.e. profitable) as it first appears. Consequently, Sacks and Marsden (1989) call for 100 per cent reimbursement of such staff.

The second key issue concerns the GPs new managerial role in relation to other members of the primary health care team. The new GP contract positively encourages the development of the practice nurse with the shift to clinic based remuneration and flexibility in the reimbursement of other types of ancillary staff. Consequently the increase in GP employed nursing staff has been exponential. In 1983 there were 3284 practice nurses employed in England and it was estimated that this number had increased to 17000 by 1990, with the spurt in growth occurring in 1989 (Healthcare Parliamentary Monitor Statistics).

The managerial future and role of community nurses (i.e. health visitors, district nurses etc.) is, at present, uncertain. Indeed, *Nursing in the Community* (1990) clearly sets out the various managerial and organisational options for community nursing. Five models were discussed – although no particular one was recommended. Briefly, these were as follows:

1 The 'Stand Alone' community trust or DMU model, where the community unit would manage all community health services and offer them to a variety of purchasers.
2 The locality management/neighbourhood nursing model (recommended in the Cumberlege Report 1986), in which mixed teams of community staff would be managed in geographical patches or around consortia of GP practices or health centres under the overall control of the community unit (trust or DMU).
3 An expanded FHSA model, in which the FHSA would assume responsibility for the provision of community services.
4 A vertical integration or outreach model, which could take a variety

of forms. For example, a combined acute/community unit which purchasing authorities could contract with for the provision of 'complete packages of care'.

5 The Primary Health Care Team (PHCT) – GP managed model, in which community services would be brought under the control and management of general practice.

Clearly community nurses are both well placed and well equipped to provide a comprehensive range of health promotion and disease prevention services within the local community (i.e. via health visitors, district nurses etc.). However, their future hangs in the balance at present, essentially due to the non-prescriptive nature of the report and the competition with practice nurses which has been strengthened with the implementation of the new GP contract. Whilst Cumberlege called for the phasing out of subsidies for practice nurses, *Promoting Better Health* and the subsequent health care reforms, although recognising the role of community nurses, have tended to favour the development of practice nurses as the way forward in terms of health promotion. In short, although community nurses health promotion role is recognised, the assumption is that GPs will be the leaders. That is to say, health promotion will become GP-centric, which is contrary to WHO directives which emphasise the crucial role of nurses.

The community nurses do not have a specified role, and even practice nurses seemingly have a secondary role *vis-a-vis* fully fledged *nurse practitioner* status. This is not new: throughout history nursing interests have been subordinated to others within the health policy arena. This tells us something about nursing which cannot be separated from a wider understanding of health policy issues and the competing interests which jostle for power within this arena. In short, nursing interests are consistently subordinated to the interests of other dominant and powerful interest groups (i.e. medical profession, general management) within health care arena. This may be the end-product of a number of factors, for example; the under-developed professional status of the nurse compared to that of other groups; and the powerlessness and absence of practical organisation of the nursing profession which often sees itself 'outside politics and political power struggles' (Clay 1987:1):

> Nursing is perhaps the most unassertive profession in the UK, yet more than ever, we need collectively to look beyond immediate problems and pre-occupations to see the forces that are active around us and tackle them.

This non-participation can further be explained by reference to the gender division in nursing, as Salvage (1985:7) notes: 'Like other women workers, nurses have low pay, low status and lack political muscle', and as Clay (1987:2) additionally points out: 'Many have children and other family commitments with all the social and cultural obstacles to active participation in political life this brings'.

A number of consequences flow from the GP based managerial model. First, the degree of autonomy the GP allows, and secondly, whether these developments replace the PHCT by a practice team (Marks 1988) with all staff directly employed by the GP. DHA based community nurses are extremely sceptical about coming under GP management or indeed any clinical management, hence the rejection by the HVA of the 'GP' and 'outreach' models. The fear is loss of autonomy and fragmentation. As Bowling (1987:631) argues, the growth of the PN: 'has angered members of the wider nursing profession who believe it is not in the professional interests of nursing to be employed by a member of another profession'. Clearly there will be a need to collaborate between the various employers, but as Robinson (1990:133) argues: '. . . agreement on the sharing of services between the GP and CN managers may prove difficult when services provided by the HA produce payments for the GP'. Furthermore, CN managers may prevent or restrict the role development of attached CNs, hence it may be easier for PNs rather than the CNs to expand and develop their role in the primary care sector.

Certainly, if the GP has to purchase HV or DN services, this may prove expensive. Hence the PN, in economic terms at least, may be a more attractive option. The DHA nurses are clearly in a difficult position and thus may prefer the 'if you can't beat 'em join 'em' mentality'. As a HV recently wrote to the HVA:

> I now view myself as a health promotion specialist having changed in March from a HV post to dare I say it . . . practice nursing. I changed for many reasons, family, health, cutbacks, limitations and sheer frustration. . . . In my new job I am actively promoting health education amongst the population. . . . I still view myself as HV first, PN second. I urge members to be adaptable and promote their role for the future (Evans 1991:28).

Furthermore, this shift towards a GP-based managerial model in which the PN plays a key role may have implications for standards of care. For example, are PNs adequately trained for such health promotion activities? HVs and DNs would argue that health promotion is built into their training programme, whereas the PN course which runs for 10 days is not compulsory. The facilitator programme may be successful in attending to PN training needs, but we have to ask whether the HV and DN training would be more appropriate in terms of a health promotion and disease prevention role. However, GPs may wish to employ more qualified PNs (e.g. HV and DN) irrespective of cost, so that more services such as sports injury clinics or home visits, may be provided and so put the practice in a stronger position for attracting patients (North and Porter 1991).

However a key question remains to be addressed concerning this managerial shift: is it effective to organise health promotion services in this way? In other words, will the work community nurses do in the home, particularly picking up the families that do not attend the surgery, and their wider role within the local community, be lost (Wrench and Irvine 1984)? Will the primary role of prevention be lost in favour of secondary screening procedures within the surgery?

Having discussed some of the implications of managerialism for primary health care prevention, it is to a consideration of the second major theme identified in the recent NHS reforms, namely, the introduction of market principles and their implications for primary health care prevention, that the paper now turns.

The introduction of 'market principles'

The key issues here concern the introduction of the 'internal market', the 'purchaser-provider' distinction within the NHS and the financial incentives contained within the new GP contract. Relationships will, from now on, be contractual in nature between, on the one hand, the 'purchasers' of health care (DHAs, FHSAs, GP fund-holders) and, on the other, the 'providers' of these services (e.g. Directly Managed Units (DMUs), Trusts and the private sector). In future, provider units (e.g. acute, community, priority care, health promotion units etc.) will have to compete with one another in the medical market-place for the service contracts of these commissioning authorities. Consequently, so the Government argues, 'money will follow the patient', and as a result – although again this is a source of considerable debate – 'consumer sovereignty' and 'choice' will be enhanced together with the quality, effectiveness, efficiency and value for money of the NHS. Of course, whilst money will indeed, to a large extent, 'follow the patient' with regard to the new GP fund-holding initiative and in respect of 'extra contractual referrals', for those who remain non-fund holding GPs, money will not actually follow but will, in effect, *precede* the patient via the DHA contracting process. This will constrain their choice of referral within the internal health care market.

Clearly the adoption of management principles and practices within the NHS – principles derived from the industrial private sector – represents a further attempt to introduce market principles into the health care system, particularly with respect to contracting for services mentioned above and the emphasis upon control of costs and value for money. However, there are more central elements in the trading relationship in the economic market place which have been introduced into the health service by the new GP contract and the White Paper proposals *Working for Patients*. First, there is the emphasis on consumer choice and sovereignty, and secondly, there is an emphasis on competition and profitability.

The emphasis upon 'consumer choice' and 'sovereignty' shows a shift in perspective away from the traditional collectivist participation model where the needs of patients as a whole are represented via agencies such as Community Health Councils (CHCs), towards a more individualistic model in which services are organised according to consumer demands (Strong and Robinson 1990). Hence the emphasis in this latter model is placed upon the informed and enterprising consumer who is free to shop around in the health care market in pursuit of the best buy. Within this market-based, 'consumer-led' model, patients are to be provided with more information concerning the range of service provision, whilst the procedures for changing GPs have become much easier. Moreover, FHSAs have now been charged with the responsibility of conducting regular consumer satisfaction surveys in order to gauge public opinion of local service provision.

More specifically, in relation to the provision of preventive services, clearly the changes may enable patients, if they wish, to choose GPs who offer a wide range of preventive services, although the actual motivation, extent and ability of patients to 'shop around' for health care appears to be fairly limited, particularly for the elderly, the chronically sick and the disabled. However, studies of patient satisfaction with general practice (Williams and Calnan 1991), have shown that the key determinants of consumer satisfaction relate to the nature and quality of the doctor-patient relationship. Indeed, doubts have been raised about whether the new changes will actually lead to an improvement in the nature and quality of the doctor-patient relationship.

Whilst health education is a crucial part of prevention, the current social organisation of the doctor/nurse/patient relationship tends to be a major obstacle to effective health education. For example, Tuckett *et al* (1985) in their study of how general practitioners and patients communicated, showed the majority of consultations were one sided and doctors did little to encourage patients to present their views and there was little discussion of the consequences of a patient's illness. However, if general practitioners and nurses are to become more effective educators they need to adopt a more patient-centred approach, show greater versatility and flexibility in their professional role, and move away from a specialist and towards a more diffuse role. The doctor and nurse would need to adopt the role of counsellor, giving the patient the reassuring advice and support in order for them to 'help themselves'. The emphasis would be on the general practitioner to shift towards the practice of a more holistic or socially oriented type of medicine.

Yet will the recent government proposals encourage such a shift? The answer to this, at least according to some commentators, is 'No'. For example, as Bartholomew (1989) states: 'The emphasis on quantifiable behaviour in the White Paper proposals could shift general practitioners from the practice of holistic or socially oriented medicine towards more medically oriented behaviour'.

There is also the question of the role of the nurse and to what extent community nursing becomes involved in prevention. In this respect, a major issue seems to be whether the practice nurse will perform an instrumental role acting as a complement, probably a subordinate, to the general practitioner or if they will act as a substitute to the doctor becoming more fully involved in health education and counselling as a *nurse practitioner*. From the patient or consumer point of view, nurses may be more accessible than doctors although little is known about the nature of the relationship between practice nurse and patient and whether it is conducive to effective health education. Early evidence from field trials (Coronary Prevention Group 1990) shows that smoking cessation advice by nurses is not very effective, at least, compared with general practitioners. Recent evidence (Coronary Prevention Group 1990) also shows that primary health care teams involved in health examinations have a very limited understanding of nutritional principles and doubts have been raised, therefore, about the value of dietary education from these sources.

However, other evidence suggests the contrary, namely that the nurse is indeed well-placed and acceptable to the patient (Anggard *et al* 1986; Bowling 1988; Fowler *et al* 1988). For example, they have been shown not to be a cheap substitute for the GP but a valuable resource (Fallon *et al* 1988) and are effective in their health promotion activities (Bowling 1981, 1985; Bowling and Farquhar 1989; Bowling and Stilwell 1988; Kenkre *et al* 1985; Robson *et al* 1989; March and Clew 1984). Considering that GPs probably do not wish to be involved and that the GPs contract may reduce the number of female doctors, the role of the nurse could provide a skilled and welcomed contact for the patient.

In short, it is unclear at present whether the increasing involvement of practice nurses in health promotion and disease prevention represents a progressive or retrograde step in the minds of consumers. Similar issues surround the concern that the number of women GPs looks set to decline after the introduction of the new contract. The Medical Womens Federation has already voiced concern that the new working arrangements have resulted in at least 20 women leaving partnerships and discouraged many women from entering general practice. Thus, whilst women, as nurses, may be more likely to be involved in health promotion in the future, the number of women GPs may decline. This has obvious implications concerning consumers' gender preferences, and whether nurses are seen as adequate substitutes for GPs. Moreover, as Tuckett *et al* (1985) found in their study of doctor-patient interaction, women were twice as likely as men to find themselves in consultations in which their expressed theories and views were disregarded by their GPs.

The emphasis upon competition is well illustrated in relation to the new GP contract which aims to increase the reliance of a doctor's income on capitation and fee for service payment. It is an attempt to improve the range and quality of services available by making doctors pay more 'performance related' (i.e. financial rewards for achieving immunisation and vaccination targets etc.). Thus, the emphasis on capitation is intended to reward the competitive GP who increases or maintains his or her market share as indicated by patient list size. It is in this sense that GPs will increasingly find themselves competing with one another within the internal market for patients.

Similarly in the White Paper, *Working for Patients*, GP fund-holders will be encouraged to compete for patients and to bargain with hospitals and other provider units, thereby creating competition between these providers of health care for GP contracts. In addition, GPs will be rewarded for maximising their profits in budgeting by ploughing savings back into the 'business'. On the other hand, profiteering and malpractice will be controlled by medical audit and by various forms of administrative and political control. In short, the effect of the introduction of market principles within primary care will be that GPs will be competing with each other, whilst, once the 'steady state' expires, GP fund-holders as purchasers will increasingly have to compete with DHAs – who in merging will remain the most powerful commissioners within the internal market – in order to obtain the best possible deal for their patients. Indeed, the power of GP fund-holders within the internal market in the first year of the NHS reforms seems likely to dramatically decline as the 'gloves come off' in the subsequent years and the market is played to the full by the DHAs.

Yet, whilst the emphasis upon health promotion and disease prevention within the NHS reforms is to be welcomed, what impact will the introduction of such market principles have on the quantity and quality of preventive care provided within primary care?

One of the implications of the new contract is that while preventive services may be more widely available (i.e. *quantity* of service provision will increase) there are doubts about the *quality* of the services provided. In this respect, much will depend on the role of the audit committees and the level of support and direction given by the FHSAs. The payment of a sessional fee for health promotion and disease prevention clinics may well lead to an increase in the number or quantity of clinics provided at the expense of quality. For example, as Forbes (1988) points out in commenting on the experience of fee for service systems in Western Europe: 'The popularity of fee for service, however, has been tempered by the side effects of this payment system. The most frequent criticism is that doctors have a clear incentive to increase the quantity of the service irrespective of any improvement in the service quality'. Also, as Robinson *et al* (1989) point out, health screening and health promotion aimed at the affluent worried well might become more attractive to general practitioners because of their revenue earning potential at the expense of less money-spinning services such as long term care for the chronic sick. This criticism applies both to the new contract and 1989 White Paper with its proposals for general practitioners to become budget holders. In addition, there is the possibility of a shift in the balance of preventive care away from routine opportunistic screening in the consultation – where those most in need of such services are reached – towards clinic based preventive activities where the financial rewards are more lucrative. In this sense the current emphasis upon the clinics industry may be another classic example of the inverse care law in operation. Moreover, the problem for GPs of achieving immunisation and vaccination targets in inner city areas, together with the difficulty of recruiting patients within such areas to health promotion clinics etc., may well act as a disincentive for inner city GPs and consequently exacerbate inequalities in service provision nationally.

Moreover the competitive ethos of the new contract, in which GPs may seek to maintain or increase their market share of patients, may lead to a diminution in consultation length, which may have a detrimental effect upon effective health education and counselling. For example as Morrell (1989) points out:

> Overall, the contract is imbued with the belief that 'good care', as it defines it, will attract more patients to the doctors providing this care, and the doctors will consequently receive greater financial rewards through a system of payment based largely on capitation. It ignores perhaps the most crucial aspect of primary care, which is concerned with the time doctors can devote to listening to and identifying their patients' problems and to provide counselling, advice, health education, and appropriate management.

This argument appears to be supported by the evidence (Calnan and Butler 1988) in that as the number of hours worked in the practice and outside the practice increases, the length of consultation decreases. Hence, the time available particularly to carry out health education in the consultation will diminish along with the quality of care. In short, the evidence suggests that the shift in the system of professional reimbursement for general practitioners away from a mix of capitation and salary (allowance) towards a mix of capitation and fee for service may lead to an increase in the provision of a range of preventive services but will also lead to a reduction in quality.

Clearly, all these changes have implications for consumer sovereignty, but what exactly are the implications of general management and market principles for the professional sovereignty of those within the primary care sector? It is to this particular issue that the paper now turns.

Implications for professional autonomy

In the United States some commentators (Haug 1973; Starr 1982; McKinlay and Arches 1985; Light and Levine 1988) have suggested that medical professional autonomy is under threat through: (i) the impact of managerialism and bureaucraticisation limiting the extent to which doctors have control over the terms, conditions and content of their work (i.e. the 'proletarianisation thesis'), and; (ii) deprofessionalisation where the 'enlightened consumer' is more knowledgeable and critical of doctors' activities (i.e. the 'deprofessionalisation thesis', see Elston [1990] for a review of these two theses). Will these processes be encouraged within the primary care sector as a result of the recent introduction of managerialism and market principles?

Certainly, in terms of the proletarianisation thesis, the recent NHS reforms might mean a reduction in autonomy for GPs in that they are now accountable to FHSAs, although of course, much will depend on the managerial stance taken by FHSAs in the future. As we have seen, FPCs have, in the past been seen merely as administrative bodies with a 'pay and rations' function. However, all this is now supposed to be changing. As June Huntingdon states in a recent *Health Services Journal* article: '*The front line between medicine and management in the family practitioner services has changed* and will continue to do so as FHSA general managers take tough decisions on resource allocation.' GPs have generally enjoyed a high degree of professional autonomy. The developments of 1990 began to establish the FHS as a managed public service. As *FHSAs . . . Today's and Tomorrow's Priorities* states: '*Existing boundaries between the clinical and the managerial have been tested and have begun to move.* The process will continue in 1991 and beyond' (1991:8).

Moreover, as Huntingdon (1990) also notes, many GPs with the 'sole trader' mentality will resist such activities, having entered general practice precisely because of the benefits it offered them in terms of independence and autonomy. New, much more detailed and specific contractual requirements, accountability, monitoring, and resource allocation according to managerially set policies and targets for primary care are alien notions indeed for GPs to have to grapple with in the post NHS reforms. Certainly there is empirical evidence to suggest that, since the introduction of the new GP contract, GP job satisfaction has declined (Calnan and Corney 1991).

Also, the information and resources that FHSA general managers will have will 'radically change the balance of power between them and GPs' (Huntington 1990:325). However, the experience of the implementation of the Griffiths recommendations suggests that influencing practitioners behaviour is easier said than done. From an economic point of view in some ways the changes have given the GP more freedom to negotiate their incomes. On the other hand they are more vulnerable to market forces and do not have the cushion of a salaried income which in part came from the allowance component of the pre-contract financial arrangements.

What of clinical autonomy? Certainly, the introduction of indicative drug budgets, the implementation of medical audit, and the increasing involvement of other professions within the primary care sector may mean that GPs will have to struggle to keep control over clinical decisions. On the other hand, the historically dominant position of the medical profession within the health care division of labour (Freidson 1970), coupled with the increasing role of GPs in the management and control of resources, may mean that they are actually more able to control the division of labour and to delegate unwanted tasks and duties to practice nurses and other members of the primary care team. Certainly, preliminary indications seem to suggest that this is happening with respect to health promotion and disease prevention tasks and duties.

This raises the question of whether nurses will be able to extend their role and if so, will this represent a challenge to GP autonomy? Certainly, the opportunities in health promotion seem to offer that possibility. The 'Fullard model' may promote role extension for the PN. As Cater and Hawthorne (1988) in their study of PN suggest:

> Nurses who work solely in practices have become involved in a wider range of duties and responsibilities than the DN. PNs listed preventative services more frequently in the description of their work than did the HA employed nurses . . . Health promotion and screening are developing areas in general practice and this appears to be the area in which PNs are developing their role.

Does this mean that GP employment is conducive to the development of nurses' professional status and autonomy? Bowling (1981:64) suggests that GP professional sovereignty may be an obstacle:

> . . . the challenge for the future appears to be how to develop an expanded role for the nurses in general practice while minimising role conflict and overlap with doctors and without conflicting with the professional interests of either group.

Thus the development of this potentially valuable role will depend on the collective demands of community nurses and supportive GP attitudes. However, it seems that the latter is still limited; the *Georgian Research Society* (1991) showed that whilst GPs wanted nurses to extend their role they did not see autonomy as a pre-requisite for this development.

Finally, what of the GPs autonomy from the patients themselves (i.e. the 'deprofessionalisation theses')? Once again it appears that the situation, at least at present, remains unclear. As the deprofessionalisation theorists argue, an increasingly 'well-informed' lay populace, and the rapid expansion of alternative medicine, may represent a challenge to the cultural authority of medicine and its monopoly over health-related knowledge (Haugh 1973; Elston 1990). Certainly, regarding the recent NHS reforms, the increased emphasis upon consumer choice and sensitivity to 'customer' needs (via consumer satisfaction surveys), together with the increased proportion of GP income derived from capitation, may mean that GPs in the future have to pay far greater heed to the concerns and wishes of their patients. Consequently, the distance between patient and doctor may be reduced. On the other hand, however, the increased managerial and administrative role of the GP, together with the constraint of time and the delegation of many (health promotion) tasks and duties to other members of the primary care team, may actually mean an increased distance between doctor and patient. Moreover, despite the recent changes, particularly those which allegedly make it easier for patients to change their GP, it seems that the extent to which patients will actually 'shop around' for health care remains fairly limited. Furthermore, as a recent study found:

> Patients tended not to think of themselves as consumers who should be wary of the quality of services offered by doctors. Rather, they preferred to trust their doctor, and therefore did not devote effort to actively seeking out information about their doctor or evaluating his or her services (Lupton *et al* 1991:559).

In short, it is far too early to judge whether the recent reforms will put the professional sovereignty of GPs at risk. Certainly, the emphasis on consumer sovereignty, managerialism and the development of primary health care teams might encourage the processes of 'deprofessionalisation' and 'proletarianisation' outlined above. However, in the latter case, if the new GP fund-holding initiative takes off, it will of course be the doctors themselves who become the managers. Indeed, this may be one strategy by which GPs slip the Gordian knot of FHSA managerial control.

Conclusion

This paper has been concerned with addressing the implications of the recent NHS reforms for primary care prevention. Yet, at a theoretical level, what exactly do these reforms mean? How are we to interpret and understand them theoretically, and what theoretical framework best explains them? It is to a consideration of these issues that the paper now turns in closing.

In his discussion of health care politics, Alford (1975) distinguishes three sets of structural interests: *dominant* (professional monopolists), *challenging* (corporate rationalisers) and *repressed* (community population). In essense, Alford argues that the medical profession represents the dominant interest group in the health service, but that they may be challenged by corporate rationalisers such as health care planners and administrators. Similarly, patient and consumer groups may also attempt to move from their repressed position in order to articulate and pursue their common interests and goals.

64 Simon J. Williams Michael Calnan, Sarah L. Cant and Joanne Coyle

Neo-Marxists are also interested in elites but, in contrast, their interest lies in relating elite groups and the welfare state to the class structure and the capitalist mode of production. From this perspective, the NHS helps maintain a healthy workforce and legitimates capitalism. Neo-Marxists also see an imminent 'crisis of the welfare state' in which demands for more resources are constrained by the imperatives of the capitalist accumulation process. In short, so the neo-Marxists argue, capitalism cannot survive with or without the welfare state (Offe 1984).

A combination of these two theoretical perspectives (i.e. the structural interests theory of Alford [1975] and neo-Marxist theories of the welfare state), suggests that the recent NHS reforms (i.e. the introduction of general management, internal markets, efficiency savings, performance indicators, disease prevention etc.) may perhaps most fruitfully be viewed as an attempt by the 'corporate rationalisers' to respond to public and professional concern about the under-funding of the NHS by the promise of greater output without significantly greater input (Harrison, Hunter and Pollitt 1990). In Alford's (1975) terms, this represents a significant challenge by the 'corporate rationalisers' to the 'dominant interests' of the medical profession; particularly through an ideological strategy which advocates the hitherto repressed interests of the 'consumer'. Furthermore, this theoretical perspective helps explain much of the medical profession's largely negative reaction and opposition to the recent NHS reforms. Harrison *et al* (1990:161) reach similar conclusions in their analysis of the '*dynamics of British health policy*'. As they state:

> Thus, we reach the conclusion that neo-Marxist theory can be used to account for the shift from ideological corporatism to competition amongst structural interests in the period 1981 to 1984. In other words, economic factors have ultimately produced a modification in the structure of elites: a growing managerial challenge to the dominance of the consultants, which is likely in its turn to bring about a weakening of the latter.

In conclusion, it is clear that the 'frontiers of control', the political philosophy and economic principles underpinning the NHS, and the boundaries of prevention are, at present, in a state of considerable flux, transition and uncertainty. If a theatrical metaphor may be used for a moment, the stage has been set and the script, in the shape of the NHS reforms, has been written. What remains to be seen is how the ensuing drama unfolds as the relevant actors play their parts and interpret their roles.

Centre for Health Service Studies,
University of Kent at Canterbury

Acknowledgements

We are grateful to the two anonymous reviewers for their helpful and constructive comments on an earlier draft of this paper.

References

Alford, R. (1975) *Health Care Politics*. Chicago: University of Chicago Press.

Allsop, J. and May, A. (1986) *The Emperor's New Clothes: Family Practitioner Committees in the 1980s*. London: King's Fund.

Anggard, E.E. *et al* (1986) Prevention and cardiovascular disease in general practice. A proposed model. *British Medical J.*, 293, 177.

Bartholomew, J. (1989) *Working for patients*. Unpublished M.Sc. dissertation, University of London.

Beattie, A. (1991) Knowledge and control in health promotion: a test case for social policy and social theory. In Gabe J., Calnan M., and Bury M. (eds) *The Sociology of the Health Service*. London: Routledge.

Bowling, A. (1981) *Delegation in General Practice*. London: Tavistock.

Bowling, A. and Stilwell, B. (1988) (eds.) *The Nurse in Family Practice*. London: Scutari Press.

Bowling, A. (1985) DHA Policy and the extended role of the nurse in primary health care. *J. Advanced Nursing*, 10, 443-54.

Bowling, A. (1987) Practice nurses and nurse practitioners. *The Practitioner*, 231, 631–3.

Burns, T. (1981) *Rediscovering Organisation: Aspects of Collaboration and Managerialism in Hospital Organisation*. Edinburgh: Unpublished paper.

Calnan, M. (1991) *Preventing Coronary Heart Disease: Prospects, Politics and Policies*. London: Routledge.

Calnan, M., and Corney, R. (1991) *Changes in Job Satisfaction amongst General Practitioners*. Centre for Health Services Studies, University of Kent: Unpublished paper.

Calnan, M. and Butler, J. (1988) The economy of time in general practice. *Social Science and Medicine*, 20, 465–71.

Cater, L. and Hawthorne, P. (1988) A survey of practice nurses in the UK in their extended roles. In Bowling, A. and Stilwell, B. (eds.) *The Nurse in General Practice*. London: Scutari Press.

Clay, T. (1987) *Nurses: Power and Politics*. London: Heinemann Nursing.

Coronary Prevention Group (1990) *Coronary Heart Disease Prevention in Primary Care: Making it Happen*. Report of a Conference. London: Wordworks.

Department of Health and Social Security (1976) *Prevention and Health: Everybody's Business*. London: HMSO.

Department of Health and Social Security (1983) *NHS Management Inquiry (Griffiths Report)*. London: DHSS.

Department of Health and Social Security (1984) *Report of the Joint Working Group on Collaboration Between FPCs and DHAs*. London: DHSS.

Department of Health (1990) *General Practice in the NHS: A New Contract*. London: HMSO.

Department of Health (1990) *Health Care Parliamentary Monitor*. London: HMSO.

66 Simon J. Williams Michael Calnan, Sarah L. Cant and Joanne Coyle

Elston, M.A. (1991) The politics of professional power: medicine in a changing health service. In: Gabe, J., Calnan, M. and Bury, M. (eds.) *The Sociology of the Health Service*. London: Routledge.

Evans, A. (1991) From health visitor to practice nurse. *Health Visitor*, 64, p. 28.

Fallon, C.W., Bhopal, J.S., Gilmour, W.H. and Bhopal, R.S. (1988) The work of the Family Practice Nurse: An audit of an Inner City Practice. *Health Bulletin*, 46, 179–81.

Forbes, J.F. (1988) Public policy and primary care in the UK. *Family Practice*, 5, 237–41.

Fowler, C. *et al* (1988) The extended role of the practice nurse in preventative healthcare. In Bowling, A. and Stilwell, B. (eds.) *The Nurse in Family Practice*. London: Scutari Press.

Fullard, E., Fowler, G. and Gray, M. (1984) Facilitating prevention in primary care. *British Medical J.*, 289, 1585–87.

Gabe, J., Calnan, M. and Bury, M. (1990) *The Sociology of the Health Service*. London: Routledge.

Georgian Research Society (1991) The attitude of GPs towards nurses: a pilot study. *British J. General Practitioners*, 41, 19–22.

Gerhardt, U. (1989) *Ideas About Illness*. London: Macmillan.

Godfrey, C. and Robinson, D. (1990) *Manipulating Consumption: Information, Law and Voluntary Controls*. Aldershot: Avebury.

Griffiths, J. (1990) 'A new GP contract for health promotion?, *Primary Health Care Management*, 1, 8–10.

Ham, C. (1985) *Health Policy in Britain*, (2nd Edition). London: Macmillan.

Haug, M. (1973) Deprofessionalization: an alternative hypothesis for the future, *Sociological Review Monograph*, 20, 195–211.

Health Education Authority (1990) *Implications for Health Promotion/Disease Prevention*. London: HEA.

Health Education Authority (1990) *Health Promotion and Implementation of the NHS White Paper*. London: HEA.

Harrison, S. (1988) *Managing the National Health Service: Shifting the Frontier?* London: Croom Helm.

Harrison, S., Hunter, D. and Pollitt, C. (1990) *The Dynamics of British Health Policy*. London: Unwin Hyman.

Hunter, D.J. (1991) Managing medicine: a response to the crisis, *Social Science and Medicine*, 32, 441–8.

Huntington, J. (1990) Change at the grass roots, *Health Services J.*, 324–5.

Huntington, J. (1990) Getting down to business, *Health Services J.*, 1359.

Kenkre, J. *et al* (1985) Nurse management of hypertension clinics in general practice assisted by a computer, *Family Practice*, 2, 17–22.

Klein, R. (1989) *The Politics of the NHS (2nd Edition)*. Longman: Harlow.

Labour Party (1991) *The Better Way to a Healthy Britain*. London.

Light, D. and Levine, S. (1988) The changing character of the medical profession, *Milbank Q.*, 66, 10–32.

Lupton, D., Donaldson, C. and Lloyd, P. (1991) Caveat emptor or blissful ignorance: patients and the consumerist ethos, *Social Science and Medicine*, 33, 559-68.

McKinlay, J. and Arches, J. (1985) Towards the proletarianization of physicians, *International J. Health Services*, 15, 161–95.

March, C.N. and Chew, C. (1984) Well man clinics in general practice. *British Medical J.*, 288.

Marks, L. (1988) *Promoting Better Health. An analysis of the government's programme for primary health care*. London: King's Fund.

Maynard, A. and Tether, P. (1989) (eds.) *The Addiction Market: Consumption, Production and Policy Development*. Aldershot: Avebury.

Morrell, D.C. (1989) The new general practitioner contract in the Health Review – what it means. *British Medical J.*, 23.

National Health Service Management Executive (1991a) *The Role of FHSAs – Today's and Tomorrow's Priorities*. London: NHSME.

National Health Service Management Executive (1991b) *Integrating Primary and Secondary Health Care*. London: NHSME.

North, N. and Porter, E. (1991) All change ahead, *Nursing Times*, 87, 57–60.

North West Thames RHA (1990) *Nursing in the Community (Roy Report)*.

Offe, C. (1984) *Contradictions of the Welfare State* (edited and translated by J. Keane). London: Hutchinson.

Robinson, G. (1990) The future of practice nurses, *British Medical J.*, 132–3.

Robinson, J. *et al* (1989) Using nurses for preventative activities with computer assisted follow-up. A randomised control trial, *British Medical J.*, 298, 433–6.

Robinson, R. (1989) New healthcare market in the NHS Review – what it means, *British Medical J.*, 298, 437-9.

Sacks, G. and Marsden, R. (1989) Evaluation of a practice-based programme of health checks: financial cost and success at risk detection. *J. Royal College of General Practitioners*, 39, 369–72.

Savage, J. (1985) *The Politics of Nursing*. London: Heinemann Nursing.

Secretaries of State for Social Services, Wales, Northern Ireland and Scotland (1987) *Promoting Better Health: The Governments Programme for Improving Primary Care*. London: HMSO (Cmnd 249).

Secretaries of State for Social Services, Wales, Northern Ireland and Scotland (1989). *Working for Patients*. London: HMSO (Cmnd 555).

Secretary of State for Health (1991) *The Health of the Nation: A Consultative Document for Health in England*. London: HMSO (Cmnd 1523).

Secretary of State for Health (1992) *The Health of the Nation: A Strategy for Health in England*. London: HMSO (Cmnd 1986).

Starr, P. (1982) *The Social Transformation of American Medicine*. New York: Basic Books.

Strong, P. and Robinson, J. (1990) *The NHS Under New Management*. Milton Keynes: Open University Press.

Tuckett, D., Boulton, M., Olson, C. and Williams, A. (1985) *Meetings Between Experts*. London: Tavistock.

Williams, S. (1986) Case studies in collaboration, *Family Practitioner Services J.*, 13, 39–43.

Williams, S.J. and Calnan, M. (1991) Key determinants of consumer satisfaction with general practice, *Family Practice*, 8, 237–42.

Williams, S.J., Calnan, M. and Cant, S. (1991) Health promotion and disease prevention in the 1990s, *Medical Sociology News*, 6, 20–9.

Wrench, J.G. and Irvine, R.C. (1984) Coronary heart disease: an account of a preventive clinic in general practice, *J. Royal College of General Practitioners*, 34, 477–81.

[36]

The Reorganization of the Medical Profession

Eliot Freidson, Ph.D. *

It requires no special perception to see that health care is going through massive changes in the United States. Before World War II it was largely a cottage industry composed of self-employed physicians working primarily in their own offices and sometimes sending their patients to hospitals where nurses and members of a few other health care occupations cared for the patients according to the doctors' orders. It was, furthermore, financed largely by charitable contributions and by the patients themselves. And while it did require machines and other tools of the trade that even then were too expensive for individual physicians to own themselves and use in their offices—making physicians somewhat dependent on hospitals for access to capital equipment as well as beds and paramedical services—health care technology was not sufficiently developed to support a large manufacturing industry. Finally, in those days the role of government was essentially passive, protecting the institutions of health care by licensing, tax, and other laws, but remaining otherwise uninvolved.

Much has changed since then, and change has accelerated since the passage of Medicare legislation. Most physicians still work in their own offices, but they have become less able to deal with their patients' ailments without the aid of services and goods that are outside their own control. Health care occupations have multiplied in large numbers and

*Professor, Department of Sociology, Faculty of Arts and Science, New York University.

form an ever more complex division of labor. More than anything else the hospital has changed, with consequences for all producers and consumers of health care. Hospitals no longer exist merely for the convenience of "attendings", and they have developed a complex administrative structure to coordinate the division of labor. Furthermore, after the federal government began financing health care, they had to develop elaborate medical record systems and complex accounting schemes. The massive expansion of health care technology, with its train of consequences for capital costs, new specialized occupations, and even new legal and ethical problems, has added to the complexities of hospital administration.

What do these changes mean? Do they have a distinct direction and are they likely to continue in that same direction indefinitely? What are their consequences for the consumers of health care? And what are the consequences for the producers? All of these questions cannot be answered in a single, short article, but surely we can gain some insight into answers by focusing on the medical profession. In the past, physicians were clearly the key producers of health care. Thus, if we focus our attention on them and on the way the changes of the past decades have affected them, we may be able to gain an especially strategic view of what has been happening. Indeed, most prophecies of the future shape of health care have emphasized changes in the role of the medical profession.

MAJOR THEORIES

In this paper, I shall review several major theories concerning the position of physicians in the health care system and their future status. I shall argue that those theories are flawed, taking too little into account to be useful guides for our understanding and distorting our view of what is happening. I shall then discuss some important but often overlooked changes in the medical profession and go on to suggest my own way of making sense of the changing position of physicians. Finally, I shall discuss some of the implications of that theory.

Professional Dominance

A useful way to grapple with the various theories that predict radical changes in the status of the medical profession within the health care system is to contrast them with the position, asserted not long ago, that the medical profession dominates the system. My phrase "professional dominance" (Freidson 1970a) was later taken up by Illich (1980) and others. However, "professional dominance" is merely a phrase and thus masks a number of different facets of the profession's position in the health care system. My usage was drawn from ecology rather than from politics, and it referred primarily to the relation of the medical profession to most other health care occupations in the division of labor. Other occupations existed under medicine's shelter, and while these occupations gained their protection from outsiders, they had to exist only on what medicine allowed them and had to give up the capacity to be independent and grow large and strong. In such ecological usage, the primary emphasis was on the legal subordination of nurses, pharmacists, inhalation therapists, and others to medical orders, sustained by the licensing system. The medical profession was portrayed as dominant in a division of labor in which other occupations were obliged to work under the supervision of physicians and take orders from them. With its exclusive license to practice medicine, prescribe controlled drugs, admit patients to hospitals, and perform other critical gatekeeping functions, the medical profession is portrayed as having a monopoly over the provision of health services, a monopoly that Berlant (1975) has emphasized at some length.

Other writers, however, have gone well beyond those limited economic and occupational aspects of the health care system in characterizing the position of the medical profession. The most sweeping characterization of the professional dominance of physicians is certainly that of Illich (1976), though Foucault and his followers (for example, Arney 1982) imply even more. Illich asserts that the medical profession creates the needs that lead people to seek their services, that it in effect influences consciousness itself so that people think of their problems as medical in character and as requiring the aid of health professionals. This power is much more than what Starr (1982) calls the "cultural authority" of medicine: it might more appropriately be called ideological or cultural hegemony, a pervasive form of intellectual dominance that controls the way people think. A somewhat less sweeping but related characterization of such hegemony is found in work by McKinlay (1973), Zola (1972), and especially Conrad and Schneider (1980) on "medicalization".

Deprofessionalization and Consumer Dominance

In contrast to those characterizing the medical profession as dominant in the health care system—on the one hand controlling access to critical aspects of health care, including the use of a variety of other occupations in the division of labor and protected by an economic monopoly, and on the other asserting control over the way people think about themselves and their problems—there are others who believe that the medical profession is in decline (for historical views, see Starr 1978 and Burnham 1982). One theory is that medicine is losing its professional status. The theory of deprofessionalization is most closely associated with the work of Haug (1973, 1975, 1977), who spoke about professions in general, even though one might guess from the substance of her analysis that she had medicine in mind more than, say, law or accounting. Betz and O'Connell (1983) advance a similar, though less complex, analysis of medicine in particular (see also Toren 1975).

The major emphasis of the theory of deprofessionalization is on the relations between professionals and consumers. Professional status presupposes that consumers have some special trust in professionals that they do not have in mere specialists. In the case of the latter, consumers actively question, even challenge those offering specialized services: they do not accept them on mere faith. Trust or faith, however, seems to depend in part on the general prestige of an occupation. It also depends in part on the degree to which the occupation has a genuine monopoly over a particular body of knowledge and skill, that is, the degree to which consumers feel they do not know enough to be able to judge the specialized service themselves and to make their own choices. According to the deprofessionalization theory, consumers' unquestioning trust diminishes as the "knowledge gap" between the medical profession and the consumer diminishes. Today's consumer is better educated and thus likely to know more about medicine, which closes the knowledge gap. Furthermore, the computerization of knowledge has made it more accessible to all, and new specialized occupations have arisen around bodies of knowledge and skills that physicians themselves are not competent to employ.

All these trends lead to the deprofessionalization of medicine—the reduction of physicians to mere secular specialists, dependent on rational, well-informed consumers who approach their services with the same questioning attitude they bring to other commodities in the marketplace. According to this theory, consumers, not physicians, will dominate health care in the future, and medicine will become just another health occupation.

Proletarianization and Managerial Dominance

Finally, there is the theory of the proletarianization of the profession, drawn from Marxism. One of the basic tenets of Marxism is the assumption that eventually all participants in the capitalist economy will be drawn into one of two opposing classes: those possessing capital or serving as the agents of capital, the bourgeoisie, and those who perform the basic productive labor of the economy but who are exploited for the cause of profit and the accumulation of capital, the working class. Marxist theorists differ in their view of the place of the professions in the present class system, some seeing them to be allied with capital and others seeing them in "contradictory class locations". Still others, however, see them as eventually joining the working class, or proletariat, losing control of their work, and becoming subject to the exploitative discipline of the managers who serve the ultimate interests of the capitalist class (Oppenheimer 1973; Larson 1980). In the case of the American medical profession in particular, McKinlay is the most recent proponent (1982), with Coburn, Torrance, and Kaufert (1983) doing much the same for the medical profession in Canada.

It is a bit difficult to be entirely clear about the application of the theory of proletarianization to the medical profession, because proletarianization itself remains unarticulated as a concept and because there is so much equivocation (McKinlay 1982, 37–38) about the degree to which the process has already occurred and the pace of change itself. Those who employ the theory, however, seem to emphasize above all the overriding importance of two changes in the position of the medical profession that have already begun.

First, they point out that more and more physicians are salaried rather than self-employed. Thus, they are losing their economic independence and assuming the wage-labor status of the proletariat. Second, more and more they practice in bureaucratically organized institutions, their work thereby becoming subject to the control of management. A similar change in status is suggested by Starr's notion of medicine's loss of "professional sovereignty", though he does not draw on Marxist theory or terminology.

THE EVIDENCE FOR THE THEORIES

Described in such a compact fashion, it is easy to see that the theories do not really address each other, that is, they do not look at the same evidence and interpret it differently so much as they look at different evidence and assert that it is the key to understanding the changing position of the medical profession. In some cases, the evidence itself is too weak to rely on as support for the theory. In other cases, the evidence is ambiguous enough to be amenable to more than one reasonable interpretation. And most important of all, a great many analytically important conditions affecting the position of the medical profession in the health care system are completely overlooked. Let us turn to examining the evidence that is relevant to assessing the theories.

The theory of professional dominance emphasizes two quite different kinds of phenomena—cultural or ideological on the one hand, and economic and legal on the other. It can be argued plausibly that they are interdependent: that the special, privileged, and authoritative position of the medical profession could not be obtained in the first place and maintained subsequently unless the profession had some "cultural authority", unless its orientation to health and illness and its knowledge and skill were widely respected. Thus, some degree of respect and trust is essential to gaining a legally supported economic monopoly from the state. However, the degree of respect and trust must be great, compared to what other occupations receive, if that monopoly places other health care occupations in a subordinate position.

Respect and trust are one thing, and cultural hegemony another. The capacity to control how people think of themselves and their problems is a far more profound form of dominance than the capacity to be dominant in a division of labor. The concept of hegemony is such that it is difficult to specify (or even imagine) the evidence one would need in order to demonstrate its presence and document its operation. Should it be asserted that one manifestation of such hegemony lies in the way that human problems are "medicalized", that is, interpreted as medical problems or diseases, the evidence available shows that there is no consistency of source—that lay groups are as prone to medicalize their problems and urge a reluctant medical profession to take jurisdiction over them as the medical profession is eager to do so on its own. This is true in part because of the social, political, and economic structure surrounding the ideology: in the nineteenth century one gained at least social and political benefits by being considered "sick" rather than "bad", and in the modern welfare state one stands a chance of getting economic benefits as well.

On balance, I do not believe that the thesis of cultural hegemony in its full-blown form can be settled by anything other than faith, which I lack. It is an idea to play with rather than a concept to address systematically and use analytically. Occupational dominance and monopoly are much easier to deal with empirically. It is clear that medicine remains the key occupation in health care: it is dominant in the health care system's division of labor, and its position is sustained by an elaborate tissue of licensing laws and quasi-legal systems of institutional licensing and accreditation of health programs. "The AMA cooperates . . . in the accreditation of over 3000 educational programs, at more than 1700 institutions, for the 26 allied health professions it recognizes" (Havighurst and King 1983, 149).

This is not to say that all in the health care system are under the doctor's orders, for dentists, optometrists, podiatrists, chiropractors, and others have operated independently of medicine in the past while others have emerged more recently. But in every case those who are licensed to practice independently of medicine in health-related matters practice in a carefully delimited sphere of activity, whether surgical, pharmacological, or technological. (For an examination of the positions of physicians' assistants and nurse practitioners, see Kissam 1975.) While the medical profession has never been completely successful in preventing independent practice in areas that border on or even compete with it, it remains successful in limiting it and preserving its own strong monopoly. There is no evidence of a trend toward weakening that monopoly, though there is a literature that urges action to do so. It would be a mistake to regard such literature as evidence of actual change instead of desire for change.

That statement contradicts the implication, if not the actual assertion, of the theory of deprofessionalization, that medicine has become or is clearly on the road to becoming just one of a multitude of health-related occupations, without a special position among them. It rests on the objective evidence of licensing laws and accreditation practices and the continued failure of efforts to change them significantly. For example, various states have passed "sunset laws", which automatically terminate "a board, commission or agency unless reauthorized or reestablished by the legislature" (Roederer and Palmer 1981, 2). In many instances, licensing boards were prime targets of sunset laws, the hope being that new licensing legislation would be written to reform the system. But as Lippincott and Begun (1982, 477) conclude, sunset laws have been a "dismal failure" in changing the situation. Thus, we find little evidence that the medical profession's legally sustained position in practice and in the division of labor is being changed so significantly as to become just one of a number of health care occupations.

If that is so, then we should expect the profession to have some position of respect and trust in the public's eye. The deprofessionalization theory asserts that there has been a loss of such a position, and indeed some evidence of a decline does exist (Betz and O'Connell 1983). If that decline really does exist, why have there not been greater changes in the medical monopoly? The answer is that the decline is only relative and has not been of sufficient magnitude to sustain any serious attacks on the profession's monopoly.

A recent comprehensive review of surveys of public "confidence" in American institutions, has shown that all major American institutions, not just medicine, have suffered a decline in public confidence over the past decades. Medicine, however, has remained the institution in which the *greatest* amount of confidence exists (Lipset and Schneider 1983). Furthermore, the public continues to be overwhelmingly "satisfied" with the quality of the medical care it receives from doctors (Health Insurance Association of America 1982, 14). None of those findings supports the idea that there has been a decline in trust of such magnitude as to support deprofessionalization processes.

Other evidence to sustain the deprofessionalization thesis is equally weak. The notion that the population has become on the average better educated than in the past is true enough, but the assumption that this reduces the "knowledge gap" between medicine and the health consumer is valid only if medical knowledge and technique have stagnated and not increased. Like science and technology, however, medical advances have been increasing exponentially, far faster than the rate of increase in lay knowledge. If anything, one should expect the "knowledge gap" to increase rather than decrease, with the computerization of new knowledge having little to do with the capacity of lay people to use or understand it. Indeed, Langwell and Moore (1982, 12) review findings that consumers exercise direct choice over less than half of the health services they consume and that only in the use of routine pediatric and obstetrical care are consumers well informed.

In all, the deprofessionalization theory makes far too much of the potential of the consumer movement. It is conceivable that consumers can keep up with medical advances, but only if they, too, specialize. This in fact is what has occurred. Various health consumer groups specialize in particular issues such as childbirth and women's health care, particular chronic illnesses or disabilities, and the like. Such groups are small, composed primarily of educated, middle-class women, and often their members are transient. The consumer movement in any case has no broad grass-roots base in the population. It is less a function of organized activities on the part of numerous consumers than it is of organized political actions by "program professionals" (McCarthy and Zald 1973; Walker 1983) who lead public interest groups. Without deprecating the value and importance of the consumer movement, one should not exaggerate its capacity to change drastically the position of the medical profession in the health care system.

It seems, then, that the evidence that the medical profession is losing its position of relative public trust, its relative supremacy in the occupational division of health labor, and its command over truly esoteric knowledge and skill is quite poor and unpersuasive. Change has indeed been taking place in each of those areas, but it has been of insufficient magnitude to have had critical effects and of insufficient duration to sustain the idea of a steady, unilinear trend into the future. As yet, we must take those characteristics of relative public trust, exclusive command over a body of specialized knowledge and skill, and dominance in the division of labor as givens and ask how other changes qualify or limit them. This is what the proletarianization thesis, if true, can answer.

The theory of proletarianization points out that there is a distinct trend toward physicians' being salaried rather than self-employed, a trend that may accelerate over the coming decade (Friedman 1983). However, an important proportion of salaried physicians is not actually in practice, instead serving as administrators, researchers, teachers, and the like, and another proportion collated in labor statistics is salaried only in the technical sense of being employees of their own professional corporations. Thus, the magnitude of this trend is certainly exaggerated in official statistics. However, there is no doubt the trend exists, even though it remains to be seen whether it will continue indefinitely until all physicians become salaried workers.

The question is what the trend means. Certainly it cannot mean loss of professional status as such, for the majority of all professions has always been employed rather than self-employed. It does mean loss of what Marxists call petit bourgeois status—a purportedly anachronistic survival of early or precapitalist times—but that is not synonymous with professional status. The assumption of the proponents of the proletarianization thesis seems to be, however, that loss of self-employed status means loss of control over the economic terms and conditions of work, which is one characteristic of the working class's relationship to capital. But in fact employment status does not, in and of itself, mean loss of economic independence. If one's position in the labor market is strong, one can specify the terms and conditions of one's employment, granting little power to the employer. Similarly, if one's position as a self-employed entrepreneur in the marketplace is weak, one is at the mercy of the consumer's terms and conditions, a position of vulnerability that the history of medicine has often documented for self-employed physicians in bad times. The mere status of being employed or self-employed tells us much too little to be analytically useful. Even if the trend toward employed status continues, it does not, in itself, imply anything of importance about the changing status of physicians. The nature of their monopoly, the supply of competitors, and the available economic resources are much more important.

The other major element cited in the theory of proletarianization is the nature of the organizations in which physicians, employed or self-employed, work. They are called bureaucracies and their operation characterized by Max Weber's ideal type of rational-legal administration. These are organizations governed by an elaborate set of written rules, keeping meticulous records, differentiated into specialized positions or offices, each with carefully defined responsibilities and organized into a pyramidal hierarchy with ranks of officials and supervisors whose function is to coordinate and control the work of those below them. Work is fragmented into small, highly specialized tasks, and discretion is minimized. In the case of medicine, it is the hospital that is invoked as such an organization, though it is noted that there is also a trend for clinics, some Health Maintenance Organizations, and other forms of potentially large-scale practice to replace individual office practice and extend bureaucratization into the community outside the hospital. The consequence of this bureaucratization is said to be the loss of professional autonomy, reducing the physician to a mere cog in a machine.

In all, there can be no doubt that there is a trend toward larger and more complex hospitals and practice organizations and toward the greater rationalization of all services, medical and otherwise. Both governmental and private pressures to reduce costs—or to prevent further rises in cost—serve as the motor for such rationalization, as do governmental regulations themselves. The basic issue is the degree to which rationalization is instituted and the form that rationalization takes, not the mere fact of rationalization. Does Weber's model actually describe that form or does it serve a special, nondescriptive function? Giddens notes that Marxist writers "characteristically accept too much of what Weber has to say about the nature and consequences of bureaucratization . . . while declaring bureaucratic domination to be a specific outcome of the class system of capitalism" (1982, 200), and he goes on to deny that individual autonomy is impossible in bureaucracy, that organizations in fact conform to the ideal type and operate accordingly, and that the worker is powerless (202–5). Indeed, even economists, who have had a notorious appetite for ideal types or abstract models, have discovered that hospitals are hardly fully rationalized organizations (Harris 1977; Pauly and Redisch 1973).

Current organizational theorists have suggested that open-system and loosely coupled system models that fit organizations such as schools and hospitals would also suit hospitals far better than Weber's ideal type. This is not to deny the value of the ideal type, but rather to caution against forgetting that it *is* an ideal type and assuming instead that it describes empirical reality.

At the foundation of the concept of proletarianization is the notion of completely alienated workers, without control over their economic circumstances, without any important voice in the policies of the organizations that employ them, subject to close and oppressive supervision, and unable to exercise significant choice in the work they do and the way they do it—in short, the stereotype of the industrial blue-collar worker. Without reference to those concrete conditions to provide focus for the collection of evidence, proletarianization is not a concept so much as a slogan. What we must ask, then, is how closely the position of physicians conforms to those characteristics in large practice organizations in general and in the hospital in particular.

Looking at the evidence on the place of the medical profession in the hospital, we must note that in the United States, trends toward employment notwithstanding, most fully qualified physicians are not employees but "attendings". They are dependent on the hospital for the care of some of their patients and the performance of some of their work, but the hospital is also dependent on them to provide patients. It is only the physician who has the right to admit patients to the hospital and to choose and take responsibility for their modes of treatment, so it is no accident that new, for-profit hospitals actively court physicians who serve a well-insured clientele to join their staffs. Furthermore, the standards of the Joint Commission on Accreditation of Hospitals, which are generally relied on by both state and federal authorities, require that the medical staff of hospitals, unlike the nursing staff or any other occupation in the hospital, be *directly* responsible to the governing board rather than to the chief executive officer (Christoffel 1982, 108–10; somewhat dated but still relevant is Southwick and Siedel 1978).

In American labor law, professional employees, among whom are employed physicians, are assigned a special craft status and marked off from ordinary employees by the special characteristic of having the legitimate right to exercise discretion on an everyday basis in the conduct of their work. Thus, physicians are in a fairly strong economic bargaining position in the hospital because they have a monopoly over the right to admit, determine treatment, and discharge patients, and it is assumed that they exercise discretion in the course of their work. Furthermore, they have direct access to the policymaking governing board, and there is in fact at present a distinct trend toward more and more hospital governing boards' including medical staff among their members (Noie, Shortell, and Morrisey 1983).

Save for the matter of supervision and control, which I shall discuss in more detail shortly, I think it can be said without fear of contradiction that the present position of physicians in hospitals and other organizations in which they work is in no reasonable way analogous to that of the blue-collar or white-collar worker in factory or firm. Most are not even employed by them, and whether employed or not they have a special, policy-relevant relationship with the governing board. They have a large amount of control over the tasks they undertake and the way they perform them. It is true that they are not wholly autonomous, but when one takes into account the operation of the invisible hand of the market in constraining the self-employed, putatively "free" professional, they never were. Neither the facts of employment nor of working in large, complex organizations constitute in and of themselves sufficiently persuasive evidence to support the use of the concept of proletarianization to characterize the position of physicians in a truly analytic fashion.

PROFESSION—AGGREGATE OR ORGANIZATION?

On the whole, I think it fair to say that all the theories I have discussed are too grand and sweeping to have much more than rhetorical and possibly political value. They are casual about providing the evidence to support their validity, and as often as not when they do provide evidence it is of dubious relevance to the analytic implications of their concepts. I suggest that at bottom their flaws stem from an inadequate conception of what a profession is in the United States, particularly the medical profession. They tend to conceptualize the profession implicitly as an aggregate of individual practitioners and not as an organized social entity. Thus, dominance is defined by the relations between individual physicians and other health care workers, or by the doctor-patient relationship; deprofessionalization by the relationship between doctors and demanding consumers; and proletarianization by the relationship between doctors and employers and managers.

While the profession is indeed composed of individuals doing their daily work with others, it is also corporate in character. The profession is organized by formal associations whose officers negotiate licensing laws, accreditation standards, and the like that establish the framework within which its individual members work. Furthermore, some important segments of the profession are not engaged in everyday practice. And finally, the profession is stratified: elite members of the profession perform special roles in professional associations and institutions and engage in critical negotiations with legislators and government officials in shaping laws and administrative procedures as well as with the governing boards of hospitals and other institutions. Other elites, as we shall see, establish, advance, and communicate the body of knowledge and skill claimed by the profession.

Thus, to conceive of the profession as a mere aggregate is to be insensitive to critical forms of functional and hierarchical differentiation within the profession and the institutions that are responsible for insulating practitioners from some of the changes that are taking place and reorganizing their relationships with each other in adaptation to other external changes. It is that organized character of the profession and the connection of its organization to state policymaking and institutional chartering that pose a major barrier to actual deprofessionalization or proletarianization. Potentially critical pressures have been cushioned by adaptive changes in the organization of the interrelations among members of the profession, changes intended to satisfy the demands of consumers, politicians, and third-party payers without sacrificing overall professional control.

CHANGES IN THE NORMS AND PRACTICE OF PROFESSIONAL CONTROL

The significance of two changes in the formal and informal rules governing economic and professional relations within the profession have not been adequately recognized. First, while competition between other occupations and the medical profession has remained seriously limited, open and public competition among practitioners *within* the profession is now possible through advertising. Previously discouraged as "unethical", advertising became possible when a Federal Trade Commission order of 1979 barred the American Medical Association from exercising formal bans against advertising. Its order was upheld on appeal by the U.S. Court of Appeals for the Second Circuit in New York and affirmed by the Supreme Court in 1982. An effort to pass federal legislation to exclude the medical profession from the jurisdiction of the Federal Trade Commission and the Sherman Antitrust Act also failed in 1983. While antitrust action to increase competition between physicians and other health practitioners seems of limited potential in spite of Dolan's (1980) enthusiasm, the increase of overt competition within the profession itself is of some importance, breaking as it does a tradition that has helped sustain the cohesion of the medical profession during its twentieth century prime.

Competition in health care has received a great deal of attention over the past ten years, during which the ideology of classical economics has been revived and reasserted as the key to solving the fiscal crisis of health care in the United States, so I need not address it in any detail here. (For a review of research on competition, see Langwell and Moore 1982.) Advertising is one form of such competition. What is more, it *publicizes* competition. Advertising is a public claim of superiority that, explicitly or implicitly, denigrates competitors. Furthermore, it appeals to the lay criteria of potential patients rather than to professional criteria. Public statements denigrating competitors were not uncommon among physicians before the twentieth century: in earlier days it was not unheard of for one physician to deprecate the diagnosis and treatment recommended by another. Nor was it uncommon to advertise that one did *not* employ unpopular cures such as bleeding or dosing with cathartics.

Open, public competition for patients inevitably means strained collegial relations. Advertising lower prices than another physician implies that the other physician charges too much. Advertising elaborate credentials such as board certification in a specialty, for example, maligns the competence of physicians without them, even though specialty boards disclaim any intent to make invidious distinctions. (See Havighurst and King 1983, 141 and Stevens 1971, 43 for a discussion of the way specialization was considered to be invidious and divisive, an issue still exercising the legal profession in the United States.) While competition for desirable patients always goes on among both employed and self-employed physicians serving the same population, with some being considerably more successful than others, professional norms that control advertising minimize invidious comparisons, prevent open warfare, and preserve a modicum of harmony and decorum within the profession.

It is too early to tell just how far the use of advertising will go in health care. Given constraints on "misleading" advertising that did not exist in earlier times, extensive advertising campaigns are far more likely to be useful to relatively large and specialized health care organizations than to individual physicians. If that should be the case, individual members of the profession will not be in public competition with each other and their relations will not become especially strained. Eliminating some of the restrictions on advertising is therefore primarily of symbolic importance, representing the collapse of one of the traditional devices the profession has used to preserve its nominal solidarity. Of far more immediate importance to the solidarity of the profession is the second of the two changes—the collapse of the norms governing the way colleagues evaluate and control each other.

An important tradition bearing on the cohesion of the profession is the norm of suspending overt, public judgment about the competence, conscientiousness, and ethicality of colleagues even though privately one may feel they have made serious errors or have been negligent (Freidson 1970b, 1980; Bosk 1979). A related norm discourages taking any action to control the behavior of errant colleagues. These norms have been displayed in a variety of situations in the past. In the courts, when malpractice suits were brought against physicians, it has often been noted that it was difficult to find physicians who would testify as experts against their colleagues. This "conspiracy of silence" has been attacked and seriously weakened over the past 20 years, and it is far more common now for physicians to testify against each other.

A related phenomenon is to be found in the activities of local and state medical association disciplinary committees and state licensing boards. In the past, they were notorious for their reluctance to pursue complaints against physicians (Derbyshire 1969). Publicity and political pressure have forced them to be considerably more active in investigating, judging, and censuring the conduct of colleagues. Indeed, in some states "informer laws" have been passed that require physicians to report gross negligence on the part of colleagues to disciplinary boards on pain of being accused of "unprofessional conduct", a charge that can lead to the suspension or loss of the license to practice.

Finally, and most importantly, we may note the implication of the establishment of a series of formal review procedures, some required by federal legislation and administrative law and some strongly encouraged by large private health insurers. For some time all hospitals accredited by the Joint Commission on Accreditation of Hospitals have been required to have committees that review aspects of the care provided by the medical staff, but neither the way committee reviews were conducted nor the substance of their findings were subjected to very close or critical scrutiny, and accreditation requirements left great leeway in their modes of operation. Indeed, it was their inadequacy in discovering and dealing with errant colleagues that led to the publicity that sparked "informer laws", as well as to other review requirements imposed by the state.

Medical research was the first target of federally mandated institutional committees that required formal review of the protection of the welfare and rights of "human subjects" (Barber et al. 1973; Gray 1975). In the late sixties, the first federal effort to control increasing costs required hospitals to establish formal utilization review committees to assess the propriety of the decisions of physicians to hospitalize their patients, followed later by legislation requiring the more elaborate Professional Standards Review Organizations. Since that time, a variety of other committees has been required, committees that focus less on the logistics of medical decisions than on their complex social, psychological, and ethical implications; the Infant Care Review Committees, which monitor the life support of deformed newborns, is a very recent example. In all of these review and disciplinary committees, active membership is either exclusively or predominantly medical.

It is not necessary to go into exhaustive detail in order to make the point that a variety of formal mechanisms has developed to examine, judge, and, if necessary, correct and control the technical and ethical standards employed by physicians in the conduct of their work. They now exist primarily in the hospital, but they are also found in large-scale ambulatory care Health Maintenance Organizations and public clinics. Their operation has certainly been facilitated by the use of computers to record and collate large masses of information that were difficult to deal with systematically in the past. Working in such committees, it is no longer possible for physicians to say, There but for the grace of God go I, or, Who am I to judge? and, save for some covert gossip with trusted colleagues, be silent. Physicians are now required to judge and take action through such committees. Furthermore, this action is *formal* in character, being a form of official supervision and control of individual practitioners' decisions. And since their activities must be on the record they cannot be merely informal, private, and advisory—indeed, they are always potentially public.

While it would be false to claim that practitioners are now stripped of all the protection that collegial relations used to provide, it can be claimed that the rules of the game have changed sufficiently in medicine to have introduced important changes in the relationship that members of the medical profession have with each other, both in the way they compete with each other in the marketplace and in the way they interact with each other at work, particularly in large, complex institutions subject to financing by the state.

Superficially, these changes might be interpreted as bureaucratization in Weber's ideal-typical sense, for they are accompanied by an increase in hierarchical positions as health care organizations grow in size, records become more and more elaborate, specific standards govern the formal evaluation of more and more work, supervision in the form of evaluation of work becomes more and more widespread, and hierarchical positions of responsibility increase in number and variety. However, in all circumstances involving the work of medicine, it is members of that profession who are in charge of setting standards, reviewing performance, and exercising supervision and control. Thus, those changes do not affect the position of the profession as a corporate body in the social as well as institutional division of labor so much as they affect the *internal* organization of the profession, in the relations among physicians. In essence, I suggest, they are creating more distinct and formal patterns of stratification within the profession than have existed in the past, with the position of the rank and file practitioner changing most markedly.

We can gain better insight into the peculiarities of that emerging position by contrasting it to that of the classic industrial proletariat. In what is now a classic though historically overdrawn portrait of proletarianization, Braverman (1974) emphasizes the process by which capitalist management "expropriated" the skills of workers. Nonworkers—that is, managers and more particularly industrial engineers—studied the production process as the workers performed it, developed new methods of selecting and performing production tasks designed to make these tasks more amenable to supervisory control, and then required the workers to do their jobs in the new way. The workers thus became mere passive tools of management, the proletariat: they were supposed to do exactly what they were told to do.

That condition is superficially analogous to what I have described for medicine today, but with a critical difference that destroys the pertinence of what is analogous. In the case of medicine, both supervision and control and the creation of "production standards" are carried out by members of the same profession as those who perform the basic, productive medical work. In the case of supervisory and managerial authority over medical work, a variety of legal and quasi-legal devices in the United States requires that the supervisors and managers of physicians also be physicians. The professional corporation, for example, is a legal form in which it is required that shareholders be only those who are practicing members of the corporation; shares, furthermore, cannot be transferred to or even inherited by lay people.

To take another example, state laws against the "corporate practice of medicine" may not prevent lay investors from owning shares in for-profit health care enterprises in many states, but the requirement is that, if the chief executive officer of the practice unit is not a physician, then the head of the medical staff must be. In factories, a truly analogous situation would be the requirement that no supervisor or manager of production could hold the position without first having received the training of an industrial worker.

It is the same for the standards that are being established to order the work of rank and file physicians. They are established by members of the profession, and not by outsiders who develop their own standards for their own reasons. Two methods of establishing standards may be noted. One is fairly common and, in fact, has a long tradition of use in negligence or malpractice suits: if a physician hospitalizes a patient for a condition that most other physicians do not believe requires hospitalization, the physician is asked to justify the deviation from the standard. The same method is employed in assessing the individual's decision to keep a patient in hospital. This method establishes a standard for evaluation by democratic professional consensus, by invoking the most common practice of all the physicians in an institution, community, region, or even nation, as the criterion by which to judge individual practices. Individuals are no longer free to do whatever their idiosyncratic judgment suggests, but the constraint on their judgment is generated by collective *collegial* practice and not by "outsiders".

A rather different method is likely to be more important over the long run, however—deriving standards for supervising and controlling practice from professionally authoritative knowledge and practice. For example, at outpatient pediatric clinics at two New York City hospitals, computers monitor the treatment of children in light of mandated treatment procedures that have been specified for 85 percent of the patients' complaints. If the computer shows that a physician has not followed them, then he or she must justify that deviation to medical superiors (Sullivan 1984). It is not that a physician cannot deviate, but that deviation must be formally justified by reference to a common body of practice that is considered to be a legitimate norm. It is conceivable that the deviant was correctly exercising discretionary judgment in an individual case, and the opportunity is provided to demonstrate its propriety. This opportunity is provided to physicians in every review context with which I am familiar. The rank and file practitioner thus has virtually statutory opportunity to use discretion in following standardized procedures and to deviate from them.

In that same New York City program of pediatric practice, it was noted that since the system was instituted there has been a sharp drop in the prescription of antibiotics for the treatment of colds and the like—a prescribing practice that has long been common among physicians and long deplored by medical authorities. If the standard procedure were to be determined by widespread medical custom, the prescription of antibiotics to treat upper respiratory infections could conceivably be a formal rule. Instead, the rule was based on the authoritative opinion of elite practitioners and the scientific findings of medical researchers.

Increasingly, elite practitioners and researchers rather than the common customs of rank and file establish the standards for medical work, much the way the standards of industrial engineers do so for industrial work. Unlike the engineers, however, those authorities are members of the same profession as the rank and file, sharing the same basic professional training but afterward going on to a different postgraduate training and a different career line within the profession. Working primarily in medical schools and teaching hospitals, they cannot be said to be outsiders expropriating the skills of practitioners. Rather, they are the ones who teach those skills to practitioners in training, and who create, expand, screen, and revise them. Their position within the medical profession as authorities who set the standards by which the work of the rank and file practitioner is evaluated and controlled becomes considerably more formal than it was in the past.

THE REINFORCEMENT OF STRATIFICATION IN MEDICINE

In essence, these new modes of evaluating and exercising control over the work of physicians are created by reinforcing and formalizing the positions of medical administrators or supervisors and of medical researchers. There is nothing new about the positions themselves. After all, chiefs of staff and heads of services or departments have existed in hospitals for as long as there have been medical staffs, and medical researchers and professors have existed as long as there have been medical schools. Originally they held part-time positions in the United States, but over the past century the trend has been toward their becoming full-time, salaried positions. More important, until recently both positions were advisory rather than authoritative. As Goss (1961) showed, while the physician-administrator's authority in such "housekeeping" matters as scheduling would be accepted by those in his or her unit, in matters involving the practice of medicine itself such authority was only advisory.

The same could be said for the recommendations of researchers and other cognitive authorities: while in their teaching and in their journal articles they may have condemned the prescription of antibiotics for upper respiratory infections as both ineffective and potentially dangerous, practitioners were free to ignore their conclusions. Now, however, in hospitals and other large practice settings, the authority of both the physician-administrator and the physician-researcher has become more extensive and definite and has become more binding on the practitioner. Formal administrative authority and formal cognitive authority analogous to "line" and "staff" authority in industry become much more definite, leaving rank and file practitioners with considerably less freedom of action than existed in the past. This does not mean that they are no longer professionals with a significant degree of discretion; rather, it means that their discretion must take into account the authoritative norms laid down by other members of their profession, that they become in some sense subordinate to a select group of their own colleagues.

In most writing on medicine, stratification within the profession has been approached largely in terms of the relative prestige and income of the specialties (Abbott 1981). But neither prestige nor, for that matter, income, tells us anything about the authority relations among members of either the profession as a whole or the specialty. The literature has largely neglected the position of academics and administrators. Indeed, the tendency has been to see them as in some sense separate professions and not "real" doctors. Alford (1975), for example, sharply distinguished practitioners as "professional monopolists" from administrators and medical school teachers and researchers, whom he clustered together with industrial, institutional, and governmental agents to constitute the "corporate rationalizers" (see also Brown 1979, 204–7). He was right to distinguish them from practitioners in that there are important differences in their aim and orientation, but wrong to separate them because all three are essential parts of the same organized profession.

Those in medical schools, teaching hospitals, and the like control, codify, refine, communicate, and augment the profession's body of knowledge and skill: their activities maintain control by the profession over knowledge and technology and discourage "expropriation" by outsiders. Those in administrative positions in practice organizations balance the necessity to carry out the collective ends of a governing board, municipality, state, firm, or whatever against the needs and desires of those who do the medical work, thereby buffering the practice of medicine against the political and economic pressures of the environment. Without physicians serving in both roles, the profession could only sustain a position that is at best like that of the crafts, dependent on its organization but at the mercy of others' technological innovations and administrative practices. Nor could it sustain the plausibility of that part of its ideology that claims to be concerned with the collective, public good.

But both researchers and administrators do have a different perspective than everyday practitioners. They are certainly more committed to the rationalization of practice (Scott 1982a, 225; 1982b) in the interest of scientific or therapeutic knowledge, on the one hand, and of more adequately serving a population or organization within the limits of available resources on the other. As Scott (1982a, 222) points out, both researchers and administrators are oriented to the "macro care" of populations, while practitioners are oriented to the "micro" or clinical care of individuals. There is therefore bound to be tension if not conflict between the practitioners of the profession and the administrators who supervise them by employing the standards that are created by the researchers (Scott 1982a, 229).

These are the major lines of cleavage within the profession, with far deeper implications for the unity of the profession as a whole than mere differences of specialty, prestige, or income. Where once all practitioners could employ their own clinical judgment to decide how to handle their individual cases independently of whatever medical school professors asserted in textbooks and researchers in journal articles, now the professors and scientists who have no firsthand knowledge of those individual cases establish guidelines that administrators who also lack such firsthand experience attempt to enforce. Where once all practitioners were fairly free to decide how to manage their relations with patients, now administrators attempt to control the pacing and scheduling of work in the interest of their organization's mission, which may regard the collective interests of all patients (or of investors or insurance funds) to be more important than the interests of individual practitioners and their relations with individual patients.

Even though there are significant escape clauses in the form of offering the practitioner an opportunity to justify deviation from administratively imposed norms, it is not hard to imagine the potential for conflict. Nor is it hard to see the organized division of interests that arises between practitioners as a whole and physician-administrators, policymakers, and researchers.

TRENDS IN THE IMMEDIATE FUTURE

Where, then, is the medical profession going? I will not hazard prophesying the far future, but I will suggest probable directions for the next decade or two. In brief, I can say that the medical profession is going where health care in general is going—toward greater rationalization and formalization. Rationalization of financing and accounting for care is fairly well advanced already and is likely to continue. Rationalization of the organization of care, however, has been slower to develop and because of both the nature of health care itself and the place of the medical profession in the division of labor it is not likely to advance so far.

But there can be no doubt that it will continue, particularly in relatively large-scale settings such as hospitals, clinics, and Health Maintenance Organizations, but also in more specialized units such as urgent care centers that are part of continuing efforts to control costs—whether to maintain profits for investors or to prevent increased demands on public funds. Rationalization will also be an important part of continuing efforts to control the quality of care and the accountability of those who provide it.

Rationalization of matters bearing on cost and health care itself is, of course, interconnected and is expressed through the social arrangements by which care is organized. Rationalizing social arrangements in health care organizations means formalizing the relationships among its participants. The health care division of labor among the various participating occupations has already been formalized. It is the medical profession that alone was able to resist formalization until recently, thereby preserving the appearance of a unified profession.

Perhaps because it resisted so successfully in the past it is likely to have to go through even more changes than other health care occupations in the immediate future. Given cost control efforts and increases in the number of physicians, it is likely that the profession's average income will decline. It is possible that the profession's prestige will decline as well, though certainly not precipitously and only modestly in relation to other professions. And it is likely that changes will continue to occur, as they have been doing during this entire century, in the periphery of medicine's jurisdictional boundaries in the health division of labor. But there is no reason to believe that medicine's basic position of dominance, its key position in the health care system, will change. It will have considerably less control over the economics of health care, however, and will have to struggle to maintain its strong voice in policymaking and in the governance of the organizations in which its members work.

I do not see changes that will actually transform rather than merely alter the position of the medical profession in either the nation or the health care system. Many of the changes to which the profession is adapting are to be welcomed as long overdue methods of providing greater protection to patients and to the public treasury, but even in those cases members of the profession formulate the standards and staff the formal positions created to administer them. While there can be no doubt that nonphysician administrators have increased in importance and will continue to play more important roles in the emerging system, there is no sign that they will gain legitimate authority to formulate standards, supervise, and control health care. That remains in the hands of medicine and its "allied health occupations".

What is far more seriously contested is control over the allocation of resources to health care. That is what lay administrators in hospitals and other large practice organizations are likely to control, in conjunction with their governing boards, and that is where the medical profession will find its greatest challenge, both in the particular institutions in which its members work and in the legislatures where politicians ultimately determine the amount and type of resources to be made available to the health care system.

To meet that challenge requires effective political organization, however, and there is the real possibility that medicine is losing its cohesion and thus its capacity for effective political organization. The formalization of professional control has led to formal distinctions between the judges and the judged, the authoritative researcher and the compliant practitioner, the superordinate and the subordinate. And even among rank and file practitioners, that large minority, if not majority, who will continue to work in small, private settings will have interests quite divergent from those working in large organizations, so that not even they may be able to act as a body. While all may be expected to join together for common action to increase the resources made available to the health care system as a whole, on which they all depend, their differences and lack of a common sense of profession may prevent them from being as effective as they were in the past.

REFERENCES

Abbott, A. (1981). "Status and Status Strain in the Professions," *American J. of Sociology* 86 (January):819–35.

Alford, R. (1975). *Health Care Politics*. Chicago: University of Chicago Press.

Arney, W. R. (1982). *Power and the Profession of Obstetrics*. Chicago: University of Chicago Press.

Barber, B.; Lally, J. J.; Makarushka, J. L.; and Sullivan, D. (1973). *Research on Human Subjects*. New York: Russell Sage Foundation.

Berlant, J. L. (1975). *Profession and Monopoly*. Berkeley: University of California Press.

Betz, M., and O'Connell, L. (1983). "Changing Doctor-Patient Relationships and the Rise in Concern for Accountability," *Social Problems* 31 (October):84–95.

Bosk, C. L. (1979). *Forgive and Remember*. Chicago: University of Chicago Press.

Braverman, H. (1974). *Labor and Monopoly Capital*. New York: Monthly Review.

Brown, E. R. (1979). *Rockefeller Medicine Men*. Berkeley: University of California Press.

Burnham, J. C. (1982). "American Medicine's Golden Age: What Happened to It?" *Science* 215 (March 19):1474–79.

Christoffel, T. (1982). *Health and the Law*. New York: The Free Press.

Coburn, D.; Torrance, G. M.; and Kaufert, J. M. (1983). "Medical Dominance in Canada in Historical Perspective: The Rise and Fall of Medicine?" *International J. of Health Services* 13 (No. 3):407–32.

Conrad, P., and Schneider, J. W. (1980). *Deviance and Medicalization*. St. Louis: C. V. Mosby Company.

Derbyshire, R. C. (1969). *Medical Licensure and Discipline in the U.S.* Baltimore: Johns Hopkins University Press.

Dolan, A. K. (1980). "Antitrust Law and Physician Dominance of Other Health Practitioners," *J. of Health Politics, Policy and Law* 4 (Winter 1980):675–90.

Freidson, E. (1970a). *Professional Dominance*. New York: Atherton Press.

________. (1970b). *Profession of Medicine*. New York: Harper and Row.

________. (1980). *Doctoring Together*. Chicago: University of Chicago Press.

Friedman, E. (1983). "Declaration of Interdependence. More and More Physicians Find Salaried Status Attractive," *Hospitals* 57 (July 1):73–80.

Giddens, A. (1982). *Profiles and Critiques in Social Theory*. Berkeley: University of California Press.

Goss, M. E. W. (1961). "Influence and Authority Among Physicians in an Outpatient Clinic," *American Sociological Review* 26 (February):39–50.

Gray, B. H. (1975). *Human Subjects in Medical Experimentation*. New York: John Wiley & Sons.

Harris, J. E. (1977). "The Internal Organization of Hospitals: Some Economic Implications," *Bell J. of Economics* 8:467–82.

Haug, M. R. (1973). "Deprofessionalization: An Alternative Hypothesis for the Future," *Sociological Review Monographs* 20:195–211.

_______. (1975). "The Deprofessionalization of Everyone?" *Sociological Focus* 3:197–213.

_______. (1977). "Computer Technology and the Obsolescence of the Concept of Profession." In *Work and Technology*, ed. M. R. Haug and J. Dofny, 215–28. Beverly Hills: Sage Publications.

Havighurst, C. C., and King, N. M. P. (1983). "Private Credentialing of Health Care Personnel: An Antitrust Perspective," *American J. of Law & Medicine* 9 (Summer):131–201; (Fall):263–334.

Health Insurance Association of America. (1982). *Health and Health Insurance: The Public's View*. Washington, D.C.: HIAA.

Illich, I. (1976). *Medical Nemesis*. New York: Pantheon Books.

_______. (1980). *Toward a History of Needs*. New York: Bantam Books.

Kissam, P. C. (1975). "Physician's Assistant and Nurse Practitioner Laws: A Study of Health Law Reform," *Kansas Law Review* 24 (Fall):1–65.

Langwell, K. M., and Moore, S. F. (1982). *A Synthesis of Research on Competition in the Financing and Delivery of Health Services*. DHHS Publication No. (PHS) 83-3327, Research Report Series. Washington, D.C.: National Center for Health Services Research.

Larson, M. S. (1980). "Proletarianization and Educated Labor," *Theory and Society* 9 (January):131–77.

Lippincott, R. C., and Begun, J. W. (1982). "Competition in the Health Sector: A Historical Perspective," *J. of Health Politics, Policy and Law* 7 (Summer):460–87.

Lipset, S. M., and Schneider, W. (1983). *The Confidence Gap*. New York: The Free Press.

McCarthy, J. D., and Zald, M. N. (1973). *The Trend of Social Movements in America: Professionalization and Resource Mobilization*. Morristown, N.J.: General Learning Press.

McKinlay, J. B. (1973). "On the Professional Regulation of Change," *Sociological Review Monographs* 20:61–84.

_______. (1982). "Toward the Proletarianization of Physicians." In *Professionals as Workers: Mental Labor in Advanced Capitalism*, ed. C. Derber, 37–62. Boston: G. K. Hall.

Noie, N. E.; Shortell, S. M.; and Morrisey, M. A. (1983). "A Survey of Hospital Medical Staffs—Part I," *Hospitals* 57 (December 1):80–84.

Oppenheimer, M. (1973). "The Proletarianization of the Professional," *Sociological Review Monographs* 20:213–27.

Pauly, M. V., and Redisch, M. (1973). "The Not-for-Profit Hospital as a Physicians' Cooperative," *American Economic Review* 63 (March): 87–99.

Roederer, D., and Palmer, P. (1981). "Sunset—Expectation and Experience." Louisville, Ky.: Council of State Governments, June.

Scott, W. R. (1982a). "Managing Professional Work: Three Models of Control for Health Organizations," *Health Services Research* 17 (Fall):213–40.

———. (1982b). "Health Care Organizations in the 1980's: The Convergence of Public and Professional Control Systems." In *Contemporary Health Services: Social Science Perspectives*, ed. A. W. Johnson, O. Grusky, and B. H. Raven, 177–95. Boston: Auburn House.

Southwick, A. F., and Siedel, G. J., III. (1978). *The Law of Hospital and Health Care Administration*. Ann Arbor: Health Administration Press.

Starr, P. (1978). "Medicine and the Waning of Professional Sovereignty," *Daedalus* 107 (Winter):175-93.

———. (1982). *The Social Transformation of American Medicine*. New York: Basic Books.

Stevens, R. (1971). *American Medicine and the Public Interest*. New Haven: Yale University Press.

Sullivan, R. (1984). "City Expanding Use of Computers to Monitor Pediatric Care," *New York Times* 133 (February 29):B24.

Toren, N. (1975). "Deprofessionalization and Its Sources," *Sociology of Work and Occupations* 2 (November):323–37.

Walker, J. L. (1983). "The Origins and Maintenance of Interest Groups in America," *American Political Science Review* 77 (June 2):390–406.

Zola, I. K. (1972). "Medicine as an Institution of Social Control," *Sociological Review* 20:487–504.

Rationalization and the Deprofessionalization of Physicians*

GEORGE RITZER, *University of Maryland*
DAVID WALCZAK, *Union College*

Abstract

The Weberian theory of rationalization, especially the concepts of formal and substantive rationality and the conflict between them, are used to analyze contemporary changes affecting the medical profession. Three major types of changes are discussed—changes in government policies, the changing nature of medical delivery systems, and changes within medical delivery systems. It is argued that these changes are impelling the medical profession away from substantive rationality and in the direction of formal rationality. Increasing formal rationality is likely to lead to greater external control over physicians and to a decline in the ability of the medical profession to distinguish itself from bureaucrats and capitalists. These changes, in turn, are likely to lead to some degree of deprofessionalization of physicians. Alternative future scenarios are also mentioned.

Sociological theories are often discussed in their own terms and in isolation from social changes. While these discussions can be useful, it is important that such theories be linked to the changing social world. The objective in this paper is to take major components of the Weberian theory of rationalization and apply them to contemporary changes in and around the paradigmatic profession—physicians. As we will see, the application of rationalization theory allows us to gain new insight into what is happening to the medical profession.

The widely known and extremely important developments affecting the medical profession include antitrust decisions, corporatization, conglomeration, bureaucratization, technological change, unionization, and the rise of McDoctors (no-appointment, walk-in medical facilities modelled after fast-food restaurants), third-party payers, HMOs (Health Main-

*We thank Andrew Abbott, Peter Abell, Bob Antonio, Jere Cohen, Peter Conrad, Kenneth Kammeyer, and anonymous referees for helpful comments on earlier drafts of this paper. Thanks also to the General Research Board at the University of Maryland for funding this project. Direct correspondence to George Ritzer, Department of Sociology, University of Maryland, College Park, MD 20742.

tenance Organizations), prospective payment systems based on pre-set DRGs (Diagnostic Related Groups), and the like.[1] Sociologists have been interested in the nature and significance of these changes as well as how they relate to the professional status of medicine. Unfortunately, the major sociological efforts in this area have not been notably strong theoretically.[2]

In addition to theoretical weaknesses, work in this area has been characterized by conflicting and contradictory conclusions and prognostications. In *The Social Transformation of American Medicine*, Paul Starr (1982) looked at many of the changes enumerated above and forecast a weakening of the sovereignty, the deprofessionalization, of medicine.[3] In contrast, Eliot Freidson (1986) in *Professional Powers* argued that the general idea of professional decline is greatly overstated.

This paper addresses itself to changes in and around medicine as well as to the debate over deprofessionalization with the conviction that they need to be analyzed from a strong theoretical perspective. In fact, they must be addressed theoretically since the changes are occurring, and are likely to continue to occur, and we do not yet have definitive empirical data.[4]

The theory employed here is derived from the work of Max Weber as well as that of a number of recent analysts of his work. What those analysts have done is to underscore the centrality of rationalization theory to Weber as well as to clarify the theory itself. Although Weber had a complex, multi-faceted sense of rationalization (Brubaker 1984; Kalberg 1980; Levine 1981), he used it most powerfully in his image of the modern western world, especially in the capitalistic economy[5,6] (Collins 1980; Weber [1927] 1981) and bureaucratic organizations (Cohen 1981; Weber [1921] 1968, pp. 956–1005), as an "iron cage" (Mitzman 1969; Tiryakian 1981) of rational structures. Weber described capitalism and bureaucracies as "two great rationalizing forces" ([1921] 1968, p. 698). In fact, Weber ([1922–3] 1958, p. 291) saw capitalism and bureaucracies[7] as involving similarly rational and methodical action, serving to reinforce one another and furthering the rationalization of the Occident.[8] In Weber's ([1921] 1968, pp. 227; 994) view, the only real rival to the bureaucrat in technical expertise and factual knowledge was the capitalist.[9]

It is our thesis that structural changes (especially as they relate to bureaucracies and capitalism) surrounding the American medical profession are leading to greater external control over it and impelling it in the direction of absorbing many rational characteristics (Relman & Reinhart 1986). This greater external control and internal rationalization are crucial factors in the deprofessionalization of physicians.[10] Such changes could have profound implications for the entire professional category since physicians have for many years been the model profession.[11]

This paper will be composed of three sections. First, we will briefly delineate those aspects of rationalization theory to be utilized in this analysis. Second, we will look at the meaning of the concept of a profession as well as medicine's position as a profession. Third, we will look at the forces that are coming to control the medical profession, impelling it in the direction of increasing rationalization and, in the process, serving to deprofessionalize physicians.

Rationalization

Taking Weber at his word, it is difficult to argue that he had an overarching theory of rationalization. He rejected the idea of "general evolutionary sequence" ([1927] 1981, p. 34). He was critical of thinkers like Hegel and Marx who he felt offered general, teleological theories of society. In his own work he tended to shy away from studies of, or proclamations about, whole societies. Instead, he tended to focus, in turn, on social structures and institutions such as bureaucracy, stratification, law, the city, religion, the polity, and the economy. Lacking a sense of the whole, he was unlikely to make global generalizations, especially about future directions. Furthermore, the rationalization process that Weber described in one social structure or institution was usually quite different from the rationalization of another structure or institution. As Weber put it, the process of rationalization assumes "unusually varied forms" ([1922–23] 1958, p. 293; see also, Weber [1920] 1958, p. 20; Weber [1904–05] 1958, p. 78) and "the history of rationalism shows a development which by no means follows parallel lines in the various departments of life" (Weber [1904–05] 1958, p. 77; see also, Brubaker 1984, p. 9; Kalberg 1980, p. 1147).

This being said, it is clear that Weber does have a deep concern for the overarching effect of one type of rationalization on the Western world (Weber [1921] 1968, p. 1156; Brubaker 1984). While rationality is used in many different ways in Weber's work, what interests us here is a process involving one of four types identified by Kalberg (1980; see also, Levine 1981), *formal rationality*.[12] Formal rationality involves, as is usually the case with Weber, a concern for actors making choices in terms of means and ends. However, in this case that choice is made in reference to universally applied rules, regulations, and laws. These, in turn, are derived from various large-scale structures, especially bureaucracies and the economy.[13] The emphasis in formal rationality is on rationality at the macro-levels—rules, regulations, laws, bureaucracies, and economies—and its impact on the conduct of individuals (Weber [1921] 1968, p. 1116).

Of the four types of rationality delineated in Kalberg's analysis, *only* formal rationality is both macro-sociological and distinctive to the West. Our concern here, then, is with the formal rationality of the Western world, especially as it is found in bureaucracies and the economy. It is primarily this type of rationalization as it is found in these sectors that is having a profound effect on the medical profession. The key point is that formally rational structures and institutions and their rules and regulations are coming to exercise increasing control over physicians, altering their character by making them more formally rational and, in turn, contributing to deprofessionalization.[14]

To help us better understand the relation between (formal) rationality and professionalization, it is necessary to introduce another of Kalberg's types of Weberian rationality—*substantive rationality*.[15] The distinctive aspect of substantive rationality is that the effort to find the most rational means to ends is shaped by a coherent set of social values. While value-driven rationality and formal rationality (determined by rules, regulations, laws, and structures) may coexist, they may also come into conflict with one another.[16] In fact, Brubaker (1984) sees an irreconcilable tension here since formal rationality is indifferent to the social values that are central to substantive rationality. The conflict between formal and substantive rationality[17] may be descriptive of the current relation between (formal) rationalization and professionalization (a specific case of substantive rationality).[18]

The professions (at least in the recent past) can be characterized by substantive rationality since professionals are led by social values to make rational choices of means to ends. These values include altruism (or the good of the client and/or collectivity rather than personal gain), autonomy, and authority over clients. The value-guided conduct that characterizes the professions may come into conflict with the rules- and regulations-guided conduct (without regard to values) that characterizes formal rationality.[19]

While we are characterizing the professions as value-rational, this does not imply an inherently positive view of them or a necessarily negative view of what is happening to them as a result of formal rationalization. While a value like altruism may lead physicians to some very laudable actions (taking the needs and interests of patients before their own), values like autonomy and authority over clients may lead them to actions that further their self-interest and adversely affect the interests of patients as well as of the society as a whole. Thus, the idea of the medical profession as being characterized by substantive rationality does *not* lead us to a romantic view of physicians prior to the spread of formal rationalization, nor does it lead us to conclude that the effects of formal rationalization are necessarily negative. What we are saying is that the spread of formal rationalization is tending to overwhelm substantive rationality and contributing to the deprofessionalization of physicians. This leads us to another aspect of our thesis—the medical profession is undergoing deprofessionalization because the differences between it and (formally rational) bureaucrats and capitalists are being eroded. If bureaucrats, capitalists, and physicians can all be best seen as formally rational, then why should the public accord physicians the distinctive label of a profession?

While setting these two types of rationalities and rational structures in opposition to one another, it is important to remember that they are Weberian ideal types with the result that in the real world all social structures are characterized by *both* formal and substantive rationalities. Thus, real bureaucracies are affected by larger values and the professions have elements of formal rationality. This, too, allows us to get away from the simplistic and romantic idea that what we are witnessing is the regrettable disappearance of the more human professions in the face of the rise of inhuman formally rational systems. Perhaps all we are seeing is more formal rationality and less substantive rationality, but even if we characterize the situation in this way, this seemingly minor shift is having profound implications for the professions. We will have occasion to return to the issue of the mix of formal and substantive rationality in bureaucracies and professions later in the paper.

Professionalization and the Medical Profession

The study of the professions has been obsessed with, and many feel distorted by, the medical profession (e.g., Arney 1982; Berlant 1975; Freidson 1970, 1975, 1980; Gelfand 1980; Larkin 1983; Starr 1982). After all, it was the medical profession that achieved unparalleled professional power, prestige, and income. All occupations that sought to professionalize took physicians as their model. Medicine was seen by sociologists as the paradigmatic profession and all other occupations were compared, implicitly or explicitly, to it.

Historically, sociologists have conceptualized professions and the process of professionalization in three basic ways (Ritzer & Walczak 1986). The process (Caplow 1954; Wilensky 1964) and structural-functional (Goode 1957; Greenwood 1957)[20] views of the professions generally, and of medicine in particular, dominated until about 1970 when the now-dominant power perspective emerged (Forsyth & Danisiewicz 1985; Freidson 1970; Hall 1983; Jamous & Peloille 1970; Johnson 1972; Klegon 1978; Larson 1977; Ritzer 1975b; Roth 1974).[21] There was an almost simultaneous critique of the process and structural-functional paradigms *and* of the supposedly distinctive characteristics of the medical profession. At a general level, the power perspective rejected the idea that the professions were distinguished by any distinctive historical stages or inherent characteristics. Rather, the view emerged that what distinguishes the professions from other occupations, either wholly or most importantly, is power (McKinlay 1973). Professions came to be seen as occupations that had the power (derived, for example, from control over uncertainty and indeterminacy [Jamous & Peloille 1970]) to win the exalted label of "profession" and once they did, they were seen as exploiting that situation to further enhance their power. More particularly, especially in the work of Eliot Freidson

(1960, 1970, 1975, 1980), the sense emerged that what truly distinguished the medical profession was its power over clients, other occupations, and the larger society.[22]

These three approaches, especially the power orientation, lead to the following definition of a profession as: "*an occupation that has had the power to have undergone a developmental process enabling it to acquire, or convince significant others (for example, clients, the law) that it has acquired a constellation of characteristics we have come to accept as denoting a profession*" (Ritzer & Walczak 1986, p. 62). The characteristics we have come to associate with the professions are, among others, the values (altruism, autonomy, and authority over clients) discussed above (as well as general systematic knowledge [Baer 1986], distinctive occupational culture and community and legal recognition). Professional ideologies (Forsyth & Danisiewicz 1985; Gieryn, Bevins & Zehr 1985) are a major source of the view among the public that these characteristics are associated with professions.

Along with a sense of the power of the professions in general, and medicine in particular, came a sense of the *fragility* of that power. That is, while power was something that professions won for themselves, they had to work hard and continually to retain it. Clients (Rothstein 1973), other occupations (Larkin 1983; Zola & Miller 1973), and the larger society (Jamous & Peloille 1970) could bestow power, but they also had the ability to limit and even withdraw that grant (Johnson 1972). The concern for the sources of the power of the professions was transformed, at least in part, into an interest in their loss of power, an interest in the process of *deprofessionalization* (Haug 1973, 1975; Rothman 1984; Toren 1975).[23] A variety of forces seemed to be at work that were causing clients, other occupations, and the larger society to curb the power of the professions. We can define deprofessionalization as *a decline in power which results in a decline in the degree to which professions possess, or are perceived to possess, a constellation of characteristics denoting a profession*. More specifically, deprofessionalization involves a decline in the possession, or perception that the professions possess, altruism, autonomy, authority over clients, general systematic knowledge, distinctive occupational culture, and community and legal recognition.

Linking this section on professionalization/deprofessionalization with the preceding section on rationalization, we are arguing that physicians (and their substantive rationality) are being profoundly affected by the spread of formal rationality and that this is contributing to some degree of deprofessionalization. At one level it is simply that formally rational structures (especially capitalistic and bureaucratic) are exercising increasing control over physicians (Kerr 1985), that more external control generally means less power, and that a decline in power is a major aspect of deprofessionalization. At another level, the distinctive substantive rationality of the medical profession (with its emphasis on values such as altruism, authority over clients, and autonomy) is being supplanted by formal rationality (with its emphasis on structures, rules, and regulations). To the degree that physicians come to be characterized by formal rationality, they will be unable to continue to lay claim effectively to the distinctive title of professional. The main thesis of this paper, then, is that the spread of formal rationality is a major cause of the deprofessionalization of physicians.[24]

Rationalization and Deprofessionalization

In this section we examine a lengthy list of changes in large-scale structures and institutions that are exerting increasing control over physicians and impelling medicine (and its substantive rationality) in the direction of greater formal rationalization and ultimately deprofessionalization. All of these changes involve an increasing impact of capitalism and/or bureaucracy on physicians. The developments to be discussed include changes in governmental policies (especially at the federal level)—antitrust decisions, Medicare and Medicaid, the development of a prospective payment system and diagnostic related groups (DRGs); structural changes in the organization of medical delivery systems—corporatization, conglomeration, free standing primary care centers ("McDoctors"), health maintenance organizations (HMOs), entrepreneurialism, and advertising; and changes within these organizations—professional managers, accounting systems and an emphasis on quantifiable costs, formalization of controls, and technological advances.

As we briefly discuss each of these changes, we will focus on how they are fostering greater formal rationality in general in medicine and, more specifically, increases in the specific components of such rationality —efficiency, predictability, calculability, (external) control, and substitution of non-human for human technology (Eisen 1978; Kalberg 1980; Ritzer 1983). The sets of changes as well as the increases in formal rationality will, in turn, be linked to the deprofessionalization of physicians, their loss of power generally and the erosion of their distinctive substantive values (autonomy, authority over clients, and altruism).

Changes in Government Policies

By their policies, federal (Feldstein 1986) and state governments have exerted increasing control over medicine and played an important role in the emergence of more formally rational medicine. One key factor in the expansion of capitalism (and bureaucratization) in medicine was the birth and development in the mid-1960s of Medicare and Medicaid, both of which provided a secure source of reimbursement to those capitalists interested in investing in the medical marketplace (Michel, Shaked & Daley 1985). Additionally, Medicare and Medicaid helped to increase the demand for medical care.[25] Congress responded to a perceived shortage of physicians by passing the Health Professions Educational Assistance Act (HPEA) in 1963 (Feldstein 1986). Increased numbers of physicians have spurred competition among physicians and one way of being more competitive is by rationalizing medical activities, that is, becoming more efficient in the delivery of medical services.

Another example of external governmental control was the 1975 Supreme Court ruling that professionals, including physicians, are subject to the provisions of the Sherman Antitrust Act. Prior to this decision, medicine (along with other professions) was seen as autonomous and self-regulating, and thus exempt from antitrust laws (Costilo 1985; Feldstein 1986; Havighurst 1983). Since 1975, a number of antitrust suits have been filed challenging the anti-competitive practices of the medical profession (e.g., restraint of innovative forms of health care, price fixing). While many of these suits have been dismissed, the effect has been to help open medicine to the formally rationalizing influence of market competition.

In the early 1980s a prospective payment system emerged, by which hospitals were paid under Medicare. By using a system of Diagnostic Related Groups (DRGs), the federal government has established the amount it will reimburse hospitals for a given medical diagnosis, no matter how long the patient is hospitalized. As a result of external control by DRGs, physicians are pressed by hospitals into becoming more efficient in their use of ancillary services and in getting patients in and out of the hospital as quickly as possible (Gray 1986).

While the prospective payment system may help stem the rising cost of medical care, it may also have the unintended consequence of contributing to the deprofessionalization of the medical profession by threatening its autonomy and shifting authority over patients away from the doctor and into the hands of third-party bureaucrats. With discussions underway to extend the DRG payment mechanism beyond Medicare to all physician services performed during hospitalization (Mitchell 1985), it is possible that DRGs will contribute to even more external control and deprofessionalization of medicine in the future.

Third-party payers (e.g., the government, Blue Cross) have grown increasingly concerned about spiralling medical costs and have sought to deal with the problem by limiting what they will pay for as well as how much they will pay for it (Michel, Shaked & Daley 1985; Vraciu 1985). Thus, a third party payer may have a policy of not paying for certain procedures, or not allowing hospitalization for certain procedures, or only paying a given amount for a procedure. Such policies clearly exert control over physicians and contribute to increasing formal rationality by bringing a great deal of calculability to the practice of medicine. The third-party payer's formally rational emphasis on money comes into conflict with the physician's substantively rational altruistic interest (at least, ideal typically) in the patient. As one physician-union leader put it (albeit somewhat romantically and unrealistically), doctors are "'the only ones who think of patients as individuals . . . not as dollar signs'" (Colburn 1985, p. 7).

Changing Nature of Medical Delivery Systems

A key and relatively recent development is the corporatization of medicine. The most notable element of this is the growth of investor-owned hospitals. For-profit hospitals are not new, but in the past they were primarily small, independent operations (Gray 1986). More recently, we have seen an increasing number of for-profit hospitals owned by publicly traded health care companies that own multiple facilities. This has contributed to the continuing decline of small, independent proprietary hospitals. Medicine is coming to be increasingly characterized by formally rational, large-scale capitalistic corporations (e.g., Humana Inc., Hospital Corp. of America) that are interested in hospitals, indeed the entire medical complex, as profit-making ventures (Ermann & Gabel 1986; Gray 1986). As more and more physicians become employees of such hospitals, it will be difficult to maintain their altruistic values in such a profit-oriented environment. The pressure to earn profits is likely to lead such hospitals to reduce the autonomy and undermine the authority of physicians. Furthermore, medical corporations are not only likely to rationalize their own hospitals, but the competitive pressures they create are also likely to force non-profit hospitals into taking similar actions.

Related to this is the growth of free standing primary care centers; "McDoctor's," or "Docs-in-the-Box," profit-oriented chains of storefront medical outlets that are modeled after fast-food chains. These are usually drop-in, no-appointment facilities that dispense medical care in much the same efficient way that McDonald's serves hamburgers. In some cases (e.g., Humana's Medfirst medical clinics), McDoctor's are owned by the large corporations that own for-profit hospitals and thereby McDoctor's become simply another arena in which the corporation's principles of formal rationality can be applied. In other cases, they may be independent chains, or even single outlets opened by an enterprising physician/entrepreneur. Even in these cases, given the McDonald's model, there is a strong inclination to rationalize operations as much as possible. Fast and efficient medical service is emphasized. There is a tendency to take only those patients with simple and easily handled medical problems. Since the work is comparatively simple, and highly routinized, less well-trained technical people can often be utilized instead of the much more costly physicians. These are highly predictable settings that look and operate much the same way from one time or place to another time or place. Procedures are elaborately developed and they exert considerable control over what employees (including physicians, where present) can and cannot do.

Another significant development is the rapid growth of Health Maintenance Organizations (HMOs) (Tarlov 1986). While these organizations take a variety of forms, all of them are business organizations in which the objective is to work within budgetary constraints, or in some cases to turn a profit. As business organizations, HMOs are under tremendous pressure to rationalize operations in order to minimize costs and maximize income. Physicians, and their norms of autonomy, authority and altruism, are affected by these pressures whether they control these HMOs or are employed in them.

Also significant is the "conglomeration" of medicine. Whether it be through expanding product lines or product-line diversification, these large medi-giants aim to integrate healthcare facilities, medical services, and insurance functions on a regional or national basis (Vraciu 1985).[26] Large corporations are not only coming to own for-profit hospitals, Mc-Doctor's, and HMOs, but they are also controlling health insurance firms, buying out hospital supply companies, and generally moving in the direction of controlling as many components of the "medical-industrial complex" as possible (e.g., nursing homes, laboratories, emergency-room services, home care, etc. [Ermann & Gabel 1984; Gray 1986; Relman 1980; Schlesinger 1985]). To compete, large, non-profit organizations like Blue Cross–Blue Shield are expanding in a similar manner. In either case, ever-larger conglomerates are increasingly impelled to rationalize their operations. This means that they are going to seek ways of becoming more efficient, predictable, and calculable, of replacing more and more workers with non-human technologies, and of exerting increasing control over employees (including physicians).

Those physicians who resist moving into various large-scale capitalistic medical organizations, are going to have to be even more entrepreneurial than they have been in the past. Physicians have, of course, always combined professionalization and entrepreneurialism, but in order to compete in today's more market-oriented medical system, physicians are going to be forced to emphasize business practices more with the result that professionalization may suffer. Further, physicians in private practice are coming to emphasize entrepreneurialism more and professionalism less by opening an array of free standing or noninstitutional health care centers including pathology labs, health promotion centers, obesity and substance abuse clinics, chains of local emergency rooms, proprietary hospitals, and nursing homes (Goldstein 1984; Gray 1986).

While good empirical data do not yet exist on the impact of entrepreneurialism on patient care decisions, there is suggestive evidence that "is adequate to confirm the common sense conclusion that investments and economic arrangements that reward physicians financially for making certain patient care decisions (e.g., ordering lab tests) will bias physicians in favor of making such decisions" (Gray 1986, p. 159). In any case, it is clearly harder for primarily entrepreneurial physicians to continue to claim to adhere to substantive rationality, especially the value of altruism. Furthermore, the demands of the capitalistic marketplace will exert greater control over an entrepreneurial physician.

One result of this control by the market is the expansion of advertising by the various agencies involved in the medical business, including even physicians in private practice. While there are still strong negative sentiments among some physicians toward advertising (Allen, Wright & Raho 1985), there is evidence to suggest that advertising is gaining acceptance in the medical profession (Darling & Bergiel 1983; Folland 1985). Here is one of the clearest examples of the erosion of the distinction between professional and capitalist, between substantive and formal rationality. Again, with physicians advertising their services on television and in the newspapers, it will be harder for them to continue to put forth an altruistic image. Patients are more likely to question the authority of physicians selling their services side-by-side with used car salespeople.

Changes Within Medical Delivery Systems

Within large-scale corporate hospitals, chains, HMOs, etc., we see the rise of professional managers and their power over physicians (Gray 1986; Quintana, Duncan & Houser 1985). In their quest to maximize profits,[27] these managers are committed to a full-scale formal rationalization of their procedures, including those procedures that apply to the medical profession. This rationalization has a profound effect on physicians, especially if they are employed by a hospital (Battistella 1985). As members of these rationalized hospitals, physicians are forced to work more efficiently, quantify many heretofore qualitative elements of their work (Starr 1982), operate in a predictable manner from one time to another, utilize advanced technologies as much as possible, and allow themselves in an increasing number of domains to be replaced by non-human technologies, and submit to external control, often by superiors who are businesspeople rather than fellow professionals.

To Weber ([1927] 1981, p. 275), the most important presupposition of a capitalist enterprise was a rational capital accounting system.[28] Such accounting systems have become very important to medical organizations, meaning that physicians are coming to be evaluated and controlled by an array of quantitative economic measures.[29] These systems are aimed at ascertaining whether the various things that physicians do are cost-effective. The formal rationality of cost-effectiveness is likely to come into conflict with the substantive rationality of the medical profession since the main basis for a decision may shift from the welfare of the patient to the cost of an undertaking. The physician is now more likely to be a rationing agent or a gatekeeper of medical services (Agich & Begley 1985; Cassel 1985).

It is feared that an emphasis on cost will tend to force medicine to abandon longshot diagnostic techniques and treatments because they cannot be legitimized on a cost basis even though, if successful, patients might benefit from such diagnosis or treatment. Another fear is that a focus on profits will tend to prevent physicians employed in for-profit hospitals from treating low-income patients and force such patients to be sent to remaining public hospitals (Starr 1982). These and other forces threaten the altruistic image of physicians.

While there is some evidence to suggest that for-profit hospitals may rationalize by providing less uncompensated care (bad debt and charity cases) and by treating a smaller proportion of uninsured patients, the data are weak and far from conclusive. For-profit hospitals may offer some services that differ from those offered by not-for-profit hospitals, but it has not been established that these services are necessarily the more profitable ones (Ermann & Gabel 1986). However, for-profits do appear to rationalize operations by employing fewer people (per bed) than not-for-profit hospitals (Ermann & Gabel 1986; Watt et al. 1986). While showing some modest increase in recent years, for-profit hospitals have not been active participants in research and teaching functions (Gray 1986).

Another factor in the formal rationalization of medicine is the profession's increasing dependence on expensive and sophisticated medical technology. Rather than controlling simple technologies as was true in the past, physicians are finding themselves in positions whereby they are more likely to be controlled (and their autonomy reduced) by advanced technologies and the technicians who design them, control them, and interpret their results. As Reiser in his book *Medicine and the Reign of Technology*, puts it: "medicine has now evolved to a point where diagnostic judgments based on 'subjective' evidence—the patient's sensations and the physician's own observations of the patient—are being supplanted by judgments based on 'objective' evidence, provided by laboratory procedures and by mechanical and electronic devices" (1978, p. ix). Technological advance, as a component of advancing rationalization, represents a threat to the professional status of medicine. The subjective, qualitative, and autonomous judgments of physicians are beginning to be replaced by the objective, quantitative results emanating from various advanced technologies. (For example, computer programs are currently being used and refined that "help" physicians diagnose illnesses.) The result of a test utilizing various advanced technologies is far more predictable, that is replicable, from one time to the next. Most importantly, these technologies are coming to exert more control over physicians.

Not only are advanced technologies coming to control physicians, they are also helping to reduce the physician's authority over patients. The patient is well aware that much of the work is being done by technologies and technicians and this serves to erode the authority of the physician in the eyes of the patient. These technologies serve to routinize, and thereby demystify, medical practice.[30,31] Furthermore, patients are increasingly able to bypass the physician altogether and go straight to the technician and in some cases even avoid the technician and go directly to the technology itself (e.g., blood pressure machines in drug stores, home pregnancy tests). All of this constitutes a threat to the idea that professional physicians possess their own distinct body of general systematic knowledge.

In addition to being a threat to professionalization in itself, advancing technology is linked to many of the other forces serving to deprofessionalize medicine. The paradigmatic physician on his/her own in private practice is not able to afford to own most of the advanced technologies that are sweeping the field. It is the capitalist enterprises and the large bureaucracies that are able to afford these technologies. In this way, the dependence on technology is linked to the bureaucratization and capitalization of medicine. In order to gain access to these technologies, physicians must subordinate themselves to, even become employees of, these organizations. Within these organizations, the high cost of modern technologies may cause administrators to become involved in decisions that in the past had been left to the physician (Shea & Margulies 1985; Watts 1985). In the past, the physician owned the (simple) technologies, or else had ready access to them in hospitals that were controlled by fellow physicians. That is now less the case, with the result that there is strong pressure in the direction of deprofessionalization.

All of the factors discussed thus far tend to put physicians increasingly in contact, and in conflict, with bureaucracies.[32] Investor-owned hospital systems, chains of McDoctor's, HMOs, and third-party payers are all huge bureaucratic systems. Bureaucracies, of course, were Weber's paradigm case of formal rationality and given our theme of the conflict between professionalization and rationalization, they become a central source of the deprofessionalization of medicine.[33] As McKinlay put it: "The single feature that most distinguishes present-day medical practice from earlier forms—indeed has altered it almost beyond recognition—is its high degree of bureaucratization" (1982, p. 39). The elements of formal rationality are expressed to an extreme degree within the bureaucracy and the physician who must work in, or deal with, bureaucracies experiences conflict over each of them. For example, the bureaucratic emphasis on efficiency often comes in conflict with what the physician feels is in the best interest of the patient. Most important is the bureaucratic notion of control from the top versus the professional norm of peer control. In huge, bureaucratic systems, those at the top of bureaucracies, and thereby those who are making decisions and issuing directives, are often nonprofessionals; bureaucrats and/or businesspeople. The control that such people are able to exercise is a profound source of the deprofessionalization of physicians.[34] While at one time physicians dominated health organizations, there is now more shared authority with administrators and even subordination of physicians to administrators (Gray 1986).

Freidson offers a somewhat different view. What Freidson (1984) emphasizes is that it is not nonprofessionals, but rather an elite group of professionals, that is coming to control other professionals. As a result, Freidson (see also, Starr 1982) sees the emergence of a stratification system within the professions involving those who create the controls, those who impose them, and those on whom they are imposed. If we accept Freidson's view, then it is the physicians on the bottom who are most likely to be deprofessionalized; to lose their autonomy and perhaps their authority over clients. But it could also be argued that higher, or even the highest, ranking physicians will experience deprofessionalization since they will be controlled, at least to some degree, by bureaucratic rules and regulations.

In fact, although he purports to disagree with the foregoing thesis on the role of bureaucratization in deprofessionalization,[35] Freidson (1984, 1985) does tend to support it when he argues that it is not bureaucratization (and control by nonprofessionals) that is crucial, but rather the "formalization of professional controls." By this he means that instead of being controlled informally, professionals are being controlled by codified technical standards. What Freidson does not recognize is that this formalization of controls is part of the broader process of formal rationalization. Formalized controls serve, among other things, to make the work of professionals more predictable and to increase external control over it.[36]

Although the views expressed in the last two paragraphs see an antithesis between bureaucratization and professionalization, there is a perspective which sees the possibility of a new social form emerging out of the interrelationship of these two processes. In this view, formal rationality need not win out over substantive rationality, but the two can interpenetrate and create a new, hybrid form of rationalization. Substantively rational medical professionals and formally rational systems will *both* be transformed by their relations with one another. If this turns out to be the case, we cannot anticipate the significant deprofessionalization described throughout this section, but the professions will be transformed by this process and it is likely that even in this eventuality some deprofessionalization is also likely to occur.

Although he is writing about lawyers in large law firms, it is necessary to briefly address Nelson's (1981) work at this point. On the surface,

Nelson's conclusions seem to contradict the basic thrust of this paper. That is, he finds that to a large degree the large law firm has resisted bureaucratization (and formal rationalization) and retained its professionalism (and substantive rationality). However, even here, Nelson found consciousness on the part of attorneys "of the need to rationalize their firms by identifying profit centers, formalizing data on the firms' operations, and establishing clear lines of communication and authority" (1981, p. 129). More importantly, he finds a clear trend toward greater formal rationalization "in *the most rationalized form of legal services organization: the large law clinic*" and its "computerized forms, centralized administration, advertising, and routinized procedures" (p. 138; italics added). Finally, although Nelson argues against the main thesis of this paper in the case of elite law practice, he seems to accept it in the case of medicine, at least as it is practiced in the modern hospital.

Another point worth mentioning is that modern bureaucracies are currently undergoing substantial change and are no longer so formally rational (DiMaggio & Powell 1983; Ouchi 1981). As the changed position of the United States in the world political economy pushes organizations in the direction of greater substantive rationality, they will link up with professionals moving into them and experiencing an increase in formal rationality. This, too, points toward lesser deprofessionalization, but deprofessionalization nonetheless.

Conclusions

The objective in this paper has been to use the effects of contemporary social changes on medicine as a case study of the applicability of the Weberian theory of rationalization to the modern social world. Our conclusion is that these formally rational social changes are leading to greater external control over, and formal rationalization of, medicine and that these, in turn, are contributing to the deprofessionalization of medicine. The dividing line between substantively rational physicians and formally rational bureaucrats and capitalists is increasingly blurred with the result that it is harder for physicians to claim the distinctive position of profession and to have that claim accepted by the public. Given the paucity of empirical data on this issue, and the conflicting nature of the data that exist, an adequate theoretical perspective is especially important in trying to understand what is currently happening to medicine. The theory of rationalization has allowed us to see clear linkages among a series of disparate social changes and to understand how they are changing the nature of medicine and contributing to the deprofessionalization of physicians.

While we have made the case for a specific scenario in this paper, several other scenarios are possible. One alternative is that new forms will emerge that combine formal and substantive rationality—new professional, bureaucratic, and capitalistic structures. These new forms that combine the two types of rationality would still tend to point in the direction of deprofessionalization, but not to the degree of this paper's main thesis. Another possibility is that rather than be controlled and changed by formal rationality, the medical profession will absorb it, control it, and emerge as powerful and as professional as ever. Still another possibility is that in the future we will witness a new form of "hyper-rationalization" combining practical, theoretical, substantive, and formal rationality and that the medical profession will control it. In this scenario, the physicians will emerge from the current period of changes with even greater power and with an even higher degree of professionalization. Although this paper's thesis is that significant deprofessionalization of physicians is likely, we will need to await the outcome of contemporary events to see which of these scenarios ultimately occurs. Whatever proves to be the case, Weberian theory is of great utility in helping us understand social changes in the medical profession and generating hypotheses about the future.

A caveat is in order. Our concern has been the deprofessionalization of American medicine. We have sought to understand and explain this development with a central aspect of the theory of rationalization. A more adequate explanation would require a comparative and/or historical analysis involving medicine in other, more-, less- or non-rationalizing societies. Such a comparative analysis would allow us to be on a far firmer ground in concluding that it is, indeed, rationalization that is the major causal factor in the deprofessionalization of medicine. It is hoped that this work may stimulate such cross-cultural and/or trans-historical research. More generally, it seems clear that we need more work seeking to link abstract sociological theories to what is happening in the social world.

Notes

1. Our focus is largely on changes in medicine in the last decade or two, but some of these changes were well under way long before the 1970s.
2. Starr's (1982) work is largely atheoretical. Freidson's (1986) work is stronger theoretically, but it is still not wholly satisfying from a theoretical point of view. For example, the Weberian theory of rationalization plays a central role in Freidson's (1986, p. 3) work (as it does in this paper), but he has an undifferentiated sense of the concept which is not informed by the work of such important neo-Weberians as Kalberg (1980), Levine (1981), and Brubaker (1984).
3. While Starr foresaw a decline, he made it clear that such "a trend is not necessarily fate" (1982, p. 449).
4. Since this is a theoretical work, a number of assertions about the medical profession are made later in the paper that lack empirical support. They are, in a sense, a series of hypotheses that need empirical testing. In some cases, that testing is being done now (e.g., Kerr's [1985] study of physicians in an HMO), while in others testing will need to be delayed until contemporary changes take a clearer form.
5. A capitalist economy is a specific case of a rational economy, "a functional organization oriented to money-prices which originate in the interest-struggles of men in the *market*" (Weber [1915] 1958, p. 331).
6. Although Weber felt that capitalism was highly rational, he believed that a socialist society

would be even more rational. Since this paper focuses on changes in American medicine, we will focus on capitalism as a rationalizing force. A similar paper on medicine in the Soviet Union would examine socialism as a rationalizing agent. In fact, this suggests the need for a comparative study that would allow us to test empirically Weber's views on this issue.

7. Of course, these are not completely distinct since large capitalistic enterprises are one of the places in which we find bureaucracies (Weber [1922–3] 1958, p. 299).

8. In the 1920 Introduction to *The Protestant Ethic and the Spirit of Capitalism*, Weber ([1920] 1958) focused on "a specially trained organization of officials" (bureaucracy) in his discussion of rationalization, but he also mentioned capitalism in the same context as "the most fateful force in our modern life."

9. While Weber may have thought of capitalism and bureaucracy as the paradigm cases of this rationalization process, in the modern world it could be argued that the fast-food restaurant, and more generally the franchise, has supplanted them as the best example of this process (Ritzer 1983). Hence, our concern in this paper could be termed the "McDonaldization" of American medicine and of the professions in general.

10. Although we are forecasting some degree of deprofessionalization of physicians, their power, status, and continuing control over a centrally important area of human existence lead us to believe that they will *not* tumble far down the professional continuum.

11. Starr makes this point in the case of physicians: "In the twentieth century, medicine has been the heroic exception that sustained the waning tradition of independent professionalism. Physicians . . . escaped from corporate and bureaucratic control . . . But the exception may now be brought into line with the governing rule" (1982, p. 420).

12. According to Kalberg, the other types are practical, theoretical, and substantive rationality. We will deal with substantive rationality shortly and with the relation between formal and substantive rationality throughout this paper. Thus, we are using only a small portion of Weber's rationalization theory and of Kalberg's (and Levine's) systematization of it. To keep the analysis manageable, and because we view the relation between formal and substantive rationality as central, we will not deal with practical and theoretical rationality, although they could be applied to this case. For example, the advances in medical technology to be discussed later in this paper could be seen as the result of increases in both practical and theoretical rationality.

13. Others are the legal and scientific spheres.

14. We do not want to seem to imply that formal rationalization, or any other type of rationalization, is a self-actuated "force" that is sweeping over the medical profession. In fact, Weber is clear that material and ideal interests drive the process of rationalization. In this case, owners of for-profit medical facilities, health insurance executives, and government bureaucrats can all be seen as pushing, in their own self-interests, the process of formal rationalization in medicine.

15. It is this distinction between formal and substantive rationality that differentiates the thesis of this paper from that of Ritzer (1975a). The latter was operating with a general sense of the process of rationalization that allowed the author to see both professionalization and bureaucratization as part of this general process. In this paper, the distinction between the two types of rationalization permits us to see the points of tension between professionalization and bureaucratization.

16. Not only may these types of rationality coexist and conflict with each other, but each may also coexist and conflict with the other two types of rationality (practical, theoretical). Further complicating matters in Weberian analysis, all four types of rationality can occur in various institutions, organizations and occupations.

17. To take one example, Weber argues that "the 'free' market is . . . an abomination to every system of fraternal ethics" ([1921] 1968, p. 637). The free market is an example of formal rationality and a system of fraternal ethics is one of the types of substantive rationality that comes into conflict with formal rationality.

18. In his study of lawyers in large law firms, Nelson (1981) also associates professionalism and value (substantive) rationality.

19. Another way of characterizing this struggle is as one between two contemporary sets of social structures. On the one hand, there are formally rational structures in which rules, regulations and laws determine the choices of means to ends made by individuals in them. On the other hand, there are substantively rational structures in which larger values shape choices of means to ends. Formally rational structures like bureaucracies and the capitalist economy are increasingly coming into conflict with substantively rational structures like the professions; a conflict from which formally rational structures are likely to emerge victorious.
20. We are combining the closely related trait and structural-functional approaches under a single heading. See Saks (1983) for an orientation that differentiates between them.
21. Just as the power approach seems to be gaining preeminence, a number of analysts (e.g., Freidson 1983; Murray, Dingwall & Eekelaar 1983; Saks 1983) have come to question this single-minded focus on power.
22. A possible fourth, micro-sociological approach (as opposed to the macro-sociological orientation of the other three approaches), may be found in Dingwall (1976).
23. Since this is a Weberian analysis, we will use the concept of deprofessionalization rather than the related, and more Marxian, notion of the *proletarianization* of the professions (Derber 1982; Oppenheimer 1973). Proletarianization is a different and more extreme view of the loss of power of the professions. While few Marxists envision a drastic descent to the level of assembly-line workers, they do see professionals, like other proletarians, increasingly needing to sell their labor time in order to have access to the means of production.
24. As we will discuss at the conclusion of this paper, other outcomes are also possible.
25. Also fueling this increased demand was the expansion of private sector medical insurance.
26. A related issue is the growing "conglomeration" of the healthcare purchaser—for example, government or business coalitions organized to negotiate mass purchases of health care (Freedman 1985).
27. While managers of non-profit hospitals are also seeking to rationalize, it is the goal of profit maximization that leads the managers of for-profit hospitals to rationalize with a vengeance.
28. It is also important to look at some of the other presuppositions of capitalism enumerated by Weber since many of them also stand in opposition to professionalization. For example, Weber ([1927] 1981, p. 276) sees the freedom of the market in general, and of the labor market in particular (Begun 1986), as one such presupposition. It could be argued that professionalization is a limitation on the labor market and therefore antithetical to capitalism. The appropriation of the means of production by the capitalist is a threat to professional power. The tendency to adopt ever more rational technologies serves to make professional activities more calculable, predictable, controllable, etc.
29. Nelson (1981) discusses how this is also occurring in the large law firm.
30. Rothman (1984) makes this point about the effect of technology, but in a study of law not medicine.
31. As a counter-position to this, Horobin (1983) argues that modern advances, while making things more determinate, have also created new areas of indeterminacy which serve to maintain the power of the medical profession.
32. See Nass (1986) for a very unusual image of this conflict from a Weberian perspective in which professionals are viewed as leaders of one-person organizations or as organizations.
33. Rothman (1984) makes a similar point about the legal profession.
34. There are some (e.g., Schlesinger 1985) who disagree with the view that increasing bureaucratization will reduce physician control.
35. And there are a number of conflicting studies on the issue of the relation between professionalization and bureaucratization (see Ritzer and Walczak 1986, pp. 205–10). Among the positions are an inherent conflict between the two, the emergence of a new organizational form that combines elements of professionalization and bureaucratization, the dominance of bureaucrats, or the dominance of professionals. More directly relevant to the thesis of this paper, in a study of physicians in an HMO, Kerr (1985) found *both* bureaucratic restraint and professional autonomy.

36. It is also the case that lower-status physicians are more likely to be controlled by these standards than the higher-status physicians who create and enforce them. Even in this instance, however, some deprofessionalization is likely to occur.

References

Agich, George J., and Charles E. Begley. 1985. "Some Problems with Pro-Competition Reforms." *Social Science and Medicine* 21:623–30.

Allen, Bruce H., Richard A. Wright, and Louis E. Raho. 1985. "Physicians and Advertising." *Journal of Health Care Marketing* 5:39–49.

Arney, William Ray. 1982. *Power and the Profession of Obstetrics*. University of Chicago Press.

ASIM Today. 1986. "The Impact of DRGs on Patient Care." American Society of Internal Medicine.

Baer, William C. 1986. "Expertise and Professional Standards." *Work and Occupations* 13:532–52.

Battistella, Roger M. 1985. "Hospital Receptivity to Market Competition: Image and Reality." *Health Care Management Review* 10:19–26.

Begun, James W. 1986. "Economic and Sociological Approaches to Professionalism." *Work and Occupations* 13:113–29.

Berlant, Jeffrey Lionel. 1975. *Profession and Monopoly: A Study of Medicine in the United States and Great Britain*. University of California Press.

Brubaker, Rogers. 1984. *The Limits of Rationality: An Essay on the Social and Moral Thought of Max Weber*. Allen & Unwin.

Caplow, Theodore. 1954. *The Sociology of Work*. University of Minnesota Press.

Cassel, Christine K. 1985. "Doctors and Allocation Decisions: A New Role in the New Medicare." *Journal of Health Politics, Policy and Law* 10:549–64.

Cohen, Ira. 1981. "Introduction to the Transaction Edition." Pp. xv–lxxxi in Max Weber, *General Economic History*. Transaction Books.

Colburn, Don. 1985. "Unionizing Doctors: Physicians Begin Banding Together to Fight for Autonomy and Control Over Medical Care." *Health-Washington Post* June 19:7.

Collins, Randall. 1980. "Weber's Last Theory of Capitalism: A Systematization." *American Sociological Review* 45:925–42.

Costilo, L. Barry. 1985. "Antitrust Enforcement in Health Care: Ten Years After the AMA Suit." *The New England Journal of Medicine* 313:901–04.

Darling, John R., and Blaise J. Bergiel. 1983. "Health Care Advertising: A Comparative Analysis." *Journal of Health Care Marketing* 3:21–28.

Derber, Charles (ed.). 1982. *Professionals as Workers: Mental Labor in Advanced Capitalism*. Hall.

DiMaggio, Paul J., and Walter W. Powell. 1983. "The Iron Cage Revisited: Institutional Isomorphism and Collective Rationality in Organizational Fields." *American Sociological Review* 48:147–60.

Dingwall, Robert. 1976. "Accomplishing Professions." *Sociological Review* 24:331–49.

Eisen, Arnold. 1978. "The Meanings and Confusions of Weberian 'Rationality.'" *British Journal of Sociology* 29:57–70.

Ermann, Dan, and Jon Gabel. 1986. "Investor-Owned Multihospital Systems: A Synthesis of Research Findings." Pp. 474–91 in *For-Profit Enterprise in Health Care*, edited by Bradford H. Gray. National Academy Press.

Feldstein, Paul J. 1986. "The Emergence of Market Competition in the U.S. Health Care System: Its Causes, Likely Structure and Implications." *Health Policy* 6:1–20.

Folland, Sherman T. 1985. "The Effects of Health Care Advertising." *Journal of Health Politics, Policy and Law* 10:329–45.

Forsyth, Patrick, and Thomas J. Danisiewicz. 1985. "Toward a Theory of Professionalization." *Work and Occupations* 12:59–76.

Freedman, Steve A. 1985. "Megacorporate Health Care: A Choice for the Future." *The New England Journal of Medicine* 312:579–82.

Freidson, Eliot. 1960. "Client Control and Medical Practice." *American Journal of Sociology* 65:374–82.

______. 1970. *The Profession of Medicine*. Dodd, Mead.

______. 1975. *Doctoring Together: A Study of Professional Social Control*. Elsevier.

______. 1980. *Patients' Views of Medical Practice*. University of Chicago Press.

______. 1983. "The Theory of the Professions: State of the Art." Pp. 19–37 in *The Sociology of the Professions: Lawyers, Doctors and Others*, edited by Robert Dingwall and Philip Lewis. Macmillan.

______. 1984. "The Changing Nature of Professional Control." *Annual Review of Sociology* 10:1–20.

______. 1985. "The Reorganization of the Medical Profession." *Medical Care Review* 42:11–35.

______. 1986. *Professional Powers: A Study in the Institutionalization of Formal Knowledge*. University of Chicago Press.

Gelfand, Toby. 1980. *Professionalizing Modern Medicine: Paris Surgeons and Medical Science and Institutions in the 18th Century*. Greenwood.

Gieryn, Thomas, George M. Bevins, and Stephen C. Zehr. 1985. "Professionalization of American Scientists: Public Science in the Creation/Evolution Trials." *American Sociological Review* 50:392–409.

Goldstein, Michael S. 1984. "Abortion as a Medical Career Choice: Entrepreneurs, Community Physicians, and Others." *Journal of Health and Social Behavior* 25:211–29.

Goode, William J. 1957. "Community within a Community: The Professions." *American Sociological Review* 22:194–200.

Gray, Bradford H. (ed.). 1986. *For-Profit Enterprise in Health Care*. National Academy Press.

Greenwood, Ernest. 1957. "Attributes of a Profession." *Social Work* 2:45–55.

Hall, Richard H. 1983. "Theoretical Trends in the Sociology of Occupations." *The Sociological Quarterly* 24:5–23.

Haug, Marie R. 1973. "Deprofessionalization: An Alternate Hypothesis for the Future." Pp. 195–211 in *Professionalization and Social Change*, edited by Paul Halmos. University of Keele.

______. 1975. "The Deprofessionalization of Everyone?" *Sociological Focus* 8:197–213.

Havighurst, Clark C. 1983. "The Doctors' Trust: Self-Regulation and the Law." *Health Affairs* 2:64–76.

Horobin, Gordon. 1983. "Professional Mystery: The Maintenance of Charisma in General Medical Practice." Pp. 84–105 in *The Sociology of the Professions: Lawyers, Doctors and Others*, edited by Robert Dingwall and Philip Lewis. Macmillan.

Jamous, H., and B. Peloille. 1970. "Changes in the French University-Hospital System." Pp. 111–52 in *Professions and Professionalization*, edited by J. A. Jackson. Cambridge University Press.

Johnson, Terence. 1972. *The Professions and Power*. Macmillan.

Kalberg, Stephen. 1980. "Max Weber's Types of Rationality: Cornerstones for the Analysis of Rationalization Processes in History." *American Journal of Sociology* 85:1145–79.

Kerr, Stephen T. 1985. "Referral in Education and Medicine: Differing Patterns of Development in Specialized Professions." *Work and Occupations* 12:416–36.

Klegon, Douglas. 1978. "The Sociology of Professions: An Emerging Perspective." *Sociology of Work and Occupations* 5:259–83.

Larkin, Gerald. 1983. *Occupational Monopoly and Modern Medicine*. Tavistock.

Larson, Magali Sarfatti. 1977. *The Rise of Professionalism: A Sociological Analysis*. University of California Press.

Levine, Donald. 1981. "Rationality and Freedom: Weber and Beyond." *Sociological Inquiry* 51:5–25.

McKinlay, John B. 1973. "On the Professional Regulation of Change." Pp. 61–84 in *Professionalization and Social Change*, edited by Paul Halmos. University of Keele.

______. 1982. "Toward the Proletarianization of Physicians." Pp. 37–62 in *Professionals as Work-*

ers: Mental Labor in Advanced Capitalism, edited by Charles Derber. Hall.
Michel, Allen, Isreal Shaked and John Daley. 1985. "The Proprietary Hospital Industry: A Financial Analysis, 1972–1982." *Social Science and Medicine* 21:235–42.
Mitchell, Janet B. 1985. "Physician DRGs." *The New England Journal of Medicine* 313:670–75.
Mitzman, Arthur. 1969. *The Iron Cage*. Universal Library.
Murray, Topsy, Robert Dingwall, and John Eekelaar. 1983. "Professionals in Bureaucracies: Solicitors in Private Practice and Local Government." Pp. 195–220 in *The Sociology of the Professions: Lawyers, Doctors and Others*, edited by Robert Dingwall and Philip Lewis. Macmillan.
Nass, Clifford I. 1986. "Bureaucracy, Technical Expertise, and Professionals: A Weberian Approach." *Sociological Theory* 4:61–70.
Nelson, Robert L. 1981. "Practice and Privilege: Social Change and the Structure of Large Law Firms." *American Bar Foundation Research Journal* 1981:97–140.
Oppenheimer, Martin. 1973. "The Proletarianization of the Professional." Pp. 213–27 in *Professionalization and Social Change*, edited by Paul Halmos. University of Keele.
Ouchi, William. 1981. *Theory Z*. Addison-Wesley.
Quintana, Jose B., W. Jack Duncan, and Howard W. Houser. 1985. "Hospital Governance and the Corporate Revolution." *Health Care Management Review* 10:63–71.
Reiser, Stanley Joel. 1978. *Medicine and the Reign of Technology*. Cambridge University Press.
Relman, Arnold S. 1980. "The New Medical-Industrial Complex." *The New England Journal of Medicine* 303:963–70.
Relman, Arnold S., and Uwe Reinhardt. 1986. "An Exchange on For-Profit Health Care." Pp. 209–23 in *For-Profit Enterprise in Health Care*, edited by Bradford H. Gray. National Academy Press.
Ritzer, George. 1975a. "Professionalization, Bureaucratization and Rationalization: The Views of Max Weber." *Social Forces* 53:627–34.
———. 1975b. "The Emerging Power Perspective in the Sociological Study of the Professions." Paper presented at the meetings of the American Sociological Association.
———. 1983. "The McDonaldization of Society." *Journal of American Culture* 6:100–07.
Ritzer, George, and David Walczak. 1986. *Working: Conflict and Change*. 3d ed. Prentice-Hall.
Roth, Julius. 1974. "Professionalism: The Sociologist's Decoy." *Sociology of Work and Occupations* 1:6–23.
Rothman, Robert. 1984. "Deprofessionalization: The Case of Law in America." *Work and Occupations* 11:183–206.
Rothstein, William. 1973. "Professionalization and Employer Demands: The Case of Homeopathy and Psychoanalysis in the United States." Pp. 159–78 in *Professionalization and Social Change*, edited by Paul Halmos. University of Keele.
Saks, Mike. 1983. "Removing the Blinkers? A Critique of Recent Contributions to the Sociology of the Professions." *The Sociological Review* 31:1–21.
Schlesinger, Mark. 1985. "The Rise of Proprietary Health Care." *Business and Health* January/February:7–12.
Shea, Steven, and David Margulies. 1985. "The Paperless Medical Record." *Social Science and Medicine* 21:741–46.
Starr, Paul. 1982. *The Social Transformation of American Medicine*. Basic Books.
Tarlov, Alvin R. 1986. "HMO Enrollment Growth and Physicians: The Third Compartment." *Health Affairs* 5:23–35.
Tiryakian, Edward A. 1981. "The Sociological Import of Metaphor: Tracking the Source of Max Weber's 'Iron Cage.'" *Sociological Inquiry* 51:27–33.
Toren, Nina. 1975. "Deprofessionalization and its Sources: A Preliminary Analysis." *Sociology of Work and Occupations* 2:323–37.
Vraciu, Robert A. 1985. "Hospital Strategies for the Eighties: A Mid-Decade Look." *Health Care Management Review* 10:9–19.
Watt, Michael J., et al. 1986. "The Comparative Economic Performance of Investor-Owned

Chain and Not-for-Profit Hospitals." *The New England Journal of Medicine* 314:89–96.
Watts, Malcolm S. M. 1985. "Some Side Effects of Science and Technology on Medical Practice." *The Western Journal of Medicine* April:545.
Weber, Max. (1904–05) 1958. *The Protestant Ethic and the Spirit of Capitalism*. Scribner's.
______. (1915) 1958. "Religious Rejections of the World and Their Directions." Pp. 323–59 in *From Max Weber*, edited by Hans H. Gerth and C. Wright Mills. Oxford University Press.
______. (1920) 1958. "Author's Introduction." Pp. 13–31 in *The Protestant Ethic and the Spirit of Capitalism*. Scribner's.
______. (1921) 1968. *Economy and Society*. 3 vols. Bedminster Press.
______. (1922–3) 1958. "The Social Psychology of the World Religions." Pp. 267–301 in *From Max Weber*, edited by Hans H. Gerth and C. Wright Mills. Oxford University Press.
______. (1927) 1981. *General Economic History*. Transaction Books.
Wilensky, Harold L. 1964. "The Professionalization of Everyone?" *American Journal of Sociology* 70:137–58.
Zola, Irving Kenneth, and Stephen J. Miller. 1973. "The Erosion of Medicine from Within." Pp. 105–16 in *The Professions and Their Prospects*, edited by Eliot Freidson. Sage.

[38]

Public Health Policy Forum

American Journal of Public Health

Reprint

Disease Control Priorities in Developing Countries: Health Policy Responses to Epidemiological Change

Dean T. Jamison, PhD, and W. Henry Mosley, MD, MPH

ABSTRACT

Health systems in developing countries are facing major challenges in the 1990s and beyond because of a growing epidemiological diversity as a consequence of rapid economic development and declining fertility. The infectious and parasitic diseases of childhood must remain a priority at the same time the chronic diseases among adults are emerging as a serious problem. Health policymakers must engage in undertaking an epidemiological and economic analysis of the major disease problems, evaluating the cost-effectiveness of alternative intervention strategies; designing health care delivery systems; and, choosing what governments can do through persuasion, taxation, regulation, and provision of services. The World Bank has commissioned studies of over two dozen diseases in developing countries which have confirmed the priority of child survival interventions and revealed that interventions for many neglected and emerging adult health problems have comparable cost-effectiveness. Most developing countries lack information about most major diseases among adults, reflecting lack of national capacities in epidemiological and economic analyses, health technology assessment, and environmental monitoring and control. There is a critical need for national and international investment in capacity building and essential national health research to build the base for health policies. (*Am J Public Health* 1991;81:15–22)

Introduction

The policy debate in international health has often been polarized around conflicting viewpoints on such issues as preventive versus curative services, selective versus comprehensive primary health care, or integrated versus vertical programs. As we approach the 21st century, it is becoming clear that framing the issues in these terms will not enlighten the policy process, primarily because it limits the options largely to actions that can be carried out directly by ministries of health. Profound social and economic transformations are projected to impact on health in the developing countries in the 1990s and beyond; implications for the epidemiological profiles of these countries will be dramatic.[2–4] A more comprehensive analytical approach is required to formulate health policies that will not only respond to but actually guide the development process to maximize its health gains, minimize its potential adverse consequences, and deal cost-effectively with the emerging quantitative importance of noncommunicable diseases.

Over the next decade there will indeed remain perhaps 30 to 40 countries in the lowest income bracket where the health problems will be dominated by the infectious and parasitic diseases of childhood along with undernutrition and high fertility.[5] Most of these are in Sub-Saharan Africa and South Asia, and intervention strategies must continue to focus on establishing basic infrastructures and delivering established, low-cost technologies.[6] At the same time, however, there will be a larger group of countries, predominantly in Latin America and East Asia, that are newly emerging into the middle income category. Most of these countries are not free of the infectious diseases, yet at the same time are beginning to face a new set of health problems related to rapid urbanization and industrialization.[3,7,8] These include: injuries, occupational diseases and, increasingly, preventable chronic diseases among an aging population.[9] Such a growing epidemiological diversity among and within countries in the developing world demands a flexible approach to international health policy formulation.

Policy Development

It is useful to consider health policy development as involving three complementary tasks: first, *identifying the major disease problems,* assessing their social and economic consequences, and evaluating the costs and effectiveness of alternative intervention strategies; second, *designing health care delivery systems* including establishing the human and physical infrastructures, providing for drugs and logistical support, and developing managerial capacities and funding mechanisms; and third, *defining and choosing what governments can do* through the full range of policy instruments that are at their disposal in the areas

Address reprint requests to either author. Dr. Jamison is with the Department of Community Health Sciences, University of California, Los Angeles, CA 90024. Dr. Mosley is with the Department of Population Dynamics, Johns Hopkins University, School of Hygiene and Public Health, Baltimore, MD 21205.

This paper, invited by the editor, draws in part on a forthcoming book edited by Jamison and Mosley[1]; it is based on work undertaken and supported by the Population, Health, and Nutrition Division of the World Bank. The views expressed in this paper are those of the authors and do not necessarily represent those of the World Bank. The authors are indebted to Drs. D. A. Henderson and A. R. Measham for valuable comments.

of persuasion, taxation, regulation and the provision of services.

Like a three-legged stool, coherent health policies require a solid foundation of technical analysis in all three areas in order to identify effective strategies and establish sustainable programs. Through the 1960s and 1970s the second task, designing institution-based delivery systems, (generally following a Western medical model) was the dominant theme in health policy formulation for the developing world. It was in this period that the policy debates centered around the relative allocation of resources for preventive versus curative services and, when disease eradication programs were being implemented, vertical versus integrated programs. The Alma Ata Conference on Primary Health Care in 1978 introduced the principle of "Health For All."[10] Conceptually this encompassed all health problems in the population, was community-based, and involved all sectors of government. Given the resource constraints in the health sector, many health professionals and donors narrowed the agenda, limiting consideration to childhood communicable diseases.[11] This led to selective primary health care programs focusing largely on population-based technical interventions such as oral rehydration therapy and immunizations for child survival[12] which, in turn, led to policy debates about the relative merits of selective versus comprehensive primary health care interventions.[13]

The third task, assessing the full array of government instruments available, particularly those outside the traditional purview of ministries of health (such as regulation and taxation) to protect and promote the health of populations is not well established in much of the developing world. The full range of instruments is, however, fully entering the public debate on policy in a number of industrialized countries. For example, in the United States the process was initiated with the publication of "Healthy People: The Surgeon General's Report on Health Promotion and Disease Prevention" in 1979 which defined a set of health goals for 1990 for infants, children, adolescents, adults, and the aged.[14] To achieve these goals, 15 priority areas for intervention were identified and grouped under three strategic approaches: preventive health services, health protection, and health promotion.[15] Preventive health services included: primary preventive interventions such as immunizations and family planning, secondary prevention for conditions like high blood pressure as well as curative services for such conditions as sexually transmitted diseases. Health protection encompassed areas where regulation and taxation would be important including toxic agent control, occupational safety, accident prevention, and fluoridation. The health promotion strategies—involving behavioral changes related to smoking, alcohol and drug abuse, diet and exercise—required government interventions not only in education but also through regulation and taxation.

The process of setting national objectives in the US has now been extended with *Healthy People 2000: National Health Promotion and Disease Prevention Objectives.*[16] Based on three years consultation with more than 300 national organizations and state health departments, the goals have been reformulated to go beyond mortality reduction: to increase the span of healthy, disability-free life; to reduce disparities in health by giving more attention to the vulnerable high risk groups such as the poor, minorities, and the elderly; and, to increase access to basic health services.[16] In this context, new priority areas have been added such as cancer screening, AIDS, preventive health services, and surveillance.

Three factors have been key to the successful mobilization of public and professional interest and debate in the United States.[17] First, there was a clear definition of the health problems of concern and their social and economic as well as medical determinants. Second, the 15 priority areas selected for health improvement were further subdivided into 227 health promotion objectives for the 1980s.[18] These detailed objectives represented precise, quantifiable management strategies which were realistic in terms of resource constraints and time frame for implementation, yet demanding enough to push the system to new levels of capability. Third, the *process* of problem identification and health policy formulation involved the broadest participation of all segments of society.[19] On the one hand, a considerable breadth of expertise was drawn from the fields of epidemiology, management sciences, economics, behavioral sciences, and communications to define the problems and issues to be addressed and propose strategic alternatives. On the other hand, there was broad political and public participation in devising solutions. The necessity of this third step (which is rare in developing countries) cannot be overemphasized: the policy formulation process should be an educational experience about the health problems for all concerned since it will be necessary to reach a wide national consensus on issues, policies and implementation strategies which will cut across many sectors including finance, trade, agriculture, transportation, industry, education, and others. It must also be emphasized that successful mobilization of debate and concern is far from sufficient, as the example of the US also, unfortunately, attests. Where the political will for public action is lacking and resources are unallocated, health outcome indicators, such as infant mortality rates among minority groups, can remain shamefully high.

A first task in a comprehensive analysis of the health sector requires an estimation of the burden of disease in the population. This should be done in a framework that considers not only the capacity of the health system to deal with these diseases but also the rapidly changing social, economic, and political context that may be influencing both the structure and organization of the health system as well as disease risks and health behaviors in the population. Because of the extraordinary diversity among developing countries, it is unrealistic and, indeed, inappropriate to come up with global policies; rather, what is presented here is a conceptual and analytical approach with illustrations of the range of factors which must be considered in any particular setting. This approach takes into account that there will be a continuing evolution of disease control priorities based on the social and economic transformations countries are undergoing with their accompanying demographic and epidemiologic transitions.[20]

The Changing Determinants of Disease

A first determinant of the changing health picture developing countries will be experiencing is the demographic transition, largely driven by the rate of fertility decline. This will produce major changes in the age structure of populations which will have a large impact on the health picture.[21] Table 1 taken from World Bank projections for the period 1985 to 2015 illustrates the changing demographic and health picture for developing countries worldwide.[22] Overall, slower growth of the childhood population coupled with declining death rates are projected to reduce the health problems of all age groups. But this is more than counterbalanced by the

TABLE 1—Health Problems of Different Age Groups

Age Group	Population in Developing Countries, millions		Deaths in Developing Countries, millions		Important Health Problems	
	1985	2015	1985	2015	Problems on the Unfinished Agenda	Neglected and Emerging Problems
Young children (0–4 years)	490	626	14.6	7.5	Diarrheal disease ARI Measles, tetanus, polio Micronutrient deficiencies Malaria	Injury
School-age Children (5–14 years)	885	1196	1.6	1.3	Schistosomiasis Geohelminth infection	Adolescent pregnancy Disability
Young adults (15–44 years)	1667	2918	5.0	6.0	Maternal mortality Malaria Excess fertility	Tuberculosis Injury AIDS STDs Mental Illness
Middle-aged (45–64 years)	474	1131	5.9	10.4		Cardiovascular disease Cancers COPD
Elderly (65+ years)	153	358	11.0	22.5		Disability Depression
TOTALS	3669	6229	37.9	47.7		

SOURCE: Jamison and Mosley, (forthcoming)[1]
NOTE: Many of the conditions for older age groups manifest themselves clinically long after the processes leading to the clinical condition have been initiated; preventive intervention will therefore need to be directed to younger ages.
AIDS: acquired immunodeficiency syndrome
STDs: sexually transmitted diseases
COPD: chronic obstructive pulmonary disease
ARI: acute respiratory infection

rapid increase in the adult and aging population. Regionally the picture is much more diverse. The population of children under age five in Latin America and Asia will increase by only 2 percent to 5 percent, respectively, in size. By contrast, this age group is projected to grow 38 percent in the Middle East and 70 percent in Sub-Saharan Africa from 1985 to 2015. Clearly the future requirements for maternal and child health services will be quite different across these regions. At the other end of the age spectrum a very different picture emerges. In all of these regions the populations over age 65 will be dramatically growing in size with projected increases ranging from 134 percent to 164 percent. This continuing growth in the older age groups is due to a phenomenon called the "momentum" of population growth; it is a consequence of the large numbers of children born in the past when fertility was high who advance through older age groups over time. The result is that essentially all developing countries will have to provide for the health needs of a rapidly increasing adult and aged population for many years into the future.[4] A broad assessment of how to meet these needs may be found in Feachem, *et al*, (forthcoming).[23] At the same time, in those countries where the fertility transition is barely underway (largely in Sub-Saharan Africa), policymakers must simultaneously plan to continue to rapidly expand maternal and child health services.

A second determinant of the changing health picture is the major social and economic trends which are transforming the risk factors themselves.[24] The most obvious indicator of these trends is the shift from rural to urban living. In 1985, barely over 30 percent of the population of the less developed regions lived in urban areas, but this pattern is changing rapidly.[25] The urban population will reach 40 percent by the year 2000 and surpass 50 percent by the year 2015. Already seven of the world's 12 megacities (population 10-million or more) are in developing countries. By the year 2000 the developing world will add six more cities to this number.

A shift from a rural subsistence economy to an urban market-oriented industrial economy is generally associated with reductions in risks to communicable diseases because of better sanitation in urban areas. At the same time, however, economic growth brings with it new health problems.[26] Very high rates of injuries related to motor vehicles, industrial accidents, and toxic chemicals (e.g., pesticides) are usually seen in developing countries because of a lack of resources and institutions to establish and enforce safety measures.[27] Undernutrition may diminish because of improved markets, only to be replaced by overnutrition with rising risks of death due to obesity, hypertension, atherosclerosis, and diabetes.[28] Rising incomes also bring changes in lifestyle including increases in smoking, alcohol use, and substance abuse, all of which are expected to increase the risk for chronic diseases.

An analysis of the tobacco-related diseases provides an excellent illustration of how a disease-oriented approach can inform health policy.[29] In the United States it is now well established that tobacco use is responsible for more than 30 percent of all cancer deaths as well as being among the strongest risk factors for chronic obstructive pulmonary disease and ischemic heart disease.[30,31] In recent years, rising rates of lung cancer associated with cigarette consumption have been observed in Japan, Singapore, and Shanghai.[32] A recent analysis by the World Bank has documented a direct relationship between tobacco consumption and higher levels of national income among developing countries.[33] This relationship is not coincidental. Rather, it is driven by promotion, pricing, tax policies, and even international trade relations. The impact of the latter is best attested by the rapid increases in cigarette consumption among young people in several east Asian countries where multinational tobacco corporations have recently opened new markets, assisted in some cases by aggressive (even coercive) trade policies of the United States Government.[34]

Taking China as an example, Peto projects that if current smoking trends continue due to a failure to introduce the array of policies necessary to reduce tobacco consumption in the next several years, an estimated two million Chinese men will die annually from tobacco-related health problems by the year 2025.[35] Cumulatively, one may anticipate 50 million tobacco-related deaths among the 500 million Chinese now under the age of 20. National policies to protect populations from tobacco-related diseases clearly must move beyond the usual realm of the health sector into areas of regulation and taxation of the industrial enterprise related to the manufacture and distribution of tobacco products and, in many countries including the United States, ultimately into a restructuring of rural economies where tobacco is produced.[36-38]

The AIDS (acquired immunodeficiency syndrome) epidemic provides another illustration of some of the links between economic development and disease transmission. In assessing the situation in Sub-Saharan Africa, Over and Piot document a strong correlation between the rate of HIV infection in 18 cities, a high ratio of males to females in urban centers and a low level of female education.[39] The implications of these findings are that AIDS transmission is facilitated by development strategies which favor males for urban employment. This generates a high demand for prostitutes; prostitution, in turn, is facilitated by low levels of female education so that women have few alternative economic opportunities open to them. An AIDS-control program must go beyond promoting the use of condoms and treating sexually transmitted diseases (STDs) and consider broader social policies relating to female education and labor force participation.

Epidemiologic Polarization

The epidemiologic transition in the developing world is neither a steady nor a uniform process. The great variations in life expectancy between countries attests to this; as of 1988, a dozen Sub-Saharan African countries still had life expectancies under 50 years, while an equal number of countries in Latin America and Asia (including China) had life expectancies of 70 years or greater.[40] Additionally, within developing countries (and developed countries as well) wide disparities in health conditions across different social classes or different regions are not uncommon. Frenk and colleagues have referred to these disparities as "epidemiologic polarization" and "epidemiological stagnation."[3,41] These disparities are not limited to the infectious diseases of infants and children but include the chronic diseases of adults as well.[7,23] A centrally important conclusion for health policy is that in most developing countries pre- and post-epidemiological transition problems will coexist.[41] As Foege and Henderson have observed, the developing countries ". . .will not have the luxury of dealing with two kinds of problems sequentially. For the remainder of this century they will be dealing with both simultaneously."[42]

The increasing burden of chronic disease is initially likely to affect the relatively more affluent and politically vocal older groups who are growing in numbers. This being the case, governments will need to take great care to assure that the infectious diseases which predominantly affect children and the poor are not neglected in the face of resource demands placed in large measure by the more affluent. The challenge is to develop equitable policies and strategies to meet these unprecedented conditions in the developing world.

Assessing Disease Control Priorities

The World Bank, as a part of an exercise to assess the cost and effectiveness of alternative intervention strategies for over two dozen acute and chronic diseases of adults and children, commissioned a series of analytical studies, each co-authored by individuals combining economic, epidemiological, and clinical expertise. Cost effectiveness was expressed in terms of dollar cost per discounted healthy life years gained (DHLY). The details of these studies are reported elsewhere.[43] Several general conclusions which emerged from this undertaking will be described here in terms of their implications for the process of policy development in developing countries.

First, while child survival interventions (immunizations, provision of antenatal and delivery care, vitamin A supplementation, improvements in domestic hygiene, oral rehydration therapy [ORT] for diarrheal diseases in high mortality environments, and antibiotic therapy for acute respiratory infections) appear to be highly cost-effective ($5-50 per DHLY), there were a range of adult health interventions which were estimated to be equally cost-effective. Among the most prominent are: anti-smoking campaigns plus tobacco taxes, passive case finding and short-course chemotherapy for tuberculosis, the targeted management of sexually transmitted diseases, cataract surgery, the use of condoms to prevent HIV transmission, and hepatitis B immunization to prevent liver cancer and cirrhosis. At the other extreme, the cost per DHLY for a number of adult diseases is so high (greater than $1000) that public policy should probably discourage their use in settings where health resources are severely constrained. Among these are coronary bypass surgery, mitral valve replacement for rheumatic heart disease, medical management for hypertension, and tertiary management of lung, liver, esophageal, and stomach cancer. With reference to cancer, it should be noted that cancer pain control appears to be a relatively cost-effective intervention for adults ($150 per DHLY) reaching the same level as: maternity care services for maternal mortality; public preventive campaigns to prevent cardiovascular disease; medical management of angina; and insulin management of insulin-dependent diabetes melitis.

This analytical approach revealed a number of neglected and emerging health problems which should be accorded far higher priority. Topping the list of emerging problems are the tobacco-related diseases which, interestingly enough, were not even mentioned in the 1980 World Bank Health Sector Report.[44] Tuberculosis appears to be the greatest "neglected" disease.[45] In 1990 there will be an estimated 8.4 million new cases and 2.7 million deaths, over two-thirds of which will be among productive adults (ages 15–59), primarily the poor. Significantly, this disease alone accounts for about 37 percent of an estimated seven million avoidable adult deaths in the developing world.

Some findings challenge the current international donor commitment to global priority setting. Provision of ORT *in low mortality environments* (at $200 per DHLY) is estimated to be about 20 times less cost effective than tuberculosis control (using passive case detection and short course chemotheraphy) or leprosy rehabilitation. Even cervical cancer screening (Papanicolaou smears) are estimated to be an equally good buy for the money. In *high mortality environments*, in contrast, ORT can be quite cost-effective, underscoring the need for analysis at the country or even district level.

A major observation from the World Bank exercise is the paucity of empirical data from a majority of the developing countries about most of the major chronic diseases of adults.[23,46] Considering that, on a global level, more than half the world's deaths due to cancers and cardiovascular diseases, three-fourths of the injury deaths, and 85 percent of the chronic obstructive pulmonary disease deaths occur in developing countries, the virtual absence of any information about the levels, trends, and determinants of these conditions for the majority of the world's population is truly tragic. Given this lack of developing country data, most of the estimates of the cost-effectiveness of interventions for the World Bank study had to be derived from research carried out in the industrialized world. While these estimates are probably reasonable in grossly illustrating the relative cost-effectiveness of alternative interventions, the actual cost-effectiveness of a particular intervention could easily vary by two- to tenfold or more in any given situation, depending on a host of local factors. For example, with interventions, like immunizations, that require total population coverage, cost-effectiveness is strongly conditioned by the underlying level of disease incidence and case fatality rates. For therapeutic interventions, cost-effectiveness is determined not only by the institutional costs of reaching the target group and then making the correct diagnosis, but also by the probability that appropriate therapy will be prescribed by the caregiver and that the patient will actually comply with the treatment regimen.[47-50] Similarly, the costs of monitoring and enforcing regulatory approaches depend upon the reach and capability of the governmental infrastructure.

Implications for National Governments

It should be clear that there is an urgent need to reassess health sector priorities in developing countries. National health policy assessment can be usefully informed with a consideration of global trends and findings such as presented above, but it must quickly evolve to a critical analysis of the local epidemiological picture cast in its social-cultural, administrative, economic, and political context. Such an approach to policy formulation must begin by assessing the full range of health problems in a society; examining broadly their demographic, social, and economic determinants; and identifying alternative courses of action in all of these areas which could improve the situation. This last step must take into consideration the costs and effectiveness of all possible instruments of government intervention including taxation and regulation as well as persuasion and the direct provision of services.[4]

Many governments will need to create new institutions and reconfigure old ones to build the capacities required for policy analysis and implementation. Among the analytical and technical capacities required are the following:

- *Demographic analysis*—These capabilities provide the fundamental underpinnings for a population-based health system. Demographic data provide the basis for designing intervention strategies as well as for assessing the impact of the disease burden on the population.
- *Epidemiological surveillance*—While some epidemiological surveillance is carried out in most developing countries, it is usually limited to selected infectious diseases. These capacities will need to be greatly strengthened as health program strategies move more toward interventions involving regulation, taxation, subsidies, and information programs in order to reduce acute and chronic disease risks by changing behaviors and improving environmental conditions.
- *Economic and financial analysis*—These capabilities will be essential to measure the cost-effectiveness of alternative intervention strategies as well as to assess the overall claim of the health sector on scarce development resources.
- *Health technology assessment and control*—Institutional capabilities in this area must include not only the assessment of the effectiveness of new drugs, vaccines or treatments, but also their costs and benefits when introduced into the health system.
- *Environmental monitoring and control*—In most developing countries capabilities in this area must be greatly expanded beyond the traditional water and sanitation activities to monitor and control (through taxation as well as regulation) a much broader range of environmental risks including air pollution, toxic wastes, traffic hazards, and other injury risks.
- *Occupational safety*—Rapid urbanization and industrialization in developing countries is often associated with risks of work-related injury five to 10 times higher than in developed countries. There is a major need to develop the capacity to monitor and control occupational health risks.

While many of these institutional capacities exist in some measure in health ministries, their functions are limited for a variety of reasons including lack of professionally qualified personnel, limited resources and, particularly, lack of enforceable statutory authority. If health systems are to be transformed to meet the challenges of the future, a high priority must be given to empowering health ministries to carry out the monitoring and regulatory tasks needed to effectively function in new areas. In addition, mechanisms need to be established that will give them an appropriate voice in tax policy. Ultimately these capacities will need to be developed at regional and local levels within countries as well as at the national level.

Implications for International Aid

Official development financing for health by bilateral and multilateral donors in 1986 amounted to $3.7 billion with the US contribution accounting for 16 percent of the total.[51] While external support represents only a small fraction of the total public and private sector health expenditures in developing countries, in fact, because much of the donor assistance is directed toward the poorest countries, its proportional impact in influencing health policies and program strategies is relatively large. This is particularly true when it promotes policies which lead to a reallocation of national resources. The impact of the donor-driven child survival initiative in promoting immunizations and oral rehydration therapy worldwide is an excellent illustration of this.[52]

TABLE 2—Instruments of Aid

	Modality of Assistance	
Objectives	Program Implementation	Capacity Strengthening
1. Service Delivery	Supports acquisition of drugs, equipment, and technical assistance, for delivery of EPI, vector control programs, hospital services, etc.	Invests in institutional development and staff training to improve efficacy of service delivery—e.g. through improved logistics and supply systems.
2. Policy Improvement	Identifies specific areas of policy improvement (e.g. tobacco advertising bans or introduction of cost-recovery mechanisms) and includes them (usually with conditionality) as part of an assistance package.	Invests in development of policy and planning departments in ministries or universities; invests in staff training and advanced education.
3. Undertaking Research (including epidemiologic, evaluational and economic analyses)	Conducts (perhaps with involvement of aid agency or expatriate staff) research or analyses to strengthen formulation of policy or delivery of service.	Invests in national (and international) capacity for undertaking research relevant to epidemiological and economic conditions of developing countries. This capacity strengthening involves both institutional and human resource development.

In looking to the future, it is useful to categorize international aid on the basis of whether its objective is to: 1) support the provision of services; 2) influence the policy environment; or 3) support research. Table 2 divides approaches to meeting these three objectives into two modalities of assistance: program implementation and capacity strengthening. Program implementation is largely oriented toward short-term results, while capacity strengthening generally requires long-term investments in institutional development. Traditionally, the dominant role of international assistance has been to provide services and related commodities where they were unavailable or inadequate; most donor support to child survival programs falls in this category. Recently, more attention is being given to structuring aid to change the policy environment, either directly, for example, by channeling more support to private and non-profit NGO (nongovernmental organizations) sectors, or indirectly by attaching conditions to aid packages, for example, by requiring cost recovery or extension of services to underserved populations. Presently only a small fraction of aid is directed toward research, much of which, in fact, is in specialized programs such as the Tropical Disease Research Program or in a few institutions like the International Center for Diarrheal Disease Research, Bangladesh.[53]

The earlier discussion has highlighted the fact that developing countries are now moving through the epidemiologic transition at very different paces and often incompletely. As a result there is a great diversity both in health conditions and in institutional capacities among and within countries.[2] This creates a far more diffuse planning environment than existed when most of these countries were still in a pre-transitional stage two or three decades earlier. No longer can a few strategic objectives command central importance for health policy. Rather, a much broader range of relatively less prominent health conditions and associated interventions will compete for resources and attention. In light of this, and given the fact that extremely little is known about the levels, trends, and determinants of the majority of diseases afflicting populations in the developing world, the conclusion is inescapable that as far as donor assistance is concerned, far higher priority should be given to research, both building research capacity and conducting research to strengthen the formulation of health policy. This, in fact, is the conclusion reached by the Commission on Health Research for Development in its recent report.[53] The Commission specifically placed a high priority on local epidemiological and operational analyses which they labeled as "Essential National Health Research" (ENHR).

Broadening the array of diseases for consideration to encompass all ages and expanding the arena of policy options to include the full range of instruments for government intervention will demand a diversity of analytical skills. National governments will require broad technical competence not only in the biomedical and clinical sciences including epidemiology but also in economics, sociology, anthropology, the management sciences, and communication. In most countries, new institutions may need to be developed. The international donor community generally, and the United States in particular, could most effectively use its limited resources in the areas of education, training, research, and technical assistance, where it has strong comparative advantage.[54] Furthermore, because most of the major disease problems are actually of global concern (e.g. tobacco-related diseases, substance abuse, AIDS, injuries, occupational diseases, cardiovascular disease, cancer, malnutrition) much could be gained through international collaborative endeavors in these disease control efforts.

Conclusion

For over a decade the international public health community has given a priority to the communicable childhood diseases. This had been appropriate. The problems are major, the technological and epidemiological tools have become powerful, and the payoff for adapting and applying what is known is high. While the implementation strategy for selective primary health care as originally proposed by Walsh and Warren may have been oversimplified and too narrowly concerned with infectious diseases, the problem-oriented, population-based conceptual approach is fundamentally correct.[11,55] Furthermore, as more and more governments have seriously addressed the problem of child survival, the range of interventions has broadened.[56] For example, diarrhea control programs have moved from simply relying on packets of oral rehydration salts to the use of homemade fluids, the dietary management of diarrhea, the promotion of personal hygiene, and use of soap. More importantly, policy recommendations supporting child survival have now expanded widely, encompassing such issues as female education and the status of women.

The rapid demographic transition that many developing countries are undergoing is now producing great epidemiological diversity among developing countries; this demands that health policymakers consider a broader range of options. Over the next 25 years it is not unreasonable to project a 50 percent to 60 percent decline in the numbers of deaths among infants and children related to advances in child health coupled with rapidly declining birth rates which will stabilize the numbers of newborns from year to year over much of the world. Overall, however, there will be a rise in the total number of deaths as the population evolves toward an older age structure. The epidemiological transition is not occurring uniformly, however, and most countries will have a large lingering burden of communicable diseases among children, particularly in Sub-Saharan Africa where the fertility transition has hardly begun. This situation will impose the greatest challenge on health systems operating under constrained resources to select the most effective and efficient means of disease prevention, case management, and rehabilitation.

It must be emphasized that extending the range of choices means not only choosing to implement new initiatives but also choosing to reduce investments of public funds in health care activities that are clearly not cost-effective. While this may be difficult, given the traditions of Western medical practice, the fundamental issues of equity as well as efficiency are involved. Efficient resource allocation is desirable in every sector. In the health sector, however, in a very direct way, unnecessary death, disability, and illness occurs if resources are committed to one intervention when another has higher health gains per unit of expenditure. The human cost of uneconomic resource allocation is very real and very large. Perhaps even more than in other sectors, then, the imperative exists for policymakers in the health sector to undertake constant assessment of intervention cost-effectiveness.

Probably the most important advance in policy formulation that could come from a disease-control strategic approach is a willingness to consider a range of options available to governments beyond the direct provision of health services. Particularly important as countries are moving through an accelerated process of economic development is the judicious use of regulation, legislation, taxation and subsidies to promote or discourage enterprises, activities, or behaviors which may have health consequences. Also, the importance of mass communication for social mobilization to promote health cannot be over-emphasized. A high priority problem demanding such multi-faceted policy intervention and global cooperation is tobacco consumption.

It is universally recognized that improved health in the broadest sense is a fundamental indicator of the development process. As the Nobel Laureate T. W. Schultz observed, ". . .the wealth of nations (has) come to be predominantly the acquired abilities of people—their education, experience, skills, and health."[57] The task of health policy is to define clear, realistic, and measurable objectives which can guide the development process toward effectively and efficiently producing good health for all. □

References

1. Jamison DT, Mosley WH: Selecting disease control priorities in developing countries. Chapter 1. *In:* Jamison DT, Mosley WH (eds): Disease Control Priorities in Developing Countries. Oxford and New York: Oxford University Press for the World Bank, forthcoming.
2. UNDP: Human Development Report 1990. New York, Toronto: Oxford University Press, 1990.
3. Frenk J, Bobadilla JL, Sepulveda J, Cervantes ML: Health transition in middle-income countries: New challenges for health care. Health Policy Plann 1989; 4:29–39.
4. Mosley WH, Jamison DT, Henderson DA: The health sector in developing countries: Prospects for the 1990s and beyond. *In:* Breslow L, *et al,* (eds): Ann Rev Public Health 11. Palo Alto, CA: Annual Reviews Press, 1990; 335–358.
5. World Health Organization: Global Estimates for Health Situation Assessment and Projections, 1990. Geneva: WHO, 1990.
6. Feachem RGA, Jamison DT, Bos ER: Changing patterns of disease and mortality in Sub-Saharan Africa. *In:* Feachem RG, Jamison DT (eds): Disease and Mortality in Sub-Saharan Africa. Oxford: Oxford University Press for the World Bank, forthcoming 1990.
7. Briscoe J, *et al:* Adult health in Brazil: Adjusting to new challenges. Report No. 7807-BR. Washington, DC: World Bank, 1989.
8. Jamison DT, Evans JR, King T, Porter I, Prescott N, Prost A: China: The Health Sector. A World Bank country study. Washington, DC: World Bank, 1984.
9. Murray CJL, Feachem RG: Adult mortality in developing countries. Trans R Soc Trop Med Hyg 1990; 84:1–2.
10. WHO/UNICEF: Primary Health Care. Geneva: WHO, 1978.
11. Walsh JA, Warren KS: Selective primary health care—An interim strategy for disease control in developing countries. N Engl J Med 1979; 301:18–28.
12. Grant JP: The State of the World's Children 1982–83. United Kingdom: Oxford University Press for UNICEF, 1982.
13. Editorial: The debate on selective or comprehensive primary health care. Soc Sci Med 1988; 26:877–878.
14. US Department of Health, Education, and Welfare/Public Health Service. Healthy people: The surgeon general's report on health promotion and disease prevention. Washington, DC: Govt Printing Office, DHEW Pub. No. (PHS) 79-55071, 1979.
15. Breslow L: Setting objectives for public health. Annual Review of Public Health 8. Palo Alto, CA: Annual Reviews Press, 1987; 289–307.
16. US Department of Health and Human Services, Public Health Service: Healthy People 2000: National Health Promotion and Disease Prevention Objectives—Conference Edition. Washington, DC: Department of Health and Human Services, 1990.
17. McGinnis J: Setting objectives for public health in the 1990s: Experience and prospects. Annual Review of Public Health 11. Palo Alto, CA: Annual Reviews Press, 1990; 231–249.
18. US Department of Health and Human Services/Public Health Service. Promoting health/preventing disease: Objectives for the nation. Washington, DC: Govt Printing Office, 1980.
19. US Department of Health and Human Services/Public Health Service. Prospects for a healthier America: Achieving the nation's health promotion objectives, Proceedings of a two-day meeting February 6–7, 1984. Washington, DC: Office of Disease Prevention and Health Promotion, November 1984.
20. Omran AR: The epidemiological transition: A theory of the epidemiology of population change. Milbank Mem Fund Q 1971; 49:509–538.
21. Kinsella K: Aging in the Third World. International Population Reports Series P-95, No. 79, Washington, DC: Department of Commerce, Bureau of the Census, September 1988.
22. Bulatao RA, Stephens PW: Demographic estimates and projections, by region, 1970–2015. *In:* Jamison DT, Mosley WH (eds): Disease Control Priorities in Developing Countries. Oxford and New York: Oxford University Press for the World Bank, forthcoming.
23. Feachem RGA, Kjellstrom T, Murray CJL, Over M, Phillips MA (eds): The Health of Adults in the Developing World. Oxford and New York: Oxford University Press for the World Bank, forthcoming.
24. Roemer MI, Roemer R: Global health, national development, and the role of government. Am J Public Health 1990; 80:1188–1192.
25. United Nations: Global estimates and projections of population by sex and age: The 1988 revision, Department of International

Economic and Social Affairs. New York: United Nations, 1989.
26. Susser M. Industrialization, urbanization and health: An epidemiological view. International Population Conference, Manila, 1981 Vol. 2. Liege, Belgium: IUSSP, 1981; 273–303.
27. Stansfield SK, Smith GS, McGreevey W: Injury. *In:* Jamison DT, Mosley WH (eds): Disease Control Priorities in Developing Countries. Oxford and New York: Oxford University Press for the World Bank, forthcoming.
28. Pearson TA, Jamison DT, Trejo-Gutierrez J: Cardiovascular disease. *In:* Jamison DT, Mosley WH (eds): Disease Control Priorities in Developing Countries. Oxford and New York: Oxford University Press for the World Bank, forthcoming.
29. Zaridze DG, Peto R (eds): Tobacco: A Major International Hazard. World Health Organization/IARC Scientific Publication No. 74. New York: Oxford University Press, 1986.
30. Ernster VL: Trends in smoking, cancer risk, and cigarette promotion. Cancer 1988; 62:1702–1712.
31. Bumgarner JR, Speizer FE: Chronic obstructive pulmonary disease. *In:* Jamison DT, Mosley WH (eds): Disease Control Priorities in Developing Countries. Oxford and New York: Oxford University Press for the World Bank, forthcoming.
32. Lee HP, Duffy SW, Day NE, Shanmugarathnam K: Recent trends in cancer incidence among Singapore Chinese. Int J Cancer 1988; 42:159–166.
33. Barnum H, Greenberg R: Cancers. *In:* Jamison DT, Mosley WH (eds): Disease Control Priorities in Developing Countries. Oxford and New York: Oxford University Press for the World Bank, forthcoming.
34. Chen TTL, Winder AI: (commentary) The opium wars revisited as US forces tobacco exports in Asia. Am J Public Health 1990; 80:659–662.
35. Peto R: Tobacco related deaths in China. Lancet 1987; 2:211.
36. Warner KE: Health and economic implications of a tobacco-free society. JAMA 1987; 258:2080–2086.
37. Warner KE: (editorial) Tobacco taxation as health policy in the third world. Am J Public Health 1990; 80:529–531.
38. Yu JJ, Mattson MF, Boyd GM, Mueller MD, Shopland DR, Pechacek TF, Cullen JW: A comparison of smoking patterns in the People's Republic of China with the United States. JAMA 1990; 264:1575–1579.
39. Over M, Piot P: HIV infection and other sexually transmitted diseases. Chapter 10. *In:* Jamison DT, Mosley WH (eds): Disease Control Priorities in Developing Countries. Oxford and New York: Oxford University Press for the World Bank, forthcoming.
40. World Bank: World Development Report 1990. New York: Oxford University Press, 1990.
41. Bobadilla JL, Frenk J, Frejka R, Lozano R, Stern C: The epidemiological transition and health priorities. Chapter 3. *In:* Jamison DT, Mosley WH (eds): Disease Control Priorities in Developing Countries. Oxford and New York: Oxford University Press for the World Bank, forthcoming.
42. Foege WH, Henderson DA: Management priorities in primary health care. *In:* Walsh JA, Warren KS (eds): Strategies for Primary Health Care. Chicago and London: University of Chicago Press, 1986; 313–321.
43. Jamison DT, Mosley WH (eds): Disease Control Priorities in Developing Countries. Oxford and New York: Oxford University Press for the World Bank, forthcoming.
44. World Bank: Health Sector Policy Paper. Washington, DC: World Bank, 1980.
45. Murray CJL, Styblo K, Rouillon A: Tuberculosis. Chapter 11. *In:* Jamison DT, Mosley WH (eds): Disease Control Priorities in Developing Countries. Oxford and New York: Oxford University Press for the World Bank, forthcoming.
46. Lopez AD: Causes of death in the industrialized and the developing countries: Estimates for 1985. Chapter 3. *In:* Jamison DT, Mosley WH (eds): Disease Control Priorities in Developing Countries. Oxford and New York: Oxford University Press for the World Bank, forthcoming.
47. Daulaire NMP: Practical issues of ARI program implementation: *In:* Gadomski A (ed): Acute Lower Respiratory Infection and Child Survival in Developing Countries: Understanding the Current Status and Directions for the 1990s. Proceedings of a workshop held in Washington, DC August 2–3, 1989. Baltimore, MD: Johns Hopkins University Institute for International Programs, 1990; 99–104.
48. Stansfield S: Potential savings through reduction of inappropriate use of pharmaceuticals in the treatment of ARI. *In:* Gadomski A (ed): Acute Lower Respiratory Infection and Child Survival in Developing Countries: Understanding the Current Status and Directions for the 1990s. Proceedings of a workshop held in Washington, DC August 2–3, 1989. Baltimore, MD: Johns Hopkins University Institute for International Programs, 1990; 193–200.
49. Mosley WH: Interactions of technology with household production of health. *In:* Towards More Efficacy in Child Survival Strategies: Understanding the Social and Private Constraints and Responsibilities. Baltimore, MD: Johns Hopkins University School of Hygiene and Public Health, 1989.
50. Leslie J: Women's time: A factor in the use of child survival technologies? Health Policy Plann 1989; 4:1–16.
51. Organization for Economic Cooperation and Development (OECD): Strengthening development cooperation for primary health care: A DAC concern. Paris: OECD, 1989.
52. Grant JP: State of the World's Children 1990. United Kingdom: Oxford University Press for UNICEF, 1990.
53. Commission on Health Research for Development: Health Research: Essential Link to Equity in Development. Oxford: Oxford University Press, 1990.
54. Committee on Foreign Affairs: Report of the Task Force on Foreign Assistance to the Committee on Foreign Affairs, US House of Representatives. Washington, DC: Govt Printing Office, 1989.
55. Mosley WH: Is there a middle way? Categorical programs for PHC. Soc Sci Med 1988; 26:907–908.
56. Warren KS: The evaluation of selective primary health care. Soc Sci Med 1988; 26:891–898.
57. Schultz TW: Investing in People: The Economics of Population Quality. Berkeley, CA: University of California Press, 1981.

Name Index